# Ocular Assessment

## THE MANUAL OF
# DIAGNOSIS
# FOR
# OFFICE
# PRACTICE

# Ocular Assessment

## THE MANUAL OF
# DIAGNOSIS
# FOR
# OFFICE
# PRACTICE

*Editor*
## BARRY J. BARRESI, O.D.
### Southern California College of Optometry

## BUTTERWORTHS
### Boston • London
### Sydney • Wellington • Durban • Toronto

**Library of Congress Cataloging in Publication Data**
Main entry under title:

Ocular assessment.

Includes index.
  1. Eye—Examination—Handbooks, manuals, etc.
2. Eye—Diseases and defects—Diagnosis—Handbooks,
manuals, etc. I. Barresi, Barry J.  [DNLM: 1. Eye
diseases—Diagnosis.  2. Optometry.  WW 141 019]
RE75.025  1983       617.7'15       83–15209
ISBN 0–409–95034–3


Butterworth Publishers
10 Tower Office Park
Woburn, MA 01801


10  9  8  7  6  5  4  3  2

Printed in the United States of America

To my parents,
Louise Barresi and Joseph Vincent Barresi, O.D.,
for their love, support, and inspiration

# Contents

# Contributors

## PRINCIPAL CONTRIBUTOR

### J. David Higgins, O.D., Ph.D.
*Private Practice, Kittery, ME*
*Assistant Professor, New England College of Optometry,*
*Boston, MA*

## CONTRIBUTING AUTHORS

### Morris Applebaum, O.D.
*Assistant Professor and Director of Clinical Training, Optometric*
*Center of Fullerton, Southern California College of Optometry,*
*Fullerton, CA*

### Barry J. Barresi, O.D.
*Assistant Professor and Director of Outreach Clinical Programs,*
*Southern California College of Optometry, Fullerton, CA*

### Larry M. DeDonato, O.D.
*Private Practice, Delano, CA*
*Assistant Professor, Southern California College of Optometry,*
*Fullerton, CA*

### Richard London, O.D., M.A.
*Assistant Professor and Associate Director of Research in Vision*
*Training, Institute for Vision Research, College of Optometry,*
*State University of New York, New York, NY*

### Robert D. Newcomb, O.D., M.P.H.
*Chief, Optometry Service, VA Outpatient Clinic, Columbus, OH*
*Clinical Assistant Professor, College of Optometry,*
*The Ohio State University, Columbus, OH*

### Lyman C. Norden, O.D., M.S.
*Chief, Optometry Section, American Lake VA Medical Center,*
*Tacoma, WA*
*Adjunct Associate Clinical Professor, College of Optometry,*
*Pacific University, Forest Grove, OR*

### Neal N. Nyman, O.D.
*Chief, Optometry Service, VA Outpatient Clinic, Los Angeles, CA*
*Associate Professor, Southern California College of Optometry,*
*Fullerton, CA*

# John W. Potter, O.D.

*Chief, Optometry Service, VA Outpatient Clinic, Las Vegas, NV*
*Assistant Professor, Southern California College of Optometry,*
*Fullerton, CA*

# Michael W. Rouse, O.D.

*Assistant Professor and Chief of Vision Therapy and Pediatrics*
*Service, Southern California College of Optometry, Fullerton, CA*

# Leo Semes, O.D.

*Assistant Professor, College of Optometry, University of Alabama,*
*Birmingham, AL*

# Preface

By his example, my father taught me that success in clinical practice comes from sincerely caring and doing your best for each patient. Early on in my formal clinical training, I also learned that in caring for patients the optometrist must be able to diagnose and solve many different clinical problems. In trying to cope with these difficult challenges, I began, as a student, to write a clinical notebook, organized by signs, symptoms, and procedures. This pocket-sized, black ring binder, a student's modest attempt to highlight salient clinical information, was the origin of this text.

What most intrigued me those years ago was that accurate diagnosis, the in-depth understanding of a patient's condition and needs, required the fluid integration of knowledge, observation, and reasoning. *Ocular Assessment* is an attempt to convey this integration and provide a practical teaching and reference source for optometry students and doctors in practice. *Ocular Assessment* does not review treatment and management of eye and vision conditions, but it does offer aid with the critical first steps of clinical assessment and diagnosis.

The first chapter in this book explains how to apply the problem-oriented system to efficiently manage an office that provides comprehensive and continuous quality patient care. Other introductory chapters show how epidemiology can contribute to the diagnostic process and explain the diagnostic principles involved in history-taking and office examination.

Following these introductory chapters, the text is divided into three parts, each providing a unique approach to the diagnostic process— Part I: Assessment of Symptoms; Part II: Assessment of Vision Conditions; Part III: Assessment of the Eye and Vision System. Chapters in all three parts are organized in the same fashion with headings that include background, history, examination, clinical significance, and selected references. Each chapter reviews the background in anatomy and pathophysiology, presents an efficient and thorough approach to history and examination, and explains how to interpret findings to reach an accurate diagnosis. Tables, line drawings, and clinical photographs are provided to complement the narrative and illustrate the range of clinical features and key diagnostic points.

Above all, this text is written for the "generalist," the doctor in office practice. I hope that *Ocular Assessment* will help you efficiently apply diagnostic reasoning, integrate new techniques into everyday practice, and encourage you to sincerely care and do your best for each patient.

Barry J. Barresi

# Acknowledgments

*From a pocket-sized notebook to a multiauthored volume, the design and substance of* Ocular Assessment *passed through several evolutionary stages. Along the way many people offered inspiration, ideas, and encouragement. Just to acknowledge a few, I extend my gratitude to my family; particularly my wife, Sandy; my teachers at Holy Cross and the New England College of Optometry; the dedicated people of Dorchester House; and my students and colleagues at the New England College of Optometry and the Southern California College of Optometry.*

*Ocular Assessment represents the team effort of hard-working authors, reviewers, typists, illustrators, and production staff. I am most grateful for Mrs. Rosemary Butterworth for her service as typist of the final manuscript and as a constant source of advice and encouragement. Some of the other people who deserve special recognition include: for manuscript reviews, Drs. Bradford W. Wild and Paul C. Ajamian; for library and referencing assistance, Patricia Carlson and staff of the M.B. Ketchum Memorial Library of the Southern California College of Optometry; for clinical photographs, Jane Stein, Dr. Arol Augsburger, Dr. John Townsend, Dr. Robert Vandervort, and Dr. Rodney Gutner; for illustrations, Andrew Baker and Richard Morrison; for typing the manuscript, Beverly Atkinson, Judy Badsteubner, Rosa Castellanos, Donna Copmen, Annabeth Curry, Richard Hawkins, and Glenda Sitland.*

*My sincere thanks go to Medical Instrument Research Associates (MIRA) of Waltham, Massachusetts, for their generous contribution, which permitted publication of color photographs taken with the Equator-Plus Lens.*

*Finally, I am most grateful to the competent editorial and production staff at Butterworths. Many individuals at Butterworths helped along the way, but I wish to extend a special thanks to Margaret Quinlin for her enthusiasm and skill in guiding this project to completion.*

# INTRODUCTION

# Barry J. Barresi
# PROBLEM ORIENTATION 1

Optometrists have a responsibility to provide comprehensive, continuous, and efficient care for their patients. This textbook primarily addresses one requirement of good patient care: effective diagnostic methods. The doctor in practice, however, regardless of dedication or skill, can care successfully for patients only if the practice is well managed. The problem-oriented system, first introduced by Dr. Lawrence Weed (1968, 1969) and later adapted for optometry, can provide a unified approach to patient care and practice administration.

To be effective, a system of practice management must reflect the principles of the clinical methods. The cornerstone of any system of practice management is a well-structured optometric record. The record format should encourage the clinician to think and act logically. The data must be organized so that the clinician's observations, actions, and analytic sense are clearly stated. Most important, the optometric record should facilitate auditing of the performance of the professional and practice support staff. Only through careful review of actual patient encounters can the optometrist identify practice deficiencies and staff incompetence; such information promotes meaningful changes in clinical methods or practice management.

The first step in implementing problem orientation is to define standards of care. This requires careful study of the character of the practice staff and patient population. A document outlining practice objectives, policies, and procedures can then be written and shared by the practice professional and support staff. Such a document, the principles of practice, can serve as a blueprint of practice administration and efficient patient care.

Many practitioners have not set down in writing what they hope to accomplish in their practice or how they expect to do it. While the practitioner with one or two support staff may not feel the need to document practice goals and policies, the optometrist in a group or clinic setting will often be overworked and dissatisfied unless the staff is well organized and shares common goals and policies. Although it is difficult to compose a document that clearly defines practice standards, such a document is essential to effective practice management. A well-conceived statement of principles of practice can bind the staff with a common commitment and means of achievement and can yield a cohesive team to provide the highest quality patient care.

A well-structured record is the cornerstone of a problem-oriented practice. The problem-oriented record (POR), an unambiguous statement of clinical actions, encourages the optometrist to deal with all of the patient's concerns, to think and act logically, and to provide appropriate and continuous care. More important, the well-structured record facilitates performance audit, thus improving the optometrist's ability to identify and correct deficiencies in the quality of patient care.

The POR has four components: the data base, problem list, plan list, and progress notes. The data base is composed of the history and findings of the examination. The key characteristic of the data base is that it is a defined universe: the optometrist decides in advance what information will be collected for comprehensive examination or for specific problems.

Two types of information are included in the data base. The minimum or defined data base (Table 1.1) is information routinely gathered from patients presenting for comprehensive examination. The problem-specific data base is information that relates to specific patient concerns or symptoms. The division between minimum and problem-specific data is reflected in the diagnostic dilemma of each patient encounter. On one hand, the optometrist may become overly concerned with a routine workup, collecting needless and redundant data. Crippled by a rigid clinical approach, the practitioner cannot progress logically to a diag-

### Table 1.1
#### Outline of the Defined Data Base, the Minimum Information to Be Collected from All Patients in the Dorchester House Eye Care Service

*History:* reason for visit, qualification and chronology of symptoms, eye history, medical history, family history.

*Patient Profile:* sex, age, occupation, usual day activities, visual demands, emotional or personality traits that may affect visual status.

*Visual Acuity:* acuities at distance and near with and without Rx, current spectacle Rx and use.

*Externals:* pupils, extraocular muscles, cover test, near-point convergence, binocular level (stereopsis versus peripheral fusion), color vision, confrontation fields.

*Refraction:* keratometry, retinoscopy, subjective, near phorias, distance phorias, gradient AC/A, accommodation amplitude.

*Physical Examination:* anterior segment, media, fundus, tonometry.

Source: Barresi and Nyman 1978.

nosis of patient symptoms or a solution of patient concerns. Or, the optometrist may become so engaged in reacting to the presenting symptoms and concerns that important screening or baseline data is not collected. Only through a balanced clinical strategy can this dilemma be resolved. By distinguishing between minimum and problem-specific data, the optometrist gains flexibility to focus on diagnosing and solving patient problems while being reminded of the minimum screening and baseline data that should be collected.

The working problem list (Table 1.2) follows collection of the data base. The list, written as numbered, short, informative titles, includes concerns of the patient or clinician and may be ocular, medical, or social in nature. It is crucial that the problems be identified at the clinician's highest level of understanding, whether by diagnosis, symptom, test, or physical finding. If the clinician is not sure of the diagnosis then the unexplained symptom or finding is listed as the problem. Question marks or tentative diagnoses are not allowed in the working problem list. As new data are collected it may be possible to increase the level of understanding and change the problem list appropriately. Problems that are well defined are also listed on the front page of the patient's record, the master problem list. On subsequent visits the master problem list serves

**Table 1.2**
**Sample Working Problem List and Corresponding Initial Plans**

*Problem 1* (Sample Diagnosis): convergence insufficiency.
*Plan.* Rx:  (A)  Brock string training b.i.d., 15-min sessions × 2 wk to improve diplopia awareness.
          (B)  Consider vectogram and aperture rule training at next visit.
          (C)  Goal: normalized NPC and other findings and eliminate symptoms.
     Ed:  Patient given handout Brock string, discuss prognosis of training, expect resolution in 4 wk, return to clinic 2 wk.

*Problem 2* (Sample Symptom): sandy feeling both eyes at end of day.
*Plan.* Dx:  Rule out lacrimal insufficiency, tear breakup time, Schirmer's test, dye dilution test, Rose Bengal staining.
     Ed:  Return to clinic 1 wk, explain lacrimal system workup.

*Problem 3* (Sample Physical Finding): lid lesion (O.D.).
*Plan.* Dx:  Photo today suspect keratoacanthoma, rule out basal cell, squamous cell carcinoma, staff ophthalmologist.
     Ed:  Return to clinic 1 wk for visit with M.D., explain reason consultation.

*Problem 4* (Sample Test Finding): vertical phoria (R. hyperphoria).
*Plan.* Dx:  Rule out fixation disparity with A.O. vectographic slide distance, Bernell lantern at near.
     Rx:  Consider Fresnel prism trial after Dx plan completed.
     Ed:  Return to clinic, explain nature phoria and possible management.

Source:  Barresi and Nyman 1978.

as a table of contents of the record. This list reminds the clinician of all the patient's problems.

In contrast, while most currently used record formats designate a space for impression or diagnosis, no rules govern the types of comments permitted. The result is scattering of information. Positive findings in the history or exam may be dealt with in an impression or diagnostic note; confusion often arises when a tentative diagnosis is included in the impression. The problem may never be evaluated appropriately nor the correct diagnosis made: for example, after an initial examination of a patient with decreased vision of unknown etiology, a practitioner may record questionable amblyopia in the impression. This label may inadvertently stick with the patient and the necessary tests or consultation to determine the cause of decreased vision may be omitted. If the problem was defined as decreased vision, then the practitioner is reminded with each patient encounter that there must be an appropriate workup to rule out organic causes of decreased vision. If the workup is negative and a cause for functional vision loss is noted, then the problem can be updated to amblyopia.

Consider the patient with multiple problems who has not been seen for a few years. Without a table of contents in the records, one is forced to review the entire chart or else to risk ignoring previous diagnostic work. In a busy practice this can quickly lead to a breakdown in the continuity of care, as with a patient with contact lenses who on initial presentation displays borderline intraocular pressure. Without a master problem list that identifies this problem and reminds the practitioner of the need for close monitoring of ocular tensions, this concern may be forgotten and the patient may receive only follow-up care for the contact lenses.

In a problem-oriented record a corresponding numbered plan must follow each problem in the working problem list (Table 1.2). The plan may include three elements: diagnostic (*dx*), therapeutic (*rx*), and patient education (*ed*). If the problem is a symptom or sign then further diagnostic studies are in order. Such a plan includes tentative diagnosis, list of rule-outs, and the diagnostic strategy, including specific tests or types of consultation. If the problem is well understood and therapy is appropriate, the associated plan includes the goals, end points, contingency plans, and details of therapy. A patient education element is included in all plans. Here the practitioner succinctly notes what the patient and family was told about the problem, any advice, explanations of planned tests or therapy, and follow-up schedules.

Unfortunately, traditional records have no system for associating plans with patient problems. Comments made in an impression may be completely ignored in the disposition. Plans may be written for problems that can only be assumed. The POR defines the practitioner's responsibility; no problems can be ignored. Properly written diagnostic plans, with a list of specific tests and rule-outs, present a clear statement of the practitioner's ability to progress logically toward a diagnosis. This information facilitates performance audit of care and alerts the practitioner to a strategy of examination that can be helpful when the patient returns for follow-up care.

Therapeutic plans that include details of goals of therapy outline the practitioner's clinical judgment and expectations. This information, of particular aid in vision-training cases, also facilitates audit and assists in providing continuous follow-up care. Patient education plans assure that the patient is respected and viewed as an active participant in his or her care. With properly written plans the practitioner's understanding of previous care is strengthened; the practitioner knows what has been done, what is being considered, and what the patient has been told. Such plans eliminate the inefficient task of rethinking an entire problem and reduce the risk of forgetting crucial aspects of the patient's problems and means of diagnosis or therapy.

With the POR, progress notes of patients returning for follow-up care are titled with the problem under consideration. The four elements of the progress notes are subjective, objective, assessment, and plans (SOAP). The subjective note includes information provided by the patient concerning the course of symptoms, compliance with therapy, understanding of patient education, and new concerns. The objective note includes the practitioner's exam findings. The assessment includes the practitioner's interpretation of the status of the problem. The plan includes any modification to the initial plan. Follow-up care can also be documented on flow sheets. Flow sheets are graphic displays of data extracted from a series of SOAP notes. For example, graphs can be kept to document changes in intraocular pressure in a patient with suspected glaucoma or convergence function in a patient with convergence insufficiency.

In contrast, traditional records of follow-up visits have no titles and may deal at random with multiple patient problems. The SOAP format (Table 1.3), however, requires that the practitioner organize data around the problem under follow-up. The source of information is coded (S) patient versus (O) exam finding. The current status of the problem (A) and new goals and details of management (P) also are stated. The result is a well-structured record clearly depicting the evolution of the patient's problems and the clinician's skill and judgment in addressing them. A well-structured progress note serves also to transmit to involved staff the practitioner's clinical judgment. It is possible that even if the same practitioner provides follow-up care, he or she may not recall how data was viewed and organized at the last visit; such risk is unnecessary when the rationale for diagnostic and therapeutic decisions made during follow-up can be retrieved from a SOAP progress note.

The POR yields a well-structured record that displays data in a logical fashion. The quality of data, however, can only be assured by careful audit. No doubt many consciencious optometrists review their work; yet

**Table 1.3**
**Sample of SOAP Note**

S  Good compliance. Has done home training with Brock string, three-dot card, lifesaver card. Lost polaroid glasses so unable to do polamirror or polaroid bar reading over last three days. Frequency of headaches seems to be decreasing to once a week.

O  CT at far with Rx 3XP
CT at near with Rx 20XP
Jump vergences near—12BO 12BI
NPC (light) 5"
P5 ±2.00 rock 14 cycles/min
P3,4-Polamirror pushups

A  Problems with 2,3, resolving well.

P  D/C Brock string. Loan-topper vectogram—5 min twice a day. Do with ±2.00 for 2 min. Other exercises remain the same.

Source:  London, Caloroso, and Barresi 1981.

this task becomes increasingly difficult. Today's optometrist must deal with expanding basic science and clinical information, a broadening scope of practice, higher expectations of consumer-oriented patients, and peer review by third-party payment, governmental, and professional regulatory agencies.

In a practice that is not problem oriented or has undefined standards of care, audit of individual and practice performance is fraught with difficulties. Without written principles of practice the efficiency of patient management suffers. The lack of written office policies can lead to confusion of staff responsibility.

In a problem-oriented practice the principles of practice provides the staff with a guidance system, a set of rules, and standards of care. Only when these ground rules are clearly defined can the needs and deficiencies of practice be identified; then meaningful change of policies and practice can be instituted to remedy past errors.

Traditional records lack rules of data organization and display and do not emphasize problem solving. Reviewing such a record is tedious. In contrast, problem-oriented records clearly reflect the four clinical actions: (1) collecting information: data base; (2) determining what is wrong with the patient: problem list; (3) managing the problem: plan list; (4) following the evolution of the problem: progress notes. Audit of a POR can then focus on important clinical behavior, thoroughness, reliability, analytic sense, and efficiency (Table 1.4).

Along with audit of individual cases, there should be an ongoing study of the overall performance of a practice. The first step in this task is the compilation of daily patient encounter logs, a compendium of patient names, chart numbers, age, sex, clinical problems, and follow-up schedule. When a log of daily patient encounters is maintained, the

**Table 1.4**
**Summary of the Problem-Oriented System Used at the**
**Dorchester House Eye Care Service**

*Problem-oriented records organize information around clinical problems and preserve the logical pathways of clinical work. The performance audit, through record review and individual observation, assures the quality of patient care and clinical teaching. The clinical index provides a perspective on the overall performance of the eye-care service.*

Problem-Oriented Records
    Data base
    Problem list
    Plan list
    Progress (SOAP) notes
Audit of Clinician's Performance
    Thoroughness
    Reliability
    Analytic sense
    Efficiency
Clinical Index
    Lists of patients with similar problems

Source: Barresi and Nyman 1978.

data can be extracted and displayed in various modes. One way of organizing the logging data is to compile a diagnostic clinical index, consisting of lists of patients filed under categories of clinical problems. For example, the practitioner may keep an index of all patients with convergence insufficiency, cataracts, or strabismus. In turn, reviewing this information may yield valuable insights into the practice character and the quality of patient care. The data can be used to (1) document the variety, relative frequency, and demographic profiles of clinical problems; (2) study series of patients with similar problems, evaluating accuracy of diagnosis and efficacy of treatment; (3) identify patients who ignore follow-up care advice; (4) plan future allocations of practice resources, staff, and equipment; and (5) determine the staff's continuing education needs.

Without a written compilation of past experiences the busy practitioner may unwittingly repeat past errors. In contrast, an ongoing retrospective analysis of patients seen can produce hard data instead of vague assumptions. Along with careful performance audit, the clinical index offers a valuable tool in assuring the continuing competence of optometrists.

When problem orientation is properly implemented, the principles of practice efficiently coordinate staff, the optometric record clearly states clinical actions, and the performance audit reveals deficiencies in the quality of patient care.

# References

Barresi BJ, Nyman NN. Implementation of the problem-oriented system in an optometric teaching clinic. Am J Optom Physiol Opt 1978;55(11):765–770.

Bjorn JC, Cross HD. Problem-oriented practice. Chicago: Modern Hospital Press, 1971.

Hurst JW, Walker HK, eds. The problem-oriented system. New York: Medcom Press, 1971.

London R, Caloroso E, Barresi BJ. Problem orientation in vision therapy. Am J Optom Physiol Opt 1981;58(5):393–399.

Sloan PG. A "problem-oriented" optometric record? Am J Optom Physiol Opt 1978;55(5):352–357.

Weed LL. Medical records that guide and teach. N Engl J Med 1968;278:593–600, 652–657.

Weed, LL. Medical records, medical education and patient care. Cleveland: Case Western Reserve, 1969.

Robert D. Newcomb
# APPLIED EPIDEMIOLOGY AND DIAGNOSIS 2

*Case 1.* The patient reads 20/20 with best correction in the right eye and 20/60 with best correction in the left. What is the diagnosis?

*Case 2.* The patient wishes to know the probability of going blind, the most likely cause of the blindness, and any preventive measures that can be taken. What do you reply?

*Case 3.* You are asked to design a vision screening program. What condition(s) do you expect to find in the population?

In all of these cases, the information provided is incomplete and does not allow for a definitive answer. One needs both epidemiologic and clinical data to answer the question with certainty, although epidemiologic data alone would allow the experienced clinician to offer educated guesses without gathering any clinical data. Awareness of pertinent epidemiologic research data and a mental checklist of possible answers based on those studies can help the experienced clinician to anticipate the more prevalent ocular problems in a patient's age, sex, and race categories. When this epidemiologic background is combined with relevant clinical data, the clinician can make an accurate and expeditious diagnosis.

## EPIDEMIOLOGY AS A RESEARCH SCIENCE

MacMahon and Pugh (1970) define epidemiology (*epi* = upon; *demos* = the population; *logos* = word or thought) as "the study of the distribution and determinants of disease frequency in man." Austin and Werner (1976) define it as "the study of how and why diseases and other conditions are distributed within the population the way they are." Daubs (1980) perhaps provides the broadest definition: "the study of man in relation to his total environment (including) not only biological but also social and behavioral factors that influence the health of humans." These definitions are certainly more descriptive of the objectives, principles, and methods of epidemiology as a research science than those traditionally found in standard college dictionaries (e.g., "the branch of medicine dealing with epidemic diseases").

In his book titled *Epidemiology and Statistics for the Ophthalmologist*, Dr. Alfred Sommer (1980) makes a particularly insightful observation about basic and applied epidemiology:

> Epidemiology has two overriding characteristics: a preference for rates rather than absolute numbers, and a peculiarly thoughtful approach to studies amounting to applied common sense.

With this in mind, it is possible to understand the unique perspective that the epidemiologist, and especially the epidemiologist who is also involved in direct patient care services, can offer in biological research projects. These research projects can be as massive and complex as the Framingham study, or as small as one doctor tabulating the number and types of various vision anomalies found in a private optometric practice.

# EPIDEMIOLOGY AS A CLINICAL SCIENCE

While it is useful to have good epidemiologic data available for the purpose of basic science research, health planning (manpower projections, construction of facilities, purchase of specialized equipment, organization of delivery systems, etc.), and the control of both acute (infectious) and chronic (degenerative) diseases, it is the need for a critical decision on patient care that underlines the value of a good literature base in clinical epidemiology. The use of sound clinical epidemiologic research assists the doctor in providing efficient and cost-effective health care because it allows for classification of patients according to established criteria for certain diseases. Optometrists are dedicated to curing and caring for patients with eye and vision problems—but this curing and caring is predicated on the ability of the doctor to differentially diagnose abnormal conditions from well-documented normal variations. Obviously, such a differentiation could not be made if valid studies had not established those norms. In visual acuity, heterophoria, intraocular pressure, cup-to-disc ratio, keratometric readings, systemic blood pressure measurement, blood glucose values—in every phase of the comprehensive optometric examination—clinical data is gathered and then analyzed according to norms established by epidemiologists sensitive to the needs of clinicians.

# DOCTORS PLAY
# THE ODDS

When a doctor of optometry examines a patient, he or she uses the results of clinical epidemiologic research to help formulate the most probable working diagnosis and then conducts tests to either substantiate or refute it. By the very nature of any clinical practice, regardless of the discipline, the clinician establishes a working diagnosis that is truly confirmed only after the recommended therapy ameliorates the patient's signs and symptoms. If the recommended therapy fails to solve the patient's problem, then further testing may be indicated, with this testing being provided either by the first practitioner or by a consultant who can offer additional testing procedures or experience with this type of problem. In the methodical process of ruling out first one potential diagnosis and then another, doctors always look for the most prevalent problems first. This logical approach to the art of diagnosis is efficient and cost effective and is based on the principles and methods of clinical epidemiologic research.

Consider the patient in Case 1 and suppose the patient is 3 years old. A mental checklist of probable causes certainly would include amblyopia ex anopsia as one of the most common causes of unilaterally reduced corrected visual acuity in this age category. But suppose the patient presented in Case 1 is 70 years old. A completely different mental checklist of probable causes should now come to mind, with cataract at the top of the list. Obviously, this does not mean that a 3-year-old child cannot have a cataract or that a 70-year-old cannot have amblyopia ex anopsia. But from an epidemiologic perspective, these conditions are age-specific; that is, they tend to be more prevalent in certain age categories than in others. When this information is combined with clinical data that indicates a unilateral rather than a bilateral reduction of corrected visual acuity, the doctor can immediately dismiss many other possible eye and vision problems and proceed to additional questions and tests to advance the working diagnosis to a definitive diagnosis.

To consider Case 2, suppose that the patient is under 5 years of age. According to the National Eye Institute, the prevalence of legal blindness in this age category is 10.5 per 100,000 population, with prenatal cataract (1.9 per 100,000), optic nerve disease (1.4 per 100,000), and retinal disease (1.0 per 100,000) as the leading causes. If the patient is in the 45- to 64-year-old age group, the prevalence of legal blindness is 211 per 100,000 population, with retinal disease (56 per 100,000), glaucoma (24 per 100,000), and optic nerve disease (23 per 100,000) as the leading causes. If the patient is over 85 years of age, the prevalence of legal blindness is 2,294 per 100,000 population, and retinal disease (646 per 100,000), cataract (492 per 100,000), and glaucoma (322 per 100,000) are the three most common causes. Here again, without even examining the patient, a doctor can use the results of sound epidemiologic research to assist in diagnosis.

In Case 3, the screening program would be designed according to the population at risk for various eye and vision disorders. A school vision screening program would be planned differently from a preinduction eye test, an occupationally related visual skills assessment, and a vision screening program in a nursing home, since each of these groups is at a different risk for various eye and vision disorders. For example, one may wish to screen for amblyopia in the first instance, myopia in the second, stereoacuity and color vision in the third, and glaucoma in the fourth. Frequently, a battery of tests is used to screen for more than one disorder, and certain clinical procedures are included or excluded in this battery of tests, depending on the age of the population to be screened and the probability of finding some of the more prevalent eye and vision disorders in this population.

All clinical health sciences, like optometry, apply epidemiologic principles, methods, and results of research protocols to prepare clinicians for the most prevalent conditions they are likely to find in certain age, sex, racial, occupational, and residential categories. Other risk factors, such as genetic predisposition and general health status, are also used to assist the clinician to analyze clinical data and formulate the proper diagnosis and treatment plan.

# PREVENTIVE HEALTH CARE

The results of epidemiologic research can be applied to prevention as well as to diagnosis of health problems. Applied epidemiology is the foundation of a new field in medicine known as *prospective medicine*. This new field was pioneered by Robbins and Hall (1970).

By employing the concept of relative risk (RR), one can estimate the likelihood of a patient dying from a certain disease process within the next 10 years based upon well-documented predisposing factors, known as risk factors. For example, suppose 100 people smoke one pack of cigarettes per day for 10 years, and 75 of them (75%) develop lung cancer. Now suppose in a matched control group (i.e., similar ages, sexes, races, living and working conditions, etc.) composed of 100 nonsmokers, 15 people (15%) develop lung cancer over the same 10-year period. The RR of developing lung cancer if cigarette smoking is a risk factor is

$$RR = \frac{75/100}{15/100} = 5.$$

The interpretation of this number, which has no units, is that the one-pack-per-day cigarette smoker is five times more likely to develop lung cancer compared to a nonsmoker. If all cigarette smokers developed lung cancer, and no nonsmokers developed it, then one could say that cigarette smoking causes lung cancer. But since there are people who smoke and do not develop lung cancer, and there are other people who do not smoke and do develop lung cancer, then cigarette smoking can only be implicated as a contributing factor (albeit a major one) that predisposes a person to developing lung cancer.

If a calculated RR value greater than 1.0 indicates a harmful risk factor (and the greater the number, the greater the risk), then a calculated RR value less than 1.0 indicates a beneficial or protective risk factor (and the lower the number, the greater the protection).

For example, in the national collaborative Diabetic Retinopathy Study (1978), the rate of visual loss in the treated group was 52 per 707 (7.4%) compared to a rate of 128 per 651 (19.6%) in the control (untreated) group after 28 months of follow-up. Therefore, for a diabetic with proliferative diabetic retinopathy, the relative risk of visual loss if with a risk factor of photocoagulation is

$$RR = \frac{52/707}{128/651} = 0.37,$$

which indicates that photocoagulation is very beneficial in preventing visual loss secondary to proliferative diabetic retinopathy. Calculated another way, the relative risk of visual loss when photocoagulation is needed but not received is

$$RR = \frac{128/651}{52/707} = 2.7,$$

which means that an untreated diabetic with proliferative diabetic retinopathy is 2.7 times as likely to suffer visual loss compared to a person with the same clinical findings who is treated.

Perhaps one day we will have detailed risk factors calculated for the leading causes of blindness in various age, sex, and racial categories, but the basic epidemiologic research in this area is scarce. To date, the best study of risk factors associated with potentially blinding eye diseases comes from the National Eye Institute's Framingham eye study, where several risk factors were identified for four leading causes of blindness in the United States (Table 2.1). These risk factors and others need to be quantified, however, and other eye diseases need to be researched.

Table 2.1
Risk Factors Associated with Four Leading Causes of Blindness

| Cause | Risk Factor |
| --- | --- |
| Senile cataract | Education |
| | Casual blood sugar |
| | Systemic blood pressure |
| | Height |
| | Vital capacity |
| | Serum phospholipid |
| | Hand strength |
| Senile macular degeneration | Systemic blood pressure |
| | Height |
| | Vital capacity |
| | Left ventricular hypertrophy |
| | Hand strength |
| | History of lung infection |
| Diabetic retinopathy | Casual blood sugar |
| | Urine sugar |
| | Other elements of diabetes |
| Ocular hypertension | Systemic blood pressure |
| | Height |
| | Casual blood sugar |
| | Pulse rate |

Source: Adapted from Kahn et al. 1977.

# EXAMPLES OF APPLIED EPIDEMIOLOGY IN OPTOMETRIC PRACTICE

The results of epidemiologic research are useful to clinicians as well as to health planners. For clinicians, epidemiologic studies

1. Document prevalences of conditions and ranges of normal biologic variations (i.e., the prevalence of amblyopia in school children; the normal range of intraocular pressure).
2. Explore associations between certain personal characteristics that may be predisposing risk factors and the clinical onset of a disease process (i.e., smoking and lung cancer).
3. Apply a scientific methodology to evaluate the beneficial as well as the detrimental effects of a new procedure or new treatment modality (i.e., the relative effects of two artificial tear preparations on "dry eye" patients).

## Descriptive Studies

As shown in Table 2.2, the overall leading causes of legal blindness in the United States in 1970 were retinal diseases (36.6 per 100,000),

Table 2.2
Incidence of Causes of Blindness in the United States

| Cause | Total | |
|---|---|---|
| | Number | Rate |
| All causes | 54,883 | 146.5 |
| Glaucoma | 6,059 | 16.2 |
| Cataract, total | 7,202 | 19.2 |
| Prenatal | 2,150 | 5.7 |
| Other | 5,052 | 13.5 |
| Retinal disease, total | 13,717 | 36.6 |
| Prenatal | 3,937 | 10.5 |
| Diabetic | 2,575 | 6.9 |
| Other | 7,205 | 19.2 |
| Retrolental fibroplasia | 1,376 | 3.7 |
| Myopia | 1,627 | 4.3 |
| Cornea or sclera | 2,584 | 6.9 |
| Uveitis | 2,822 | 7.5 |
| Optic nerve disease | 5,042 | 13.5 |
| Multiple affections | 2,405 | 6.4 |
| Other | 5,946 | 15.9 |
| Unknown | 6,103 | 16.3 |

cataract (19.2 per 100,000), and glaucoma (16.2 per 100,000). Aware that these three diseases account for 49% of all cases of legal blindness in the United States, the conscientious optometrist will perform ophthalmoscopy, biomicroscopy, and tonometry for all patients presenting for routine vision care, regardless of the patient's chief complaint.

## Correlation Studies

As shown in Figure 2.1, the distribution of myopic and hyperopic refractive errors is about equal in the 6- to 11-year-old age group. Myopia is most prevalent in the 12- to 17-year-old age category, and hyperopia is most prevalent in the 65- to 74-year-old age category.

This information is important to the optometrist since it helps predict the need for future vision examinations and the interval at which those examinations should be conducted. It is important also because it establishes population "norms" against which the doctor's own patient population can be compared.

## Clinical Trials

Table 2.3 summarizes patients in the National Eye Institute's Diabetic Retinopathy Study (DRS) who had various stages of proliferative diabetic retinopathy.

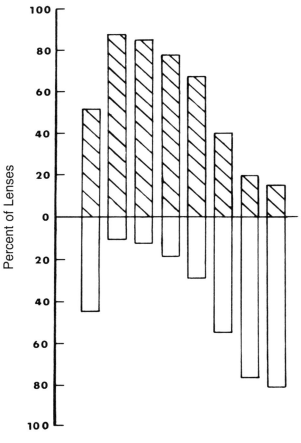

**FIGURE 2.1.**
Percentage of population age 4–74 years with
minus spherical equivalence (for myopia) or
plus spherical equivalence (for hyperopia) in
their present glasses or contact lenses by age.
(United States, 1971–1972).

As indicated by the figures, those eyes treated with appropriate photocoagulation therapy had a significantly better resultant visual acuity than those not treated. Studies such as this demonstrate the efficacy of new treatment modalities and the proper timing of their applications.

**Table 2.3**
**Percentage of Eyes with Visual Acuity <5/200 or High-Risk**
**Characteristics Present or Photos Ungradable at FVO4, for Eyes**
**with Specified Characteristics in Baseline Fundus Photographs**

| Status at IVO1 | Untreated | Treated | z Value |
|---|---|---|---|
| No new vessels | 15.3 (235) | 8.8 (240) | 2.2 |
| NVE < 1/2 disc area (no NVD) without hemorrhage | 19.4 (129) | 8.5 (117) | 2.4 |
| NVE < 1/2 disc area (no NVD) with hemorrhage | 28.6 (21) | 9.4 (32) | 1.8 |
| NVE ≥ 1/2 disc area (no NVD) without hemorrhage | 24.5 (151) | 12.2 (156) | 2.8 |
| NVD < standard photo 10A (± NVE) without hemorrhage | 58.7 (150) | 21.9 (151) | 6.5 |

Note: Number of eyes in group at first pretreatment visit [IVO1] in parentheses.
Source: Diabetic Retinopathy Study Research Group 1978.

The DRS proved scientifically that patients with proliferative diabetic retinopathy should have appropriate photocoagulation therapy to prevent blindness.

# CONCLUSION

In this textbook, the optometric clinician will be introduced to the concept of methodical differential diagnosis based on sound epidemiologic and proved clinical research. The contributing authors have stressed the importance of differential diagnosis with each clinical entity, since this is the most crucial part of caring for and curing patients. Doctors may disagree on fine points of therapy for a given eye or vision disorder, but that disagreement comes only after there is agreement on the exact diagnosis.

# References

Austin DF, Werner SB. Epidemiology for the health sciences. Springfield, Ill.: Charles C Thomas, 1976:60.

Bennett RG, Blondin M, Ruskiewicz J. Incidence and prevalance of selected visual conditions. J Am Optom Assoc 1982;53:647–656.

Daubs JG. Epidemiology. In: Newcomb RD, Jolley JL, eds. Public health and community optometry. Springfield, Ill.: Charles C Thomas, 1980;3:22.

Dawber TR, Kannel WB, Lyell L. An approach to longitudinal studies in a community: the Framingham study. Ann NY Acad Sci 1963;107:539–566.

The Diabetic Retinopathy Study Research Group. Photocoagulation treatment of proliferative diabetic retinopathy: the second report of diabetic retinopathy study findings. Ophthalmology 1978; 85:82–106.

Hall JH, Zwemer JD. Prospective medicine. Indianapolis: Methodist Hospital of Indiana, 1979.

Kahn HA, et al. The Framingham eye study. Am J Epidemiol 1977;106(1):17–32, 33–41.

MacMahon B, Pugh TF. Epidemiology: principles and methods. Boston: Little, Brown, 1970:1.

Robbins LC, Hall JH. How to practice prospective medicine. Indianapolis: Methodist Hospital of Indiana, 1970:8.

Sommer, A. Epidemiology and statistics for the ophthalmologist. New York: Oxford University Press, 1980:3.

U.S. Department of Health, Education and Welfare. Statistics on blindness in the model reporting area, 1969–70. Publication NO. (NIH) 73-427, Washington, D.C.: HEW, 1973.

# Barry J. Barresi
# DIAGNOSTIC PRINCIPLES 3

The Greek root of diagnosis means to know through. The goal of diagnosis is to understand the full dimension of etiologic, structural, and functional aspects of a patient's condition. The disciplined clinician strives to "know through" by the orderly application of knowledge, observation, and reasoning to assess the patient's problems and needs.

## BACKGROUND

When a clinician detects a manifestation of ocular disease or visual dysfunction, only a "tip of the iceberg" has been identified. Below the surface lies a series of events leading to the clinically recognizable manifestation. These antecedent events and typical sequelae represent the natural history of a clinical condition.

The tip of the iceberg may be manifest at different times in the natural history. The patient may present with risk factors only or with a preclinical state of only subtle manifestations. Etiology often indicates the sequence and time course of events leading to disease. For example, infectious disease progresses from risk factors to signs and symptoms more rapidly than chronic disease but less rapidly than traumatic disease. Regardless of etiology, early recognition permits earlier and more efficacious treatment.

The clinician with a prospective viewpoint extends the diagnostic investigation to the early events of "at risk." Promoting health practices, such as not smoking, is another step in disease prevention. Other examples of prospective diagnosis include counseling patients regarding proper lighting; safe work environment; eye protection to prevent vision dysfunction or eye injury; and prevention of stroke by referral of patients who exhibit retinal emboli, transient ischemic attacks, or hypertension. The notion of natural history must be kept in mind during the course of diagnostic investigation. Is a condition at an end stage and the patient a candidate for rehabilitation? Is a condition likely to evolve because of the presence of certain risk factors?

Diagnostic investigation typically begins with history taking and continues with the examination of vision function and ocular health. In history taking, pathophysiology, epidemiologic, and psychosocial aspects of symptoms guide the clinician's choice of questions and interpretations of patient responses. Questions are used to qualify symptoms and screen for vision and health conditions. Disciplined reasoning helps focus attention on relevant history and overlooks the false lead. Reasoning is again used to form a differential diagnosis and an examination strategy.

Knowledge of distinctions between normal and abnormal vision function and ocular morphology also guides the examination strategy. Clinical observations then are focused to qualify specific signs of vision dysfunctions or ocular disease without neglecting important baseline screening data. Throughout the history and examination, passive observation and aimless data collection should be avoided; rather, the astute clinician is an active observer, reasoning with each procedure, continually interpreting data and fine-tuning the examination strategy.

Clinical observation in history taking and examination, if disciplined and systematic, can yield a better understanding of the structural, functional, and etiologic aspects of diagnosis. A unified way of observing can be applied to both case history and examination. Knowing what questions to ask, where to look, and what to look for can be unified by investigating seven elements: site, quality, time, change, cause, effect, and relation to parts of the whole. Whether the task is interviewing a patient with vision loss, evaluating accommodation, or examining the cornea, the strategy of diagnostic investigation includes these seven elements:

- *Site:* Localizing the source of a symptom, which part of the visual system is deficient in function, or what structure or tissue is abnormal.
- *Quality:* Grading the severity of a symptom, a visual dysfunction, or a disease process.
- *Time:* Characterizing the onset, duration, and frequency of symptoms and signs.
- *Change:* Determining the variability over time, and the nature of exacerbating or alleviating conditions of symptoms and signs.
- *Cause:* Identifying associated symptoms and signs of similar etiology or predisposing conditions.
- *Effect:* Gauging consequences and possible sequelae of symptoms, dysfunctions, or abnormalities.
- *Whole and parts:* Relating specific symptoms and patient profile, regional signs, and component parts.

A unified approach to observation is helpful in deciding what questions to ask, where to look, and what to look for. But the process of diagnostic investigation also requires knowing *how* to ask questions and *how* to look. Skill in interviewing patients and using instruments and procedures is essential if clinical observations are to be objective, precise, and reliable.

# HISTORY

History taking is the premier skill of the astute and successful clinician. The encounter in which the clinician first talks and listens to the patient often sets the tone and character of the doctor/patient relationship. The history provides important information on the nature of the patient's problems, current health status, and the impact of current problems on the patient's daily life. Information gathered in the history assists in forming a workup strategy, diagnosing the patient's problems, and selecting effective management. Successful history taking means communicating effectively and asking the right questions.

Effective communication is a demanding task for patient and doctor. Ideally, the patient wants the problem solved, has realistic expectations, and is trusting and cooperative. Ideally, the doctor is primarily concerned with the patient's well-being, minimizes self-interest, and is understanding and caring. The presence or absence of these attitudes often determines the quality of communication and the caring relationship. The challenge for the clinician is to convey a caring attitude while encouraging the patient to contribute to the communication process.

Conditions of the interview are important. An office atmosphere of warmth and friendliness encourages open communication. An examination room offering comfort and privacy helps put both the patient and the doctor at ease. Attentiveness and a friendly greeting convey concern and a desire to help. If the doctor remains alert and attentive and is not distracted by note taking or interruptions, the patient feels important and perceives that the doctor cares, will listen, and will understand his problems.

The technique of questioning is another element of communication skills. Some considerations are appropriate initial questions, use of open versus direct questioning, interview bias, question loading, and closure.

Once the patient is welcomed and seated, it is time for an introductory question. The question should be sufficiently open to elicit as accurately as possible the patient's true reason for the visit: "What brings you here today?" or "Why did you come today?" Encourage the patient to talk by attentive silence or use of facilitating comments that reflect concern. Consider the patient's perspective. Don't necessarily accept the comment, "I'm just here for a routine eye examination." Consider why the patient is here. Is it fear, a specific visual problem, loneliness, or a need for reassurance?

Open questions should be balanced by more direct questions. After the patient has had the opportunity to describe the symptoms, then direct questioning can elucidate the meaning of the response. Patients often use vague words such as eye strain, blur, or headache. Direct questions refine descriptions and can fill in any gaps in the characterization of complaints.

Be careful with direct questioning to avoid the use of yes/no, biased, and loaded questions. Yes/no questions waste time and convey little information. Little is learned from the patient if the doctor does most of the talking. Biased questions lead on the suggestible patient. Rather than the question, "Does your eye ache more at night?" ask "Is there any time when your eye aches more?" Above all, don't rattle out a long list of questions. Such question loading is cold, inefficient, and yields little helpful information.

Most often, the interview flows smoothly into the examination; however, some patients may be uneasy, lonely, or fearful and will talk incessantly. These patients probably need attention more than others, but when your patience is taxed, move on and start a test procedure.

Given conditions conducive to open communication and a good technique of questioning, the clinician still needs a goal—what information is needed? What questions to ask? While specific approaches to selected symptoms and problems are discussed in following chapters, some general comments are appropriate here.

If the patient is presenting for a periodic or initial comprehensive examination, the general approach is to investigate the chief complaint and presenting symptoms, personal eye history, medical history, family history, and patient profile.

# Chief Complaint and Presenting Symptoms

What is the chief complaint? What is the cause? What does it mean to the patient? These are the underlying questions to consider as the chief complaint is investigated. First, ask the patient to explain the reason for the visit (e.g., what brings you here today?). As the patient talks of concerns or symptoms note the manner of presentation. Is the patient apprehensive, oversensitive, calm, or possibly exaggerating? Along with being sensitive to the patient's emotional reaction to symptoms and the motivation for the visit, carefully steer the interview so that any complaints can be precisely summarized in the patient's record. If the reason for the visit is a symptom, then categorize the site, time, change, cause, effect, and relation to the whole.

- *Site and quality:* Localize the source and severity of the complaint; remain alert to the precision of terms.

> *Example:* What do you mean by blurred vision?
> What do you mean by tearing?

- *Time and change:* Establish the time of onset, frequency, pattern of occurrence, and relation to particular tasks.
  *Example:* When did you notice something was wrong?
  When does it bother you?
- *Change and cause:* Determine variability and nature of associated problems. Consider differential diagnosis of symptom to formulate more specific questions.
  *Example:* What do you do about the problem
  Does anything make it better or worse?
  Any associated problems?
- *Effect, whole and part:* Determine the consequences of chief complaint and if any other eye or vision problems are present.
  *Example:* Does this problem bother you at work, at study?
  Any other problems? Vision? Pain? Red eye? Double vision?

Careful qualification of any presenting symptom is, of course, important, but a more basic goal is to uncover the patient's true motive for the visit. The question you do not directly ask the patient, but keep in the back of your mind during the interview is, "What do you want me to do for you?" Does the patient want relief for a symptom or reassurance of good vision and health? Is the patient concerned about the consequences of diabetes, hypertension, glaucoma, or other problems? Being able to uncover the patient's hidden agenda is the mark of the exceptional clinician.

Do not expect to completely qualify the chief complaint and uncover all the patient's motives early in the exam. Often it is helpful to revisit the presenting symptoms and concerns. That is, after more information from the history and examination is gathered, and a better understanding of the patient's background and emotions are known, the issues discussed earlier are investigated further. Possibly the patient had initially misunderstood some questions because of imprecise words. Maybe the patient was initially more reticent, forgetful, or just did not trust you enough. Often, given a second opportunity to explain the symptoms and reason for visit, the patient will offer new and valuable information. Sometimes the most important issues are revealed by the patient when unsolicited. For example, just as you are finishing the exam or as you leave the room the patient offhandedly comments, "By the way . . ." or, "I forgot to mention . . ." or, "You should know . . ." Listen carefully, the patient may now be revealing the motivating concerns.

Consider again the beginning of the history; when the chief complaint and presenting symptom are first characterized, make sure to succinctly note in the patient record a chronologic profile of symptoms and concerns. The next step is to investigate past eye history, current and past medical history, and family history.

# Eye History

A good perspective of the patient's past eye problems and care helps interpret current problems. Past eye problems that may increase the risk of future problems may also be uncovered. Any past eye problems? Any injury? Any operation? Any eye diseases or red eye? Medicine for the eyes?

Questions about the patient's last eye exam and problems at that time should include: How did your last eye exam turn out? Date of first prescription? Number of prescription changes? Date of last prescription? Have you worn contact lenses? How do you use your glasses?

Some standard questions to reveal other symptoms should be asked. Do you have a problem with vision or eye strain? Do you ever see double? Do you have eye pain? Flashes of light in your vision? These are just a few; avoid an excessive list and, considering the patient's age and vision status, select questions likely to yield information. Questions to evaluate specific parts of the vision system are discussed in Part III.

# Medical History

Assessment of general health should focus on systemic conditions that may manifest in the eye and vision system. In addition, coordinating care necessitates familiarity with the nature of the patient's personal health care. In certain settings, a review of organ systems is fitting. Appropriate questions include: How is your health? How do you feel in general? Any medical problems? Allergies to anything? Allergies to any medicine? High blood pressure? Diabetes? Last general physical exam?

A good drug history is extremely helpful. The easiest way is to ask the patient when the appointment is made to bring a list of all prescription and nonprescription medications currently in use. At the exam time, find out drug names, doses, uses, and whether there have been any adverse reactions to drugs. Ask also about smoking and alcohol or other substance abuse.

An obstetric history is important to rule out congenital disorders. Birth and neonate history is particularly important in the diagnosis of strabismus and perceptual disorders.

# Family History

The goal here is to determine the presence of any familial eye and systemic disorders and to ascertain the patient's genetic predisposition for eye manifestations. On occasion, in the course of the examination, certain findings may warrant a more thorough study of family data and pedigree. To qualify the history it may be desirable to examine the patient's siblings or parents and to ask the patient whether there is any family incidence of blindness or eye diseases, glaucoma, eye operations, common illnesses, diabetes, or high blood pressure.

## Patient Profile

Asking about occupation, hobbies, interests, and community life is of considerable importance in understanding patient problems and providing effective care. Getting to know patients as people and as active individuals in a community may start with the history but should underline the duration of the patient encounter.

What kind of job do you have? How do you spend your days? Tasks, physical exertion, mental stress, visual demands, all should be evaluated. Be alert to patients who are exposed to occupational eye or health hazards. Do you wear protective eyeglasses? Protective clothing or equipment?

Beyond occupation, have some appreciation for the patient's usual daily activities, hobbies, and interests. Here the goal is not just to evaluate vision status, but to extend an interest in the patient as a unique human being. Discussing hobbies and interests provides insight into the patient's personality and a measure of mental health.

The visually impaired patient being evaluated for low vision deserves the most thorough assessment of functional status and needs. The frail elderly person or child with learning problems also deserves special attention.

Throughout the assessment of the chief complaint, past eye and medical history, family history, and patient profile, take care to avoid the pitfalls of precision of terms and patient reliability. Using jargon can confuse the patient, who may not admit or realize the misinterpretation. Uncritically accepting the patient's use of certain terms can lead one astray: always qualify. For example: What do you mean by blur? By double vision?

Listen to what the patient is saying and watch how he says it. A patient's history may be unreliable because of denial that stems from personal fears or social pressures. Accepting as reliable a patient's self-diagnosis or results of previous care may also mislead the unwary clinician.

The tough challenge is to interview the patient in a way that will yield all this information in a relaxed and easy manner and still communicate your sincere concern and desire to help.

# EXAMINATION

The challenge to efficient and thorough observation is to balance examination for baseline data and problem-specific data. The clinician must systematically assess the eye and vision system and collect data to assess normal and abnormal structure and function. In conjunction with systematic assessment of the vision system, the clinician must also be able to concentrate on parts of the examination that will more likely yield findings critical to the diagnosis. In this way, every exam is unique to that patient. Each exam must take into account the patient's age, occupation, personal profile, presenting history, and health status.

The diagnostic methods presented in this text are examples of problem-specific approaches to diagnosis based upon a specific symptom, vision condition, or structure of the eye and vision system. The minimum or baseline aspect of an examination can be summarized by four objectives: health, refraction, binocularity, perceptual skills (Table 3.1).

The first priority, assessment of health, is based on observation of morphologic and functional signs. Some changes in structure or appearance of tissue can be observed solely with gross observation and without the aid of an instrument. Other signs can only be uncovered and adequately studied with special optical aids and illumination, such as a biomicroscope, ophthalmoscope, or techniques such as radiography, computed axial tomography, or ultrasonography.

Observing functional signs is an important adjunct to assessing morphologic signs. The patient's sense of vision can be studied by measurements of visual acuity, contrast sensitivity, color vision, visual fields, and electrodiagnostic techniques. Some of the cardinal signs important to the assessment of ocular health are organized in Part I by symptom,

## Table 3.1
## General Examination Procedures

| Health Assessment | Refractive Assessment | Perceptual Skills | Binocular Assessment |
|---|---|---|---|
| General observation | Visual acuity (unaided) | Screening battery for | Visual acuity |
| Visual acuity (best corrected) | Pinhole and stenopathic slit | a. Perceptual motor coordination | Cover tests |
| Monocular color vision testing | Keratometry | b. Laterality/ directionality | Near-point convergence |
| Pupil studies | Retinoscopy or objective refractor | c. Visual perception discrimination | Oculomotility studies |
| Oculomotility studies | Subjective refraction | d. Visual motor integration | Associated and disassociated phoria measures |
| External exam | | e. Auditory perceptual discrimination | Vergence testing |
| Biomicroscopy | | | Negative relative accommodation |
| Tonometry | | | Positive relative accommodation |
| Ophthalmoscopy | | | Dynamic retinoscopy |
| Blood pressure measurement | | | Accommodative amplitude |
| | | | Range of clear vision |
| | | | Accommodative facility |
| | | | Fusion and stereopsis tests |

Part II by vision condition, or Part III by the part of the eye and vision system.

The other objective in examination relates to vision conditions and vision performance. The task here is to sufficiently assess the signs of vision disorders to permit accurate diagnosis and guide effective treatment. Here the techniques of observation can be as elementary and direct as a cover test or require sophisticated instruments and test materials.

Regardless of the specific test employed by the examiner, the strategy of observation can be guided by the seven unifying elements: site, quality, time, change, cause, effect, and whole versus parts.

Another aid to observation is to strive to record findings in descriptive terms and avoid undue interpretation. The temptation is great to record an interpretation of the findings or note a tentative diagnosis. First describe what you see. Use of clinical drawings is particularly valuable to train the observer's eye and document morphology, as with the use of optic disc or corneal drawings.

# CLINICAL SIGNIFICANCE

The goal of ocular assessment is to reach as complete an understanding of the patient's needs and clinical condition as possible. While the clinician strives for a definitive diagnosis of structure, function, and etiology, often data is not complete or consultation is required. Defining the patient's clinical problems should accurately reflect the clinician's level of understanding. Speculation and guesswork has no place in the working problem list of the problem-oriented record. Available evidence may justify labeling the patient problem at many different levels, such as an unexplained symptom, unexplained test finding, unexplained physical finding, or when the problem is better understood as a diagnosis. If a problem is unexplained upon initial assessment, then a strategy for further diagnostic investigation or consultation and possible diagnostic rule-outs can be recorded in the appropriate plan list in the patient's record.

The diagnostic thought process is somewhat analogous to juggling while climbing a ladder. The clinician keeps juggling background knowledge, observation skills, and diagnostic reasoning while climbing the steps on an abstraction ladder. At the first steps of abstraction, the clinician may recognize only that something is abnormal: the patient has acute eye pain, high exophoria at near, or anisocoria. As the clinician continues with history and examination, additional evidence may justify more steps up the ladder and a diagnosis can be reached, and such symptoms may indicate acute iritis, convergence insufficiency syndrome, or Horner's pupil.

According to Engel and Morgan (1976), the diagnostic thought process can, for the sake of analysis, be divided into these six steps:

1.   Differentiate between a normal variant and an abnormal clinical finding.
2.   Specify location and quality of any structural abnormality. For example, depending upon the sophistication of the examiner, a patient with retinitis pigmentosa could be labeled as having (a) an internal eye problem, (b) a retinal problem, (c) pigmented lesions of the peripheral retina, or (d) retinal pigment epithelium problem. Each label is more precise, progressing from gross anatomic structures to an ocular cellular layer.
3.   Specify and qualify functional abnormality and correlate with structural problems. For example, for an elderly patient with the functional change of myopic shift, the structural change of nuclear sclerosis should be ruled out and correlated.
4.   Determine the etiology of any structural or functional abnormality. Is the disorder neoplastic, traumatic, infectious, genetic, or degenerative? This step is particularly notable in ocular manifestations of systemic conditions. For example, diagnostic investigation of a patient with anisocoria may proceed up several steps of the ladder: the ocular diagnosis of Horner's syndrome, systemic diagnosis of apical lung tumor, the etiologic diagnosis of smoking-induced carcinoma.
5.   Formulate the diagnostic or problem label justifiable by evidence on hand. Select the precise terms that are no more or no less, not too general, and not too specific. The formulation is predicted on the data available, the guidance of epidemiology and personal clinical experience, and the intuition of clinical judgment.
6.   Determine the patient's illness and the effect of the clinical problem on the patient's physical, mental, and social well-being. Remember that patients with the same diagnosis need different treatment. The differences in the needs of patients with facultative hyperopia, learning problems, cataracts, or impaired vision are particularly noteworthy.

The experienced clinician may find this discussion of unifying elements in observation and steps in the diagnostic process as somewhat academic. This is understandable since with years of experience comes wisdom and a growing appreciation of intuition and the art of clinical practice, but there are many pitfalls in our path. Keeping in touch with the rapid advances in the knowledge base of visual, health, and clinical sciences is difficult. Furthermore, personal knowledge can become distorted by inaccurate clinical observations or undisciplined reasoning. To avoid these pitfalls one must keep in mind the interdependence of knowledge, observation, and reasoning in the quest to "know through" a patient's problems and needs.

Seven unifying elements have been introduced to discipline the observation process in history taking and office examination. These observations, however disciplined and thorough, must be contrasted and interpreted with past clinical experience and current understanding of anatomy and pathophysiology.

Also introduced in this chapter is the six-step process in diagnostic reasoning. The sophisticated diagnostician may seem to proceed through these processes and up the abstraction ladder with ease. The thesis here, however, is that grace and acumen in diagnosis come only after drilling on the discipline of diagnostic reasoning. When this discipline is so practiced as to be ingrained, the clinician has the freedom to practice the art of caring for patients.

# References

Ball GV. Symptoms in eye examination. London: Butterworths, 1982.

Engel G, Morgan WL. Interviewing the patient. Philadelphia: W.B. Saunders, 1976.

Gregg JR. How to communicate in optometric practice. Philadelphia: Chilton, 1969.

# I
# ASSESSMENT
# OF SYMPTOMS

# Barry J. Barresi
# J. David Higgins
# VISION LOSS 4

*A disturbance of central vision often is reported as blurred, faded, veiled, smudged, curtainlike, or blackout effects.*

# BACKGROUND

Vision is a highly complex sense, of which the resolution of high contrast Snellen targets is only one dimension. In clinical practice, vision loss typically refers to disturbances of central vision manifested by reduced Snellen visual acuity.

One schema for classifying the mechanisms of vision loss is to consider the structural site of the cause of failure. A schema of five causitive sites of vision loss can be considered: motility, optical, retinochoroid, and neural. A fifth element, referred to here as diagnosis by exclusion, refers to psychogenic vision loss and amblyopia. Vision loss can be categorized in many fashions. This five-part schema, however, is particularly helpful in organizing the diagnostic investigation of vision loss. History and examination can be systematically applied to sequentially unmask the cause of vision loss, from the front to the back of the vision system.

## Motility-Related Loss

Nystagmus, eccentric fixation, and strabismus can compromise the proper alignment and steady fixation of the eyes. Disorders of binocular efficiency may also manifest with blurred vision caused by instability of accommodation.

## Optical Loss

Opacities of the ocular media may distort, scatter, or actually block the transmission of light to the retinal photoreceptors. Ametropias and accommodation inaccuracy can cause sufficient defocus to reduce visual acuity.

An uneven, spotty tear film caused by dry eye, mucous debris, or viscous ophthalmic solutions impair visual optics. The roughened corneal surface with keratitis also disturbs vision. Colored halos, ghost images, and hazy vision owing to diffraction occur with increased turbidity of transmitting tissues. Corneal edema, for example, can result from contact lens overwear, acute glaucoma, or primary corneal diseases. Incipient cataracts and the cell and flare of uveitis or vitritis also cause light scatter and vision disturbance. Dystrophic or acquired corneal deposits, cataract, vitreous hemorrhage, and intraocular masses can block light and cause more pronounced vision loss.

Presenting ametropias may represent normal changes in refraction and the need for a new correction. With fluctuations in refractive status, always be suspicious of changes caused by drugs, diabetes, and ocular disease (see Chapters 10, 11, and

35

12). Likewise, while accommodative loss occurs with aging, accommodative spasm and insufficiency can result from a variety of functional and organic etiologies (see Chapter 13).

## Retinochoroidal Loss

Retinochoroidal vision loss is caused by (a) disturbances in the macula, such as opacities in the neural layer or cellular disruption in retina or choroid; and (b) by obstacles in the line of sight, such as mass lesions or retinal detachment (see Chapter 30).

The macula is subject to primary retinal disorders of inflammation, degeneration, hemorrhage, edema, and infarction, and to a secondary response to choroidal disease. While retinal hemorrhage and edema may in some way act to impair light transmission to the sensory layer, the resulting cellular disruption, which impairs photoreceptors and retinal neuron activity, is probably the more notable mechanism of vision loss.

Retinochoroidal inflammation can represent a response to infection, trauma, poisons, drugs, and radiation. Macular degeneration, whether dystrophic or senescent, is often slowly progressive. More dramatic vision loss can occur with disciform senile macular degeneration. Retinal vascular disease, often a reflection of systematic disease, can result in acute macular edema, hemorrhage, exudation, or infarction. Retinal detachment usually results from retinal breaks, but occasionally is secondary to tumors. Choroidal melanomas can extend through the macula and block the line of sight, resulting in a dramatic moving curtain of vision loss.

## Neural Loss

Vision can fail because of impaired neural conduction from the retina through pathways to the occipital cortex or from damage to the cortical receiving areas. Congenital defects, such as optic disc hypoplasia, coloboma, and optic pits are not uncommon. Optic nerve conduction declines with inflammation, compression, ischemia, and so forth, with a consequent loss in pupillary response, red green color vision, and central vision. In most cases of postchiasmal disease, the patient is not aware of defects in visual fields but reports mobility or reading problems. With regional brain disease, other associated neurologic signs and symptoms are of more concern than the vision loss (see Chapters 32 and 33).

## Diagnosis by Exclusion Loss

If the search for motility, optical, retinochoroidal, and neural causes fails to explain the severity or type of vision loss, then amblyopia and psychogenic conditions can be considered. Although conversion disorders, malingering, depression, and amblyopia often exhibit cardinal features, all organic causes must first be excluded: diagnosis by exclusion.

Amblyopia is distinguished by association with light deprivation, constant strabismus, or long-standing uncorrected refractive error. Congenital cataract is one condition that will result in light deprivation amblyopia. When amblyopia of disuse or suppression is unilateral, the nonfixating strabismic eye, more hyperopic, or more astigmatic eye is affected. Bilateral amblyopia can occur with uncorrected high refractive, particularly astigmatic, errors (Chapter 12).

Malingering and conversion disorders are the last options to consider in diagnosis by exclusion. Differentiating between malingering, a deliberate attempt to mislead the examiner, and conversion disorder, an unconscious conversion of an idea or fantasy into a physical symptom, may be difficult. A malingering response is usually triggered by desire for compensation or retribution. The conversion of a mental symptom into vision loss is not limited to patients with major syndromes, such as schizophrenia, affective disorder, or somatization disorder (hysteria). Rather, the psychological symptom of vision loss may present in isolation. Differential diagnosis is complicated further by psychological symptoms that precede or are concomitant with organic disease.

## Diagnostic Strategy

The five-site schema of mechanism of vision loss offers a logical, front-to-back approach to differential diagnosis. Thus, the first step is to judge the causative site of vision loss, or with multiple coexisting causes, to determine the respective contribution of each cause to the severity of vision loss.

Another diagnostic schema for vision loss is to group causes on the basis of the symptoms' time course or presence of pain. For example, with gradual vision loss, certain conditions come to mind, such as cataract and macular degeneration. One of the diagnostic challenges here is to differentiate between coexisting causes. The clinician, when assessing gradual vision loss, must continually reflect on whether the lesion or abnormality is consistent with the type or severity of vision loss. An example of poor practice is to ascribe gradual vision loss and 20/40 acuity in an elderly patient to "probable macular degenera-

tion" when the view through a small pupil or lens opacity actually does not allow sufficient resolution to make the diagnosis. Even if some macular changes are observed with the ophthalmoscope, more findings are needed. For example, complaints of slow onset of reading difficulty in dim light, relatively symmetrical degrees of reduced acuity, delayed photostress recovery, and negative findings on tests for neural conduction defects would all strengthen the hypothesis that the observed macular changes are responsible. Similarly, observing lens opacities with the slit lamp does not necessarily explain all levels of reduced acuity; the history and other findings should again be corroborative.

The category of sudden vision loss includes many conditions that require emergency or urgent treatment. The particular diagnostic challenge here is appropriate and prompt triage. Effective treatment that restores sight or prevents further loss is often available. Reception office staff must be informed of the critical nature of this complaint.

The differential diagnosis of transient vision loss deserves considerable attention. Here the challenge is the differential diagnosis of conditions that threaten loss of sight, physical disability, and death. These conditions are discussed in Chapter 6.

# HISTORY

Qualifying the type of vision loss and comparing the effect on each eye is the first step in diagnosis. How is the vision loss described by the patient? Blur, dim-out, curtain or veil-like, and blackout are just some of many possible descriptions. Precision of terms is most important. Often the patient's notion of blur or double vision differs from the examiner's conception. Encouraging the patient to elaborate on the nature of loss can help avoid misunderstanding of terms. The effect on each

eye must be gauged. Is the loss unilateral, or if bilateral, which eye was affected first?

Vision loss owing to macular edema usually presents with distorted vision, or metamorphopsia. General blur is most often of refractive origin. Macular scotomas are often positive, spot, or smudge-like, while with optic nerve disease the patient is only aware of an indistinct area in the field.

Suspicion of occult optic nerve disease is raised by complaints of loss in subjective contrast, despite good Snellen acuity, and a feeling that colors are not as vivid as they used to be. The patient may thus complain that vision seems to be faded or dim. The complaint of impaired depth perception also suggests an optic nerve conduction defect. While stereopsis usually is normal, the Pulfrich phenomenon of unequal optic nerve conduction time alters perception of moving objects. Difficulty in judging the distance between stable objects can be caused by loss of binocular input in patients with bitemporal chiasmal defects.

Evaluating the time course includes determining when the loss was first noted and how the patient became aware of the loss. Was the loss transient, sudden, or gradual? This distinction can be quite valuable to differential diagnosis. While the complaint of transient loss is a reliable aid, the report of gradual versus sudden loss must be interpreted with caution. Many patients who report sudden vision loss are in fact reporting suddenly noted gradual vision loss recently observed in some circumstance where the better seeing eye was covered. Care must be taken to avoid deception by some unusual circumstances. For example, often patients with obviously congenital vision loss will associate some event in adolescence, including accident, with the vision loss.

The circumstances of onset and time course of vision loss should be investigated. Was the onset of vision coincident with new visual demands, family or work stress, illness, injury, drug use, or other physical symptoms? Do certain conditions exacerbate or alleviate the vision loss? If, for example, the problem is viewing distance, near vision may be more adversely affected by presbyopia, accommodative problems, posterior subcapsular cataracts, and hyperopic refractive shifts. Illumination difficulties may result in reduced vision at night from cataracts, myopia, amblyopia, and tapetoretinal degenerations. Reduced vision is more pronounced in daylight, with cone dystrophies or light scatter from cortical cata-

racts. Certain viewing conditions may increase blur when monocular vision loss occurs with latent nystagmus.

Two important differentiating associated symptoms are pain or red eye. Eye or head pain can occur with acute glaucoma, temporal arteritis, optic neuritis, and cranial mass lesions. Most often, vision loss with eye pain and red eye suggests external inflammation or injury that has affected visual optics, usually corneal abrasion or keratitis, but also uveitis. In contrast, painless vision loss, if sudden, suggests retinal vascular etiology or, if truly gradual, degeneration, either optical (corneal dystrophy or cataracts), retinochoroidal (macular dystrophy or senile changes), or neural (toxic or compressive lesion).

Selected examples of other associations with vision loss include colored halos with corneal edema, photopsia or floaters with retinal breaks, scintillating scotomas with migraine, dizziness with hypotension or vertebrobasilar transient ischemia, and hemiplegia and paresthesias with carotid transient ischemia. A curious association is the exacerbation of vision loss or other neural disturbances with increased body temperature from exercise or hot baths, the so-called Uhthoff's sign of demyelinating disease.

Past eye history can provide valuable clues regarding the nature of vision loss and previous eye and vision care. The patient's point of view must be considered in a history of previous eye problems, injury, and surgery. The value of records of previous examinations seems underestimated. More precise information of acuity, and refractive and health status frequently can illuminate the critical diagnostic finding.

The medical history can uncover systemic associations with vision loss. Vision loss is a symptom that deserves the most extensive review of systems and drug use. Associations between vision loss and systemic disease are so pervasive that every case of vision loss should be investigated with a high index of suspicion for underlying systemic etiologies. Knowledge of the patient's current source of primary medical care is most important. When was the last visit to a primary care physician? What conditions are under care and what treatments are being used? Again, it is often best to obtain records or call the physician, as the patient often is not totally reliable in describing the status of treatment. This information is an aid to diagnosis and to subsequent coordination of health care.

Family history can also identify patients at risk for certain etiologies of vision loss. Familiar risk factors are quite extensive, but most notable are retinal detachment, glaucoma, and corneal and macular dystrophies. Family history should include a thorough history of blindness, vision disorders, and selected medical problems such as diabetes and hypertension.

Investigating the patient profile can provide insights into precipitating events and functional consequences of vision loss. A patient can be overcome by the fear of blindness. These fears may lead to exacerbation or even repression of symptoms. How does the patient cope with the vision loss on the job or at home? Is the patient a candidate for ophthalmic surgery or low vision rehabilitation? Is the patient realistic about the future?

Assessment of the patient profile, as is the case with many aspects of the history, continues through the course of the examination. Observation of the patient's general behavior can help gauge the patient's emotional reaction to the visual symptoms and the causative illness. Clues suggesting malingering include stoicism or a passive resistance to testing. The malingerer may become agitated when inconsistencies in findings are pointed out. In contrast, the patient with conversion disorder usually enjoys the attention given in the examination. But like the malingerer, inconsistencies in findings and symptoms dominate the presentation.

# EXAMINATION

## Vision Acuity

Measurement of visual acuity is the principal procedure used to qualify the severity of central vision loss. Measurement of vision acuity also can provide clues to diagnosis. Compare distance and near acuities. Besides the obvious different presentation of accommodative and refractive errors (see Chapters 10–13) the distance/near acuity should be within two Snellen lines. When distance and near visual acuities are not consistent, suspect posterior subcapsular cataracts (PSC) or psychogenic loss. Vision acuity measurements that vary with ambient illumination occur more frequently with scatter effects and opacities of the ocular media. Compare monocular and binocular acuity. Monocular visual acuity will be reduced with latent nystagmus, decompensating hyperopia, and oblique astigmatism. Binocular visual acuity reduction or suppressions suggest monofixation, vergence, or accommodative disorders.

Skipping of letters usually is caused by uncorrected astigmatism or meridional amblyopia, but if the patient skips or has difficulty consistently with one-half of the Snellen chart, then a hemianopic field defect may be present. Some behavioral clues, particularly in children, include squinting, peeking over occluders, and resistance to occlusion, and suggest vision difficulty.

## Pupil Testing

An afferent pupil defect or reduced pupil cycle time indicates a neural conduction impairment and optic nerve disease as the cause of vision loss. Pupillary measurements of conduction impairment are surprisingly sensitive indications of optic nerve disease and are particularly helpful diagnostically when the clinician is faced with coexisting pathologies in the eye with vision loss.

Observation of pupillary escape, Marcus Gunn pupil, with the swinging flashlight is well known and is reviewed in Chapter 8. The test of pupil cycle time is less well appreciated but also is of assistance (see Chapter 31).

## Refraction

Conventional strategy and techniques will determine the optimal lens correction and best corrected acuity (Chapters 10–12).

## Motility and Binocular Assessment

Reduced acuity can occur with nystagmus (Chapter 19), eccentric fixation, strabismus, and amblyopia (Chapter 16). Diagnosis of vision loss owing to these problems usually is straightforward; however, the presentation of monofixation syndrome or small angle strabismus can be more subtle.

## Color Vision

Color vision testing is particularly useful for differentiating between cases of central scotoma caused by macular disease versus optic nerve disease. While many patients with 20/200 acuity owing to macular disease can still recognize the pseudoisochromatic plates, the patient with occult optic nerve disease and 20/20 acuity may fail the test dramatically.

Because of the frequency of congenital color defects and value of color testing in the diagnosis of vision loss, it is good practice to obtain a baseline monocular color vision test on an initial examination.

## Red Desaturation Testing

Another method to probe color vision is use of red stimuli to qualify papillomacular bundle impairment, a region frequently impaired in neurologic lesions (see Chapter 31).

## Photostress Testing

Measuring the cone adaption time is useful in differentiating macular (retinochoroidal) versus another causative site of vision loss. The procedure involves using a bright light to bleach photopigments, and then the two eyes are compared in their recovery to the original visual acuities (see Chapter 30).

## Visual Fields

Testing of the visual fields is of critical importance in the differential diagnosis of neural vision loss. While macular vision loss exhibits depression of the central fields and is best detected with the Amsler grid, other signs make the diagnosis of macular vision loss (photostress, color vision, ophthalmoscopy). With neural vision loss, testing of patient visual fields is needed to localize the neural site, such as optic nerve, chiasm, optic tracts, and occipital cortex. Neural disorders and use of visual fields testing is elaborated in Chapters 28, 31, and 32.

## Physical Evaluation

In most cases of vision loss, diagnosis is based on the history, refraction, and physical examination of the eye with slit lamp and ophthalmoscopy. Applying these procedures to assessment of the eye and the causes of vision loss is elaborated later in this text.

# CLINICAL SIGNIFICANCE

The first maxim of clinical practice is *never* to allow reduced visual acuity to go unexplained. The purpose of this chapter is to guide the clinician along the first steps in the differential diagnosis of vision loss. One of the first steps is to differentiate between mobility, optical, retinochoroidal, neural, and exclusionary causes of vision loss. The reader can then turn to the appropriate sections in the following chapters for guidance in reaching a more precise structural, etiologic, and functional diagnosis.

# Barry J. Barresi
## J. David Higgins

# OCULAR DISCOMFORT 5

*Ocular discomfort arises from or localizes in the eye or adjacent tissues. Presenting symptoms vary and range in severity from nonspecific asthenopia to compelling pain.*

## BACKGROUND

Sensation of the eye and surrounding structures is mediated by the trigeminal sensory complex. Peripherally, three major divisions arise from the gasserian ganglion: ophthalmic, maxillary, and mandibular. From the gasserian ganglion, sensory fibers proceed to the brain stem sensory nuclei, ascend to the thalamus, and finally project to the sensory cortex. Pain of peripheral origin may be well localized at the site of origin or referred from a distant structure, either intracranial or extracranial.

Pain receptors in the skin and ocular tissues can be stimulated by physical or chemical irritation, compression, distention, or tissue ischemia. Inflammation, trauma, mass lesions, vascular disturbances, or muscle fatigue may be the underlying cause. The severity of the pain is somewhat a function of the potency and duration of the pain stimulus. Patients, however, can differ markedly in their emotional reaction and description of discomfort.

## HISTORY

Patients may volunteer the complaint of discomfort or may acknowledge discomfort only after a specific question is raised. At some point, ask "Do you ever have eye pain? Do your eyes feel comfortable?" The clinician should be wary of assuming that if the symptom is only mentioned by the patient in a casual manner that it is of minor consequence. It may be that the patient is reticent because of fear of the consequences. Whenever the symptom of discomfort is uncovered, always strive for

precision of descriptive terms and a judgment of severity.

Discomfort may be described by innumerable terms or phrases. Most symptoms, however, will fall in one of three categories: asthenopia, superficial irritation, or frank pain.

*Asthenopia* is a general term for mild nonspecific ocular discomfort. The complaint is chronic, described as mild aches, pulling, drawing sensations, fatiguability, or reduced stamina with visual tasks. Se-

43

verity of the discomfort typically increases through the course of a day. Often asthenopia is precipitated by prolonged close work or a concentrated visual effort at distance such as with driving or watching a movie. In addition, these annoying sensations often are aggravated by illness, physical exertion, change in environment, or the emotional stresses of a new job or studying for an exam.

A superficial *ocular irritation* may be characterized as itching, burning, sandy, gritty, dry, scratchy, heavy lids, or a foreign body sensation. Often the irritation is aggravated by smoke, dust, wind, and hot, dry weather or prolonged use of the eyes.

The annoyance of ocular irritation and asthenopia contrasts with the compelling presentation of definite *eye pain or ache.* The complaint may be described as deep, dull, sharp, jabbing, painful pressure, or like a "headache in the eye." Often, severe ocular pain is accompanied by photophobia, tears, and, if particularly strong, nausea and vomiting.

A strategy of diagnostic investigation includes:

• *Site and quality:* As best as possible qualify the discomfort and localize the site. Does the discomfort arise from the external or internal eye, the orbit, the face or jaw?

• *Time and change:* Establish the chronology of onset, frequency, pattern of occurrence, and relationship to particular tasks or circumstances. During this interview the clinician may note that an eye ache is intensified by such varied activities as looking at bright lights, pressure on the globe or lacrimal sac, bending over, or eye movements. Each of these associations can guide differential diagnosis.

• *Change and associations:* Determine variability and nature of associated problems. Most important, note if the discomfort is associated with vision disturbances or red eye. If so, what is

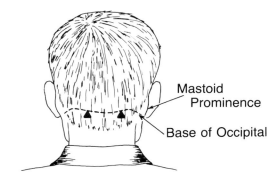

▲ = Greater Occipital Nerve – half way from midline to mastoid prominence

**FIGURE 5.1.**
**Greater occipital nerve neuralgia. Undue tenderness on palpation under the occipital prominences in the retromastoid fossa is the key to the diagnosis.**

the severity and nature of the association? For example, does vision blur before, during, or following the eye ache?

What does the patient do to relieve the problem—stop reading, splash cold water into the eyes, or rest and take aspirin? Does anything make the complaint worse? Relevant associations with ocular discomfort are almost endless and are dictated by consideration of the entities in Table 5.1 and the section on clinical significance.

• *Effect, whole and parts:* Consider the whole patient.

Openness is important; the patient must be made to feel free to describe any aspect of recent health that might bear on the problem. How does the complaint relate to the patient's profile of personality, health status, occupation, and family history? A patient's age also is significant in suggesting diagnostic categories. For example, giant cell arteritis, aneurysm, or carotid insufficiency as a cause of fronto-orbital pain would almost be unheard of in a child, whereas one would not entertain the possibility of a demyelinating neuralgia or subacute retrobulbar neuritis in an elderly patient.

Depending on the findings of inquiry to this point, the remaining eye, medical, and family history can proceed with specific causes of ocular discomfort kept in mind (see Tables 5.1 to 5.4 for guidance and appropriate chapters for special discussions).

**Table 5.1**
**Causes of Ocular Discomfort**

*Asthenopia: Mild nonspecific discomfort*

| | |
|---|---|
| Vision | 1. Uncorrected or improper correction of refractive error |
| | 2. Accommodative dysfunction |
| | 3. Binocular instability or inefficiency, particularly convergence insufficiency |
| | 4. Dazzling and glare in normal eye or eye with media opacities |
| | 5. Insufficient or annoying illumination |
| Local disease | 1. Mild dry eye, infrequent blinking |
| Psychogenic | 1. Conversion reaction |
| | 2. Malingering |
| | 3. Normal eye sensation with neurotic depression |
| | 4. Chronic tension states |

*Irritation: Moderate superficial discomfort*

| | |
|---|---|
| Local disease | 1. External inflammation or foreign body of lids, conjunctiva, or cornea |
| | 2. Structural lid problems, ectropion, entropion, lagophthalmos, trichiasis |
| | 3. Lacrimal disease, dry eye, corneal erosions |
| | 4. Mild inflammation of uveal tract or sclera |
| | 5. Overuse of nonprescription eye drops |
| Psychogenic | 1. Conversion reaction |
| | 2. Malingering |

*Pain: Local eye pain or periorbital ache*

| | |
|---|---|
| Local disease | 1. External inflammation or foreign body of lids, conjunctiva, or cornea |
| | 2. Structural lid problems, ectropion, entropion, lagophthalmos, trichiasis |
| | 3. Lacrimal disease and dry eye |
| | 4. Inflammation of uveal tract, episclera, or sclera |
| | 5. Corneal basement membrane dystrophies and recurrent erosions |
| | 6. Retrobubar neuritis |
| | 7. Acute or subacute angle-closure glaucoma |
| | 8. Orbital inflammation or mass lesion |
| | 9. Orbital tendonitis |
| Disease of adjacent structures | 1. Dental disease |
| | 2. Sinusitis |
| | 3. Temporal mandibular joint syndrome |
| | 4. Nasal trauma or surgery |
| | 5. Postherpetic pain |

**Table 5.1**
*(continued)*

| | |
|---|---|
| Neurophthalmic | 1. Greater occipital nerve neuralgia<br>2. Idiopathic benign neuralgia<br>3. Compressive lesion of nerve V<br>4. Tic douloureux<br>5. Tolosa Hunt syndrome<br>6. Diabetic third nerve infarct<br>7. Nasopharyngioma |
| Systemic | 1. Migraine<br>2. Viral myalgia<br>3. Aneurysm<br>4. Giant cell arteritis<br>5. Atypical cluster headache<br>6. Severe carotid insufficiency |
| Psychogenic | 1. Conversion reaction<br>2. Malingering |

# EXAMINATION

Essential aspects of the workup for ocular discomfort include vision analysis; gross inspection and palpation; pupil testing; assessment of extraocular movements and function of cranial nerves V, VII, and VIII; functional testing of lacrimal system; biomicroscopy of anterior segment; tonometry; and ophthalmoscopy. More specific guidance in diagnostic examination is presented in the chapters on vision conditions and vision systems.

# CLINICAL SIGNIFICANCE

## Asthenopic Profile

Hyperopia is the most common cause of refractive asthenopia. Symptoms are precipitated by increasing age and increasing accommodative effort. Asthenopic symptoms also can be related to astigmatism if uncorrected or improperly corrected. Myopia is not typically thought of as a cause of asthenopia; however, overcorrection, squinting with undercorrection, or a tendency for neck straining with close working distances can cause asthenopia or tension headaches.

Inefficient binocularity can lead to significant asthenopic complaints. While convergence insufficiency often is the culprit, accommodative problems, hetero-phorias, and intermittent strabismus must be ruled out.

Occupation and work environment must be always considered in any case of asthenopia. Insufficient or glaring illumination, poor ventilation, boring or highly demanding tasks, prolonged posture, and infrequent blinking are some elements to consider. The study or work environment may also have psychological consequences. For example, is asthenopia associated with the use of a computer terminal screen caused by vision strain or the mental stress of a complicated task and pressing demands for increased productivity?

Neurotic depression can be a primary cause of asthenopia or overlay and can ex-

**Table 5.2**
**Periorbital Ache in Normal Eye: Common Causes**

| Cause | Characteristics |
|---|---|
| *Greater Occipital Nerve Neuralgia* (see Figure 5.1) | 1. Referred pain from neck, usually with ipsilateral cervical tenderness<br>2. May be sharp but more likely a dull ache "wrapping around" from back of head<br>3. Undue tenderness on palpation under the occipital prominences in the retromastoid fossa (key to the diagnosis)<br>4. Associated history of whiplash, cervical arthritis, chronic muscle tension, rigidity (as with parkinsonism) |
| *Idiopathic Benign Neuralgia* | 1. Infrequent attacks of lightning pain in the eye, or short stabbing pain behind the eye<br>2. Quite common but with no known cause<br>3. Assess for normal fifth nerve function on both sides |
| *Sinus Headache* | 1. Usually with frontal or ethmoid infection<br>2. May be acute and severe<br>3. Typically worse in morning and with bending<br>4. Eye may be tender and mildly photophobic<br>5. Associations of nasal discharge, fever, malaise<br>6. Focal sensitivity to percussion over the sinus<br>7. Transillumination of frontal sinus |
| *Migraine Attack* | 1. Pulsing, nausea, photophobia, and classic prodrome<br>2. Predisposing events (birth control pills, skipping meals)<br>3. Acute transiently abates with valsalva maneuver<br>4. Normal mental status |
| *Viral Myalgia* | 1. Diagnosis by exclusion<br>2. Associations, other myalgias, chills, upper respiratory infection, malaise<br>3. Ache may be slightly worse with eye movement<br>4. *Alert:* Same symptoms may precede retrobulbar neuritis; keep in touch with patient, expect clearing in week or reexamine |

**Table 5.3**
**Periorbital Ache in Normal Eye: Most Serious Causes**

| Cause | Characteristics |
|-------|-----------------|
| *Aneurysm* | 1. Rare in children; most common in middle-aged women<br>2. Sharp brow pain most characteristic<br>3. Check for periorbital hypoaesthesia with wisp of cotton; check corneal reflexes<br>4. May precede or accompany minimal and variable field defects or third nerve signs; check EOMs, pupils, and lid position closely<br>5. Auscultate eye and retromastoid fossa for bruit<br>6. Inquire as to cervical rigidity<br>7. Check for pyramidal signs/Babinski reflex<br>8. If suspicious, refer to neurology |
| *Mass Compressing Nerve V* | 1. Cerebello pontine angle tumor most common cause<br>2. Look for stigmata of neurofibromatosis<br>3. Pain may be neuralgialike on occasion<br>4. Compare corneal reflexes and periorbital sensation<br>5. Check facial muscles and hearing ipsilaterally<br>6. Look for cerebellar signs: ipsilateral listing on Romberg; ipsilateral gaze nystagmus, finger dysmetria, dysdiachokinesis<br>7. Refer to neurology if suspicious |
| *Giant Cell Arteritis* | 1. Rare under age 65<br>2. Look for signs of cranial arteritis: erythema, hair loss, tenderness, nodularity, and absence of temporal artery pulse<br>3. Inquire as to systemic symptoms: night sweats, fatigue, diminished appetite, claudication, polymyalgia<br>4. Look for ocular ischemia: TIAs, cotton-wool spots, disc hemorrhage, conjunctival tortuosity, gutter ulcer<br>5. Get ESR as soon as possible and refer to internal medicine |

acerbate a concurrent physiologic cause. Conversion reactions and malingering must also be kept in mind as a diagnosis of exclusion. Often the profile of psychogenic asthenopia includes a history of general fatiguability, physical inactivity, poor diet, smoking, and excessive use of caffeine. Other somatic complaints usually abound: insomnia, low back pain, functional stomach complaints, or concern with urinary frequency.

## Irritation Profile

Mild irritation may be due to the asthenopia causes and prolonged use of the eyes,

### Table 5.4
### Periorbital Ache in Normal Eye: Rare Causes

| Cause | Characteristics |
|---|---|
| Tic Douloureux | 1. Infrequent ache or lancinating eye pain may precede full-blown syndrome<br>2. Suspect if more localized to below the eye in middle-aged or elderly women |
| Nasal Injury or Surgery | 1. Neuralgias localized to orbit not an uncommon complication |
| Postherpetic Neuralgia or Harbinger of Zoster | 1. History of ophthalmic shingles<br>2. Suspect impending attack if ipsilateral paresthesias, hypoesthesia, or early vessicles on forehead in elderly patient<br>3. Conjunctiva may be red in premonitory stage |
| Fifth Nerve Demyelination with Multiple Sclerosis | 1. Don't diagnose tic douloureux in young people with periorbital neuralgia<br>2. Compare periorbital sensation to wisps of cotton<br>3. Inquire as to historical symptoms characteristic of demyelinating disease |
| Subacute Retrobulbar Neuritis | 1. Ache often increases on extreme EOMs<br>2. Look for color desaturation, arcuate field defects, slit defects in retinal nerve fiber layer, and historical evidence of multiple sclerosis |
| Meningioma/Early Superior Orbital Fissure Syndrome | 1. Check fields, fifth nerve, EOMs, and signs of minimal proptosis/venous congestion<br>2. Palpate for hyperostosis in temporal fossa area in middle-aged women where suspicion of sphenoid ridge meningioma exists |
| Orbital Myositis/Tenonitis/SO Tendonitis | 1. Sharp ache much worse with EOMs<br>2. If tenosynovitis of superior oblique, pain worse with vertical gaze when eye abducted and may be tender to palpation to trochlear area<br>3. Lid may be puffy |

**Table 5.4**
*(continued)*

| Cause | Characteristics |
|---|---|
| | 4. Do exophthalmometry and inquire as to other myalgias and symptoms of collagen disease and trichinosis |
| *Atypical Cluster Headache/ Paratrigeminal Neuralgia* | 1. Crescendo onset of severe recurrent nocturnal or early morning eye aches, usually in males<br>2. Inquire as to rhinorrhea, conjunctival erythema, and ptosis |
| *Tolosa Hunt Syndrome* | 1. History of recurrent painful third nerve palsy; may be malaise and increased ESR rate<br>2. Diagnosis usually possible by orbital venography<br>3. Quick response to steroids and characteristic history<br>4. Pain may precede palsy |
| *Harbinger of Diabetic Third Nerve Infarct* | 1. Smoldering retroorbital pain of a day or two may precede any third nerve sign<br>2. Undiagnosable at this stage but communicate suspicion to known diabetics |
| *Severe Carotid Insufficiency* | 1. Rare (5% cases)<br>2. Requires 90% stenosis<br>3. Suspect in elderly patient with atherosclerotic risk factors<br>4. Listen for bruit over carotids and eyes<br>5. Inquire as to TIAs<br>6. Look for signs of ocular ischemia<br>7. Do ophthalmodynamometry |
| *Occult Carotid-Cavernous Fistula* | 1. May occur without trauma in elderly person with desiccating aneurysm owing to atherosclerosis<br>2. Proptosis and congestion may be minimal or bilateral<br>3. Look for globe pulsation with exophthalmometer, increased IOP, pulse of IOP, and presence of ocular bruit |
| *Referred Pain from Falx* | 1. Look for parietal/occipital lobe symptomatology and do visual field test in patients with slowly progressive ache, especially middle-aged women |

**Table 5.4**
*(continued)*

| Cause | Characteristics |
|---|---|
| *Nasopharyngioma* | 1. Suspect especially with pain more localized to maxillary region in elderly person, especially a male<br>2. Look for a Horner's pupil and partial sixth nerve paresis<br>3. Inquire as to ear pain, blocked or popping ears, epistaxis, oropharyngeal numbness, dysarthria, dysphagia<br>4. *A serious malignancy* |

but take care to rule out causes such as inflammation, lid problems, and dry eye. Complaints that are worse in the morning suggest staphylococcal blepharitis, recurrent erosion, and nocturnal lagophthalmos. Greater discomfort at night suggests dry eye, spastic entropion, senile ectropion, or contact lens overwear syndrome. Symptoms can help guide assessment, but external and slit lamp signs most often lead to diagnosis (see Chapters 21, 22, 24, and 25 on the external eye).

## Pain Profile

Eye ache can ensue from external problems such as sicca, anterior segment inflammation, corneal erosions, exposure keratitis, and corneal or lid foreign bodies. Anterior uveitis, scleritis, and closed-angle glaucoma, acute or subacute, can cause a truly compelling eye pain.

With a thorough examination of the adnexa and the globe, ruling out the common causes of eye pain is a relatively easy task. One must be certain, of course, to consider ocular disease in which the eye may seem, from a casual inspection, to be relatively quiet. Be alert to subacute angle closure, posterior scleritis, healing recurrent erosion, or chronic pars planitis.

On occasion, the cause of periorbital ache is not uncovered by routine examination. In these cases the vision analysis and health assessment is negative; the eye apparently is normal. Tables 5.2, 5.3, and 5.4 outline a threefold approach to diagnosing the cause of occult eye ache in the normal eye: first, attempt to confirm the most common causes of the complaint (Table 5.2); second, always rule out the most serious causes (Table 5.3); third, if the diagnosis is still not clear, consider the rarer causes (Table 5.4).

If after thorough consideration of both the overt and occult causes of eye ache a specific diagnosis is still not at hand, the patient should be informed that while the complaint of eye ache in a healthy appearing eye is usually benign and self-limited, it occasionally has a serious cause. Any change in the symptoms should immediately be reported and reevaluated. If the acute pain still persists after one week, a consultation with a neurologist, solely on the basis of a suspicious headache, is indicated.

# References

Bode DD. Ocular pain secondary to occipital neuritis. Ann Ophthalmol 1979; 11:589–594.

Kaseras G, Crisp AH. Symptoms without signs in outpatients attending ophthalmology clinics. Br J Ophthalmol 1978;62:340–343.

Russell RW. Symposium on the symptom of pain in ophthalmology. Trans Ophthalmol Soc UK 1980;100:251–252.

Ryan RE, Ryan RE Jr. Headache of nasal origin. Headache 1979;19:173–179.

J. David Higgins

# EPISODIC NEUROVISUAL DISTURBANCES 6

*The hallmark episodic neurologic disturbance of ocular importance is amaurosis fugax, the sudden diminution of vision in part or all of the visual field of one or both eyes, followed by complete recovery over the next several minutes to hours.*

## BACKGROUND

The preeminent causes of transient loss of vision have an ischemic basis of vascular disease in the large arteries serving the eyes and/or visual radiations (Figure 6.1). Thromboembolic disease now accounts for approximately two-thirds of all strokes. This percentage is likely to increase as earlier and more aggressive control of hypertension decreases the contribution of cerebral hemorrhage and lacunar disease to stroke data. Many intracerebral infarcts are now known to be caused by tight stenosis, thrombosis, and embolization from extracranial sites. This realization has led to the increased importance of recognizing early warning signs since in many cases surgical or medical treatment is effective in preventing stroke.

In some cases of severe multifocal atheromatous disease, a transient ischemic attack (TIA) may reflect global insufficiency. Most episodes, however, are thought to reflect platelet aggregation and embolization caused by local flow turbulence and endothelial disruption, as within an ulcerated atheroma or with cardiac valve disease (Figure 6.2). These episodes are associated with focal neurologic disturbances; the character of such disturbances depends on the exact vessel that is temporarily occluded.

## HISTORY

The single most important feature of TIA owing to embolic disease is the abruptness of onset of the focal neurologic deficit. This serves to distinguish it from most other causes of visual fluctuations.

TIAs affecting vision may be monocular (transient monocular blindness, or TMB) or binocular, in which case they usually are hemianopic, affecting corresponding fields in both eyes; or they may be total, affecting both halves of the visual field (cortical blindness).

Patients suffering from transient hemianopia often mistakenly blame the eye

53

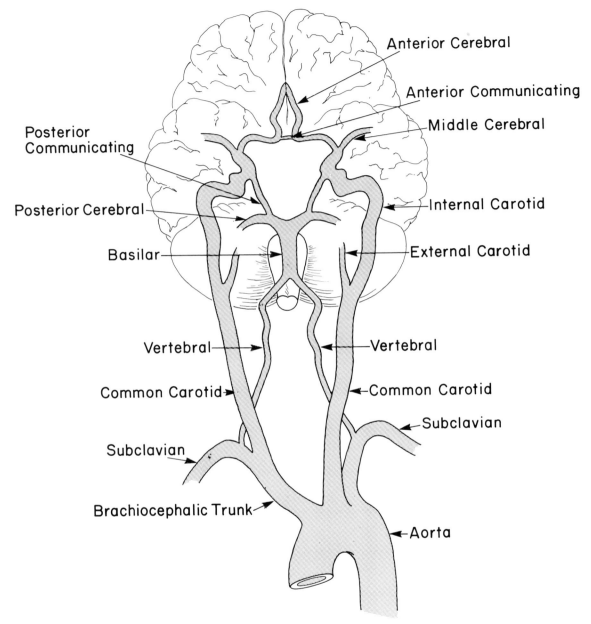

FIGURE 6.1.

Circulation to the brain. The eye and much of the cerebral hemispheres
are supplied by branches of the internal carotid arteries. The posterior
fossa and occipital lobes are supplied by branches of the vertebrobasilar
system. Note the origin of the vertebral arteries from the subclavians.

**Pathogenesis of Thrombosis and Embolism**

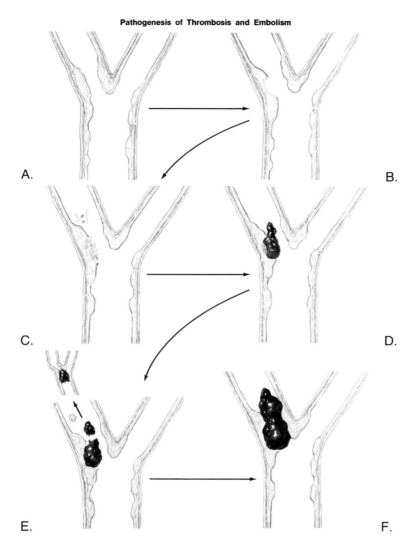

A.

B.

C.

D.

E.

F.

**FIGURE 6.2.**
Mechanisms of transient ischemic attack. *A.* Formation of atherosclerotic plaque at bifurcation. *B.* Ulcer formation with loss of intimal continuity. *C.* Platelet-fibrin aggregation and embolization. *D.* Thrombus formation at site. *E.* Subsequent embolization. *F.* Total occlusion caused by thrombus. In addition, necrosis of the plaque and embolization of the contents may occur, or a subplaque hemorrhage itself may obliterate the lumen.

on the side of the affected hemifield. When questioned, however, the patient usually becomes uncertain of whether the eye or the ipsilateral hemifield was in fact involved. This is in sharp contrast to the true TMB, where the patient usually is adamant that it was the eye itself, often actually covering each eye during the episode for verification. The distinction is important since TMB argues strongly for an ipsilateral carotid disease where transient hemianopia implies vertebrobasilar disease.

In general, vertebrobasilar attacks last less than a couple of minutes and may be associated with a brief headache. Carotid episodes usually last at least several minutes and are only rarely accompanied by headache. Additionally, the vertebral arteries are prone to compression with hyperextension and head turning in the presence of cervical arthritis (Figure 6.3). Thus, an episode of apparent right visual field fading, during painting of a ceiling for example, suggests vertebral artery disease, even if the patient is not sure of whether the right eye or field was affected.

Much more significant in localization of the vascular territory are questions concerning other "spells" (Table 6.1). Carotid territory spells usually are hemispheric, whereas vertebrobasilar spells often involve both sides of the brain stem/cerebellum, producing characteristic bilateral symptoms. Patients commonly seem unaware of, and may deny, nonvisual spells such as difficulty finding words or a short episode of dysarthria; it is helpful therefore to have the spouse present as he or she often is painfully aware of such episodes. The occurrence of other TIAs in addition to the transient visual failure always argues for prompt referral to a neurologist.

Transient monocular visual failure may be total or altitudinal. When total, the suddenness of onset is often emphasized by the patient (as if "milk splashed in my eye"). Other episodes are described as if a white or gray curtain came over the vision, usually from below and often stopping at the midline to involve only the inferior field— a description pathognomonic of ciliary artery nonperfusion to the optic nerve. The single most common transient hemispheric attack (THA) to occur in carotid artery disease is a short episode of numbness in the contralateral hand. This should always be inquired about in suspect cases, as should the occurrence of spells in general. The most common TIAs in vertebrobasilar disease probably are true vertigo and perioral paresthesia.

Many patients describe less ominous fluctuations in vision that do not resemble the classic symptoms just described. With such patients it is wise to be suspicious when multiple risk factors for atheromatous disease are present (elderly; male; premature arcus; black; obese; history of hypertension, diabetes, hyperlipidemia, hypothyroidism, smoking, coronary artery disease, completed strokes, etc.). Some nonatheromatous causes of episodic visual fluctuation are given in Table 6.2.

The general principles of history taking are the same as with any symptom. It is most important to secure in detail all relevant facts associated with the episode. Once the patient has been given free rein to relate the event in his own words, directed questions may be asked. A brief episode of nausea, sweating, and circular collapse of the field argue for a syncopeal reaction; whereas anxiety, tingling, and shortness of breath suggest a hyperventilatory episode, for example. Slow onset and spread of the disturbance are extremely uncharacteristic of ischemic events but are the rule in migraine. Inquiries as to the general status of the patient are critical. For example, dyspnea and cyanosis in a heavy smoker suggest polycythemia; whereas malaise, night sweats, and polymyalgia in an elderly patient suggest inflammatory occlusive disease owing to giant cell arteritis. In general, the history is guided by a consideration of the possibilities given in Table 6.2 as well as the possibility of atheromatous disease.

Extravascular Compression of Vertebral Arteries

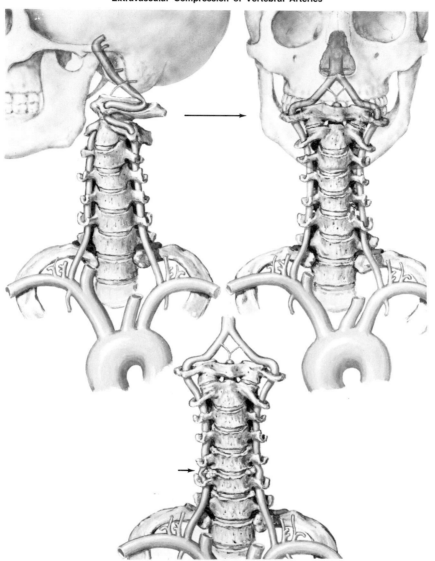

**FIGURE 6.3.**
Physiologic angulation and narrowing of left vertebral artery on head turn
(*upper left*) and normalization of flow with return of head (*upper right*).
Symptoms of vertebrobasilar insufficiency may occur with head turns
when collateral flow is poor and/or injury or degeneration results in
osteophytic changes compromising the lumen (*bottom*).

Table 6.1
Carotid versus Vertebrobasilar TIAs

| Carotid Territory | Vertebrobasilar Territory |
|---|---|
| May last minutes to an hour or more | Characteristically short-lived (minutes) |
| Headache rare | Headache common |
| Often occurs on arising | May occur on arising, on neck rotation, or on exercise of arm (subclavian steal) |
| Visual symptoms usually ipsilateral prominent and positive (curtainlike) | Visual symptoms hemianopic and vaguer |
| *Other Spells:* | *Other Spells:* |
| Contralateral hand/arm/face numbness/clumsiness | Unconsciousness |
| Contralateral weakness | Diplopia/vertigo |
| Aphasia if dominant side involved | Dysarthria/dysphagia |
| | Sensory symptoms often bilateral, especially perioral paresthesia |
| | Leg weakness/ataxia |

# EXAMINATION

An essential part of the exam when atheromatous disease is suspected is a search for these signs of ocular ischemia:

1. Low tension cupping/peripapillary atrophy/disc hemorrhage in one eye
2. Asymmetrical arcus senilis (less visible on the stenotic side)
3. Distinctly lower IOP and IOP pulse on tonometry ipsilaterally
4. CRA/CRV occlusion or optic nerve infarct
5. Unilateral signs of retinal ischemia: increased venous diameter and nicking (general stasis); cotton-wool spots and splinter hemorrhages (acute ischemia); diabeticlike retinopathy in one eye (chronic severe stasis)
6. Retinal emboli
7. Anterior segment ischemia: rubeosis with or without glaucoma; iris atrophy; conjunctival tortuosity; cataract; marginal corneal degeneration

A most significant sign is the presence of retinal emboli. Usually these represent flat crystals of cholesterol ester (Hollenhorst plaques) that have broken off an atheromatous plaque to lodge in the vessel wall at an arterial bifurcation. In most cases these are an incidental finding, since only rarely do they obstruct flow and produce symptoms. Their glistening orange appearance is unmistakable, however, and always signifies a proximal source of embolization (Figure 6.4). Rarely, one may have the opportunity to see a patient during TMB, in which case the presence of platelet-fibrin plugs may be observed in the arterial tree (Figure 6.5).

Part of the workup of any elderly patient without the benefit of a recent physical exam should include an office assessment of the vascular status. This becomes a necessity when such a patient has given suggestive evidence of recent failing (lethargy, facial asymmetry, decreased mental status, etc.) or presents with signs or symptoms of ocular ischemia (Figure 6.6). The first step of the evaluation is to

**Table 6.2**
**Nonatheromatous Causes of Episodic Visual Fluctuation**

| Cause | Characteristics |
|---|---|
| Cardiac Emboli | Atrial fibrillation, rheumatic valve disease, mitral valve prolapse, endocarditis, after occult myocardial infarction, atrial myxoma. |
| Migraine Equivalents | Slower onset of field defect, usually with a photoptic annulus of shimmer; the disturbance typically spreads centripetally to fade in the peripheral field in 15–25 minutes. |
| Migraine Mimickers | Seizure owing to tumor; ischemia from AV malformation, but also platelet emboli from heart or great vessels can simulate migraine. If new onset of aura on estrogens, the preparation should be discontinued. |
| Transient Global Hypotension | "Iris diaphragm" collapse of the visual field with dizziness, and often paresthesias; heart block/arrhythmia, orthostatic hypotension, presyncope, autonomic neuropathy, beta blockers, hyperventilation, hyperviscosity syndromes, multifocal atheromatous disease. |
| Visual Fading in Bright Light | Digitalis, demyelinating disease, but also severe carotid stenosis. |
| Visual Fading with Exercise/ Overheating | Advanced demyelinating disease. |
| Variation with Blinking | Mucus, dry eyes, floaters. |
| Morning Corneal Edema | Fuchs' dystrophy and Chandler's syndrome. |
| Variations with Illumination | As with SMD and cataracts. |
| Pseudomyopia | As with diabetes, sulfonamides, diuretics. |
| Accommodative Spasm | Chiefly on looking near to far. |
| Subacute Angle Closure | Misty vision, halos, injection, ache. |
| Severe Papilledema | Multiple fadings of vision with changes in posture. |
| Porphyria | Usually with other signs of encephalopathy. |

**Table 6.2**
*(continued)*

| Cause | Characteristics |
|---|---|
| *Arteritis* | Chiefly giant cell in elderly, but also Takayasu's disease, syphilis, and especially collagen arteritis (lupus, polyarteritis, scleroderma, etc.). |
| *Hyperviscosity Syndrome* | Leukemias, polycythemias, myelomas, macroglobulinemias. |
| *Impending CRA, CRV, or Ciliary Artery Occlusion* | — |
| *Optic Nerve Sheath Meningioma* | Unilateral visual fading on eccentric gaze. |
| *Severe Hypoglycemia* | Heat waves, spots, or migraine equivalent in patient having episodes of fatigue, tremor, dizziness, sweats, etc. |
| *Digitalis Toxicity* | Snowy vision, green or yellow mist, defective color vision, fading in bright light, prolonged after-images, hallucinations. Symptoms may be episodic; check for bradycardia, arrhythmia, headache, loss of appetite, nausea, lethargy. |

obtain brachial blood pressures in both arms. A difference of 20% in the systolics suggests subclavian artery stenosis. Significant stenosis in this artery prior to the origin of the vertebral artery (Figure 6.1) may result in *retrograde* vertebral flow (away from the brain) to serve the subclavian when the demand for blood is high in the arm, as during exercise. The symptoms of such a "subclavian steal" generally will be those seen in vertebrobasilar disease.

The next step is to evaluate carotid flow. The common carotid artery in the neck runs approximately from the clavicle to under the angle of the jaw. By far the most frequent site of stenosis is at the bifurcation of the internal and external carotid under the angle of the jaw (Figure 6.7).

The pulses should be compared on both sides.

Next, the artery should be auscultated for evidence of turbulent blood flow, that is, an audible bruit. To accomplish this the bell stethoscope attachment should be used and is lightly placed over the artery just under the angle of the jaw. The neck should be slightly extended and the face turned slightly away from the side being examined. The room should be very quiet and the examiner should listen closely for at least 20 seconds, moving the bell slightly up and down the artery while the patient holds a breath from time to time. Bruits are often recorded as "soft" when they mimic a blowing sound with each systole and "harsh" if the sound is more like a buzz. This may be graded "trace" if barely

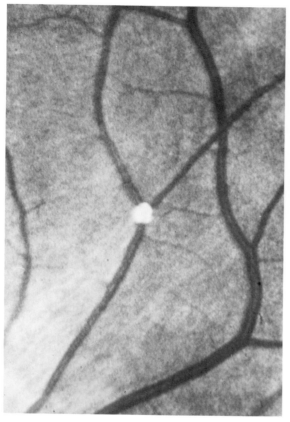

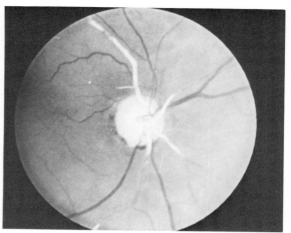

**FIGURE 6.5.**
**Platelet-fibrin emboli during an attack of**
**amaurosis fugax.**
Reprinted by permission of the publisher,
from O'Connor PR. Retinal vascular disease.
New York, Famous Teachings in Modern
Medicine, Medcom Inc., 1974.

**FIGURE 6.4.**
**Hollenhorst plaque lodged at arterial bifurcation**
**without obstructing flow. This observation**
**requires search for a proximal source of**
**embolization.**
Reprinted by permission of the publisher,
from O'Connor PR. Retinal vascular disease.
New York, Famous Teachings in Modern
Medicine, Medcom Inc., 1974.

audible to 4+ if extremely loud. Venous hum, which is sometimes heard in children or in high flow states (hyperthyroidism, cerebral arteriovenous malformation), should not be confused with a cervical arterial bruit, as it is continuous and usually disappears when the breath is held. Ca-

rotid bruits are almost invariably loudest near the bifurcation and should diminish as the bell is moved toward the heart, unlike a valve murmur that radiates into the neck. Subclavian bruits also may radiate up the neck, but are best heard in the supraclavicular fossa.

A stenotic lesion higher up in the internal carotid artery may be better heard by placing the bell over the closed lid and having the patient gently open the other eye, fixate, and open the mouth to reduce lid muscle noise.

One should also evaluate flow in the external carotid distribution. Because of anastomoses between the internal and external carotid systems, patients with complete internal carotid stenoses may have no bruits but may have increased flow in the external carotid system ipsilaterally to aid the intracranial circulation through recurrent collaterals. Thus, an increased

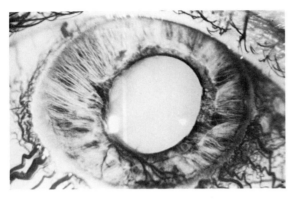

**FIGURE 6.6.**
Anterior segment ischemia following carotid ligation for aneurysm. With this type of "red eye" always suspect severe atheromatous disease or carotid-cavernous fistula.
Reprinted by permission of the publisher, from O'Connor PR. Retinal vascular disease. New York, Famous Teachings in Modern Medicine, Medcom Inc., 1974.

pulse or prominence felt in the temporal artery just in front of the ear on the suspect side is a suggestive finding. One important anastomosis between the external and internal carotid systems is the angular artery at the upper inner canthus.

With severe internal carotid stenosis, blood flow in this artery may reverse its usual direction such that flow is inward through the ophthalmic artery to feed the internal carotid system. This is best studied with doppler flow studies, but can often be detected simply by noting whether briefly compressing the temporal artery extinguishes the brow pulse. Such a finding is never normal.

Ophthalmodynamometry (ODM),* although a relatively noninvasive technique of measuring central retinal artery (CRA) pressure, suffers from poor sensitivity; it will often miss even a 70% stenosis where ulceration may be associated with dangerous embolization. In general, positive ODM findings indicate poor collateral flow to the eye coupled with high-grade or complete carotid stenosis. In this case, the patient may no longer be a surgical candidate. Here even light digital pressure on the globe may be seen to cause central retinal artery pulsation. Thermography, doppler flow studies, digital subtraction IV angiography, and ultrasound are fast becoming more sensitive noninvasive alternatives to angiography than ophthalmodynamometry.

# CLINICAL SIGNIFICANCE

The chief significance of transient visual failure is the increased possibility of stroke. Untreated, about one-third of symptomatic patients go on to develop a completed stroke over the next 3 years. One-third continue with just TIAs, and one-third become asymptomatic owing to improved collateral flow or complete stenosis with termination of embolic episodes. In general, the prognosis is better with treatment; however, the first TMB, TMB plus other TIAs, an escalating series of more frequent TIAs, and any TIA combined with any single positive physical sign (bruit, low IOP/IOP pulse, retinal emboli, etc.) signify the possibility of more imminent stroke. Prompt referral is indicated in such cases.

It is also critical to inquire as to symptoms of temporal arteritis in any elderly patient complaining of transient visual failure. Thus malaise, fatigue, myalgia, night sweats, fever, and especially signs of cranial involvement (tenderness, boring headache, nodularity, lack of pulse, ery-

---

* For an excellent discussion of ophthalmodynamometry, see Gay (1967) in the reference section.

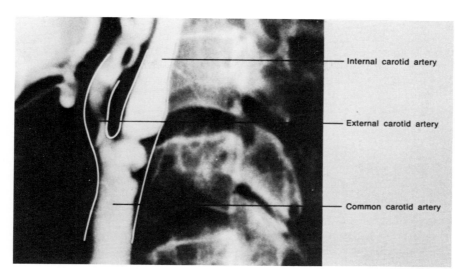

**FIGURE 6.7.**
Ulcerated atheroma at origin of internal carotid artery on angiography.
Ophthalmodynamometry would be unlikely to detect this sort of lesion
despite its potential for embolization.
Reprinted by permission from the publisher, from O'Connor PR.
Retinal vascular disease. New York, Famous Teachings in Modern
Medicine, Medcom Inc., 1974.

thema, or claudication in the distribution of the temporal artery) require an immediate sedimentation rate (Westergren method). About one-third of irreversible optic nerve infarcts caused by this disease are in fact preceded by some sort of transient visual failure. Patients with giant cell arteritis may also have cervical bruits, which however, are usually loudest as one moves downward from the bifurcation toward the supraclavicular fossa. Thus, if a careful history is not obtained from these patients, an inflammatory subclavian stenosis may stimulate a carotid TIA, and the patient may lose his eyesight for lack of prompt treatment with steroids. Patients threatened with imminent blindness are also more likely to show signs of acute retinal ischemia than those with carotid stenosis (e.g., disc hemorrhage, cotton-wool spots, or even optic disc edema).

The heart must also be considered in any patient complaining of transient vi-

sual obscuration, especially when the patient is not of advanced age. Also consider collagen vascular disease in middle age or before, especially in women. Global insufficiency owing to arrhythmia or heart block may be accompanied by a gray-out or "iris diaphragm" circular collapse of the visual field, usually accompanied by other symptoms such as faintness or drop attacks. Often, however, cardiac symptoms are focal and reflect embolization.

A frequent cause of cardiac embolization is atrial fibrillation, a relatively common cause of stroke in women. This should be suggested by an irregular pulse rate over 110 in a patient aware of palpitations. Referral of these patients is of obvious value.

Rheumatic valve disease is suggested by history and the presence of a murmur, especially in a young person with TIAs. Such valves provide a nidus for platelet aggregation and for infection. Embolization from septic valves (subacute bacterial endocarditis) is a serious complication. Usually, the patient is suffering from malaise, chills, myalgias, demonstrates a progressive murmur, and may show petechial hemorrhages in the nail beds, mucous membranes, or retina. When retinal hemorrhages have a white center (Roth's spots), always suspect this disease. It is more common in the elderly, but is also to be suspected in anyone with a history of rheumatic fever, mitral valve prolapse, the immunosuppressed, and drug addicts. The patient should be hospitalized immediately.

Mitral valve prolapse, although common, is not as benign as once believed and is a recognized cause, albeit rare, of sudden death from arrhythmia. It is also productive of platelet emboli, which may either simulate classic migraine or produce a TMB. It is to be suspected especially in younger patients with these symptoms and is sometimes associated with sunken chest and is common in hyperthyroidism. A late systolic murmur or midsystolic click in such a patient should always produce a referral for an echocardiogram. TIAs from mitral valve prolapse may occur in as many as one-fifth of the patients, tend to last only 10 to 45 seconds, and often occur on standing. Atypical Eales's disease is an occasional complication of recurrent embolization. Mitral valve prolapse of significant severity is frequently seen in Marfan's and Ehlers-Danlos syndromes, as well as in pseudoxanthoma elasticum. All three of these disorders have other significant eye signs.

Myocardial infarction frequently is occult, and loss of endothelial integrity provides a focus for platelet aggregation and embolization. Thus, any patients with TIAs reporting a recent suggestive episode (chest/arm pain, dyspnea, sweating, nausea, etc.) should be referred for an electrocardiogram (ECG) and cardiac enzyme testing. A rare cardiac tumor, atrial myxoma, is a recognized cause of TMB in young people and is caused by embolization.

Because of the multiple cardiac origins of emboli, any patient without physical evidence and risk factors for atherosclerotic disease suffering from episodic visual failure probably deserves referral to the internist. Patients with clear-cut physical evidence of a tight stenosis and suggestive symptoms and who are otherwise healthy may be referred to a vascular surgeon. Patients with atypical migrainelike seizures are usually best evaluated by a neurologist. Patients with vague symptoms and no physical evidence of stenosis are often simply placed on antiplatelet therapy (aspirin, persantine, sulfinpyrazone) by the family physician rather than face the risk of angiography. If the patient seems able to tolerate endarterectomy, however, it is probably wise to do at least further noninvasive testing for tight stenosis as outlined in the section on examination. If these tests are suggestive, the patient should be referred for further workup to a major vascular center where femoral artery catheterization for selective angiography is now associated with only a 2% risk of significant complications, and carotid endarterectomy has a risk of only 0.5%.

Patients with clear symptoms of vertebrobasilar artery disease also deserve a vascular workup. Even though these arteries are surgically inaccessible, multifocal atheromatous disease usually is present, and carotid bruits are often heard, providing evidence of underlying disease. Opening up the arch or subclavian or carotid arteries may result in better perfusion via collateral flow and improve the patient's condition.

In summary, a variety of causes may underlie transient visual failure. While some are trivial, others are of the most serious nature. It is often the eye doctor whom the patient first consults and who must make the initial assessment. Proper consideration of the causes listed in Table 6.2 will often have great import for the ultimate management and outcome of the case.

# References

Ackerman RH. A prospective on noninvasive diagnosis of carotid disease. Neurology 1979;29:615–622.

Anonymous. Tonometer helps predict stroke risk. JAMA 1975;231:457, 462.

Barnet HJM, et al. Further evidence relating mitral-valve prolapse to cerebral ischemic events. N Engl J Med 1980; 302:139–144.

Barresi BJ. Stroke, identifying the patient at risk. J Am Optom Assoc 1978; 49:794–800.

Caltrider ND, et al. Retinal emboli in patients with mitral valve prolapse. Am J Ophthalmol 1980;90:534–539.

Canadian Cooperative Study Group. A randomized trial of aspirin and sulfinpyrazone in threatened stroke. N Engl J Med 1978;299:53–59.

Enoch JM, Campos EC, Bedell HE. Visual resolution in a patient exhibiting a visual fatigue or saturation-like effect. Arch Ophthalmol 1979;97:76–78.

Forlan AJ. Unilateral visual loss in bright light: an unusual symptom of carotid artery occlusive disease. Arch Neurol 1979;36:675–676.

Gay AJ. Clinical ophthalmodynanometry. In: Gay AJ. Clinical concepts in neuro-ophthalmology. Int Ophthalmol Clin 1967;7(4):729–744.

Heyman A, et al. Risk of stroke in asymptomatic persons with cervical arterial bruits: a population study in Evans County, Georgia. N Engl J Med 1980; 302:838–841.

Hollenhorst RW. Significance of bright plaques in the retinal arteries. JAMA 1961;178:23–29.

Mehalic T, Farchat SM. Vertebral artery injury from chiropractic manipulation of the neck. Surg Neurol 1974;2:125–129.

Roseman RH, et al. Relation of corneal arcus to cardiovascular risk factors and the incidence of coronary disease. N Engl J Med 1974;291:1322–1324.

Savino PJ, Glaser JS, Cassady J. Retinal stroke: is the patient at risk? Arch Ophthalmol 1977;95:1185–1189.

Wolf PA, Dawber TR, Thomas HE. Epidemiological assessment of chronic atrial fibrillation and risk of stroke: the Framingham study. Neurology 1978; 28:977–979.

# Barry J. Barresi
# PHOTOPSIA 7

*Photopsia is a spontaneous flash or spark of light.*

## BACKGROUND

Photopsia is caused by stimulation of nerves along the visual pathway. Stimulation can occur with mechanical forces such as compression or traction or from episodic ischemia. Pressure on the globe, quick eye movements, and coughing can cause photopsia in the healthy, usually dark-adapted eye. Vitreoretinal traction, retinal breaks, intraocular neoplasm, and inflammation can cause mechanical retinal stimulation and elicit photopsia. Vitreoretinal traction that causes photopsia frequently is precipitated by posterior vitreous detachment.

Less commonly, moving microemboli of the retina or venous stasis of an impending central retinal vein occlusion can cause photopsia. The sudden vision loss of ischemic optic neuropathy can be preceded, from hours to days, by photopsia.

Migraine is the most common cause of episodic visual pathway ischemia, with consequent photopsia. Photopsia may accompany classic migraine headaches or present as an isolated migraine equivalent. Infrequently, cranial mass lesions can, by mechanical forces or by diverting blood supply, produce migrainelike photopsia. Clinical differentiation between migraine and occipital lobe arteriovenous malformation can be particularly difficult.

In the elderly, and less commonly in the middle-aged patient, visual pathway ischemia can occur with aortic arch syndrome and extracranial occlusive disease of the external carotids or vertebrobasilar arteries. Photopsia may precede or occur between episodes of monocular blindness of the carotid transient ischemic attack or the episodes of bilateral vision loss of vertebrobasilar TIAs.

## HISTORY

The patient history that is most helpful is elicited by methodical pursuit of specific information, as in the following list.

1. Qualify the symptoms. Allow the patient to describe the details of the visual disturbance. Often patients are frightened or baffled by this curious event and have difficulty verbalizing the complaint. Even so, attempt to record the details of the event in the patient's own words. Define the type of

photopsia, fast or slow, flickering, sparks, streaks, or spectrums. Identify, if possible, which eye is involved and the position and movement of the disturbance in the visual field.

2.  Temporal sequence. Determine the date of the first episode and circumstance of onset. Is photopsia evoked by eye motion or pressure? Is it noted only when quickly standing up or turning the head? If episodic, how often does it occur? Do any changes in the pattern of disturbances occur over time?

3.  Associated symptoms. Determine if any prodromal, coincident, or subsequent symptoms are present. Again, allow the patient freedom in choosing terms. Does the patient know when an episode of flashes is coming? Are any problems noted at the same time or after the photopsia occurs? Clarify each associated symptom, being particularly alert to visual disturbances, floaters, blur, metamorphopsia, blackouts, and diplopia. Rule out any episodic neurologic disturbances, such as headaches, light-headedness, vertigo, abnormal sensations, or motor deficits. Be alert to the temporal sequence and laterality of associated symptoms.

4.  Eye history. Identify any history of eye disease or vision disturbances. Question the patient to determine presence of retinal break risk factors: high myopia, aphakia, blunt trauma, ocular inflammation, and peripheral retinal degeneration.

5.  Medical history. Include a careful survey of current medical problems and medications. Specifically investigate the history of migraine headaches or migraine equivalents. Rule out stroke and retinal vascular disease risk factors, hypertension, diabetes, hyperlipidemic blood dyscrasias, and heart disease.

6.  Family history. Identify relatives with vision loss, particularly retinal detachment. Is there any family history of cranial mass lesions, stroke, or heart disease?

# EXAMINATION

The diagnostic investigation of photopsia has a two-pronged strategy. The practitioner should rule out vitreoretinal disease with tests of visual acuity, visual fields, and examination with biomicroscopy and indirect ophthalmoscopy, and rule out neuroophthalmologic deficits with tests of visual acuity, pupils, ocular movements, and visual fields.

Examine the fundus to assure the optic disks are flat with normal color and the vessels normal with no venous stasis, arteriole occlusion, or emboli. Study the retinal background to rule out hemorrhage, inflammation, tumors, breaks, detachments, and peripheral retinal degeneration. Be particularly alert to lattice degeneration with holes (see Chapter 30).

## Ophthalmoscopy

Characterize location, size, and shape of any vitreous opacities. Be alert to a ring-like opacity in front of the optic disk or macula typical of posterior vitreous detachment. Look for vitreous hemorrhage and cell pigment in the retrolental space.

## Visual Fields

When compressive intracranial lesions or episodic ischemia are suspected, careful study of the patient's visual field is of the utmost importance. Qualifying the visual field defects can often assist in localizing the site of the neurologic lesion (see Chapter 32). Subtle peripheral retinal detachment, retinal schisis, or branch retinal vessel occlusion, overlooked in ophthalmoscopy, may be demonstrated with visual field testing.

# CLINICAL SIGNIFICANCE

Isolated photopsia elicited by coughing or digital pressure and with no associated symptoms can occur in a healthy eye. Photopsia elicited by ocular movement may be innocuous, but if light flashes can be evoked by repeated ocular movement, then suspect vitreoretinal traction most likely precipitated by a posterior vitreous detachment. In contrast, photopsia caused by compressive lesions or ischemia is not evoked by ocular movement.

Monocular photopsia followed by spots in the vision strongly suggests vitreojretinal traction. Floaters that follow photopsia may represent vitreal blood, inflammatory exudates, or torn retinal tissue. Torn retinal tissue, being positioned close to the retina, is noted by the patient as being sharply outlined gray or black structures. Retinal tissue torn from the rim of the optic disk during a posterior vitreous detachment typically yields a central annular floater.

If the photopsia is stable in the visual field, noting the position can help localize the causative retinal lesion. Retinal photopsia projects in the visual field opposite the meridian of retinal pathology. Since the temporal retina is a more frequent site of lattice degeneration and retinal breaks, nasal field photopsia arouses more suspicion of vitreoretinal disease. In contrast, central photopsia suggests impending posterior vitreous separation with resultant traction or vitreoretinal adhesion in the posterior pole.

Photopsia that is not well localized or moves through the visual field is more suggestive of compressive lesions or ischemia.

Fast flickering scintillations of silvery zigzag sensations of 10- to 30-minute duration are most frequently due to migraine. Most often, migraine photopsia is accompanied by other migraine symptoms (see Chapter 9). In classic migraine, the photopsia aura of "watery vision" or "heat waves" with rapid flicker heralds the onset of a contralateral headache.

Rarely, migrainelike photopsia is caused by cerebral AV malformations, tumors, or TIAs.

Vascular steal owing to cerebral AV malformations may mimic migraine attacks for years prior to a disastrous subarachnoid hemorrhage. Typically, the visual photopsia seizures of cerebral AV malformations and tumors produce a slow-frequency flicker rather than the rapid shimmer of migraine. Semiformed geometric photopsias, like a cracked-ice appearance, point to these serious lesions. Care must be taken to assess any suspicious headaches, visual field defects, and other neurologic signs that suggest cerebral tumors and AV malformations as migraine mimickers (see Chapters 9, 31, and 32).

The episodic sensory and motor deficits caused by transient ischemic attacks may infrequently be accompanied by photopsia. Bright sparks that appear first slightly temporarily, streak outward, start and stop, and vanish in the periphery suggest passage of retinal emboli. If emboli are suspected, question for evidence of cardiovascular embolic disease, or with elderly patients, for temporal arteritis. In younger patients, atrial fibrillation, rheumatic valve disease, atrial myxoma, and mitral valve prolapse may all produce migrainelike symptoms or amaurosis fugax (see Chapter 6).

Photopsia may be innocuous or herald

vision- or life-threatening disease. All patients with this complaint deserve a thorough examination to rule out retinal or neuroophthalmologic disease. Of most importance is a careful peripheral retina examination.

# References

Barresi BJ. Stroke, identifying the patient at risk. J Am Optom Assoc 1978; 49:794–800.

Morse PH, et al. Light flashes as a clue to retinal disease. Arch Ophthalmol 1974;91:179–180.

Tolentino, FI. Vitreoretinal disorders: diagnosis and management. Philadelphia: W.B. Saunders, 1976.

Troost BT, Newton TH. Occipital lobe arteriovenous malformations. Arch Ophthalmol 1975;93:250–256.

Wiley RG. Scintillating scotoma without headache. Ann Ophthalmol 1979; 11:581–585.

J. David Higgins **8**

# DIPLOPIA

*Diplopia describes the symptom of double vision.*

## BACKGROUND

Diplopia most commonly reflects a deviation from binocular alignment caused by neuromuscular lesions at or peripheral to nuclei of cranial nerves III, IV, or VI. No matter how slowly progressive a lesion may be, the symptom of diplopia is "all or none," although it may vary with position of gaze, time of day, and other conditions. Neu-rologic lesions cause paroxysmal onset of clear-cut diplopia that is somewhat disabling—faulty localization, ocular vertigo, and perhaps even nausea. This is in marked contrast to less serious causes, which often casually present with symptoms that are more vague.

## HISTORY

When the patient complains of persistent or intermittent diplopia, first establish whether it is monocular or binocular. It is best not to ask initially whether it disappears when one eye is covered, but to ask the less leading question, "Can you do anything to clear up the double vision?" If it cannot be determined that episodic diplopia is monocular by history, a good question to ask is in what situations the diplopia is noticed and whether it seems more like a ghost image. Monocular causes of diplopia almost always produce a ghost image. With a ghost image, the viewing situation often will be revealing, such as oblique gaze through bifocals, a window, or rear view mirror. The ocular cause that most commonly produces symptoms is the viewing of bright objects in the dark, such as headlights or a television in a darkened room. Diffractive images from cataracts, floaters, and irregular astigmatism (keratoconus, blebs, pterygiums) are common. More obvious causes might manifest as retinal detachment, polycoria, an ectopic lens, or a decentered contact lens. It might be pointed out here that surgical or orthoptic intervention in patients with anomalous retinal correspondence (ARC) never produces monocular diplopia.

Binocular causes of vaguely appreciated diplopia usually are not serious and include decompensating phorias, convergence insufficiency, physiologic diplopia in the neurotic, and occasionally transient loss of sensory adaptation in older ARC patients in conditions of reduced vision, such as at night. Such patients do not rush to the doctor's office with a definite onset of the condition as do those suffering from neurologic insults.

Loss of central fusion occasionally occurs after head trauma, stroke, and myocardial infarction. Here the diplopia will manifest even with small deviations, fusion being possible only through a very small range of prismatic correction. This is more common in the elderly or debilitated, especially after prolonged occlusion owing to delayed extraction of an opaque cataract. Horror fusion is due to aniseikonia and is extremely rare. The exception may be a case where a preexisting binocular muscle imbalance has been aggravated by a major change in the prescription to one eye, such as following an attempt to fully correct a uniocular myopic shift secondary to nuclear sclerosis. The symptom merits attention to base curves, center thickness, vertex distance magnification considerations, or use of a contact lens.

The hallmark of neurologic lesions is sudden onset of any incomitant binocular deviation (see Chapter 19).

Acute neurologic oculomotor palsies are serious; about one-third of such patients do not survive 5 years. History is the same as that for any neurologic complaint and includes the following information:

1. Onset: acute/insidious; antecedent trauma; on awakening versus active, etc.

2. Course: improving/worsening; intermittent; better/worse in morning, etc.

3. Company: pain, numbness, proptosis malaise, brain stem signs, etc.

4. General health: thyroid disease, alcoholism, hypertension, diabetes, etc.

5. Muscular associations: bulbar signs (chewing, swallowing, speaking, facial, shoulder, or neck weakness); or proximal signs (weakness climbing stairs, getting out of chairs, holding arms up as in brushing hair)

6. Previous focal neurologic symptoms in young suggesting demyelination: leg weakness, optic neuritis, paresthesias, sphincter problems, L'hermitte's sign, etc.

7. Symptoms of giant cell arteritis in elderly: malaise, fever, night sweats, claudication, weight loss, headache, proximal morning myalgias, etc.

8. Signs of inflammation: prior upper respiratory illness, stiff neck, headache, fever, etc.

9. Symptoms of increased intracranial pressure: headache on arising, irritation/lethargy, vomiting, bradycardia, loss of venous pulse, etc.

# CLINICAL SIGNIFICANCE

The list of neurologic causes of diplopia is nearly endless; it will suffice here to state that all sixth nerve palsies look much the same—it is the company and the special studies that make the difference. The differential diagnosis of cranial nerve palsies requires an interested and experienced doctor knowledgeable in a wide range of areas. For most patients, including those for whom the etiology is much in doubt, the neurologist is usually the best choice of referral. This is not to say that one should not perform a full neuro-ophthal-mologic workup. Experience shows the information gathered on initial patient presentation to be invaluable in managing the patient and measuring the clinical course. For example, if a vague and episodic diplopia presents in a case of apparent adult onset intermittent exotropia, the securing of a history of closing one eye in bright sunlight since childhood strongly argues against aggressive invasive and risky diagnostic workup. On the other hand, sending a patient to the neurologist with a probable diagnosis of an uncomplicated stroke when several cotton-wool spots, malaise, and jaw claudication are overlooked may result in too easy accep-tance of the incorrect diagnosis, and fur-ther morbidity from unsuspected temporal arteritis may result.

# References

Glaser JS. Infranuclear disorders of eye movement. In: Glaser JS. Neuro-oph-thalmology. Hagerstown, Md.: Harper & Row, 1978;245–284.

Keane JR. Ocular skew deviation. Arch Neurol 1975;32:185–190.

Records R. Monocular diplopia. Surv Ophthalmol 1980;24:303–306.

# J. David Higgins
# HEADACHE 9

*Pain localized in the cranium, occipital-nucchal region, and upper half of the face is generally referred to as headache.*

## BACKGROUND

Headache is the most common and important nonvisual complaint attributed to the eyes, and perhaps the most difficult to manage expertly. Pain in the head derives from only a limited number of sources, which usually are extracranial: the eyes, teeth, sinuses, blood vessels, and, most commonly, the facial, jaw, scalp, and neck muscles. Intracranial origin of pain derives from traction, inflammation, or swelling of the meninges, blood vessels, or alteration of messages along the fifth nerve. Numerous conditions can arouse pain from these sites. Headache types profiled in this chapter include sinus, muscle tension, temporomandibular joint dysfunction, ocular, cranial, systemic, temporal arteritis, migraine, and cluster.

## HISTORY

First allow the patient to tell the story without much direction. At some point ask the patient, "How have you been feeling?" and "Is there anything else, no matter how trivial or seemingly unrelated, that has been bothering you over the last weeks/months?" Since the character of many headaches is similar, often the key to diagnosis is the presence of significant associated signs and symptoms (the "company"). Thus, the patient informing you that she has stopped menstruating and has gained weight will obviously change the entire significance of the general complaint of headache. Often patients simply do not volunteer such related conditions either because they forget, are embarrassed, or do not think that it is relevant to the eye doctor's task. These types of complaints are usually missed with the standard checklist history; so take special care to elicit them.

After obtaining the patient's story, the second stage is to ask general questions as to the onset, location, quality, severity, progression, what helps, what hurts, and so on. Even here, the more general "Tell me as best you can about how your headache feels" is better than "Do you have throbbing headaches?" After this stage the diagnosis is often suspected, and the examiner may ask more directed questions to confirm suspicions.

# CLINICAL SIGNIFICANCE

With a good history and exam it usually is possible to diagnose the specific type of headache. In some cases this will lead to a cure, as for the sinus headache. Often, however, a chronic history of headaches is present, and the diagnosis will be muscle tension or vascular or mixed headaches. Here the key is to reassure the patient that a serious cause does not exist and to explain to the patient the mechanism of the headache and the available methods to help control its frequency and severity. In some cases the patient will not be convinced of the absence of serious pathology and a referral for inexpensive, noninvasive tests such as sinus and skull films and electroencephalogram is indicated more to satisfy the patient than the doctor. It is always appropriate to tell the patient to "keep in touch" and to advise a return visit if a change in the headache character or other new symptoms arise.

In some cases, headache even of benign etiology may be so frequent or severe that the symptom itself becomes a significant cause of morbidity, resulting in missed work or inability to manage the household. In these cases, referral to a pain or headache clinic is often indicated. The staff at these centers are more likely to have the expertise, time, and willingness to treat chronic pain patients.

It is not good practice to leave the symptom of headache unresolved, or to tell the patient only "It's not your eyes." Every headache has a cause; it is a symptom of specific functional or organic dysfunction in all cases. In the case of relatively acute onset of headache or change in character of headache in a patient past 45 years of age, the motto must be that every headache has a specific cause that must be uncovered.

The headache profiles that follow focus on specific categories of headache. In some cases, however, the headache will not be easily classified. Here the task is to seek out salient aspects of the headache that suggest a greater or lesser index of suspicion; such indicators (Higgins 1981) are listed here:

1. Except for catastrophes such as subarachnoid hemorrhage, the severity of a headache usually bears little relation to its significance.

2. Relief by aspirin is not a reliable indication that a headache is benign.

3. Progression of the headache is the key to its significance; beware of the headache that is more frequent, more severe, more localized, a change in character.

4. Bifrontal or binucchal headaches of some duration are usually tension headaches.

5. Excepting migraine and TMJ syndrome, a unilateral focus is always food for thought.

6. Any occipital headache with nucchal rigidity suggests meningeal irritation; ask patient to bend neck.

7. Early morning onset is common for many benign headaches (e.g., vascular or tension associated with depression). When of recent onset, however, increased intracranial pressure must be considered.

8. Localized skull sensations (paresthesias) between headaches suggest a mass, especially meningioma in middle-aged women; palpate for hyperostosis (a bump).

9. Increasing thoracic venous pressure (coughing, lifting, straining at stool) often transiently relieves vascular headaches, but worsens those associated with increased intracranial pressure.

10. Onset or change in the character of headache in a patient over 45 years almost always has a specific etiology and is not the ordinary vascular or tension headache.

11. When questioned carefully, patients complaining of recent headaches frequently admit to always being headache-prone.

12. It is often revealing in cases of chronic headache to ask patients what they feel is the cause of the headache.

13. The evaluation of a headache must always be tempered by an evaluation of the patient's psyche. Inquire as to occupational/family stress or depression and look for corroborating signs, such as ingestion of antacids, nail biting, lack of expression or spontaneous movement.

14. The Catch 22 is that a variety of intracranial insults may produce both headache and psychic changes affecting intellectual function and emotional lability. Systemic lupus erythematosus is an excellent example of a disease in which the complaints of headache in a patient with bizarre behavior may be ignored by the physician.

15. Fortunately, headaches associated with intracranial disease nearly always reveal at least one significant associated finding besides headache if a thorough history/exam is conducted.

16. Always make the patient feel free to call you if an unexplained headache should persist, get worse, or become associated with a new symptom.

# Sinus Headaches

*Pain localized to or referred from disease in the paranasal air sinuses is described as sinus headache.*

## BACKGROUND

Many patients with chronic congestion, such as smokers or those with allergies, incorrectly blame their sinuses as the cause of their headaches. Most of these patients suffer from tension headache. Obstructive sinus disease by itself is a rare cause of headache unless actual infection coexists.

In considering the sinuses as a cause of headache, recall their anatomy and zones of referred pain. In general, pain from frontal and ethmoid sinus disease is referred to the periorbital and brow areas, the sphenoid retroorbitally or to the vertex, and the maxillary usually infraorbitally. Acute severe eye ache is the most common presentation of true sinus infection seen in the optometrist's office.

## HISTORY AND EXAMINATION

Most patients with sinus headache show clear evidence of infection with thick mucopurulent nasal discharge, some malaise, and often fever. As vascular headaches are also often secondary to occult fevers, it is worthwhile to take the temperature of any patient with recent onset of headaches, especially when accompanied by malaise. These patients may also complain of mild periorbital edema, photophobia, or ocular tenderness. All except the maxillary sinus drain better when the patient is standing, so symptoms tend to be worse on arising except for exacerbations later in the day typical of maxillary sinus disease. Sinus headache tends to be steady with pulsations appearing when cardiac output is increased, as during exercise or upon standing abruptly. Bending over or blowing the nose often causes a sudden major intensification of the symptoms, and alcohol ingestion notoriously makes the condition worse.

Besides the history and looking for signs of congestion and toxicity, it is helpful to percuss the frontal and maxillary sinuses, checking for undue sensitivity to a tap by the tip of the examiner's fingers over the suspected sinus. Both the frontal and maxillary sinuses are also able to be transilluminated, the frontal by slipping the tip of the transilluminator into the orbit just under the superciliary ridge, and the maxillary by placing the transilluminator in the patient's mouth. In either case it is necessary to wait a few moments in the darkened room in order to appreciate whether a fluid level exists, blocking the normal red glow that should be seen over these areas.

# CLINICAL SIGNIFICANCE

As the orbit may directly transmit sinus infection to the brain, the optometrist must be alert to significant lid edema, ocular tenderness, and conjunctival congestion as early signs of cellulitis. This is especially true in children, in whom ethmoiditis is the leading cause of orbital cellulitis. Additionally, when any signs of orbital fracture exist secondary to blunt trauma (numbness, diplopia, crepitus) the coexistence of sinusitis is of concern. In diabetes, even the slightest hint of cellulitis accompanying nasosinus infection should signal the possibility of mucormycosis, which has a potentially devastating tendency to lead to cavernous sinus thrombosis and the death of the patient. Look for black crusting in the nasopharynx if this disease is suspected.

Acute sinusitis usually resolves without sequelae. Patients with significant sinus disease should be under the care of a primary care physician.

The chief significance of sinus headache is to recognize and distinguish it from other more serious causes of acute severe periorbital ache. The most common serious misdiagnosis occurs with chronic maxillary pain caused by nasopharyngioma. Suspicious company might include pain near the ear, blocking and popping of the eustachian tubes, oropharyngeal numbness, dysarthria, dysphagia, epistaxis, and/or fifth nerve hypoesthesia. The most common ocular signs of this serious malignancy are Horner's syndrome and sixth nerve paresis. It is most common in elderly men but may occur anytime.

# Muscle Tension Headaches

*Muscle tension headache is pain caused by spasm and secondary metabolic changes owing to sustained contraction in scalp, neck, facial, and jaw muscles.*

## BACKGROUND

Muscle contraction is by far the most frequent cause of headache, accounting for approximately 70% of all headaches. Tension headache is a chronic syndrome, often developing in the teens, and usually reflects a maladaptive habit of excessive contraction of the small muscles of the head and scalp, most commonly in the occipitocervical or frontal regions. These muscles do not have the ability for sustained contraction seen in larger postural muscles. The resulting early fatigue takes place similar to writer's cramp: a fatigued muscle cannot maintain its membrane potential, with the result that a vicious circle takes place, that is, more spasm with further exacerbation of the ischemia, producing even more spasm with liberation of lactic acid, cramping, edema, and inflammation.

## HISTORY AND EXAMINATION

Anyone who has experienced a brow ache from squinting in bright sunlight can attest to the cramplike quality of this headache. Often, patients will describe the headache as a steady bandlike compression, often noting some local tenderness or even paresthesia in the scalp and neck. Like a back spasm, tension headache can attain alarming severity and far outlast the precipitating circumstances, often still being present on awakening the next day. Many patients with chronic tension headache will admit to always being aware of background discomfort that simply intensifies in times of stress or concentrated effort, such as prolonged reading. Patients with a bifrontal focus will often assume a painlike appearance during the history with excessive corrugator or frontalis wrinkling being manifest. Patients with an occipital nucchal focus are often aware of bracing and stiffness in the region. When the greater occipital nerve becomes inflamed, the ache will commonly radiate to the ipsilateral eye; checking for undue tenderness under the base of the skull in the retromastoid fossa is almost diagnostic of this complication.

Patients with tension headache often suffer from mixed (vascular and tension)

### Table 9.1
### Patterns of Depression

| Type of Complaint | Incidence (%) |
| --- | --- |
| **Physical** | |
| Sleep disturbances | 97 |
| Early awakening | 87 |
| Headache | 84 |
| Dyspnea | 76 |
| Constipation | 76 |
| Loss of weight | 74 |
| Trouble getting to sleep | 73 |
| Weakness and fatigue | 70 |
| Urinary frequency | 70 |
| Spells or dizziness | 70 |
| Appetite disturbances | 70 |
| Decreased libido | 63 |
| Cardiovascular disturbances | 60 |
| Sexual disturbances | 60 |
| Palpitations | 59 |
| Paresthesias | 53 |
| Nausea | 48 |
| Menstrual changes | 41 |
| **Emotional** | |
| Blue, low spirits, sadness | 90 |
| Crying | 80 |
| Feelings of guilt, hopelessness, unworthiness, unreality | 65 |
| Anxious or irritable | 65 |
| Anxiety | 60 |
| Fear of insanity, physical disease, death, rumination over the past, present, future | 50 |
| **Psychic** | |
| "Morning worst time of day" | 95 |
| Poor concentration | 91 |
| No interest, no ambition | 75 |
| Indecisiveness | 75 |
| Poor memory | 71 |
| Suicidal thoughts, death wishes | 35 |

Source: Diamand and D'Allesio 1978.

headache and describe in detail an excruciating episode of migraine while claiming to have headaches almost daily. On questioning they will admit that the "sick" headache occurs only occasionally. Interestingly, during a migraine these patients often are aware of localized areas of tenderness in the scalp muscles.

Tension headache is most rampant in two classes of patients: the anxious and the depressed. The patient with neurotic anxiety is usually the more obvious to the examiner, and the patient is aware of the relationship between headache onset and situational stress. It is the depressed patient, however, who may mask the condition and who represents the more important entity. A history of chronic early morning headache with difficulty getting to sleep and early awakening is characteristic of a spectrum of somatic complaints (Table 9.1). Other causes of early morning headache of course must be considered, such as raised intracranial pressure, migraine, sinus disease, the cervical myalgia of temporal arteritis, posterior fossa ischemia in the elderly, hypoglycemia, headache from cervical arthritis, and severe hypertension. Especially in the elderly where depression may be a disease with a fatal outcome, it is necessary to ask leading questions such as, "Do you find it difficult to do the housework now?" "Do you get out?" "Do you enjoy your meals?" "How is your sleeping?" or even to the point of asking directly whether they have been depressed or "blue" lately.

# CLINICAL SIGNIFICANCE

Finally, do not overlook the possibility of structural disease underlying the complaint. Recent whiplash, occipital nerve neuralgia, vertebrobasilar ischemia, cervical arthritis, inflammatory myalgias, temporal arteritis, meningeal irritation (nucchal rigidity), and the rigidity of parkinsonism and its more serious look-alikes may all be at the heart of cervical tension headaches. When symptoms are worse during sleep or on awakening, a small towel rolled up under the nape of the neck is helpful in patients with cervical disorders. Especially in the elderly patient, one must refrain from diagnosing a functional cause when the headache is of relatively recent onset. While depression and the causes listed above apply, so do more serious causes, and the diagnosis of uncomplicated tension headache in this age group is likely to be wrong and to delay the true diagnosis.

# Temporomandibular Joint Dysfunction

*The headache of temporomandibular joint dysfunction is attributable to excessive muscle tension in the jaw or secondary inflammation from mechanical stress of the temporomandibular joint.*

## BACKGROUND

Disease in the teeth is a rare cause of headache presenting to eye practitioners. Temporomandibular joint (TMJ) dysfunction is not rare, however, and its characteristics should be recognized. These patients sometimes suffer from an abnormality of the bite and have had recent dental work, such as a bridge or braces, as a predisposing factor. In most cases, the headache is predominantly a functional malady and a variety of the tension headache.

## HISTORY AND EXAMINATION

The headache is steady and crampy, usually occurring on one side anywhere in the temporal region from the orbit to the ear. Often these patients suffer from bruxism and tend to wake up with some stiffness of the jaw. At other times, the headache may be situational as an habitual response to life's stresses: the jaw-clenching response of "bearing down," for example.

Like any tension headache, it may last for relatively long periods, even to the extent of always being present in the background. Most patients are aware of difficulty in opening the jaw wide, a lateral deviation often being noted, with an audible click sometimes being manifest on full jaw extension.

## CLINICAL SIGNIFICANCE

TMJ headache typically is not recognized as such by patients or doctors. Since it presents as a suspicious unilateral headache, accurate diagnosis may save the patient an expensive and unnecessary workup.

# Ocular Headache

*Ocular headache accompanies sustained concentrated visual tasks and is relieved upon correction of a refractive error or oculomotor imbalance.*

## BACKGROUND

The question of "eye strain" as a cause of headache is not given much weight by most headache authorities. To the eye practitioner, however, toward whom such patients tend to gravitate, "oculogenic" headache seems relatively common.

It is doubtful that the headache accompanying use of the eyes has any specific ocular mechanism. The one exception may be headaches occurring in high hyperopia, as the brow ache of drug-induced ciliary spasm is similar to that seen in this patient population. A "pulling" or "drawing" sensation can also be appreciated by introducing prism before the eyes, and occasionally patients with clinically manifest vertical phorias will also have similar complaints. By and large, however, the headache of eye strain tends to have the character of simple muscle tension headache and is commonly localized to the brow region. In many cases this is due to squinting, especially in against-the-rule astigmatism where habitual use of excessive orbicularis tone, as if to steepen the vertical corneal meridian, is often accompanied by headache. In other cases, the sustained fixed postures and mental concentration associated with prolonged near-point tasks may be instrumental. For example, video display terminal operators frequently complain of headache. This is due more commonly to poor contrast, sustained fixed posture of extending the neck to look through the bifocals, veiling glare, and so forth, than to uncorrected refractive error itself. Hygiene should be stressed in such cases. Often, headaches attributed to use of the eyes occur with a change of task demands at work or school, and may reflect stress related to the intellectual demands per se, rather than use of the eyes.

The bulk of the population generally does not develop headaches with use of the eyes, despite the frequency of low refractive errors and moderate muscle and accommodative imbalances. This is best appreciated at the onset of presbyopia where accommodative instability, blurred vision, and often esophoria are typically heralded by the complaint that the patient's "arms are not long enough," and only rarely as headache.

## HISTORY AND EXAMINATION

Very often the patient who complains of headache attendant to the use of the eyes will admit to a chronic history of headache and suffers from neurotic anxiety depression. These "headachy" patients often describe in detail other asthenopic symptoms and tend to be photophobic; mildly blepharospastic; show inattentive jumpy pursuits; tolerate ophthalmoscopy poorly, with frequent blinking and even need for "rest"; and often show deficient upgaze and convergence—a pattern of behavior that may be labeled "ocular neurasthenia." Such patients often show undue sensitivity to normal somatic sensations and often have a relatively high frequency of physician visits, especially for functional stomach disorders, for which they may be taking antispasmotics, minor tranquilizers, or antidepressants.

When dealing with such patients, it is best not to promise total relief of the headache with a small prescription change, but instead explain that the eyestrain is only one factor producing the headaches. The patient with chronic muscle tension headaches attributed to use of the eyes is unlikely to experience total relief with any prescription; such patients tend to be "negative placebo reactors," developing new complaints even with trivial changes in their prescription. In the case of low plus lenses it is best to carry a small inventory of "loaners" before prescribing to these patients.

# CLINICAL SIGNIFICANCE

It is important to consider other conditions that may be associated with an apparent eyestrain headache. The sustained neck-flexed posture of many office workers, often combined with overuse of coffee, tea, cola, and smoking, may present as an afternoon office headache attributed to the eyes; it is often accompanied by low backache. In nervous children, one should inquire as to whether the child often fails to eat lunch and then experiences afternoon headache of a vascular quality caused by hypoglycemia. Some children will also develop vascular headaches after consuming chocolate milk in the cafeteria and often do not feel well upon arriving home from school. In adolescent newly menstruating females, the possibility of headache owing to anemia may mask as an eyestrain headache.

Be alert for easy acceptance of a small refractive error as a cause of headaches, and consider a variety of other possibilities. The headache-prone patient often seems more sensitive to small refractive errors; if no alternative cause can be found for the headache, prescribing a refractive change that can visually be appreciated by the patient is often effective.

Finally, patients suffering from the "posttraumatic" syndrome will often consult the optometrist. These patients often have suffered a relatively mild concussion or whiplash but bitterly complain of continuing symptoms long after the accident. Dizziness, nausea, accommodative instability, photophobia, and even blepharospasm are common associated symptoms. Such patients are likely to be viewed as crocks or malingerers by the physician unsuccessful in managing the complaints. Indeed, the patient's anger at the continuing disability may become a significant factor and need addressing itself. Weakness in the accessory nerve (shoulder shrugs and head turning against resistance), swallowing difficulty, or true positional vertigo, however, argue for the existence of a bona fide organic syndrome, albeit a poorly understood one. This is therapeutic and should be explained to the patient. Sympathy and referral for trial of amitripyline are about all that can be offered. Although persistent, the difficulties usually resolve, sometimes taking up to 2 years to do so. Standard measures to alleviate the photophobia and accommodate spasms should, of course, be offered.

# Primary Intracranial Disease Headaches

*Cranial headaches result from disease inside the cranium.*

## BACKGROUND

Pain-sensitive structures inside the cranium include the major blood vessels (chiefly those at the base of the brain), the large venous sinuses, and the dura. Traction on these structures from tumors, aneurysms, and abscesses will cause headache. In general, lesions above the tentorium are referred frontally, while those below radiate occipitonucchally. Increased intracranial pressure from cerebral edema or hydrocephalus typically causes generalized headache.

Occasionally, disruption of conduction along sensory nerves produces neuralgialike pain in the referral zone. For example, fifth nerve demyelinization in multiple sclerosis may present with episodic tic-douloureux-like stabs of pain in or under one eye. The location of pain in intracranial disease is not always a reliable clue to the site of the lesion; for example, meningiomas of the falx, causing occipital field defect, may refer pain to an area about the eye.

## HISTORY AND EXAMINATION

Acute onset of severe headache is characteristic of the explosive intracranial disease that occurs with subdural, subrachnoid, and intracerebral hemorrhages. Occipital nucchal headache with cervical rigidity and a positive Kernig's sign denotes significant meningeal irritation owing to the grave causes listed above, as well as to acute meningitis or abscess. In most cases, patients with such catastrophes suffer from obtundation and a variety of focal central nervous system (CNS) signs and do not present in office practice.

Occasionally, however, a patient with paroxysmal onset of migraine localized to the periorbital region will present in the office as an emergency. In these patients,

the neurologic status will be normal except, perhaps, for premonitory aura. The patient may be irritable, photophobic, nauseous, and pale, but should not show projectile vomiting. The pulsatile nature of the headache, accompanied by normal mental status, vital signs, and especially the absence of pupillary and third nerve findings, orbital bruits, and periorbital numbness, suggests migraine. Have the patient perform a valsalva maneuver to see if the headache transiently abates. If so, the diagnosis probably is migraine; if it worsens, an evolving neurologic catastrophe is suggested.

Unfortunately, most subacute intracranial lesions present with nonspecific headache that may be relieved by aspirin or other analgesics. Be suspicious when headache progressively becomes more frequent, severe, well localized, resistant to analgesics, occurs for the first time, or changes its character in a patient not normally accustomed to the symptom. In localized headache, with or without associated scalp paresthesia, consider the possibility of meningioma (Figure 9.1). These tumors are most common in middle-aged women and may produce a bump when underlying hyperostosis exists; palpate the skull.

The key to the diagnosis of intracranial disease is in the company it keeps more than in the nature of the headache. When headache is the only symptom, it is unlikely that there is a CNS lesion. This presupposes that the optometrist is alert to relevant complaints and performs a brief neurologic screen similar to that performed by other primary care practitioners. The reader is referred to the standard neurologic sources listed at the end of this chapter. In general, posterior fossa disease produces focal CNS deficits early in the course, and the reader is specifically directed to Chapter 19 for a discussion of the many subtle defects in the eye movement system that should be sought. Supratentorial lesions are less likely to be symptomatic early on, and the reader is directed to Chapter 32 for a discussion of regional symptomatology associated with lesions in or near the sensory visual system.

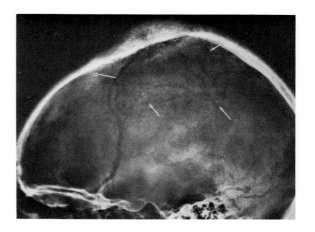

**FIGURE 9.1.**
**Hyperostosis palpable as a bump on top of the skull in a 47-year-old woman with a meningioma. Groove for the middle meningeal artery is enlarged (*a*), as are the draining diplopic veins (*arrows*).**
Reprinted by permission of the publisher, from Wood EH, Taveras JS, and Tenner MS. The brain and the eye. Chicago: Yearbook Medical Publishers, 1975. Copyright 1975, The American College of Radiology.

# CLINICAL SIGNIFICANCE

Raised intracranial pressure from any cause is almost always accompanied by moderately severe headache that tends to be worst in the morning or after lying down. Increasing venous pressure such as in lifting, coughing, and straining at stool invariably worsen the headache (whereas a valsalva maneuver transiently helps a vascular headache). General symptoms are often of an emotional (irritability/lethargy) or vegetative (bradycardia, hypertension, vomiting) nature. Except in pseudotumor cerebri, one or more focal symptoms usu-

ally will be manifest at the time the patient presents with raised intracranial pressure from space-occupying lesions or encephalitis.

Early disc signs are loss of the venous pulse and the normal ganglion cell striations, usually appreciated best with red-free light in the arcuate zones just above and below the nerve. Peripapillary retinal edema and telangiectatic vessels on the disc are also early signs that distinguish true edema from that caused by disc drusen or other congenitally anomalous discs.

Enlargement of the blind spot and fluorescein leakage are not early signs. In one series, all patients with documented raised intracranial pressure were without venous pulses even when no other prominent signs of disc edema were present (80%–90% of normal patients show spontaneous pulsations). Since many other causes of disc edema besides intracranial hypertension exist (congestive heart failure, for example, being the most common), a variety of other areas must be considered if no focal CNS symptoms exist (Chapter 31). Be alert to the typical cranial-facial appearance of Paget's disease in the elderly as a cause of brain and/or optic nerve compression in a headachy person; this disease is sometimes accompanied by angioid streaks.

Inflammatory CNS disease only rarely presents in office eye practice. Abscess or subacute meningitis should be suspected when CNS signs and symptoms are accompanied by nucchal rigidity, fever, or evidence of predisposing conditions such as otitis or subacute bacterial endocarditis.

Ischemic headaches in older patients probably are attributable to giant cell arteritis or large vessel stenosis. Transient symptoms in the carotid artery territory are well known and are only rarely accompanied by headache. Headache as a sign of posterior fossa ischemia is relatively common, however, and may be accompanied by only minor symptomatology, which is often not recognized as a spell by the patient. These patients often deny short episodes of memory lapses, dizziness, dysarthria, ataxia, and transient paresthesias and weakness. Diplopia and transient field defects are, of course, more obvious to the patient.

The elderly are especially prone to subdural hemorrhage, since the bridging emissary veins exiting the brain become relatively unsupported on their way to the skull table because of senile cerebral atrophy. This presentation is usually secondary to trauma, even trivial, and the headache is often explosive; however, the entity of "chronic subdural hematoma" also exists. Here, chronic rebleeding eventually produces a clot, which presents as a progressing supratentorial mass weeks or even months after trauma. Therefore, headache and mild dementia in the elderly must always prompt questions relating to antecedent trauma. The ultimate disaster in these patients is a downward pressure gradient herniating the temporal lobe, uncus, or hippocampus through the tentorium to crush the brain stem. Anisocoria in bright light is the key early sign (Hutchinson's pupil) of third nerve trunk failure owing to this complication (see Chapter 18, Figure 18.3). If present in this type of patient, immediate hospitalization is in order.

# Headache and Systemic Conditions

*Systemic headache refers to pain in the head secondary to generalized dysfunction.*

## BACKGROUND

Headache is probably the single most common complaint reflecting metabolic, febrile, toxic, and many other systemic alterations. In most cases, however, the headache is not the most important symptom, and other complaints are relied upon for diagnosis. When headache dominates the symptomatology, however, the patient with an occult systemic disorder may present to the eye practitioner.

## HISTORY AND EXAMINATION

Although it is not expected that a full review of systems be part of the eye exam, it must be stressed that all patients must be asked how they have been feeling in general and whether anything besides their eyes has been bothering them recently. This is especially critical when headache is of relatively recent onset. A patient with mononucleosis is likely to complain of headache and perhaps burning of the eyes; the patient is less likely to volunteer symptoms related to sore throat, recent fatigue, and enlarged cervical lymph nodes. It is exactly this type of company that should be sought by the alert practitioner, as it is the basis of the diagnosis.

The most common headache type associated with systemic conditions is the secondary vascular headache, which is sensitive to head movement, may throb, and is often associated with irritation such that the patient prefers to lie in a quiet, dark room. As with common migraine, the pain temporarily abates during a valsalva maneuver ("Take a deep breath and try and blow out forcibly while keeping your mouth, nose, and throat closed"). In common migraine, however, much of the pain derives from extracranial vasodilation, and digital pressure on both temporal arteries will usually temporarily reduce the pain. In secondary intracranial vasodilation, such as that caused by viremia, compressing the temporal arteries usually is ineffective.

The reader should review standard medical texts for full discussion of those more important conditions where headache may be a prominent feature. Be especially familiar with those conditions that have specific eye company in addition to headache, as these disorders are more frequent than primary intracranial disease. For example, a headachy patient with a Horner's pupil and weight loss, coughing, and shoulder pain, may lead to a diagnosis of apical lung cancer in a patient about to be given eyeglasses.

# CLINICAL SIGNIFICANCE

Outside of simple constipation (often not volunteered), inflammatory disease is the most common type of disorder associated with headache. Here an irritable throbbing ache sensitive to head motion often occurs, representing a vascular headache associated with mild occult fever or systemic toxins. Malaise, loss of appetite, fatigue, myalgias, and other toxic effects may coexist. Many important and chronic conditions are associated with low-grade fever that may not be recognized by the patient. Thus, questions as to afternoon and evening chills and sleep awakening sweats are part of the approach to a new onset of vascularlike headaches; the importance of simply taking the patient's temperature cannot be overstressed. Although often associated with minor illness, important conditions such as chronic infectious disease (tuberculosis), inflammatory disease (lupus), and neoplastic disease (lymphoma) may present with occult fever and produce headache as a prominent early complaint.

Anemia is also associated with secondary vascular headache and should be suspected in newly menstruating females, menopausal-aged women with gynecologic problems, and in patients with signs and symptoms of pernicious anemia. Laboratory work is thus suggested by pallor, fatigue, increased pulse rate, systolic hypertension, and spooning of fingernails.

Hypoglycemia also produces headaches with a vascular quality and should be suggested by "hungry headaches," especially late in the afternoon or with early morning awakening following sugary bedtime snacks, and especially when those are combined with alcohol consumption. These patients may note other accompaniments such as irritability, tremor, sweating, light-headedness, a racing mind, or even focal neurologic episodes such as vertigo or migrainelike photopsias.

Endocrinologic disease may also cause headache, especially thyroid disorders and Addison's disease. All patients with symptoms and signs of hypothyroidism and significant headache should have a field exam for temporal field diminutions suggesting panhypopituitarism secondary to a pituitary adenoma (Figure 9.2, and in Chapter 31, Figure 31.14).

Essential hypertension as a cause of early morning headache is much overstressed. Certainly the existence of hypertensive encephalopathy owing to abrupt and marked increase in blood pressure (e.g., kidney failure or renal artery stenosis) is often associated with headache. Also not to be overlooked is pheochromocytoma, where an adrenalin-secreting tumor may be associated with spells of severe pulsing headache, anxiety, pallor, sweating, and tremor. The optometrist should be aware of the signs of neurofibromatoses with which it may be associated (Figure 9.3). Moderate hypertension associated with headache and disc edema without significant accompanying hypertensive retinopathy is more prudently viewed as "hypertension associated with posterior fossa mass" until proved otherwise.

Ischemia/anoxia as the cause of headache has already been discussed in the section on intracranial disease and is sometimes an important antecedent of stroke in the elderly. In younger patients, ischemic headache may represent a collagen arteritis, or a hyperviscosity syndrome, such as in multiple myeloma or polycythemia, which may underlie headaches in heavy smokers. The anoxic headache of the stuffy bedroom is probably a universally recognized example of this mechanism. Headache caused simply by pulling the bedcovers over one's head is known as "turtle headache" and is surprisingly common in those oversleeping in daylight.

One should not forget that medicines themselves are important causes of headache, especially vasodilators and estrogens, so the *Physicians' Desk Reference* will occasionally have to be consulted. Psychiatric patients taking monoamine oxi-

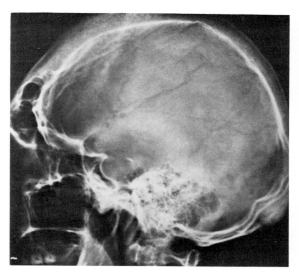

**FIGURE 9.2.**
Chiasmal masses often present with isolated headache. Note marked "ballooning of the sella" and enlargement of the frontal sinuses owing to pituitary adenoma in acromegaly. Also see Figure 33.13.
Reprinted by permission of the publisher, from Wood EH, Taveras JS, and Tenner MS. The brain and the eye. Chicago: Yearbook Medical Publishers, 1975. Copyright 1975, The American College of Radiology.

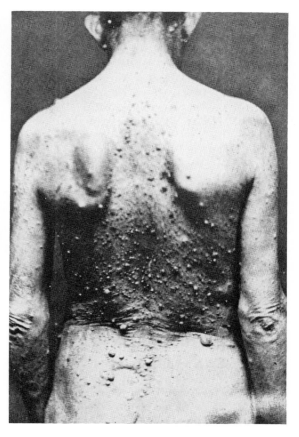

**FIGURE 9.3.**
Neurofibromas are characteristically most numerous in the axillary and truncal regions, as in this patient with von Recklinghausen's disease.
Courtesy Dr. P.I. Yakovlev. Reprinted by permission of the publisher, from Merritt HH. A textbook of neurology. Philadelphia: Lea & Febiger, 1973; 5th ed.

dase inhibitors are especially prone to develop significant episodes of hypertension and headache associated with ingestion of sympathetic amines (e.g., tyrosine in cheese or phenylephrine in eye drops). As with tricyclic antidepressants, one should avoid dilating these patients with sympathomimetics. Digitalis and its derivatives also commonly produce headache when blood levels are only mildly elevated above the therapeutic level. Since this represents a potential emergency, it is important to recall that snowy vision, yellow green vision, difficulty adjusting to illumination changes, and complicated photopsias, including hallucinations, are key symptoms of toxicity. Other notables are lethargy, nausea, bradycardia, and arrhythmias. If suspected, proper referral may save a life.

Toxic substances associated with the work environment, especially aromatic petroleum by-products and carbon monoxide, cannot be fully discussed, but the practitioner should be alert to this possibility in headache associated with the workplace. Ironically, headache patients often consume intemperate amounts of nicotine, caffeine, and alcohol and present to the optometrist hoping to find a cure for their headaches.

# Temporal Arteritis Headache

*Such headache is described as pain in the head, face, or neck secondary to inflammation, claudication, or myalgia produced by giant cell arteritis.*

## BACKGROUND

Giant cell arteritis is a systemic disease characterized by multifocal granulomatous inflammation of unknown etiology, occurring principally in larger arteries throughout the body. It typically strikes elderly patients and has a mild female preponderance.

## HISTORY AND EXAMINATION

When prominent arteritis exists in the cranial vessels the disease is usually obvious, with severe boring headache anywhere from the eye to the neck, but often in the distribution of the temporal artery, which may be erythematous, tender, firm, and pulseless (Figure 9.4). Ischemic muscle pain may be evident, as on chewing (jaw claudication). Since the ophthalmic artery is commonly involved in cranial arteritis, signs of stasis such as enlarged veins, cotton-wool spots, and transient ischemic attacks may be seen; permanent loss of vision from central retinal artery occlusion or, more commonly, short ciliary artery occlusion (ischemic optic neuropathy), are real possibilities.

Giant cell arteritis with a prominent cranial focus should not be missed. Unfortunately, the cranial involvement may remain occult at the time of visual disaster. This inflammatory vasculitis may strike in any distribution—peripheral, coronary, aortic arch, and vertebrobasilar.

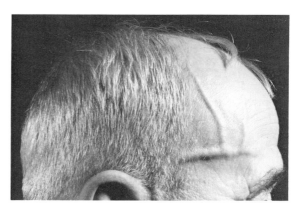

**FIGURE 9.4.**
Increased prominence of temporal artery and its branches in giant cell arteritis. Prominence is also seen in severe carotid stenosis where a supranormal pulse may be evident, unlike in temporal arteritis.
Reprinted by permission of the publisher, from Healy LA and Wilske KR. The systemic manifestations of temporal arteritis. New York: Grune & Stratton, 1979.

The ophthalmic artery is the only commonly involved artery in the carotid distribution. Systemic symptoms include coldness, paresthesias, or claudication in any distribution (e.g., angina or calf cramps on walking), malaise, fatigue, diminished appetite, low-grade fever (often with night sweats), and especially proximal muscle myalgia (usually most prominent in the cervical-shoulder area on arising); this latter pain is also often characterized as a "headache" by the patient. Any elderly patient whose general condition seems to be deteriorating should always be specifically questioned as to the existence of these constitutional symptoms.

About one-third of the patients with temporal arteritis experience optic nerve infarct preceded by TIAs. Since involvement of the aortic arch or subclavian vessels may produce a bruit radiating into the neck, it is crucial to take a full history and to avoid premature assumption of atherosclerotic carotid stenosis as the cause of amaurosis fugax.

# CLINICAL SIGNIFICANCE

Untreated, giant cell arteritis commonly produces significant disability. Blindness may occur in as many as 50% of the patients whose treatment is delayed.

Oculomotor paresis is also relatively common. When this disease is suspected, an ESR (Westergren method) should be taken promptly. If signs and symptoms are convincing in the presence of a normal ESR (extremely rare), a temporal artery biopsy may be necessary to make a definitive diagnosis. Temporal artery biopsy has, however, occasionally resulted in stroke in patients harboring significant carotid stenosis, as it provides important collateral circulation to the CNS in such patients. Biopsy does, however, provide incontrovertible evidence to justify long-term steroid treatment and its attendant complications.

Although ischemic optic neuropathy usually is associated with large vessel disease, the appearance of a totally infarcted disc where the swelling is extremely pale, and little or no hemorrhaging exists, should always suggest giant cell arteritis in the elderly patient (Figure 9.5). Delaying steroid treatment in such patients may result in the catastrophe of bilateral blindness. Indeed, many authorities feel patients with signs of ocular ischemia should be hospitalized, with the legs raised, given IV fluids, and started on 500 mg of IV methylprednisolone every 12 hours for the

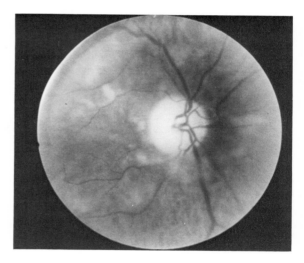

**FIGURE 9.5.**
Pale edema of the optic nerve with cotton-wool spots in retina. These signs of acute ischemia in two vascular distributions suggest a vasculitis. Patient was a 78-year-old woman with classic signs of temporal arteritis and a sedimentation rate of 131 mm/hr by the Westergren method.
Reprinted by permission of the publisher, from Donin JF and Keane JR. Diagnostic problems in neuro-ophthalmology. New York, Famous Teachings in Modern Medicine, Medcom Inc., 1973.

first 3 days to minimize a bilateral visual catastrophe. In addition, patients must be strongly encouraged to continue steroid treatment until the ESR remains totally normalized with the medication tapered to zero. This may take many months, during which time the patient is likely to feel totally asymptomatic, and noncompliance is a real possibility. Because of its protean complications, temporal arteritis should always be considered in any case of relatively acute onset of physical or mental deterioration in the elderly.

# Migraine Headache

*Migraine is paroxysmal severe headache that is periodic, often unilateral and throbbing at onset, and usually accompanied by nausea, photophobia, and general irritation. When preceded by focal neurologic dysfunction, the attack is referred to as a classic migraine. The majority of sufferers do not have such a premonitory aura, in which case the headache is referred to as common migraine.*

## BACKGROUND

In the final analysis, the actual mechanism of both common and classic migraine is unknown. While intracranial vasoconstriction and capillary steal via opening of AV shunts precede the headache and are temporarily related to the aura, it is unlikely that pure ischemia underlies the slow spread of the neurologic defect so typical of migraine; it may "trigger" the aura, however. Furthermore, while both intra- and extracranial vasodilation may occur on the involved side during the headache, producing these changes experimentally is not necessarily accompanied by headache in a nonsusceptible population. The pain itself probably requires additional factors such as vessel wall edema, release of pain-producing substances, and perhaps even cerebral edema as the irritability, nausea, photophobia, and sensitivity of the migraine headache to movement are all characteristic of postconcussion headache.

An ever-expanding array of biochemical, autonomic, psychological, vascular, and other anomalies set the migraine population statistically apart from nonsufferers. For example, EEG abnormalities are two to six times more frequent in this group. Additionally, increased platelet aggregation and release of the vasoactive amine 5-hydroxytryptamine just prior to the headache is characteristic of many sufferers. It is not surprising, therefore, that a wide variety of insults are capable of provoking an attack: psychological (compulsive personality, stress), hygienic (fatigue, poor eating habits), hormonal (birth control pills, onset of menstruation), sensory (flickering lights), and biochemical (tyrosine in cheese, $\beta$-phenylethylalamine in chocolate, octopamine in citrus).

# HISTORY AND EXAMINATION

Migraine headache occurs in about 8% of the general population, with a noteworthy female preponderance after puberty. It is second in prevalence only to tension headache, with which it is commonly associated. Most women with vascular headache notice some remission during pregnancy, and in any case there is a general tendency for the headaches to diminish with age. In a small subset of women, the attacks are characteristically premenstrual. It is common to note a worsening of the disease with estrogen ingestion.

In the absence of focal aura, even common migraine may be preceded by vague vegetative premonitions such as water retention, anxiety, mood changes, pallor, and sweating. In a straightforward case the headache is periodic; paroxysmal in onset, often in the morning; often beginning with a unilateral periorbital focus and a throbbing quality lasting at least several hours to days. At maximum intensity, the patient is usually somewhat incapacitated, irritable, photophobic, nauseous, and resistant to movement of the head or exertion, thus similar in all respects to the secondary vascular headache of a "hangover." In the downhill phase there often is some scalp tenderness, a tendency to sleep, diuresis, and a feeling of warmth and well being. Most affected patients can name a close family relative with this disorder. In contrast to tension headache, the patient with migraine is seldom vague about describing the details of the last headache and what he or she was doing at the time of onset.

The disease usually makes its appearance during adolescence, but may be heralded in childhood by periodic gastrointestinal distress in which the headache eventually becomes the more prominent component. Such children, as is generally true of people with migraine, are more likely to suffer from accommodative spasm and motion sickness. The combination of seeing the blackboard blurry on looking up from close work plus malaise and headache on coming home from school often results in a visit to the optometrist. Such children often may be taking antispasmotics for their "functional stomach disorder" as well, highlighting the broader range of autonomic instability in migraine. Childhood migraine often evolves into severe classic migraine and is more strongly associated with EEG abnormalities. If severe, phenytoin (Dilantin) and blue-tinted lenses may benefit this subgroup of patients with migraine, especially if abnormal photic driving of the EEG can be demonstrated. In childhood migraine an extended trial of abstinence from chocolate is always indicated.

When preceded by a stereotypical aura, the diagnosis is usually obvious to the doctor, if not to the patient. In the absence of a distinct aura, sudden onset of severe periorbital headache still may cause the patient to present as an emergency. The diagnosis is usually suggested by the pulsatile nature of the headache and other characteristic accompaniments. It is helpful to remember in such cases that the pain should temporarily abate during a valsalva maneuver, following which it may intensify briefly. If it worsens, consider a space-occupying intracranial lesion. Additionally, if the ache is not transiently helped by brief temporal artery compression, consider a secondary vascular headache.

The aura of classic migraine may involve any system, such as proximally spreading finger paresthesia, hemiparesis, vertigo, or diplopia owing to a skew deviation, but for the optometrist, the visual aura is the most frequently seen and important characteristic. Although exceptions exist, the following are the characteristics that are most consistent with a relatively benign diagnosis of classic migraine:

1. Onset: insidious, then becoming more apparent, as opposed to the sudden onset of the full deficit in vascular disease.
2. Character: a central zone of indistinct vision, "watery" vision, "heat waves," usually accompanied by a sensation of rapid flicker; an incomplete annulus of shimmer may sometimes mark the indistinct zone, which may develop into a frank scotoma.
3. Duration: 15 to 25 minutes is true of the great majority of auras.
4. Progression: centripetal; the indistinct zone slowly expands peripherally into one hemifield of both eyes before gradually fading.
5. Relation of aura to the headache: should precede the headache with the display in the contralateral field when the headache is unilateral.

# CLINICAL SIGNIFICANCE

Even nonsusceptible patients occasionally can be prone to acute vascular headache if there is chance association of enough predisposing conditions or the presence of systemic illness. The following factors predispose to migraine and secondary vascular headache:

1. Bright flash/flickering light
2. Stress/chronic muscle tension/hyperventilation
3. Fatigue/sleeping late/afternoon naps
4. Hot baths/overheating/excessive sun exposure
5. Hunger/episodic hypoglycemia
6. Violent exercise/severe episodic hypertension
7. Fever/toxicity/anemia
8. Ischemia/anoxia/close rooms
9. Preceding menstruation/water retention
10. Estrogen preparations
11. Vasoactive medications for angina/hypertension
12. Toxic vapors, hydrocarbons, carbon monoxide

Migraine and vascular headaches may occur as a reaction to consumption of certain foods:

- Ripened aged cheeses (e.g., cheddar)
- Chocolate
- Red meats with nitrites (bologna, hot dogs, etc.)
- Monosodium glutamate
- Alcohol, especially red wines
- Excessive tea, colas, nicotine, and especially coffee

Foods that generally have a less significant vasoactive effect are:

- Fermented, pickled, and marinated foods (wine vinegar, yogurt, sour cream, fresh raised breads, doughnuts, etc.)
- More than one glass of citrus juice per day
- Excessively salty foods (corned beef, chips, nuts)
- Miscellaneous (bananas, chicken liver, canned figs, avocados, and macadamia nuts)

In general, however, migraine is a chronic-recurrent disease. Although significantly associated with other signs of autonomic and vasomotor instability (e.g., Raynaud's phenomenon, vasospastic angina), it is unlikely that reported associations of the disease with increased risk of myocardial infarction, stroke, and of collagen disease are of clinically significant statistical weight. The disease may thus be regarded as benign save for its effect on quality of life. The chief clinical significance of migraine is with regard to classic migraine, in which several other conditions must be considered.

Usually a history of stereotyped episodes will make the practitioner comfortable with the diagnosis of classic migraine; even here one is more comfortable when the aura and/or headache occasionally changes sides. A significant change in the patient's stereotyped aura, sudden onset at full intensity, slow frequency flicker (1– 2 Hz), semiformed geometric quality (e.g., "kaleidoscopic" appearance), lack of centripetal spread, abnormal duration, and the absence of headache or headache beginning during the aura are all signs that suggest the possibility of a more serious cause.

Vascular steal from cerebral AV malformation is the greatest mimicker of migraine (Figure 9.6). There are records of patients who suffered stereotyped "migraine attacks" for years prior to a disastrous subarachnoid hemorrhage. Usually, however, at least one component on the aura is atypical for migraine and is noted in a thorough history. All suspicious presentations should therefore undergo auscultation with the bell stethoscope placed over the occipital-parietal regions, closed lids, and retromastoid fossas to listen for a bruit. Occasionally, a patient may be aware of a noise in the head synchronous with the pulse. Additionally, a careful field exam should be performed to determine whether a persisting scotomatous defect exists in the locale of the aura. If the presentation is truly suspicious, a referral to a neurology department for angiography is indicated.

Since the most common presenting sign of brain tumor is seizure, it is well to remember that a mass in the optic radiations or occipital lobes may be entirely asymptomatic, except for the presence of visual photopic seizures that may mimic the migraine aura. Here, too, the perimeter may be invaluable in detecting a neg-

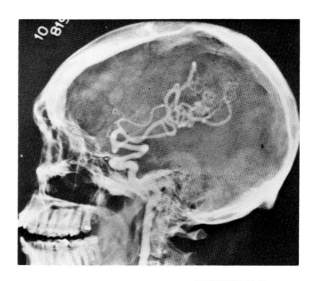

**FIGURE 9.6.**
Arteriovenous malformation in left parietal lobe of a 32-year-old man with a long history of episodic photopsias simulating migraine. Reprinted by permission of the publisher, from Cogan D. Neurology of the visual system. Springfield, Ill.: Charles C Thomas, 1966.

ative field defect. Both tumors and AV malformations often are associated with slow-frequency flicker rather than the rapid shimmer of migraine. Semiformed geometric photopsias (cracked-ice appearance) should also lead one to suspect these lesions. Furthermore, cerebral photopsias are never staccatolike and thus should never be confused with a retinal photopsia caused by vitreoretinal traction.

The most frequent atypical migraine presentation, however, has its onset in the elderly, where the display often occurs without headache or nausea ("migraine equivalent"). Probably the episode is not triggered by the same functional ischemic (vasoconstriction) mechanism as in the young. Nevertheless, the more consistent the aura fits with the stereotyped pattern previously discussed, the more likely it is to be benign. These patients, however, should be questioned as to other spells, evidence of cardiovascular embolic disease and, of course, temporal arteritis. The major vessels and skull should also be auscultated and a detailed field exam performed in the area of the aura.

The patient taking a digitalis derivative should be queried as to headache, nausea, and lassitude, and the pulse should be checked for bradycardia and signs of arrhythmia; such signs indicate digitalis toxicity, which can quickly lead to a fatal outcome. Visual hallucinations also occur in digitalis toxicity and may be mistaken for a psychotic episode.

In younger patients with suspicious auras, one must always consider the heart as a source of emboli. Atrial fibrillation, rheumatic valve disease, occult myocardial infarction, atrial myxoma, and especially mitral valve prolapse may produce migrainelike symptoms or amaurosis fugax. Refer to Chapter 6 for a discussion of these entities.

Episodic hypoglycemia is commonly responsible for lowering the migraine threshold in infrequent sufferers. Ask whether any suspect foods were eaten prior to the episode. An "anxiety attack" accompanied by hyperventilation also frequently triggers an episode of focal migraine in those normally not predisposed. In females taking birth control pills or older women taking estrogens for hot flashes, a change in the character of the usual aura or a fresh onset of focal neurologic auras demands immediate discontinuation of the preparation, as this has been one of the few clear warning signs observed of impending stroke in this population. The frequently observed exacerbation of the headache itself by estrogens is, however, apparently benign, as long as the patient is willing to tolerate the headaches.

Often no cause can be found for the onset of atypical classic migraine in an adult, and the clinician becomes more comfortable with the diagnosis as the disease evolves into a periodic stereotyped pattern. Despite its rare occurrence, the optometrist should never be comfortable with a monocular visual disturbance (ocular migraine) or that associated with third nerve signs (ophthalmoplegic migraine), especially in an adult. These patients should be referred to the neurologist, as should anyone with a truly atypical presentation.

Once the more serious mimickers of migraine are ruled out, the approach to classic migraine is similar to that of common migraine. The associations listed at the beginning of this section should be pointed out to the patient; this is done best by constructing a list to use as an office handout. A referral to a headache clinic or specialist is in order when migraine is recalcitrant to previous therapy and significantly affects quality of life; a great variety of new therapeutic approaches currently are available.

# Cluster Headache

*Cluster is a subtype of vascular headache characterized by epochs of frequent, brief, extremely severe, unilateral boring headache in the periorbital-temporal region, accompanied by ipsilateral rhinorrhea and conjunctival congestion.*

## BACKGROUND

The precise pathophysiology of cluster headache is unknown. It differs from migraine in its marked male predominance (8:1), onset in adulthood, lack of family history, and absence of subjective pulsation. Unlike migraine, no change in serotonin levels accompanies the headache, although blood histamine levels in many sufferers are found to be elevated. Sufferers are supersensitive to small doses of vasodilators (e.g., histamine, nitroglycerin), but only during the headache-prone period, and the headache always occurs only on the affected side. Blood flow and thermography demonstrate diminished flow in the area of the angular, supraorbital, and frontal arteries, which anastomose with the intracranial circulation via the ophthalmic artery. During the headache, however, there is an increased intraocular pressure pulse, and dilation of the ophthalmic artery has been observed.

## HISTORY AND EXAMINATION

In the usual case, this distinctive headache is characterized by periods of headache proneness in which headache may occur one or more times a day (the cluster), followed by a period of complete refractoriness that may last a year or more. The headache tends to be excruciating, with a nighttime predilection (most commonly 90 minutes after retiring) and unilateral orbital focus; it is the only benign headache of an intensity to be commonly associated with rocking and pacing. Besides the characteristic nasal congestion, conjunctival erythema and tearing, a transient or even permanent Horner's syndrome may accompany or follow. The headache is short lived, almost never going beyond 45 minutes in duration. Affected patients tend to be hard-driving substance abusers, but during the headache epoch abstention from alcohol is almost universal because of its tendency to provoke the headache. Sufferers tend to have a strongly masculine, leonine profile (square jaw, deep facial furrows, leathery skin, etc.) (Figure 9.7); affected females are reported to be masculine-appearing as well.

When affected, females are more likely to suffer from a chronic form of the syndrome (chronic paroxysmal hemicrania), in which attacks are very frequent and are not associated with periods of remission. These patients often are not controlled by the usual prophylactic medications and do well on aspirin and, especially, indomethacin.

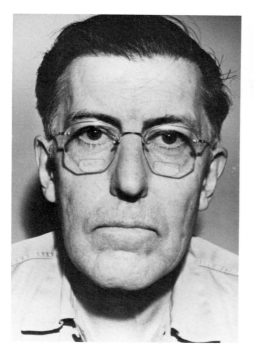 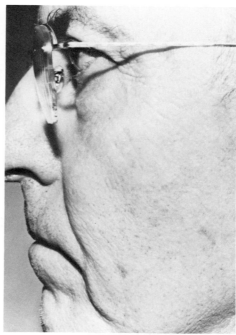

FIGURE 9.7.

Face in cluster headache. Note prominent square jaw, deep facial furrows and leathery *peau d'orange* appearance of skin (see also Figure 20.26). Reprinted by permission of the publisher, from Diamond S and Dallesio DJ. The practicing physician's approach to headache. Baltimore: Williams & Wilkins, 1978; 2nd ed.

# CLINICAL SIGNIFICANCE

This headache has several points of significance for the optometrist. First, because of the red eye, cluster headache may be confused from history with an attack of angle closure glaucoma if the patient has not been seen during an episode. If the angle is suspicious it is best to do a provocative test, and of course to closely question the patient as to the details of the attack (abrupt onset of severe periocular pain ceasing suddenly in 35 minutes is not likely to be angle closure glaucoma).

Second, any patient with a paradrine unreactive Horner's pupil (postganglionic lesion) should always be questioned as to clusterlike headaches; such third-neuron

Horner's syndromes appearing without company are virtually always benign when there is a classic history of cluster.

Third, the eye doctor should never diagnose cluster headache on the basis of only one or two attacks. This type of presentation may herald other entities, such as herpes zoster, cavernous sinus inflammation (Tolosa-Hunt syndrome), or more serious disease such as a paratrigeminal mass, nasopharyngioma, or posterior communicating artery aneurysm. Without history of at least several stereotyped attacks, it is always necessary to search for company, such as periorbital numbness or decreased corneal reflex, signs of incomitancy, pupillary/lid third nerve signs, listening for an orbital bruit with the bell stethoscope, and so forth. Finally, it is absolutely necessary to diagnose this headache, as specific therapy is usually highly effective, and untreated cluster headache has even led to suicide. Management of cluster should be by the headache specialist.

# References

Bickerstaff E. Neurological complications of oral contraceptives. New York: Oxford University Press, 1975.

Cohen K. Sinutabs for cluster headaches. N Engl J Med 1980;303:107–108. (Letter)

Denny-Brown, D. Handbook of neurological testing and case recording. Cambridge, Mass.: Harvard University Press, 1974.

Diamond S, Dalessio DJ. The practicing physician's approach to headache. Baltimore: Williams & Wilkins, 1978, 2nd ed.

Glaser JS. Neuro-ophthalmology. Hagerstown, Md.: Harper & Row, 1978.

Graham JR. Cluster headache. Paper read at International Symposium on Headache. Chicago, October, 1969.

Greedan JF, Domino L. Headache. N Engl J Med 1980;303:221. (Letter)

Hanington E. The headache book. Westport, Conn.: Technomic, 1981.

Hayreh, SS. Anterior ischemic optic neuropathy. New York: Springer-Verlag, 1975.

Healy LA, Wilske KR. The systemic manifestations of temporal arteritis. New York: Grune & Stratton, 1979.

Higgins JD. Headache. Rev Opt 1981; 4:130–139.

Huber, A. Eye signs and symptoms in brain tumors. St. Louis: Mosby, 1976, 3rd ed.

Kairys DJ, Tibbets C, Saliba K. A standard optometric headache history. J Am Optom Assoc 1983;54:165–176.

Karseras G, Crisp AH. Symptoms with signs in outpatients attending ophthalmology clinics. Br J Ophthalmol 1978;62:340–343.

Katzman R. Clinical approach to dementia. In: Smith JL, ed. Neuro-ophthalmology, focus 1980. New York: Masson, 1979;35:341–346.

Kudrow L. Cluster headache: diagnosis and management. Headache 1979; 19:142–150.

Levin BE. The clinical significance of spontaneous pulsations of the retinal vein. Arch Neurol 1978;35:37–40.

Louis S. A bedside test for determining the subtypes of vascular headaches. Headache 1981;21:87–88.

Mathews WB. Practical neurology. Oxford: Blackwell Scientific, 1975.

Reik L Jr., Hale M. The temporolmandibular joint pain-dysfunction syndrome: a frequent cause of headache. Headache 1981;21:151–156.

Ryan RE, Ryan RE Jr. Headache of nasal origin. Headache 1979;19:173–179.

Singer, F. Paget's disease of bone. New York: Plenum, 1977.

Smith JR, Landan SA. Smoker's polycythemia. N Engl J Med 1978;298:6–10.

Thompson, HS. Topics in neuro-ophthalmology. Baltimore: Williams & Wilkins, 1979.

Tyler GS, McNeely HE, Dick ML. Treatment of posttraumatic headache with amitriptyline. Headache 1980;20:213–216.

Walker HK, Hall WD, Hurst JW. Clinical methods. Woburn, Mass.: Butterworth, 1980.

Walsh, TJ. Neuro-ophthalmology: clinical signs and symptoms. Philadelphia: Lea & Febiger, 1978.

# II
# ASSESSMENT OF VISION CONDITIONS

# J. David Higgins
# HYPEROPIA 10

*In the unaccommodated hyperopic eye, a virtual object located at a point behind the eye (the far point) is clearly imaged on the retina, while all objects in real space are focused behind the plane of the retina. The retinal image suffers from increasing dioptric blur as an object approaches from optical infinity; that is, the eye is "too short" or the optics are "too weak." Such a static system is, however, only characteristic of an eye with no accommodative facility, such as in senility or with cycloplegia.*

*In most youthful eyes, hyperopia is facultative. Accommodation adds enough optical power to properly image objects on the retina and provides clear comfortable binocular vision at all reasonable viewing distances. When accommodation is not sufficient to provide consistent vision because of high hyperopia or advancing age, hyperopia is absolute.*

*When plus lenses are added in front of youthful hyperopic eyes the patient is able to relax an equal dioptric amount of ciliary tone and still see clearly. Since all previous efforts to see have been associated with a lifelong history of ciliary muscle contraction, most youthful patients are not able to relax completely their ciliary muscles, and some ciliary tonus remains. The incomplete amount of hyperopia thus revealed in subjective refraction is termed* manifest *hyperopia. The residual amount of voluntarily irrelaxable tonus is revealed by cycloplegia and is termed* latent *hyperopia.*

# BACKGROUND

As in myopia, the lower hyperopic errors probably reflect multifactored inheritance and tend to behave as if autosomally dominant, with the very high errors behaving as if recessive. Compared to those of the myope, hyperopic eyes are smaller and have more positive-angle lambda, shallower anterior chambers, and smaller scleral canals. Often the hyperopic optic disc looks smaller than the myopic optic disc, is more erythematous, and tends to have a smaller but deeper cup with centrally emerging vessels. In some families, a small scleral canal precipitates physiologic block of axoplasmic flow through the lamina cribrosa. As a result, axons swell and optic disc margins blur. Such optic discs tend to develop drusen later in life. Since the magnification of fundus detail with the direct ophthalmoscope is diminished in high hyperopia, it is often difficult to tell whether an optic disc is slightly hypoplastic or whether the effect is optical. In addition, novice observers often have difficulty gauging vessel calibre in hyperopic eyes.

Small, highly hyperopic eyes often do not obtain perfect 20/20 vision upon refraction. Whether this reflects a purely ocular condition associated with the development of the optic cup or a combined central nervous system (CNS) defect is unknown. Hyperopia tends to predominate in numerous retardation syndromes, with the notable exception of Down's syndrome.

In high hyperopia, substandard acuity may represent mild bilateral refractive amblyopia if accommodation has not been sufficient to produce consistent retinal clarity. Even more important is the consistent association of small degrees of hyperopic anisometropia (as low as 1 diopter) with some degree of unilateral refractive amblyopia. As opposed to myopic anisometropia, where the more ametropic eye usually obtains retinal clarity at close fixation distances, the hyperopic anisometrope will always accommodate for the least hyperopic eye; thus the more ametropic eye consistently fails to obtain retinal focus. This factor, along with central suppression, probably accounts for the presence of the amblyopia. In many of these eyes, a small microtropia may escape detection. Here the prescription of spectacles alone has little effect on the amblyopia since patching is also necessary. The condition often is familial.

Significant degrees of amblyopia are associated with the development of more clinically observable squints. Constant accommodation predisposes children with facultative hyperopia to esophoria; the eso deviation at near and far depends on the static distance phoria, the amount of hyperopia, and the magnitude of the accommodative convergence/accommodation (ACA) ratio. Although accommodative strabismus may be manifest early in life, for some unknown reason these children tend to retain fusion for the first 2 or 3 years of life before developing intermittent, then constant, esotropia. When a child of this age shows intermittent esotropia, such as when tired, it is best not to delay examination. These cases can rapidly evolve into constant unilateral esotropia with amblyopia even when only of several weeks' duration. If treatment is delayed, regaining fusion may be difficult even when a spectacle prescription eliminates most of the turn.

# HISTORY

Except in very high errors, hyperopia usually presents with visual or asthenopic symptoms during reading. Symptoms result from the increased demand on accommodation or, with esophoria, from the demands of fusion. Hyeropic children who retain fusion past the age of 4 tend to do well until adolescence, when increased reading demands and smaller sized print precipitate symptoms. If no symptoms are noted at this stage, the patient either is not inclined to read or is sufficiently compensated to carry on asymptomatically until the prepresbyopic years. At this point, decreasing accommodative amplitude produces symptoms of blurred vision at near range, sometimes spasms of accommodation upon looking up from reading, and asthenopia only occasionally. Obviously, not every patient will fall into these infant, adolescent, and prepresbyopic patterns, as some children with high hyperopia sometimes will present in the early school years, and those with a moderate amount of hyperopia may become symptomatic upon leaving school when occupational demands require more reading than was attempted previously.

Besides the obvious complaint of blurred vision at close range, youthful hyperopic patients tend to present with asthenopic symptoms, including headache during prolonged reading. The headache of hyperopia may occasionally represent true ciliary muscle ischemia, but this is unlikely unless significant spasm exists. In most patients, headache probably reflects the increased concentration required by marginal focus, accommodative instability, or the need for voluntary vergences to overcome an esophoria and maintain fusion. In this light, the headache, usually bifrontal, probably is a simple tension headache occurring in patients somewhat prone to excessive scalp contraction during stressful tasks. Occurring especially in highly hyperopic children is a peculiar "glowering" expression that often accompanies close viewing, with obvious frontalis and corrigator wrinkling, underscoring the effort to see. Even with significant near esophoria it is rare for patients to have diplopia during reading, as accommodation is more likely to relax with consequent blurred vision. Patients with significant hyperopia and esophoria occasionally note that they can maintain accurate accommodation by closing one eye and allowing the eye to turn without diplopia.

Significant accommodative spasm in hyperopes usually is associated with occupational tasks requiring prolonged close viewing combined with situational stress or neurotic anxiety. Mild spasm on looking up from reading is quite common in symptomatic hyperopia, however, especially when accompanied by esophoria at near range.

When symptoms of blurred vision associated with hyperopia have a relatively acute onset it is necessary to consider the cause. Often this will be nothing more than the normal development of absolute hyperopia in patients in their late thirties or early forties, who often decompensate and note symptom onset over a period of a few months. This is especially true when occupational demands create a need for more intense close work and the symptoms, once noted by the patient, will be fixated on and given exaggerated significance. It is easy to forget that such patients may be quite naive and need reassurance that their symptoms are a normal expected change. Also common in this age group is the abrupt noting of symptoms following ingestion of minor cycloplegics, such as in many of the commonly used tranquilizers, antidepressants, antihistamines, and antispasmodics. Although the amplitude of accommodation may only be minimally affected, the increased accommodative effort may produce an esophoria responsible for the near symptoms. More serious causes of accommodative paresis that may result in the sudden onset of symptoms via the unmasking of a preexisting facultative hyperopia are discussed in Chapter 13.

# EXAMINATION

Cycloplegic refraction in children is indicated by a presenting history of intermittent strabismus, detection of an eso deviation, a reduced acceptance of the plus sign found in retinoscopy, and other signs of latent hyperopia.

In most cases, two drops of 1% cyclopentolate instilled 5 minutes apart produce adequate cycloplegia in 40 minutes. If an intermittent strabismus is suspected from the patient's history, or if the retinoscopic exam still shows variable reflexes with suspiciously low plus acceptance subjectively, full cycloplegia with atropine is indicated. While usually suspected from retinoscopy, it is not uncommon for young adults to demonstrate 4 to 5 diopters of hyperopia when perhaps only 1 diopter can be manifest subjectively. Such patients are usually symptomatic, have resisted glasses in the past, or deny any interest in reading.

In very young children it is always a good idea to be suspicious when hyperopia is unequal by a diopter or more, even when the errors are relatively low. This is especially true when the child is too young to obtain visions, when lack of fixation precludes a good cover test, when the more hyperopic eye recovers slowly from an esophoria from behind cover, or when the parents cannot be relied on to observe the presence of a squint. It is better to err on the side of prescribing in these cases. A useful test is to disassociate the eyes with a 15-diopter prism and look for a strong unilateral fixation preference with a Hirschberg test; if obtained, spectacles should be prescribed. In such children with anisometropic hyperopia, it is necessary to rely heavily on the retinoscope, as the more hyperopic eye routinely will reject most of the excess plus. A standard binocular balance is often impossible at this age, especially if amblyopia exists.

In slightly older children with hyperopic anisometropia, a difference in visual acuity of more than one or two lines usually signifies microtropia or monofixation, even when the cover test appears negative. In such cases it is useful to repeat the unilateral covering of the "good" eye while simultaneously giving instructions assuring intense fixation. Often a telltale outward flick of several prism diopters will then be seen. If not, central suppression to the Bagolini or the Worth four dot flashlight at 10 feet is suggestive, as is 60 to 80 arc seconds of stereo on the Wirt test. Random dot stereo in microtropia, however, will usually show no stereopsis or greatly diminished performance in the area of 400 arc seconds. Such children need to undergo a short trial of patching in ad-dition to wearing glasses to be sure of recovery from the amblyopia. It is always wise to get a second view of the optic disc in a more hyperopic eye associated with amblyopia, since the entity of optic nerve hypoplasia may be present, which occasionally has serious accompaniments (see Chapter 31).

In older children, surprisingly low degrees of hyperopia are sometimes accompanied by asthenopic symptoms following reading. When accompanied by even small esophorias, the symptoms are usually truly related to a need for spectacles or base-in training. Even here it is sometimes wise to see what a little time will do, especially if the symptoms are of recent onset and associated with a period of malaise, such as in recovering from illness or coping with stress associated with family problems, school, or peer pressure.

When not accompanied by esophoria, near symptoms in low hyperopia absolutely demand that the practitioner directly measure the amplitude of accommodation via the pushup method to rule out a paresis. Assuming the amplitude is normal, it is wise to demand excessive documentation of a need for plus with extensive near point testing such as in measuring the lag, negative relative accommodation/positive relative accommodation (NRA/PRA), and accommodative facility. Even here, deficient performance is most typical of anxiety and depression associated with tension headaches. Functional stomach and other somatic complaints often are documented by multiple visits to doctors.

In older prepresbyopic patients the exam is quite straightforward and usually is addressed to the simple complaint of blurred near vision rather than asthenopia. Even in this age group, be alert to signs of residual latent hyperopia, such as more plus in retinoscopy versus manifest refraction, more plus at near than expected for age, residual esophoria, blur in the base in duction at distance, or increased plus acceptance in binocular versus monocular refraction.

Usually it is not necessary to cycloplege patients over the age of 30 unless sudden onset of variably blurred distance vision suggests a spasm. It is possible, if one wishes, to manifest a little more hyperopia by allowing the patient to view the chart for several minutes in a mildly fogged state, or under a small base-in prism. Usually the quickest method to gauge the extent of the total hyperopia is to rely on the prescription that balances the near point findings—that produces an NRA slightly in excess of the PRA, or lenses half a diopter or so less than those that eliminate the lag in a near crossed cylinder or duochrome test. Failure to do so often results in under-prescribing, with the patient returning in 6 to 12 months with the recurrent complaint of "short arms." Usually more latent hyperopia is discovered on rerefraction.

Unilateral hyperopic shifts are distinctly rare in normal eyes. When accompanied by substandard vision or metamorphopsia, it is best to consider that the photoreceptors have suddenly been moved forward, as from an orbital mass, detachment of the retinal pigment epithelium (RPE) in the elderly or, as is most common, because of a central serous choroidopathy where a "smudge" partially obscures central vision. In this latter condition, light reflected from the choroid may mask the refractive change to the retinoscope despite a clear hyperopic shift subjectively.

# CLINICAL SIGNIFICANCE

The clinical significance of hyperopia is several-fold. First, it is essential to recognize its role in the development of accommodative esotropia in young children and in the entities of refractive and microstrabismic amblyopia when the errors are unequal.

Second, the presence of hyperopia when accompanied by asthenopic symptoms always demands an investigation for other possible causes of the asthenopia (e.g., dry eye or reduced tear break up times) before accepting the refractive error as the cause.

Third, a careful history and exam is required in younger patients to determine whether symptoms of decreased school performance are really related to a need for glasses.

Finally, in some patients the apparent onset of symptomatic hyperopia may reflect a more serious cause affecting the third nerve and the accommodative status or the axial length of the globe.

In the usual case of low hyperopia, however, patients tend to present later in life with definite visual symptoms related to near point tasks, and the refraction and its interpretation are quite straightforward. Prescribing for hyperopia can require considerable expertise and experience as compared to myopia. As this is not within the scope of this book, the reader should consult the available literature on this topic.

# References

Borish IM. Clinical refraction. Chicago: Professional Press, 1970;3rd ed.

Duke-Elder W. Duke-Elder's practice of refraction. New York: Churchill Livingstone, 1978;9th ed. 37–43.

Manor RS. Use of special glasses in the treatment of spasm of the near reflex. Ann Ophthalmol 1979;11:903–905.

Safir A. Refraction and clinical optics. Hagerstown, Md.: Harper & Row, 1980.

Wright KW, Walonker F, Edelman P. 10-diopter fixation test for amblyopia. Arch Ophthalmol 1981;99:1242–1246.

# J. David Higgins
# MYOPIA 11

*Myopia describes a refractive error in which a real object at a certain point in space, the far point, is perfectly imaged on the retina of the unaccommodated eye, while more distant objects are focused anterior to the retina and cause the symptom of blurred distance vision. Myopia may be predominantly axial, refractive, or both.*

## BACKGROUND

The incidence of myopia varies among populations, ranging from near zero in more illiterate cultures to as high as 70% in Japanese colleges. Near work is not the sole factor in the etiology of myopia; for example, moderate uncorrected hyperopes require more accommodation for near, yet quite consistently retain their hyperopia throughout life. Those destined for myopic progression tend to be myopic at preschool age or demonstrate only low hyperopia of one-half diopter or so.

Myopia of more than 6 diopters occurs in about 2% of myopes, is usually axial, tends to manifest early in life, and tends to progress more with accompanying vitreoretinal degenerations. High myopia usually demonstrates autosomal recessive inheritance and occasionally is related to inherited enzyme defects affecting connective tissue in general, such as Marfan's syndrome, homocystinuria, Ehlers-Danlos syndrome, and the Weill-Marchesani syndrome. High myopia is also associated with prematurity and the use of oxygen with or without signs of retrolental fibro-

plasia. Females tend to be more commonly affected.

In contrast to the predominance of the axial component seen in high myopia, the vast majority of low and moderate myopias tends to reflect an unhappy association of numerous optical factors. Low and moderate myopia thus reflect multifactorial inheritance and often behave as if autosomally dominant.

There is little doubt that the typical progression often noted clinically in early adolescence is, at least in part, related to near work in a susceptible population. The reported successes in halting the progression via the use of antiaccommodative devices, such as atropine and bifocals, have yet to be shown effective for the most important subgroup, pathologically progressive high myopia. For the youngster with low myopia, the treatment would still seem to be worse than the disease given the recent improvements in contact lens materials if glasses are seen as a cosmetic problem.

As a group, myopic eyes tend to demonstrate several anatomic features: large globe size, which may simulate exophthalmos; deeper anterior chambers; and larger entrance pupils. The optic nerve tends to appear paler and larger than in hyperopia and more often demonstrates increased diameter of the physiologic cup, with exposure of the lamina. In higher myopia a conus may be present, especially when coupled with astigmatism, in which case oblique entrance of the optic nerve is often noted. Circumpapillary conus with reduced vision should suggest hypoplastic nerves and a search for accompaniments.

In addition, edema of the myopic disc can be more difficult to observe, and myopic discs are less commonly subject to pseudopapilledema and drusen deposition.

A retina that is stretching is the probable cause of reduced dark adaptation and color perception differences, which are sometimes noted by patients with anisometropic myopia. Bilateral high myopes commonly note the difficult seeing at night. Since the intraocular pressure (IOP) induced shear or stretching force on the coats of the eye is proportional to the radius of the eye's curvature, any eye with a somewhat elongated vitreous cavity is subject to higher stretching forces. Accommodation creates a temporary rise in intravitreal pressure; thus, with regard to reading, larger eyes possibly suffer more adverse effects with further ballooning of the coats of the eye and increase in myopia. Why some eyes elongate and others do not is unknown, despite extensive research on this subject.

Since the lamina cribrosa lies closer to the plane of the retina in myopia, cupping tends to be more shallow than in hyperopia. The optometrist must be alert to the hazard of shallow "saucerization" of such discs, which would indicate glaucomatous decompensation. Myopic eyes also seem somewhat more prone to field loss. Additionally, the more highly myopic eyes tend to be associated with low ocular rigidity, such that the tensions tend to be underestimated when measured with Schiøtz's tonometer. When forced to use a Schiøtz on such eyes, it is best to take the pressure using both the 5.5- and 10-g weights and then resort to published tables (Kolker and Hetherington 1976) to "factor out" the rigidity variable.

# HISTORY AND EXAMINATION

In low myopia, squinting may be associated with worsening of tension headaches in those so prone. Occasionally, the onset of myopia aggravates the symptoms of a preexisting convergence insufficiency. In the usual case, however, the history and examination are not problematic, with a relatively straightforward refraction corroborating the myopic basis of the complaint of blurred distance vision.

In infants and small children the history focuses on the more objective signs of squinting, failure to recognize the parents across the room, and so forth. Simply observing the eyes may be helpful in diagnosing high myopia, as in noting their increased prominence or a pseudoesotropic appearance owing to negative angle lambdas, which are more likely in such patients. In small children, cycloplegic retinoscopy is invaluable when the examination proves difficult otherwise. High myopia in premature infants exposed to oxygen should suggest the possibility of retrolental fibroplasia, and indirect ophthalmoscopy becomes indicated.

With an abnormal body habitus, inherited connective tissue disorders should be considered. The most common, Marfan's syndrome, would be evident in one of the parents, since it is autosomally dominant; however, an elongated appearance with excessive arm span is also characteristic of homocystinuria, especially if the child is blond and pale with malar erythema or telangiectasia. Both Marfan's syndrome and homocystinua have important systemic and ocular complications, such as retinal detachment and dislocated lenses. Homocystinuria is associated with mental retardation in half the cases. Intervention with diet and vitamin $B_6$ therapy may be helpful. The iris in homocystinuria may partially transilluminate, erroneously suggesting phenylketonuria, incomplete albinism, or even pigment dispersion syndrome if the chamber is excessively deep.

High myopia occasionally may represent infantile glaucoma, especially in a colicky child with photophobia and tearing. If the cornea is not obviously hazy, a transparent ruler is helpful in measuring visible corneal diameter, as the infant's fixation of an interesting object need not be obstructed.

School-aged children do not usually present special problems in refraction, except that the restricted viewing conditions of the phoropter can be associated with mild accommodative spasm and overestimation of the degree of myopia. This is suggested by the relatively mild degree of blurring on the entrance acuities compared to the refraction, and by the tendency of the subjective refraction to demand too many lens changes to clear up the last two or three lines on the chart. Overreliance on the duochrome test often results in an overcorrection in children. When in doubt, resort to the trial frame. A more common and alarming result of this mild spasm tendency in children occurs when one fails to obtain good vision in the phoropter, with the result indicated by the retinoscope. Adding half a diopter or so more minus may still yield only 20/25 to 20/30 vision. Before venturing further, it is often beneficial simply to hold the retinoscopically suggested trial lenses in front of the child's eyes, as often this alone yields 20/20 vision and avoids a time-consuming workup for nonexistent entities.

Adolescent children occasionally pose problems that test the refractive skills of the examiner. Commonly, a complaint of blurred distance vision in school turns out to be of an episodic nature, especially upon the shifting of gaze from prolonged close work to the blackboard. Such a tendency to spasm often results in poor vision when the child is tested in a vision screening because of proximal accommodation in the instrument. This is a common reason for teenagers to fail the drivers' vision screening test. Such mild spastic tendencies, occurring frequently in young girls, are generally harmless. The refractionist should concentrate attention on near-point testing. These children often show accommodative instabilities with or without esophoria, and a careful refraction will often demonstrate some degree of hyperopia. When the refraction shows tendencies for spasm, such as varying reflexes in retinoscopy, it is best to use cycloplegia, since occasionally the degree of hyperopia found is surprisingly high. Careful questioning may reveal a source of stress in the home or school. Finally, mild accommodative spasms when accompanied by episodic headache and functional stomach disorders often herald a more clear-cut migraine syndrome to follow in later adolescence.

Other more serious causes of myopic shifts seen in children include keratoconus, juvenile onset diabetes, and, rarely, a nephrotic syndrome. Nephrotic syndrome might present with lower lid edema or be evident from the fundus or blood pressure measurement.

Refraction in adults is generally straightforward. Sudden onset of myopia may occasionally reflect spasm in those doing intense close work, and in these patients cycloplegia will often demonstrate a surprising degree of latent hyperopia. Occasionally, such a spasm will reflect accidental instillation of a miotic, which may occur with nurses or gardeners; organic phosphate insecticides have strong anticholinesterase properties. It is important in cases of suspected spasm to obtain an actual measurement of the amplitude of accommodation prior to cycloplegia, as the two measurements will combine to indicate whether the spasm is associated with a simultaneous paresis of accommodation. This sort of pseudomyopia is characteristic of the sudden onset of diabetes, but it may represent a neurologic syndrome that heralds the onset of other bulbar palsies, such as botulism or reflecting pinealoma.

Ciliary-body edema will also produce pseudomyopia and represents an uncommon idiosyncratic response to sulfonamides, thiazide and carbonic anhydrase diuretics, and occasionally to digitalis. Pseudomyopia usually is not accompanied by fluctuating vision or retinoscopic reflexes, small pupils, or esophoria; it is not abolished by cycloplegia.

The most common cause of atypical myopic shifts, however, occurs in the elderly and reflects the process of nuclear sclerosis. In these patients one must refrain from prescribing for small refractive changes. The dioptric improvement noted on the high-contrast, high-frequency acuity chart often will not be appreciated in daily living where low-frequency attentuation owing to light scattering is more important to quality of sight. Furthermore, an elderly patient may have a difficult time adjusting to the new spectacle magnifications, especially if the change is greater in one eye. It is often best to insist on a clear subjective improvement with a trial lens in a lighted room before prescribing changes.

It is also prudent to reevaluate the depth of the anterior chambers from time to time in patients whose lenses are swelling. In addition, the slit lamp examination should corroborate the suspected lens changes, or another cause, such as a diabetic myopic shift, must be sought.

The entity of night myopia occasionally attains clinical significance. Blurred vision while driving at night is a common presenting complaint that indicates that myopia has progressed. Empty field accommodation, the Purkinje shift, positive spherical aberration, and decreased depth of field with nighttime mydriasis all combine to produce a further myopic shift of variable proportions, which will be more manifest to the myope. Vision in absolute hyperopia may actually improve, as elderly low hyperopes often find they see better by taking off their glasses when driving at night. Occasionally, when an occupational need exists, such as long-distance trucking, it is necessary to assess and prescribe specifically for night myopia by using trial lenses over the patient's habitual spectacles. A caveat is that stationary nyctalopias often are accompanied by myopia. A good question to ask is whether the patient can identify the well-known constellations in the night sky; if not, or when a positive and family history exists, an electroretinogram (ERG) and dark adaptometry should be obtained.

# CLINICAL SIGNIFICANCE

In general, the significance of myopia is no more than the blurred vision that requires spectacle or contact lens prescription; however, always consider systemic and ocular associations, pseudomyopia, and spasm. It is especially prudent to proceed methodically in the case of sudden myopic shift.

Myopia associated with spasm is common in adolescent females, but even these cases require attention to psychological stress, the near-point status, and the neurologic status. Pseudomyopia associated with drugs and ciliary-body edema usually is easily diagnosed, as the effect is not dose dependent and generally occurs promptly upon starting therapy.

Myopic shifts in diabetes usually imply that blood sugar is significantly elevated and a simple fasting blood sugar test will be positive. When such patients are being seen for the first time, the examiner might not have access to a previous refraction and can miss the presentation entirely. It is prudent, therefore, to ask specifically about weight loss, fatigue, thirst, and family history. The myopic shift of nuclear sclerosis in the elderly is well known to practitioners. Surprisingly, these patients may comment more about their renewed ability to read fine print than their blurred distance vision. Prescribing for myopia shifts demands astute clinical judgment.

Finally, any patient with significant axial myopia should undergo a peripheral retinal exam at least every other year. Such patients should also be informed as to the symptoms of fresh retinal tears, since early prophylaxis is much preferred to the uncertainties of retinal detachment surgery. The most important propensity for retinal detachment in myopes undoubtedly is associated with Stickler's disease. Here, unlike its usual sporadic occurrence, the high myopia is dominantly inherited. Affected siblings are likely to show a variety of skeletal dysplasias, the most characteristic of which is a flattened midface, often accompanied by cleft palate. In such children, the vitreous looks suspiciously optically empty and there may be membranes, pigmentary retinal changes, and presenile cataract.

# References

Birnbaum MH, ed. Symposium: perspectives on myopia. Am J Optom Physiol Opt 1981;58:515–569.

Bovino JA, Marcus DF. The mechanism of transient myopia induced by sulfonamide therapy. Am J Ophthalmol 1982;94:44–102.

Daub J, Shotwell AJ. Optical prophylaxis for environmental myopia: an epidemiological assessment of short term effects. Am J Optom Phyiol Opt 1983;60:316–320.

Kelly T, Chatfield C, Tustin G. Clinical assessment of the arrest of myopia. Br J Ophthalmol 1975;59:529–538.

Kolker A. Hetherington J. Beeker and Shaffer's diagnosis and therapy of the glaucomas. St. Louis: C.V. Mosby, 1976;449–461.

Michaels, DD. Visual optics and refraction: a clinical approach. St. Louis: C.V. Mosby, 1980;2nd ed.

Sorsby, A. Emmetropia and its aberrations; a study in the correlation of the optical components of the eye. London: Her Majesty's Stationery Office, 1957.

Symposium: clinical management of physiologic myopia. Ophthalmology (Rochester) 1979;86:679–712.

# J. David Higgins
# ASTIGMATISM 12

*Astigmatism is an optical anomaly with unequal refraction of light in different meridians of the eye. A distant point source of light produces two major, but perpendicular, focal lines near the retina. When one line is focused on the retina the condition is simple* astigmatism, either myopic or hyperopic, depending on whether the other focal line falls in front of the retina or behind. When both focal lines fall in front of or behind the retina the condition is compound *myopic or hyperopic* astigmatism. In mixed *astigmatism, one line falls in front and the other behind the retina.*

## BACKGROUND

Most significant astigmatic errors result from a flex in the cornea producing a regular toric refracting surface with two major meridians or axes of symmetry. A keratometric reflection off a toric cornea is not distorted except, perhaps, for an elliptical elongation corresponding to the major and minor axes of astigmatism, which are always 90% apart in regular astigmatisms. When the more powerful refracting meridian is vertical, the astigmatism is "with-the-rule"; when horizontal, it is "against-the-rule." When the major and minor meridians are more than 30° off the horizontal and vertical, the astigmatism is oblique. Any interruption in surface quality or aberration of the cosine-squared law of a toric surface will produce noticeable distortions in the reflected image and represents irregular astigmatism.

A certain amount of astigmatism can be due to intraocular optical aberrations, such as tilting of the lens. This astigmatism averages 0.50 diopters against-the-rule with a standard deviation of $\pm 0.37$ diopters, regardless of spherical refractive error, age, or angle lambda. In many eyes, this internal astigmatism is counterbalanced by nearly equal and opposite with-the-rule corneal astigmatism.

Approximately 70% to 90% of young children demonstrate some degree of with-the-rule corneal astigmatism. With aging, however, a flattening of the vertical corneal meridian occurs, with senile eyes showing a marked preponderance of against-the-rule corneas.

The causes of astigmatism are varied and not well understood. In most cases, it is surprising that the various meridional radii of corneal curvature are usually within a few hundredths of a millimeter. Low degree of astigmatism probably represents simple developmental variation.

High astigmatism often is associated with a more notable malformation of the eye, as the optic discs in such eyes often show an oblique entrance, with ectasia of the inferior nasal fundus producing physiologic bitemporal field depressions, not to be confused with a chiasmal lesion.

Astigmatism can be acquired and usually is due to corneal insults, such as deformation from a chalazion or traction from limbal wound healing, as after cataract extraction. Scarring, especially when associated with surface irregularities, is likely to produce irregular astigmatism and markedly reduce vision. This is best appreciated in considering Fuchs' dystrophy, where vision remains surprisingly good despite the scattering and hazy appearance of the cornea. When blebs produce surface irregularities observable with the keratometer, however, vision falls markedly. Other examples of surface irregularities producing visual decrement are pterygia and the wetting defects of sicca, where vision will vary with the blink. The two most frequently seen causes of irregular astigmatism, however, are those caused by contact lens abuse and the corneal ectasias, chiefly keratoconus. Patients with scleral buckles often undergo large astigmatic changes, underscoring the importance of careful refraction.

Acquired internal astigmatism of moderate degree occurs occasionally in elderly patients with cortical or subcapsular lens opacities and again underscores the need to refract accurately such patients before assuming their vision is uncorrectable. Tilting of the lens, as in early subluxation, will also produce astigmatic changes, as is most commonly seen in Marfan's syndrome and in homocystinuria.

A serious cause of unequal meridional refraction is a ciliary-body mass. Sector paresis of the ciliary body and iris is often seen after trauma, but it also occurs in Adie's syndrome, neurosyphilis, and secondary to photocoagulation. These eyes may show an astigmatic shift on accommodation for close vision. Thus, anyone complaining of unexplained blurring at the near point, and with a flat sector visible in the pupil, may deserve a separate refraction at the reading distance and a search for the cause.

Uncorrected astigmatism in high degrees is associated with amblyopia, as the retina never has the benefit of a clear image (regardless of viewing distance). Significant amblyopia arises mainly when such astigmatism is unilateral—probably owing to coexistent central suppression, with or without a clinically measurable tropia. Refractive amblyopia associated with bilateral astigmatism does exist, however, since it is possible to demonstrate lower resolution in the more ametropic meridian, even after spectacle correction. It is rare, even in the presence of bilateral errors in the range of 6 to 8 diopters, to see corrected visions worse than 20/40, and the vision usually improves further after only a short trial of wearing glasses, even in children past the age of 6 years.

Considering this association with amblyopia, remember that high astigmatism is the most faithfully transmitted of all ametropias, behaving as if autosomally dominant. Thus, seeing a child or mother with such a condition would prompt a question as to whether there are other siblings at home as, statistically, one-half will be similarly affected.

# HISTORY

There are no specific symptoms for astigmatism, and the full range of asthenopic complaints may be expected. Unless there has been a recent increase in visual demands, it is best to look for other causes of eye fatigue when symptoms are of recent onset. In general, however, asthenopic symptoms are common, may predominate over visual ones, and often occur when reading unless myopic astigmatism exists.

In this respect, against-the-rule astigmatism is the biggest culprit, especially when combined with even low degrees of hyperopia. Such patients may unconsciously increase orbicularis tone against the vertical limbi to steepen the vertical meridian and obtain clearer vision. Many will not admit to squinting, but telltale brow ache after one-half hour's reading implicates this form of muscle tension headache. When symptoms are clear, prescriptions for errors as low as 0.50 to 0.75 diopters for against-the-rule astigmatism are perfectly legitimate.

# EXAMINATION

Several signs during the examination suggest astigmatism and are helpful when dealing with difficult refractions in young children.

An oval appearance to the pupil or optic disc is characteristic of high astigmatism, with the long axis of the pupil corresponding to the more myopic meridian. A qualitatively special kind of distortion is also noted in examining the fundus of high astigmatism; this is difficult to describe but is known to most experienced examiners. A blur of disc and vessel detail in a specific orientation and not in others, which reverses when the ophthalmoscopic lens power is altered, is specific for astigmatism, as is linear elongation of the foveal reflex.

In obtaining entrance acuities, the phenomenon of scattering is typical of astigmatism, as when the patient may read two-thirds of the 20/30 line, but also one-third of the 20/25 line and yet miss one-third of the 20/40 line. Additionally, a one-line improvement of the binocular acuities over the monocular acuities is suggestive of astigmatism, especially oblique. This phenomenon is, however, also typical of decompensating hyperopia and some cases of macular degeneration, especially cystoid.

Another interesting aspect of the astigmatic exam is the marked individual variation in uncorrected acuities. While in one patient an error of 0.75 diopter may reduce vision to 20/30, another may have several diopters and laboriously read the same line. Often in children only a little improvement in acuities is noted upon testing through the correction lenses, and the examiner may doubt the refraction. It is best with any evidence of poor school work or other symptoms to correct these moderate to large errors. A second visit usually results in a more precise subjective refraction corroborating the original findings and producing a more distinct difference in the corrected versus uncorrected acuities. With larger errors, the keratometer can be employed to estimate the total astigmatism by referring the readings to the spectacle plane and combining this with the expected value of 0.50 diopter against the rule for internal astigmatism.

Although not mentioned in the literature, retinoscopy in some larger pupils will repeatedly overestimate with-the-rule astigmatism and underestimate against-the-rule astigmatism; this may be an occasional factor underlying a discrepancy between the keratometer readings and the retinoscopic result.

In children, a spectacle prescription for high bilateral astigmatism usually is sufficient to overcome an associated amblyopia. When unilateral, however, one should also look for microstrabismus with a cover or 4-prism-diopter-base-out test, as well as signs of central suppression. In such eyes it is often necessary to patch for improvement of the amblyopia.

Since bilateral astigmatism of moderate to high degree is characteristic of partial albinism, it is well to consider this cause when corrected visions remain 20/40 or worse. These children may be only moderately fair and do tan slightly as they get older; however, they are distinctly fairer than the parents and unaffected siblings since the disease is autosomally recessive. While the fundus is always at least suspiciously blond, the keys to diagnosis are a poorly developed macula (e.g., absent reflex, little pigmentation, and arterioles infringing on the fovea), poor stereo performance, and mild to moderate iris transillumination. The latter is best noted in a darkened room with a slit beam directed straight on through the pupil. Such transillumination may occur in phenyketonuria, homocystinuria, and in the pigment dispersion sometimes associated with secondary glaucoma.

Acquired astigmatism is usually suspected when a significant astigmatic change is noted, especially in one eye. In the absence of a previous refractive history, be suspicious when the amount and axes of astigmatism are distinctly asymmetrical between the eyes. When caused by corneal deformation, usually some degree of irregular astigmatism is noted in retinoscopy and confirmed by distortion of the mires on keratometry. In the absence of obvious causes, such as that associated with contact lens abuse or those readily apparent to the slit lamp, such a change usually reflects a chalazion, another mass in the upper lid, or keratoconus.

A common problem in office practice is to distinguish between irregular astigmatism associated with contact lens wear and early progressive keratoconus. In general, a reduction in myopia and associated with-the-rule changes in a patient without strong personal or family history of atophy suggests mechanical deformation. This is especially true if overwear and evidence of significant edema or thick or large high-riding lenses exist. In addition, a stationary lens resting on the lower lid or a dirty silicone lens may produce such corneal deformations in susceptible persons. Make sure that another cause for reduced vision, besides the small amount of kera-tometric distortion, does not exist. Thus, a good internal exam is called for, as well as noting that the vision approaches normal via overrefraction or through a pinhole to eliminate the optical effects of the corneal irregularity.

Be especially suspicious of the cause of unilateral astigmatism not explained by the keratometric readings. If the patient is unusually long-boned, a partial subluxation of the lens associated with Marfan's syndrome (dominant) or homocystinuria (recessive) would have to be considered. In a lightly pigmented child with psychomotor retardation and malar erythema, finding a urinary excess of homocystine may lead to dietary measures that may ameliorate progressive mental deterioration. Other causes will often be obvious, such as sector plegia associated with trauma, Adie's syndrome, or even a ciliary-body mass. This latter reason makes it necessary to gonioscope the angle and to use the scleral depressor with the indirect ophthalmoscope to examine the ciliary body and its environs. Occasionally, such a finding may also represent neurologically significant partial internal third-nerve palsy, as was once common in neurosyphillis; even an aneurysm may be at the root of the problem.

In most astigmatic patients the examination is quite straightforward. The retinoscope usually is more sensitive in estimating the amount and axis of astigmatism than the degree of spherical ametropia and may be relied upon heavily in children for this purpose. When excessive reliance on the retinoscope is necessary, it is wise to carry out a straddling procedure. This is accomplished by sweeping 45° to each side of the tentative minus cylinder axis using the plane mirror and resetting the axis alignment slightly away from any "with" motion so seen and again checking for neutrality. If necessary, the process is repeated until no further changes are indicated.

In infants, there usually is considerable difficulty in holding lenses before the eyes for retinoscopy. All refractionists should be proficient in spiraling techniques with the streak retinoscope to avoid missing large refractive errors (Copeland 1970). This procedure requires cycloplegia, although accommodation can usually be stabilized by working in total darkness as well.

The cross-cylinder test is more popular for subjective confirmation nowadays than the astigmatic dial or fan chart, probably because it is less confusing, more rapid, and not as sensitive to improper spheres set in place in the refractor. It is not unusual, however, to see patients reject the retinoscopic finding in favor of the habitual correction using this test. When this is suspected, it is necessary to remind the patient to ignore any distortion of the letters and to concentrate only on the task of identifying them using a threshold line.

In some cases it may be necessary to directly measure the acuities comparing the observed retinoscopic change versus the habitual prescription. When these steps are taken, the retinoscopic findings usually are found to represent the more accurate refraction. Hand-held cross cylinders also are invaluable, as one may quickly introduce them when the degree of visual impairment calls for a more powerful cross cylinder to accomplish the test properly. They are, of course, very helpful in large spherical ametropias, which require use of the trial frame or overrefraction clips incorporating the pantoscopic tilt to be worn by the patient. Serious error in the astigmatic component can result if the pantoscope tilt is not considered. A tilt of even 8° will produce an astigmatic change of 0.5 diopter in a 5-diopter sphere.

# CLINICAL SIGNIFICANCE

Besides producing blurred vision or asthenopic complaints, the significance of astigmatism is several-fold. First, except in the presence of unusually high anisometropic astigmatism or an accompanying strabismus, an associated amblyopia usually is mild and responds to a spectacle prescription. If the vision is more reduced or does not respond, then another more serious cause of reduced vision should be sought. Second, since high astigmatism often is familial, it is prudent to suggest a visit for any children in the family who

have never been examined. Third, unusual astigmatic presentations suggest the possibility of acquired astigmatism, which may have a variety of causes—both corneal and internal.

The diagnosis of astigmatism forces a judgment: is the refractive error responsible for the patient's complaints? Making this clinical judgment and selecting a comfortable wearing prescription are the more difficult and interesting areas of the art of refractive treatment. Unfortunately, they are not within the scope of this book.

# References

Baldwin WR, Mills D. A longitudinal study of corneal astigmatism and total astigmatism. Am J Optom Physiol Opt 1981; 58:206–211.

Bear JC, Avrum R. Cylindrical refractive error: a population study in western Newfoundland. Am J Optom Physiol Opt 1983;60:39–45.

Borish IM. Clinical refraction. Chicago: Professional Press, 1970; 3rd ed.

Cobb SR, MacDonald CF. Resolution acuity in astigmats: evidence for a critical period in the human visual system. Br J Physiol Opt 1978;32:38–49.

Copeland JC. Streak retinoscopy. In: Sloan AE, Manual of refraction. Boston: Little, Brown, 1970; 2nd ed.

Karseras AG, Crisp AH. Symptoms without signs in outpatients attending ophthalmology clinics. Br J Ophthalmol 1978;62:340–343.

Milder B, Rubin ML. The fine art of prescribing glasses without making a spectacle out of yourself. Gainesville, Fla.: Triad Scientific Publishers, 1978.

Pappas CJ, Anderson DR, Briese FW. Is the autorefractor reading closest to manifest refraction? Arch Ophthalmol 1978;96(6):997–998.

Rengstorff RH. Astigmatism after contact lens wear. Am J Optom Physiol Opt 1977;54(11):787–791.

# Richard London
# ACCOMMODATION 13

*Accommodation is the dioptric adjustment of the eye to obtain sharpness for the target of regard. Accommodation is effected. by changes in the shape of the crystalline lens. Problems affecting the accommodative system may present as a decrease in total amount of available accommodation, a lag of accommodation too far beyond the plane of regard, an inability to sustain accommodation for a prolonged period, difficulty in rapidly adjusting accommodation for changes of viewing distance, accommodative spasm, or imbalance in the accommodation/convergence relationship. Each problem presents with characteristic findings.*

*Deficiency of accommodation is absent or reduced ability to accommodate. The synonyms absence of accommodation, absolute presbyopia, paralysis of accommodation, insufficiency of accommodation, and ill-sustained accommodation all fit under this general heading.*

*Infacility of accommodation is an inability to readily alter accommodative response to a dioptric change in stimulus, usually manifested as a sluggish accommodative response to change in fixation distance. Synonyms are inflexible accommodation and accommodative inertia.*

*Spasm of accommodation is a clonic cramp resulting from overstimulation of the ciliary muscle. Synonymous terms are hyperaccommodation, hypertonic accommodation, and pseudomyopia. Less common is a tonic cramp, which may present as a structural rather than functional disorder.*

## BACKGROUND

Criteria of deficiency of accommodation are more than 2 diopters below Donders' expecteds, or more than 0.50 diopter difference between the eyes. Hoffstetter's formula, 15 minus ¼ age, is the minimum expected accommodation available.

Age is an extremely important factor in determining the cause of deficient accommodation. The 45-year-old who can no longer hold the telephone book far enough away to read and has an otherwise unremarkable ocular examination probably is entering presbyopia. This is referred to as a static accommodative insufficiency since innervation is normal, the problem being in the lack of response by the lens or ciliary body. A dynamic accommodative deficiency is of more concern, as is a unilateral decrease in accommodation.

Nerve supply for accommodation arises from both divisions of the autonomic nervous system. The parasympathetic innervation arises from the Edinger-Westphal nucleus and runs superficially along with the third nerve, finally entering the eye as the short ciliary nerves. These simultaneously innervate the ciliary muscle and the iris sphincter. Sympathetic innervation originates in the hypothalamus and runs to the ciliospinal center of Budge, synapsing with the preganglionic neuron, which runs to the superior cervical ganglion. There it synapses with the postganglionic neuron, which travels along the internal carotid plexus and enters the eye as the long ciliary nerve. Parasympathetic innervation is the more potent of the two systems, being responsible for positive accommodation and pupil miosis. Negative accommodation and mydriasis are a combined result of parasympathetic relaxation and sympathetic stimulation. The balance between these two innervations may be represented as the resting or dark focus of the eye. This means that under conditions of degraded visual stimulation, such as at night or during adverse weather conditions, the eye will maintain a certain resting level of accommodation. This is reported by the patient as night myopia and often requires an additional prescription of $-0.50$ to $-1.00$ for night driving.

Bilateral dynamic insufficiency may result from a lesion in the Edinger-Westphal nucleus in the midbrain. Lesions of the fascicular and peripheral branches of the oculomotor nerve result in a unilateral reduction in accommodation and usually a dilated, fixed pupil. Recent illnesses, notably mumps, measles, influenza, scarlet fever, whooping cough, tonsillitis, anemia, encephalitis, and diphtheria may reduce amplitude or sustaining ability of the accommodative response. Especially important in children is the ingestion of lead, which may also lead to behavioral and mental changes, sluggish pupils, and a lead line along the base of the gums. Glaucoma may produce accommodative insufficiency in children and young adults through secondary ciliary-body atrophy. In adults, common causes for reduced accommodation are anemia, encephalitis, multiple sclerosis, myotonic dystrophy, possibly myasthenia gravis, lactation, and trauma to the craniocervical region (especially whiplash). Diabetes mellitus may cause a transient paresis or paralysis of accommodation, as well as changes in refraction. This is most common after insulin treatment has been started. Pineal tumors leading to Parinaud's syndrome may result in a reduced accommodative response occurring weeks before decreased pupillary light response, leading to an inverse Argyll Robertson pupil. Choroidal metastasis may involve the ciliary plexus if it spreads in the suprachoroidal space. Drugs also can lead to bilateral accommodative decreases (see Table 13.1). Alcohol reduces accommodation when the dosage is at the toxic level. Parkinsonian drugs such as trihexyphenidyl (Artane or Lystrone), ganglion-blocking drugs affecting the ciliary ganglion, and any CNS stimulant or tranquilizers, such as phenothiazides, negatively affect accommodation. Antihistamines may slightly reduce accommodation. Cycloplegics such as atropine, scopolamine, and homatropine all produce internal ophthalmoplegia. Care must be taken to check for these ingredients in skin ointments and systemic over-the-counter medications used by patients. Marijuana is reported to decrease accommodation.

Unilateral causes of decreased accommodation are numerous and occasionally quite serious. A difference of more than 0.5 diopter between the eyes may be significant. Trauma resulting in a tear of the iris sphincter or the zonules of Zinn, or a posterior displacement of the ciliary attachment usually is easily seen with the slit lamp. Blunt trauma may initially result in miosis and accommodative spasm followed by pupil dilation and accommodative paresis. Accommodation usually returns within 2 months; the pupil does not recover as well. Iridocyclitis, with the accompanying red, often painful eye, cells and flare, and irregular pupil may decrease accommodation. Ciliary-body aplasia should also be considered. Herpes

zoster scars along the forehead and tip of the nose indicate ocular involvement of the nasociliary nerve. A sinus problem may lead to a unilateral decrease in accommodation without affecting pupillary responses. These patients often present with early-morning headaches, made worse with a prone posture. Test by percussing and transilluminating the sinuses. Antihistamine therapy may return accommodative function to equality. Focal infections such as those caused by dental caries may temporarily reduce accommodation unilaterally, as may dental injections used during treatment.

It is frequently stated that spasm of

### Table 13.1
### Nonfunctional Causes of Accommodative Problems

| Bilateral* | Unilateral |
|---|---|
| *Drugs* | *Local eye disease* |
| Alcohol | Iridocyclitis |
| Artane | Glaucoma |
| Lystrone | Choroidal metastasis |
| Ganglion blockers | Tear in iris sphincter |
| Phenothiazides | Blunt trauma |
| Antihistamines | Ciliary-body aplasia |
| Cycloplegics | Scleritis |
| CNS stimulants | Adie's syndrome |
| Marijuana | |
| Cholinergic drug(s) | |
| Morphine(s) | |
| Digitalis(s) | |
| Sulfonamides and carbonic anhydrase(s) inhibitors | |
| *General disease: Adults* | *General disease: Adults* |
| Anemia | Sinusitis |
| Encephalitis(e) | Dental caries |
| Diabetes mellitus | Trigeminal neuralgia(s) (tic douloureux) |
| Multiple sclerosis | Posterior communicating artery aneurysm |
| Myotonic dystrophy | Parkinsonism |
| Myasthenia gravis | Wilson's disease |
| Malaria | Midbrain lesions |
| Typhoid | |
| Fatigue cramp-ciliary(s) | |
| Toxemia | |
| Syphilis(s) | |
| Botulism | |

**Table 13.1**
*(continued)*

| Bilateral* | Unilateral |
|---|---|
| *General disease: Children* | |
| Anemia | |
| Mumps | |
| Measles | |
| Influenza(e) | |
| Scarlet fever | |
| Whooping cough | |
| Tonsillitis | |
| Encephalitis(e) | |
| Diphtheria | |
| Meningitis(s) | |
| Lead and arsenic poisoning | |
| *Neuro-ophthalmic* | *Neuro-ophthalmic* |
| Lesion in Edinger-Westphal syndrome | Fascicular nerve III lesion |
| Trauma to craniocervical region (whiplash) | Herpes zoster |
| Pineal tumor | Horner's syndrome |
| Parinaud's syndrome | |
| Polyneuropathy | |
| Anterior poliomyelitis | |

Note: s = spasm; e = either spasm or deficiency; no qualifier = deficiency.
*Bilateral problem may start unilaterally.

accommodation is usually secondary to a neurotic hysterical disposition. In fact, the vast majority of cases are functional, and often present in a group commonly associated with hysterical amblyopia: adolescent children (especially girls) with excessive pressure over school performance and visual acuity that does not respond readily to correction. An interesting variant of hysterical presentation is the "spasm" of the near reflex. In this presentation, the patient manifests a spasm of the entire near triad: accommodation, convergence, and miosis.

Factors that appear to increase the likelihood of accommodative spasm are compound hyperopic or mixed astigmatism, and simple or latent hyperopia especially if anisometropic. Patients exhibiting distance exophoria who have been slightly overminused in the binocular state, or who use accommodative-convergence to maintain binocularity, may show mild spasm. Interestingly, prepresbyopes and groups with subnormal accommodative ability also tend to show accommodative spasm, especially when looking up following prolonged near work. Some patients may show "accommodative esophoria," demonstrating an increasing esoposture as demanding, near work is attempted.

Accommodative spasm crises may be symptomatic of local inflammation as well as CNS lesions. Uniocular spasms are always more suspect. History should address questions concerning blunt trauma, ocular inflammation such as scleritis, iritis, and uveitis. Slit lamp exam should focus on signs of trauma such as Vossius ring, corneal scars, and inflammatory signs, such as cells and flare in the anterior chamber and cells in the vitreous.

Destructive lesions leading to accommodative paresis may begin as irritative lesions with resultant spasms. Cyclic oculomotor palsy, sympathetic paralysis, and syphilis also lead to excessive accommodation.

Drugs may produce bilateral accommodative spasm. Cholinergic drugs such as eserine and pilocarpine may produce marked spasm, especially in young adults and children. Epinephrine, therefore, is preferable to pilocarpine in glaucoma therapy in young patients. Other anticholinesterase drugs, such as those found in garden poisons, also may result in accommodative crises. Excessive doses of vitamin $B_1$ (thiamine) may increase accommodative amplitude in the elderly, as may caffeine to a lesser degree. Sulfonamides may also lead to excessive accommodation or pseudomyopia.

# HISTORY AND EXAMINATION

Asthenopia following near work is a frequent cause of concern for these patients. Headaches may occur around the brow region. Ask the patient, "Do the headaches develop toward the end of the day?" If they do, the next question should address itself to whether the headaches are present in the absence of prolonged near work: "Do you suffer the headaches on weekends or holidays?" Headache resulting from prolonged static posture should also be considered. The general state of health should be carefully probed since these patients frequently exhibit general fatigue toward the end of the day. If the answer is affirmative, it is important to determine if both the fatigue and near point problems are of recent onset. Photophobia, tearing, burning, frequent eye rubbing, inability to concentrate, trauma, diplopia, and "an arm too short to hold reading material at a viewable distance" may be symptomatic of accommodative deficiency.

A problem-specific data base for accommodative complaints is presented below, in a routine examination sequence. Several aspects of accommodation should be tested: amplitude, stability, posture, and facility.

Pupillary reflexes must be carefully considered to rule out pathology. Check for aberrant regeneration during versions or with optokinetic nystagmus (OKN). Concomitancy should be established by cover testing since excessive spasm may present as an esotropia, and many neurologic insults may affect accommodation.

Orbital and retromastoid bruits may be listened for with the bell portion of the stethoscope. The slip lamp provides important information about trauma and inflammation. In addition, blepharitis may be observed in these patients as a sequel to rubbing their eyes in a futile attempt to achieve clarity.

The amplitude of accommodation is determined either by the push-up or minus lens technique. It must be remembered that a low positive relative accommodation (PRA)—less than 1.75 diopters is suspect—may be reflective of an accommodative-convergence problem (low base in ranges). Thus, when investigating the patency of the accommodative system, monocular testing must always be included. Tests of lag of accommodation or plus acceptance are good indicators of the relative plane of focus and accommodative accuracy for a target of regard. The fused cross-cylinder test (14B) net expected findings is +0.75 diopters or less, unless there is a need for additional plus at near. An objective correlate of this test is provided by dynamic retinoscopy.

MEM (monocular estimation method) retinoscopy has proven to be a quick and accurate measure of the amount of accommodation free of convergence for a given plane (posture). A lag of more than +0.75 diopters or a difference of more than 0.50 diopter when probing each eye is considered significant.

Acuity is the first clue to the possibility of spasm. Vision is usually 20/60 to 20/

100 monocularly, although it occasionally may be worse. During the subjective the patient may require an unusually high number of minus lenses to obtain equality in the duochrome (bichrome) test, or to go from 20/30 to 20/20. Binocular refraction either by Turville or American Optical (AO) vectograph usually manifests more plus. The minus lens amplitude of accommodation, or the PRA over the best acuity lenses is likely to be reduced. Phoria findings may show an eso deviation at distance (always a sign of concern if the patient had previously been orthophoric. Consider other signs of increased intracranial pressure before accepting a simple spastic etiology). Fused cross-cylinder findings may show a minus projection, and MEM retinoscopy is likely to reveal an against motion. Static retinoscopy tends to show a variable reflex. Small amounts of against-the-rule cylinder are often subjectively desired. Cyclogel 1% instilled in two drops 5 minutes apart following one drop of 0.5% Alcaine usually will produce a lessening of the spasm, a decrease in eso deviation, and more plus in the retinoscopy. In darkly pigmented patients, however, or in the presence of a major spasm, atropine may be needed for relaxation. In lieu of the use of cycloplegics, several techniques may be attempted to determine the actual refractive error. Allowing the patient to sit undisturbed behind mild fogging lenses is known as the delayed subjective technique. Some patients under conditions of fog may actually accommodate in an attempt to clear the chart. Base-in prism added to the above procedure may assist relaxation. The near retinoscopy technique of Mohindra (1977) may reveal more plus than a static, especially if the spasm is mild. An attempt to break the spasm by means of accommodative flexibility training with ±2.00 flippers for 1 week prior to refraction may be successful in mild cases.

The basic strategy for accommodative facility testing is to rapidly alternate the flexion and relaxation of the accommodative response. This may be accomplished by altering viewing distance, in which case convergence is also altered, or by maintaining the plane of convergence and altering the accommodative stimulus by means of lenses. The preferred method employs ±2.00 lenses in a pair of flippers. The patient views a 20/30 line of letters held at 16 inches. The examiner flips the lenses from plus to minus as the patient reads aloud from the chart, thus demonstrating that clarity has been achieved. The test is performed monocularly to check accommodation, and binocularly, introducing accommodative-convergence demands. Less than 12 cycles in a minute, or a difference of more than two cycles per eye, is considered inadequate.

When flippers are not available, it is possible to measure the response time performance needed to shift fixation from far to near in continuing cycles. This testing condition has the advantage of placing the patient in a more normal environment. Accomodative infacility patients usually do not show plus acceptance on fused cross cylinder or MEM. A pattern of unsteady centric fixation is often noted on visuoscopy.

# CLINICAL SIGNIFICANCE

## Accommodative Infacility

*Accommodative infacility* frequently is found in young patients who complain of not being able to see the blackboard after near point activities or vice versa. Frequently, these patients have a history of academic underachievement. Older prepresbyopes also may report blur or decreased distance acuity as a result of accommodative infacility. In addition, they may report a prolonged time span prior to clearing near targets. An example is the patient who is experiencing difficulty in reading the speedometer while driving down the highway. Asthenopia at near is common, along with frequent eye rubbing and blinking. Micropsia may occasionally be reported. Patients who present a neurotic profile may also show difficulties with accommodative facility.

Amblyopes, particularly those with eccentric fixation, manifest accommodative infacility, since accommodative control is exercised by the fovea, an area whose function is depressed in amblyopes.

Some patients experience more difficulty in changing fixation from far to near (or plus to minus) lenses. These patients may be demonstrating early signs of accommodative paresis; hence the importance of measuring amplitude and asking about recent illness, symptoms of increased intracranial pressure, and midbrain lesions. A more common presentation is blur going from near to far (minus to plus lens), which often is caused by a mild spasm.

## Spasm

Chief complaints of spasm usually are asthenopia, especially with frontal brow ache, and decreased vision at distance, and perhaps at near point, following sustained close work. Discomfort may be noted on rotation of the globes.

Photophobia, an inability to concentrate, macropsia, and diplopia are occasionally encountered. In cases of excessive spasm in patients with high AC/A ratios, an accommodative esotropia may develop. This sequel is of special concern for parents who notice a child's eye turning in occasionally at near point. This will usually not resolve on its own, but often progresses to a constant squint at the far point as well as at near. An esotropia owing to spasm of the near reflex may present unilaterally, thus mimicking a sixth nerve palsy, or bilaterally, mimicking a crossed fixation type of esotropia. In these cases, attempted lateral gaze results in a further miosis in the ipsilateral pupil. Care must be taken, however, to inquire about recent illnesses such as meningitis, encephalitis, labyrinthine irritation, myasthenia gravis, or trauma, all of which may have similar presentations.

## Deficiency

When a decrease in accommodation is accompanied by a unilateral, dilated pupil in the eye in question, a differential diagnosis between Adie's tonic pupil and a third nerve problem must be undertaken. The patient with Adie's pupil is likely to be a healthy young woman with a complaint of tonic accommodation rather than enlarged pupil. Deep tendon reflexes may also be reduced. A near response may be elicited by having the patient look at her own thumb for 15 to 20 seconds. The third nerve pupil will show no response to light, even under a slip lamp, nor to accommodation. A ptosis and exotropia of the affected eye are also usually present in third nerve disease. Aneurysm of the posterior communicating artery should be considered if any aberrant regeneration, noncomitancy, or orbital bruit is noted (see Chapter 18).

Clearly, the concern in accommodative-deficient patients is the determination of cause. Cases with suspected systemic involvement should be referred for diagnostic consultation.

# References

Beiber JC. Why nearpoint retinoscopy with children? Optom Wkly 1974;65:54–57;78–82.

Duke-Elder S. Neuro-ophthalmology. V. XII In: Duke-Elder S. System of ophthalmology. St. Louis: C.V. Mosby, 1971.

Hoffman LG, Rouse MW. Referral recommendations for binocular functions and/or developmental perceptual difficulties. J Am Optom Assoc 1980; 45(2):119–125.

Mohindra I. A noncycloplegic refraction technique for infants and young children. J Am Optom Assoc 1977;48 (4):518–523.

Morgan MW. The clinical aspects of accommodation and convergence. Am J Optom Arch Am Acad Optom 1944;21 (8):301–313.

Rouse MW, London R, Allen D. An evaluation of the monocular estimate method (MEM) of dynamic retinoscopy. Am J Optom Physiol Opt 1982;59:234–239.

Walsh FB, Hoyt WF. Clinical neuro-ophthalmology. Baltimore: Williams & Wilkins, 1969;3rd ed.,1:544–551.

# Richard London
# VERGENCE 14

*Vergence dysfunctions are usually classified as excessive or insufficient at distance or near. This leads to four common classifications: convergence excess, convergence insufficiency, divergence excess, and divergence insufficiency. To these must be added basic exo and eso conditions.*

*Convergence insufficiency is the condition in which the exo deviation, either phoria or tropia, is greater for near vision than for distance vision. No commonly accepted cutoff criteria for the difference between distance and near deviation are available. A reasonable starting point is 10 prism diopters of difference between the two measures to be considered other than a basic deviation.*

*Divergence excess is the condition in which the exo deviation, either phoria or tropia, is greater at distance than at near. For practical purposes a minimum difference of 10 prism diopters between the two measurements should be obtained to be considered other than a basic exo deviation.*

*Basic exo is the condition in which an exo deviation, either phoria or tropia, is approximately equal in magnitude at distance and near. For practical purposes, less than 10 prism diopters of difference between the two measures is considered a basic deviation.*

*Convergence excess is the condition in which an eso deviation, either phoria or tropia, is greater at near than at distance. For practical purposes, a 10-prism diopter difference between the two measures is required for this classification.*

*Divergence insufficiency is the condition in which an eso deviation, either phoria or tropia, is greater at distance than at near. For practical purposes, a difference of 10 prism diopters between the measures is necessary for this classification.*

*Basic eso is the condition in which an eso deviation, either phoria or tropia, is approximately equal in magnitude. For practical purposes, less than 10 prism diopters of difference between the two measures is considered a basic eso deviation.*

# BACKGROUND

Four components have been identified in convergence reflex movements: tonic, accommodative, fusional, and proximal. *Tonic convergence* is the adductive movement of each eye from the anatomic to the physiologic position of rest. Since the anatomic position of rest is outward, an exo patient manifests low tonicity, while an eso patient manifests high tonicity. This aspect of convergence is responsible for the disassociated heterophoria and will be discussed in the chapter on fixation disparity and heterophoria.

*Accommodative convergence* is the alteration in the vergence posture of the eyes directly attributable to a change in accommodative response. Recording of this relationship is in terms of an accommodative-convergence/accommodation or AC/A ratio. This relationship is considered to be generally constant for an individual. Variation of the ratio is most common on the gradient test and usually is attributable to a difference in the stimulus lens used for testing. Owing to the visual systems' ability to lag accommodation, the accommodative response may not correspond directly to the 1.00-diopter plus lens frequently used in the gradient test. Since the normal lag of accommodation is +0.75 diopter, the system may absorb almost the entire stimulus lens without altering accommodative response. It is therefore recommended that a −1.00-diopter lens be used in the gradient test.

The other method of clinical determination of AC/A is the calculation method,* which compares dissociated phorias at distance and near. The low correlation between these two methods is due to the effect of proximal vergence on the near phoria.

Unlike fusional vergence, accommo-dative convergence is usually not considered effective in the elimination of anomalous retinal correspondence (ARC). Lenses may be used to stimulate accommodative-convergence, however, and reduce the demand on fusional vergence to the point that the system is able to overcome the demand.

*Convergence accommodation* is the amount of accommodative response induced by innervation to the vergence system. Its existence has been accepted for decades, along with certain characteristics such as the decline of the convergence accommodation/convergence (CA/C) ratio with age; however, no routine clinical probes of the CA/C ratio had been developed to allow for the ready incorporation of convergence accommodation data in case analysis. Carroll (1982) and Schor and Narayan (1982) have independently reported clinical methods for determining the CA/C ratio. Their findings suggest that when the slopes of the AC/A and CA/C ratios are similar (e.g., 8/1 and 1/8, respectively), fusional vergence demands arrived at from measures of the dissociated phoria and AC/A ratio are underestimated.

The reasoning behind this is that when a subject accommodates for target of regard, the vergence system changes with respect to the AC/A ratio. If this adjustment does not allow the patient to bifixate, fusional vergence must compensate. Changing the fusional vergence affects accommodation through the CA/C ratio, however, potentially resulting in a blurred image (closed feedback loop) and necessitating further focusing adjustments. This cycle continues until a point of equilibrium is found. Schor and Narayan (1982) suggest that the mean AC/A value commonly given as 3.6/1 may aid in pro-

---

* AC/A = $PD + M (H_n - H_f)$, where $PD$ = interpupillary distance in cm., $M$ = near test distance in meters, $H_n$ = objective angle at near, and $H_f$ = objective angle at far. Eso has positive (+) value; exo has negative (−) value.

viding stability between accommodative and convergence interactions.

High CA/C ratios may account for some occult causes of asthenopia under binocular viewing conditions, such as accommodative insufficiency in young, healthy patients.

*Fusional vergence* (or disparity vergence) is the movement of the eyes from the physiologic position of rest to the ortho demand position. It is a motor effort of the eyes initiated by a desire to establish sensory fusion. Volition plays a role in the institution of this response in respect to the desire to fuse disparate images. Most commonly, the amplitude of fusional vergence is measured in the horizontal plane by requiring the patient to maintain single, clear, binocular vision while prisms of increasing power are added in the base-in and base-out directions until first blur or break of the target. Measures may also be obtained in the vertical plane.

Strabismic patients who demonstrate anomalous retinal correspondence may change to normal correspondence if they are able to align their visual axes. This covariation of the angle of anomaly appears to be a result of fusional vergence.

Convergence elicited by the awareness of the nearness of an object is termed *proximal convergence.* Proximal factors may affect measurements any time contrived space instruments, such as the phoropter or stereoscopes, are employed. It must, therefore, be remembered that any simulated (reduced) space instruments that attempt to compensate for distance by means of lenses are likely to produce less reliable results than corresponding free space measures. Some patients are extremely sensitive to looking through any instrument apertures. This may accentuate eso or convergence excess findings, or reduce exo or convergent insufficiency findings. These patients are likely to show very different results on vergence tests administered in and out of the phoropter.

A commonly accepted mean value of proximal convergence is 1.25 p.d./D. How-

ever, Ogle, Martens, and Dyer (1967) found variations among the four basic patterns of oculomotor imbalances. Their means were:

| | |
|---|---|
| Convergence insufficiency | 1.2 p.d./D |
| Convergence excess | 3.6 p.d./D |
| Divergence insufficiency | 1.7 p.d./D |
| Divergence excess | 3.0 p.d./D |

The magnitude of these responses suggests that proximal convergence may be a significant entity in evaluation of binocular functioning.

Unlike the components of reflex convergence, *voluntary convergence* is initiated solely by volition, and therefore is not dependent upon a visual stimulus. It is the only disjunctive movement of the eyes that can be produced at will. During the early stages of orthoptics, voluntary convergence can supplement fusional convergence and aid the patient in developing the "feel" of convergence. The amplitude of voluntary convergence may be as much as twice that of involuntary convergence. Separate higher cortical pathways are used for efferent stimulation of voluntary and involuntary convergence. Thus, cerebral lesions may damage one while the other remains intact. Afferent stimulation of convergence shares a final common pathway. Although the anatomic substrates for vergence movements have never been precisely defined, they appear to originate in the anterior occipital area, descend to the pretectal area and subsequently to the oculomotor nucleus, midbrain, and pons. The efferent pathway involves the paramedian pontine tegmentum, midbrain tegmentum, and pretectum.

The vergence system is intimately related to the accommodative system, and disorders in one frequently affect the other. Patients with insufficient or inefficient accommodation often also present with inadequate convergence.

Hyperkinetic innervation leading to spasms of convergence or habitual excessive convergence is found in about one-sixth of ophthalmic patients. Three major etiologies are found in convergence excess patients. Most common is the group with a high AC/A ratio. The increase in convergence is associated with an overreaction of the whole near triad. The second etiology, primary convergence excess, often is due to spasm. Again, accommodation may be excessive due either to an increase in tonic innervation or to convergence-induced accommodation. Pathologic etiologies must be ruled out. Parinaud's syndrome presents with clonic spasms in primary gaze and tonic spasms in up gaze. Check for pupil anomalies. Retraction nystagmus, most easily seen on downward translation of optokinetic nystagmus targets, is essentially diagnostic of Parinaud's. Any condition leading to CNS irritation may result in a primary convergence spasm. Encephalitis will be accompanied by nystagmus. Questions related to meningitis should be addressed: does the patient have any occipital/nuchal headaches, stiff neck or Konig's sign? Trauma and labyrinthine fistulas leading to increased labyrinthine pressure are possible causes. Oculogyric crises in myasthenia gravis may present as convergent spasm. Hysteria or neuroses can cause a generalized hyperexcitable nervous system and excessive convergence. Local reflex irritation from dental problems or sinus inflammation can result in over- or underconvergence. Alcohol can lead to esophoria, and with sufficient ingestion "seeing double" is not an uncommon occurrence. Systemic syphilis and Wernicke's encephalopathy should also be considered in the differential diagnosis. Secondary convergence excess, the third major etiology, may occur as a sequel to compensation for a long-standing divergence excess.

Development of an eso deviation at distance in a previously orthophoric patient, or increase in the magnitude of deviation in an esophoric patient, is always a source of great concern. Testing and questions should be directed at signs of increased intracranial pressure.

# HISTORY

Convergence insufficiency is a very common visual condition in young adults who have near-point demands at school or office. The primary concerns usually result from symptoms rather than poor cosmesis. This is due to convergence insufficiency deviations being typically latent, present only in near tasks with few people viewing the eyes, and because the patient with a manifest turn learns to close or cover one eye in an effort to eliminate the binocular dysfunction. Occlusion of the eye masks the anomaly and reduces the symptoms. Reports of intermittent diplopia at near may be elicited by asking the patient, "Do the words appear to run together or move around when you are reading?" The patient may have compensated for diplopia by occlusion by turning the head to use the nose as an occluder or by adjusting the posture when reading. When writing, letters may be repeated within words. Even more noticeable is difficulty in aligning numbers within columns, making arithmetic burdensome. Other vague symptoms of asthenopia may be noted at distance as well as near. Vision may be blurred at either viewing distance. Near work cannot be sustained for long periods of time. Interestingly, patients with marked convergence insufficiencies may be completely free of symptoms. Questions should then be directed as to how much reading or near work is actually attempted. Patients may eliminate symptoms by avoidance of near work.

Migrainous patients often manifest a convergence insufficiency. Some reports have indicated that vision therapy along with appropriate refractive correction may lessen the frequency and severity of the headaches. It is suggested that these patients be forewarned that in initial stages of therapy a headache may be stimulated.

Patients taking drugs that facilitate accommodation may also show a convergence insufficiency. Hysterical or psychogenic causes may be the source of convergence problems. Anxiety neurosis or maladjustments to daily life may be sufficient to aggravate the condition. Differential diagnosis of serious organic causes must include encephalitis, endocrine disorders, intranasal disease, diphtheria, and occlusive vascular disease. Functional cases are more likely to have both eyes equally affected and, in addition, have accommodative defects. Further consideration must be give to differentiate medial rectus weakness as presented in myasthenia gravis or multiple sclerosis. Inquire concerning other signs of myasthenia such as diplopia, ptosis, or general fatigue—all worse at the end of the day. Cogan (1956) has classified anterior internuclear ophthalmoplegia as a condition in which a lesion of the medial longitudinal fasciculus near the area of the third nerve nucleus results in a reduction in convergence, along with defective adduction and an enhanced end-point nystagmus of the abducting eye. Although this definition is not universally accepted, it is agreed that a bilateral internuclear ophthalmoplegia in a young, healthy patient is pathognomonic of multiple sclerosis, and this condition is often accompanied by a convergence insufficiency. We have seen multiple sclerosis present as an apparently simple case of convergence insufficiency in a young woman who did not respond as expected to vision therapy. Questions should be directed at Uhthoffs' sign, Lhermitte's sign, paresthesia in the extremities at the end of physical activity, previous transient visual decrease (lasting days to a week) in one eye that resolved on its own, and other signs of retrobulbar neuritis, such as pain on movement of the eyes, that raise the suspicion of multiple sclerosis.

Complaints of divergence excess intermittent tropia usually are cosmetic. Generally, it is only when the deviation extends to near that asthenopic symptoms develop. In contrast, the phoric patient may have blurred vision at distance as a result of using accommodation to assist convergence, a pulling sensation around the eyes, and intermittent diplopia as well as asthenopia. Both phoric and tropic types of divergent excess patients are likely to close one eye when out in the sun; interestingly, it may not be the eye receiving the most glare. It is possible that the bright light makes suppression difficult, and so a stronger, mechanical occlusion of the eyes is brought about. An interesting review of possible divergence excess etiologies is covered by Cooper (1977). The deviation may manifest at any time but is usually noted before age 2, and frequently exacerbated around age 6. Following this period, the deviation may become latent and reappear at college age. Typically, the patient is unaware that the eye is turned out, but upon questioning the patient may reply that the eye "feels" different when it is out than when straight. Often the patient will need to blink in order to reestablish fusion. Deviation of the eye is most likely to occur when the patient is daydreaming, inattentive, fatigued, ill, or taking medications for illness. If a task demands stereopsis, the eyes usually straighten with facility. This dual ability may actually represent a functional advantage for the intermittent exotrope, since panoramic view may be greater when deviated, and normal fusional vergence ranges can be applied when the task demands. Any or all of the symptoms listed for the other exo deviations may be experienced by the basic exo patient: diplopia, asthenopia, frontal headaches, blurred vision, and a pulling sensation around the eyes. In fact, an apparent divergence excess may well be a basic exo case, which has learned to lock in fusional vergence at near.

Convergence excess patients suffer eye strain and frontal or occipital headaches following near work. Frequently enough discomfort is experienced to force curtailment of near activities. Intermittent blur and diplopia are common. All these symptoms tend to be worse at the end of the day or when ill or fatigued. Work may be held exceptionally close, presumably to overburden the system and induce suppression, which will eliminate symptoms.

Intermittent horizontal diplopia at distance is a frequent complaint of patients with divergence insufficiency. Nighttime driving is often the time of occurrence, making this symptom dangerous as well as annoying. Intermittent blurring at distance as well as asthenopia and headache may also be experienced.

Basic eso patients may experience any of the symptoms of the other eso deviations.

# EXAMINATION

Regardless of the etiology of convergence insufficiency, certain visual analysis findings indicate vergence difficulties. Reduction in the near point of convergence has been considered the hallmark of convergence insufficiency. Some authors have labeled a near point of greater than 9.5 cm from the cornea as absolute insufficiency. Practically, a near point break of 5 cm and recovery of 8 cm is considered the acceptable limits in asymptomatic patients. It is strongly recommended that the near point target be nonaccommodative in order to separate fusional vergence from the assistance of accommodative-convergence. Penlights have the advantages of being nonaccommodative as well as permitting the examiner to observe the Hirschberg reflex during testing. Furthermore, the penlight target makes it very easy for even a young child to note subjective diplopia. Measures of the near point of convergence may be repeated several times to check for fatigue effects. Another way to enhance the diagnostic potential of this test is to compare the near point obtained with a white light with one taken with a red glass placed over one of the patient's eyes. This lens causes a sensory fusional insult and demonstrates the ability of the visual system to overcome stress. A difference of more than 3 cm between the two near point measurements is prognostic of a potentially symptomatic patient. During visual training, a progressive reduction in the interval between the two findings is expected.

Many of the following diagnostic tests have free-space and in-instrument (or contrived space) counterparts. While the in-instrument measures provide ease of measurement, they suffer from the effects of proximal convergence. Free-space tests are more akin to the actual performance of the system in daily activities. Methods of phoria measurement are numerous. Cover testing is the most common free-space method, while the Maddox rod or von Graefe tests in the phoropter are frequently used instrument procedures. Expected findings in convergence insufficiency patients are orthophoria to slight exophoria at distance, and a marked exophoria (at least 10 prism diopters greater) at near. The calculated AC/A ratio is therefore low. In-instrument smooth vergence base-out ranges of less than 14/18/7 are considered at risk. Sheard's criterion that the opposing vergence blur should be twice the phoria has been found to be a useful discriminator of symptomatic exo patients. Many practitioners consider the recovery finding, the attempt of the visual system to reestablish fusion once it has been interrupted, to be most indicative of a comfortable zone of vision.

Free-space measures of vergence ranges typically concentrate on vergence facility, which essentially repeated fusional recovery. Expecteds for jump vergence facility of 12 prism diopters base-out, 6 prism diopters base-in at distance, and 15 prism diopters base-out, 12 base-in at near have been found useful. Base-in prism is abruptly inserted before one eye of the patient as fixation is maintained on a 20/30 vertical line of letters. Both singleness and clarity of letters must be obtained, then the prism is removed and the patient allowed to return to the ortho demand position. This procedure must be successfully repeated four times (cycles) in 30 seconds to pass. The base-out vergence is then measured.

For young children, the use of the random dot E as the fixation target eliminates some of the unreliability of reports of clarity. In this modification, the child must distinguish the random dot E from the dummy target following insertion of the prism, thus indicating bifoveal fusion. Another test of vergence facility uses prisms placed in a set of flippers exactly as used in the accommodative facility testing. No return is allowed to the ortho demand posture during testing. Four prism diopters base-in and 8 base-out at distance, 8 prism diopters base-in and 8 base-out at near must be fused 8 to 10 cycles per minute. A 20/30 line of print is the viewed target.

Suppression is often found at near in convergence insufficiency cases. In severe cases, this may be seen during phoropter base-out vergence testing when only one target, which appears to move toward the suppressed eye, is seen. For example, if the left eye is suppressed only the right eye will see the target. In the base-out smooth vergence test, the right eye will view the adducting target as moving to the left, that is, toward the suppressed eye. Diplopia may not be noticed during nearpoint of convergence or abrupt vergence testing, indicating suppression. A dramatic demonstration of suppression is the Pola-Mirror test. Wearing a pair of polaroid glasses, the patient views himself in a mirror at 50 cm (therefore optically at 1 meter) and reports whether both eyes are seen simultaneously. Suppression is indicated if one eye is blacked out. The mirror may be moved closer to the patient to check suppression during convergence. With

children, a variation of this test, the vis-à-vis test, controls for over-dependence on subjective reports. In this test, the examiner and patient both wear polaroids and sit facing each other. The examiner closes one eye and asks the child to point at which eye is closed. Failure to do so indicates an inability to see that eye and therefore suppression. Bar readers are also effective demonstrators of suppression. Stereoacuity at near may be reduced as a result of the tendency to suppress.

Fixation disparity measures should be obtained. Any manifest deviation may contribute to fusional convergence problems. Presbyopes frequently show moderate exophoria at near owing to their add, yet despite inadequate compensating vergence they are asymptomatic. The probable reason is that these presbyopes show a flatter fixation disparity curve than the nonpresbyope, and this finding is more indicative of actual functioning in near work than the phoria.

Owing to the frequent occurrence of accommodative problems concurrent with convergence insufficiency, accommodative amplitudes and facility testing should not be neglected. MEM retinoscopy may reveal an against motion, possibly indicating that accommodative-convergence is being used to assist fusional vergences. An alternative explanation for this finding is that it results from convergence-induced accommodation.

Two methods may be recommended for the clinical determination of the CA/C ratio. Following a fused cross-cylinder measurement the test may be repeated with either 6 or 12 prism diopters base-in prism split before the eyes. The prism power used becomes the denominator of the ratio and the difference between the two net findings becomes the numerator. For example, if 6 prism diopters base-in is used, and the fused cross-cylinder finding changes from +0.50D with no prism to +1.00D with prism in place, the stimulus CA/C ratio would be 0.5/6. Similarly, MEM retinoscopy may be performed with and without prism in place to arrive at the CA/C ratio in the same manner. This latter method is preferable when objective measures are desirable.

When history is suggestive of multiple sclerosis, check color vision, pupillary responses, and visual fields. Optokinetic nystagmus testing with the drum or flag is indispensable in eliciting subtle internuclear ophthalmophagia. Under binocular conditions the optokinetic target is moved first to the right and then to the left. Observation of a relative lag of the adducting eye (implicating the medial rectus) during the saccadic response suggests an internuclear ophthalmoplegia. If this response is bilateral, the diagnosis of multiple sclerosis is highly suspect.

There appears to be a significant difference in the signs as well as the symptoms between patients with exophoria and intermittent exotropic divergence excess. While the phoria patient is likely to have reduced positive fusional amplitudes at distance, reduced distance stereoacuity, and blurred distance vision, the intermittent exotrope usually is no different from the orthophoric patient in these measures. Both groups also tend to have normal near points of convergence. Amblyopia is not present, presumably because the patients are usually binocular at near and only intermittently diverged at distance.

Phoric patients tend to have smooth base-out ranges at distance of less than 7/15/8. The distance jump vergence criterion of 12 prism diopters base-out, 6 prism diopters base-in, 4 cycles in 30 seconds usually is not passed. Flipper prisms expecteds using 4 base-in, 8 base-out are 8 to 10 cycles per minute. In both abrupt vergence tests, the patient fixates a 20/30 line of print. Extreme difficulty is noted on attempts at cheiroscopic tracings. Suppression may be noted at distance on the American Optical (AO) vectographic chart. The AC/A ratio is usually normal.

Intermittent exotropes of the divergence excess type manifest a very different cluster of signs. On cover testing, these patients show an average deviation of 30 prism diopters at distance and 10 prism diopters at near. If the patient is instructed to fixate a target beyond 20 feet, the distance angle increases. A significant number of these patients may simply simulate divergence excess. If patched for 30 to 45 minutes, the near deviation may increase markedly, changing the diagnosis to basic exotropia. Excess convergence innervation, accommodative-convergence, or a greater near stimulus to fusion owing to larger retinal images or brighter targets, are likely causes for masking the near deviation. The significance of differentially diagnosing true from simulated divergence excess is important only if surgical intervention is considered. Initially, the AC/A may be quite variable, but following training it usually stabilizes as normal or slightly high.

Secondary vertical deviations, manifest only along with the tropia, are found in about one-half of these patients. These vertical deviations have little effect on therapy since they are eliminated when a vergence movement places the eyes into the primary position. It is very difficult, however, to differentiate primary from secondary vertical deviations since both are measured during fusion-free posture of the eyes. Primary vertical deviation may severely impede attempts at fusion and usually necessitates prismatic corrections. Flom (1963) recommends the following procedure for identifying vertical components in patients who cannot voluntarily converge their eyes into alignment. Minus lenses are held over the manifest correction and a cover test is performed. The lens power is increased until orthophoria is achieved. Since the stimulated accommodative-convergence affects only the horizontal vergence, any residual vertical deviation in primary gaze represents a primary deviation and should be corrected with compensating prism prior to beginning orthoptics. If the patient can temporally align his eyes by fusional or voluntary vergence, an associated phoria may be measured. If the associated phoria is present vertically, it is a primary deviation and should be corrected.

When normal fusion is interrupted, a pattern of either deep suppression or harmonious anomalous retinal correspondence is evidenced in divergence excess patients. Normal retinal correspondence is present when the eyes are straight. Myopia, especially anisomyopia, and anisoastigmia have a very high incidence among divergence excess patients. Meticulous attention should be given to arriving at proper refractive correction prior to therapy. Binocular refraction is strongly recommended, either Turville infinity balance or AO vectograph, as the cylinder axis may change 6 to 8 degrees as the eyes adduct from the deviated to primary position.

Reduced near point of convergence, reduced positive fusional amplitudes, decreased stereoacuity, suppression, and any of the other findings of the other exo deviations may be shared by the basic exo case.

Patients with convergence excess show reduced base-in vergences, usually less than 11/19/10 at near. Percival's criterion, modified to use the break-point rather than blur-point, has been reported to be a useful discriminator of symptomatic eso patients. Jump (abrupt) vergence criteria of 15 prism diopter base-out, 4 cycles in 30 seconds usually is not met. Prism flipper screening criterion with 8 prism diopter base-out, 8 base-in is 8 to 10 cycles per minute. Jump vergence tests are more similar to dynamic situations in daily experience than smooth vergence tests and should be included in the visual analysis. Comparison of a near point of convergence measured with a penlight target, and a near point of convergence with the same target and a red glass held over one of the patient's eyes should be within 3 cm. Originally developed to test convergence insufficiency patients, this method has also been shown to be effective in predicting symptomatic eso patients.

Stereopsis is often reduced in convergence excess patients. Testing with ±2.00-diopter flippers shows a failure to clear −2.00 diopters presented binocularly. This is due to inadequate base-in range combined with a high AC/A. Plus acceptance is usually found on dynamic retinoscopy, the fused cross cylinder test, and NRA/PRA comparison.

When a previously orthophoric patient develops an esophoria at distance, or there is an increase in magnitude in an esophoric patient, increased intracranial pressure must be ruled out. Cover testing in primary, left, and right fields of gaze measures concomitancy. Alternatively red glass or Maddox rod diplopia fields or a Hess-Lancaster test may be performed. Abduction will be limited in one field if a sixth nerve palsy is present. Spontaneous venous pulsation must be meticulously sought since its presence in either eye would contraindicate any spinal fluid pressure greater than 200 mm of water. Ophthalmoscopy must rule out any signs of papilledema. Careful history concerning nausea, vertigo, or headaches upon awakening, exacerbated by bending over, should be specifically addressed. Visual fields are also useful for differential diagnosis. Any supranuclear lesion near the posterior media longitudinal fasciculus or fourth verticle can give rise to eso at distance. Multiple sclerosis also may present with an eso at distance.

# CLINICAL SIGNIFICANCE

It should be recognized that patients likely to develop symptoms owing to poor fusional vergence ranges are frequently those whose ranges are just short of adequate. Patients with very poor ranges adapt by developing a squint (strabismus), suppression, occlude one eye, or avoid work at the affected distance. Slightly inadequate ranges are not perceived as an insurmountable drawback to the patient, and great effort is placed on maintenance of single binocular vision—often resulting in symptoms of discomfort.

Refractive errors may be associated with convergence insufficiency. Uncorrected myopia is the most common. Hyperopes and presbyopes following their initial correction with subsequent reduction of accommodative assistance to convergence may have insufficient positive fusional vergence. The connection between symptomatic accommodative and vergence dysfunctions is so common that even in undeniable cases of convergence insufficiency the accommodative system should be carefully checked for problems and concurrently treated if judged abnormal.

Uncorrected hyperopes and myopes who have recently obtained a first prescription frequently demonstrate near esophoria owing to excessive accommodation. Pre-presbyopes who attempt to use diminishing accommodation also manifest convergence excess, although less frequently. If accommodation is too stressful, the patient may underaccommodate resulting in a secondary convergence insufficiency. A plus lens correction will permit more accurate focussing and, as a result, reduce the convergence insufficiency. Young children, usually in the third or fourth grade, who are beginning near work in earnest may experience near symptoms, as may college students and clinical workers who have just changed to more demanding near point jobs. Any interference of vision, such as media opacities or poor illumination, may induce excessive accommodation in an effort to clear the material and lead to secondary vergence problems.

# References

Capobianco NM. The subjective measurement of the near point of convergence and its significance in the diagnosis of convergence insufficiency. Am Orthoptic J 1952;2:40–46.

Cogan DG. Neurology of the ocular muscles. Springfield, Ill: Charles C Thomas, 1956;131.

Cooper J. Intermittent exotropia of the divergence excess type. J Am Optom Assoc 1977;48:1261–1273.

Duke-Elder S. Ocular motility and strabismus. V. VI. In: Duke-Elder S. System of Opthalmology. St. Louis: C.V. Mosby, 1973.

Flom BC. Treatment of binocular vision. In: Hirsch MJ, Wick RE, eds. Vision of children. Philadelphia: Chilton, 1963;6:173–196.

Morgan MW. The clinical aspects of accommodation and convergence. Am J Optom Arch Am Acad Optom 1944; 21:301–313.

Ogle KN, Martens TG, Dyer JA. Oculomotor imbalances in binocular vision and fixation disparity. Philadelphia; Lea and Febiger, 1967.

Schor CM, Ciuffreda KG, eds. Vergence eye movements: basic and clinical aspects. Woburn; Butterworths, 1983.

Schor CM, Narayan V. Graphical analysis of prism adaptation, convergence accommodation, and accommodative convergence. Am J Optom Physiol Opt 1982;59:774–784.

Sheedy JE, Saladin JJ. Association of symptoms with measures of oculomotor deficiencies. Am J Optom Physiol Opt 1978;55:670–676.

Sheedy JE, Saladin JJ. Exophoria of near in presbyopia. Am J Optom Physiol Opt 1975;52:474–481.

Richard London

# FIXATION DISPARITY AND HETEROPHORIA 15

*Fixation disparity is a manifest deviation (under associated viewing conditions) of the eyes in which the disparate image of the fixation point falls within Panum's area, allowing central sensory fusion. Synonymous terms are retinal slip and fusion disparity.*

*Heterophoria is a condition in which bifixation is maintained through the aid of fusional reflexes. Only when there is interference with the stimulus to fusion (dissociated viewing conditions) does an eye deviate. It is, therefore, a latent misalignment of the eyes. Synonymous terms are phoria and latent squint.*

## BACKGROUND

Oculomotor deviations may result in a misalignment of the primary line of sight of the eyes, which may be manifest or latent. When corrective reflexes succeed in maintaining binocular fusion the deviation is termed *heterophoria*. If binocular alignment cannot be established a strabismus is present (Chapter 16). Inconsistent success in maintenance of binocularity is termed *intermittent strabismus*.

Sensorimotor misalignment under associated viewing conditions with maintenance of central fusion results in fixation disparity. This phenomenon demonstrates that binocularly seen directional values may differ from those seen monocularly. The change from binocular to monocular viewing conditions stimulates a change in duction equal to the fixation disparity. Errors of convergence leading to fixation disparity are quite small, usually not exceeding 10 minutes of arc, and only very rarely up to 25 minutes (approximately 0.25 to 0.75 prism diopters on the retina).

Schor (1980) suggests that two vergence components are represented on the fixation disparity curve (Figure 15.1). The flatter, central portion of the curve represents a slow neural integrator, while the steeper slopes at the extremes of the curve show the characteristics of a fast neural integrator. Fixation disparity itself may frequently be a normal characteristic of the vergence system, a steady state error serving as a reminder to the fast component controller to compensate for decay of vergence. This is possible because the error signal needed to activate vergence is less

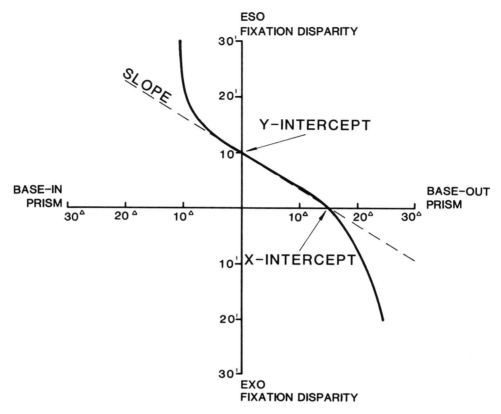

**FIGURE 15.1.**
Fixation disparity curve.

than 28 seconds of arc, far less than the size of Panum's fusional area at the fovea, which is at least 10 minutes of arc.

In heterophoria the eyes are binocularly maintained on the fixation point through the use of fusional reflexes. It is only when these reflexes are interrupted by dissociation that the ocular deviation becomes manifest. Fundamentally, the difference between heterophoria and strabismus is quantitative, depending on the patient's ability to compensate.

Etiologically, phorias may have an anatomic basis, such as the placement of the muscle insertions, or a neural basis, such as excessive innervation or spasm or a paresis.

A majority of patients who are heterophoric also show a fixation disparity, usually in the same direction as the phoria, although occasionally they may be in opposite directions. Fixation disparity magnitude, however, cannot be determined by the magnitude of the heterophoria. Prism needed to neutralize the fixation disparity may be more than the phoria in esodeviations, while it is almost always less than the phoria in exodeviations.

# HISTORY

While some authors have stated that the phoria itself may cause symptoms, it is more likely that the neuromuscular stress placed upon these reflexes results in discomfort and that the integrity of fusional reflexes must be fully investigated. Nonetheless, certain symptomatic complaints are common to phoria patients. Questions should address problems such as frontal or occipital headaches, diplopia, blurring of vision, and words running together when reading. If these complaints are due to near phorias they are usually worse at the end of a workday and better on weekends or vacations. Youngsters with phorias greater at far may have difficulty judging distances in fast ball sports. Adults with the same condition may have difficulty driving, especially when parallel parking.

Most bothersome of all is the vertical phoria. Fusional ranges are much reduced vertically, and patients may adopt a head tilt to compensate. Cyclophorias are associated with hyperphorias, as the patient attempts to use torsional fusion to assist vertical ranges. Ocular pain, headache, vertical diplopia, rapid fatigue, and hyperemia of the lids may be presenting symptoms. Of more concern are reports of vertigo, nausea, tilting of the room, and even vomiting—all frequently associated with labyrinthine disturbances as well as ocular imbalances. Ask if the symptoms resolve upon monocular occlusion. A positive answer would suggest an ocular cause, either phoria/vergence or aniseikonia. This test may be used in all cases of suspected binocular-related problems. Question whether the patient tends to close one eye or occlude an eye with the nose by turning the head during near-point tasks.

Appearance of symptoms depends also on physical and psychological variables. Periods of illness or mental stress may aggravate phoria symptoms.

Esophoria is common in the young, as is hyperopia. It has been reported to be typical in energetic or nervous patients with central overactivity.

Esophores have the disturbing tendency to fall asleep while reading, book open in their lap. Overconvergence is reported to be most marked at the beginning of sentences. Esos are reported to overestimate distances and, therefore, may be prone to bumping cars while parking.

An esophoria at distance greater than 6 prism diopters or one that had not been previously measured may be cause for grave concern. Careful examination must concentrate on differential diagnosis of increased intracranial pressure and thyroid dysfunction. Check for concomitancy and look for signs of disc edema. Special care should be taken to look for a spontaneous venous pulsation, which would rule out intracranial pressure as a cause. Question the patient about recent headaches, especially upon awakening and whether headache is worse when bending over, coughing, or straining at stool. If in doubt, recheck the phoria in a few days since pressure increases usually result in a rapid increase in the phoria.

Exophoria tends to increase with age in frequency and degree, as does myopia. Exophores commonly close one eye in sunlight, frequently not the eye into which the sun is shining. Frontal headaches, words running together, and diplopia are frequent complaints. Accommodation is often used to assist faulty vergence. In these cases, symptoms of accommodative infacility or spasm are common. Exophores are reported to underestimate distances, and therefore may reach early to catch a ball, or swing ahead of a pitch.

Many systemic pathologies may affect the phoria or fixation disparity. Myasthenia gravis may result in a periodic increase in the phoria in any direction. Ask if the symptoms are worse at the end of the day along with an associated general extremity weakness or ptosis. Cogan's lid twitch and checking prolonged up-gaze capability as the patient observes the examiner's finger are good in-office tests for myasthenia. Intravenous tensilon may reduce the phoria as well as the other symptoms.

Multiple sclerosis may present with convergence insufficiency and high exo at near, or an increasingly decompensating eso deviation at distance. Ask about Uhthoff's sign, paresthesias after long walks, retro-orbital pain, unexplained, transient monocular visual decrease. Test monocular color vision, Lhermitte's sign, and use OKN to check for a bilateral internuclear ophthalmoplegia (see Chapter 19).

# EXAMINATION

## Fixation Disparity

Since the magnitude of fixation disparity is too small to be routinely detected on unilateral (associated) cover testing, special equipment must normally be used in its determination. While the amount of fixation disparity may vary at different fixation distances, most symptomatic patients have near-point complaints, so that many clinically available near tests have been developed. All of these tests consist of a binocular fusion stimulus and two additional targets each viewed by one eye. The monocularly viewed targets are most commonly polarized vernier lines to increase the sensitivity for fine alignment. Remember that many variables may affect fixation disparity: lighting, size and placement of the fusion lock, and length of the vernier lines.

Two methods have been developed for clinical use. Most commonly, the polarized vernier lines are in fixed physical alignment, and the patient must report any offset (Figure 15.2). Compensating prism is then inserted before the eye until alignment of the targets is established. The amount of this prism is termed the associated phoria* and is equivalent to the X-intercept on a fixation disparity graph (Fig. 15.1). Fusion locks may be peripheral with a blanked out central area, which encour-ages retinal slippage, or they may be placed centrally to simulate normal viewing conditions.

A recently available instrument, the disparometer (Figure 15.3), allows direct

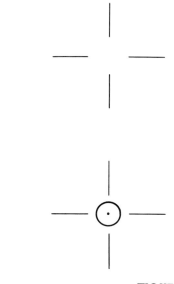

**FIGURE 15.2.**
Measurement of associated phoria. Compensating prism inserted before the eye until alignment. Amount is equivalent to the *x*-intercept on fixation disparity curve. Fusion locks may be peripheral *(top)* or central *(bottom).*

---

\* An interesting combination of mutually exclusive terms since a phoria is the ocular alignment under dissociated conditions.

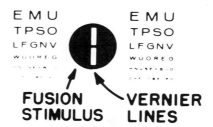

A

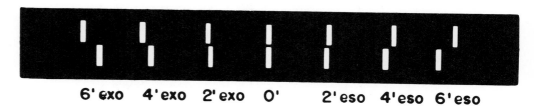

B

6' exo   4' exo   2' exo   0'   2' eso   4' eso   6' eso

FIGURE 15.3.
*A.* Target used for direct measurement of fixation disparity. *B.* Each vernier line is seen by one eye. The lower line is displaced until it is seen aligned with the stationary upper line.

measurement of the fixation disparity type, slope, and *X*- and *Y*-intercepts to be clinically determined in the course of a routine examination. Rather than use prism to neutralize the associated phoria, the disparometer presents the patient with a series of discrete-interval vernier disparities and requires the patient to identify the one that appears aligned. This is the *Y*-intercept, or actual fixation disparity (Figure 15.1). Fusional stress is then induced by the insertion of prism base-in or base-out, and the fixation disparity again measured. A curve can also be generated by the use of plus and minus lenses rather than prism. The point at which the fixation disparity is eliminated by the prism or lens is the *X*-intercept, or associated phoria.

Values of fixation disparity usually increase slowly with small prism vergence demand, and rapidly as the demand increases. At some point the system can no longer compensate and diplopia is experienced, marking the end point of the graph. Generating curves in this manner leads to four characteristic types (Figure 15.4). This classification has clinical significance for potential symptomatology and for therapy sequence, which is covered below. A fifth observed type is a U-shaped curve found in patients who have learned to use fusional vergence but have not obtained fusional accuracy. These patients overshoot the target with base-out stimulus becoming eso relative to the demand.

As prism is added, the amount of fixation disparity changes. The rapidity of this change is referred to as the slope. The most important portion of the slope for our consideration is the area between the *Y*- and *X*-intercept, that is, between the fixation disparity and the associated phoria. Some clinicians use the area 3-prism diopters on either side of the *Y*-intercept as the basis for determining the slope. A slope greater than 45° (or 1 minute/prism diopter) serves as a practical guide for the separation of potentially symptomatic patients (steeper slope) and asymptomatic patients (flatter slope). The midpoint of the flat portion of the curve is the center of symmetry.

A flat slope around the *Y*-intercept (the

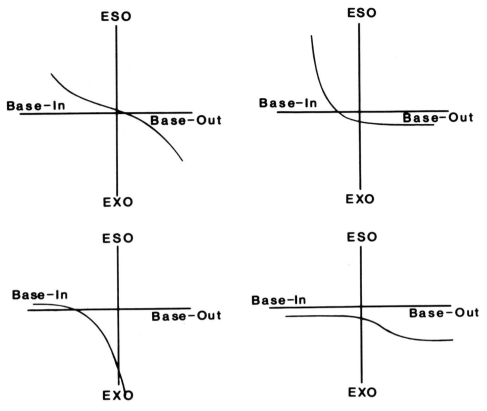

**FIGURE 15.4.**

Four types of fixation disparity curves (Ogle classification): Type I *(upper left)*, Type II *(upper right)*, Type III *(lower left)*, Type IV *(lower right)*.

actual fixation disparity measure) may suggest that the fixation disparity may be functioning as a positive purposeful error, which drives the fusional vergence system. In this instance, the fixation disparity is not likely to produce symptoms. A steep slope between the $Y$-intercept and the $X$-intercept (the associated phoria) may suggest binocular stress. In these cases the visual system appears ready to accept prism to reduce the fixation disparity. No level of disparity is maintained as stress is reduced by prism; that is, the fixation disparity rapidly approaches zero.

Accommodative infacility or inaccuracy may result in a curve that is irregular. A period of accommodative training may result in a smoother curve, allowing clearer interpretation of the actual fixation disparity.

Flom (1969) has suggested that the flick movement seen on unilateral cover testing with a larger magnitude on alternate cover testing may occasionally be a fixation disparity rather than a small angle strabismus (see Chapter 16). This is possible due to a "stretching" of Panum's fusional area. To differentiate between the two conditions, a 4-prism diopter base-out prism is inserted before the preferred eye. In strabismus, a version movement is noted in the nonpreferred eye, but no compensating vergence movement occurs. In the other "flick" cases, the prism may result in no movement in the nonpreferred eye, or, if a version did take place, a vergence returns the eye to the original position, that is, less than a 4-Δ vergence. These flick cases may be demonstrating a large fixation disparity or unharmonious ARC with a small angle of anomaly.

There is some evidence that fixation disparity curves variables may be related to symptoms in small-angle strabismics (monofixators) in much the same way as they are with patients having normal binocular vision.

Stereoacuity is often reduced in cases of fixation disparity when using either linear or random dot targets. This may be the first objective clue to the clinician to check further for fixation disparity. A small central suppression may also be evident. Turville infinity balance test simultaneously measures exo and vertical "associated phoria" along with the balance of accommodation.

# Heterophoria

A plethora of tests have been developed to test for heterophoria. All must dissociate the eyes prior to measurement. Cover testing is not only a quick method, but has the distinct advantage of being an objective measurement, requiring only careful fixation on the part of the patient. Unilateral testing should precede the alternate cover test so the patient's alignment under associated viewing conditions may be viewed prior to dissociation. Targets should present the patient with an exact point of focus. The intersection of horizontal and vertical lines in letters such as L or F make excellent distance targets. Small, accommodatively demanding near targets are critical for accurate measurement. Checks for A or V patterns may be made by tilting the patient's head downward and upward and remeasuring the phoria.

Popular in-instrument tests are the von Graefe and Maddox rod tests. The von Graefe should be done by the flash method to prevent peripheral fusion. Esophoria may be increased and exophoria decreased

with these phoropter measurements, probably owing to proximal convergence. The Maddox rod may be used in free space combined with either a Maddox scale at distance, or modified Thorington card at near. These techniques are especially useful in cases of hyperphoria, which may be of too small a degree to observe on cover testing. Two readings may be obtained, one when the patient first views a target, and later as the patient's fusion is interrupted for a more prolonged period. Also useful at near point is the Maddox wing, which gives an assessment of horizontal, vertical, and cyclo deviations.

Refraction in cases of high phorias should be performed under binocular conditions since cylinder axes may change up to 8 degrees when undergoing binocular fusion. Three binocular techniques are most common: the Turville, AO vectograph, and the Mallet system, all having some advantages.

Anisophoria, essentially a nonconcomitant phoria, is most commonly an A or V pattern, but may vary in any field of gaze. A Maddox rod, cover, or red glass in the nine positions of gaze or Hess-Lancaster test will determine the variance in phoria.

Visual acuity taken binocularly may be poorer than monocular acuity when phoria control is poor. Often this is due to either employment of accommodation to assist vergence or to suppression.

In cases of exophoria controlled by use of accommodative-convergence an accommodative infacility or spasm may be observed. Accommodative facility testing with ± 2.00 flippers is useful. MEM retinoscopy may reveal an against motion.

A near point of convergence taken with a penlight target and repeated with a red glass held over one eye of the patient is useful in determining likelihood of symptoms. The red glass interferes with sensory fusion, which can negatively affect motor fusion in cases with fragile binocularity. A receded near point with the red glass of more than 3 cm may be indicative of fragile binocularity associated with symptoms.

# CLINICAL SIGNIFICANCE

Following the determination of the magnitude and direction of the phoria or fixation disparity, a prescription of prism, lenses, or vision therapy must be determined for symptomatic patients. The clinician must be careful, however, to ascertain whether the patient is asymptomatic simply because of avoidance of stressful tasks such as reading.

Many techniques have been suggested for the prescription of prism in heterophoria. Most popular are Percival's and Sheard's criteria. A recent study has suggested that failure to meet Sheard's criterion may be effective in determining symptomatic exophores, while a failure to meet a break-point Percival's suggests problems for an esophore. This study, however, does not address the problem of reducing symptoms based upon prescription arrived at using these two criteria.

When both horizontal and vertical components are present it is difficult to judge whether one is secondary to the other. Measurement of the imbalance during associated viewing conditions helps identify the primary imbalance.

In cases of double hyperphoria (alternating sursumduction), the fixation disparity again provides an easy method for checking the oculomotor imbalance (see Chapter 16).

Most current authors favor prescriptions based on fixation disparity findings. If the hypothesis that fixation disparity is a purposeful error is correct, then no prescription would be required for asymptomatic patients. This position is supported by the view that fixation disparity represents "play" in the system, a built-in tolerance for error or the point of greatest binocular summation. Some other clinicians do not share this view and suggest that if objective testing uncovers deficiency in binocular alignment, then prescription should follow to restore prime efficiency. If this is not done, they ask, then, why measure these variables in the asymptomatic patient?

Differences between the magnitudes of associated and dissociated phorias may be the result of a slow fusional vergence response, which is activated only under conditions of binocular fusion. Slow fusional vergence appears to be an adaptive mechanism responsible for vergence (prism) adaptation and the flatter portions of the fixation disparity curve. It is possible that slow fusional vergence is the source of binocular comfort in heterophoric patients, and conversely, that asthenopia in heterophores is due to deficient adaptive mechanisms under binocular conditions. Since the variable of slow fusional vergence is operative only under associated viewing conditions, the fixation disparity curve may be a more valid criterion for prescribing than the dissociated phoria.

Of the four relevant variables of the fixation disparity curve described in the examination section, the slope is most related to slow fusional vergence or prism adaptation. A flat slope indicates good oculomotor balance, while one greater than 45° suggests likelihood of symptoms. For patients with steep slopes, prism may be prescribed, which allows them to operate on a flatter portion of the curve. The curve usually flattens before the X-intercept, and, therefore, the prescription is usually less than the associated phoria. Vision therapy appears to develop slow fusional vergence. This results in a flattening of the slope for patients with no flat portion on the curve (certain type I patients); therefore, a period of vision therapy is recommended prior to determination of a need for prescription in these cases. Remember that lenses also may reduce the fixation disparity, and the effectiveness of lenses may be judged by remeasurement of the curve.

Another variable used to determine prescription is the X-intercept, or the amount of prism (or lens) needed to reduce the fixation disparity to zero. This has been the most common clinical determinant (due to instrumentation) of need for prism, yet Sheedy and Saladin (1978) have found the presence of associated phoria to be of little prognostic value with respect to symptoms. This is likely due to the fact that many curves with different slopes can be drawn through the same $X$-intercept (Figure 15.5). Similarly, many curves may be generated through a common $Y$-intercept. Since the majority of asymptomatic patients demonstrate some degree of fixation disparity, it is likely that the reduction of the misalignment to zero is neither necessary nor desirable.

Fixation disparity curves have been divided by Ogle into four types (Figure 15.4). Type I is the most common (approximately 60% of the population) and is best correlated with asymptomatic patients. Type II (25%) cases demonstrate greater fixation disparity errors for divergence than for convergence. A personal observation is that there are two possibly distinct variations of the type II curve: one that maintains a constant eso fixation disparity, and another that crosses the $X$-axis and flattens in the exo range. It seems that many of these "cross-over" Type II cases will reveal as type I if the base-out prism demand is further increased. Type III patients (10%) show a rapid increase in fixation disparity for convergence and a flat slope for divergence. Type IV patients (2 to 5%) have lower amplitudes than type I, and type IV is observed in patients with subnormal binocularity. Symptoms are most likely to occur in the latter three groups. Sheedy and Saladin (1978) have found this classification to be the best discriminator of symptomatic and nonsymptomatic patients.

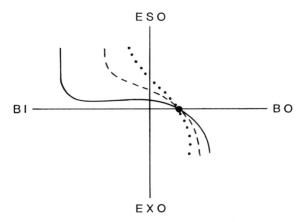

**FIGURE 15.5.**
**Three fixation disparity curves. Note the three different slopes with same x- intercept (associated phoria).**

Fixation disparity, that is, the $Y$-intercept, is measured initially with no prism in place. Ten minutes of arc is a separation point for acceptable retinal slippage; however, smaller eso disparities may produce symptoms.

Paradoxical fixation disparity, that is, a fixation disparity in the direction opposite to the phoria, is found in approximately one-third of patients. Although frequently found in postorthoptics patients, it may also occur spontaneously. Schor (1982) suggests these patients may have learned to overcompensate for their heterophoria with slow fusional vergence. The steady-state error then would serve as a reminder to compensate for the overshoot.

# References

Flom BC. Treatment of binocular vision. In: Hirsch MJ, Wick RE, eds. Vision of children. Philadelphia: Chilton, 1963;6:173–196.

Ogle KN, Martens TG, Dyer JA. Oculomotor imbalance in binocular vision and fixation disparity. Philadelphia: Lea and Febiger, 1967.

Schor CM. Analysis of tonic and accommodative vergence disorders of binocular vision. Am J Optom Physiol Opt 1983;60:1–14.

Schor CM. Fixation disparity: a steady state error of disparity-induced vergence. Am J Optom Physiol Opt 1980;57:618–631.

Schor CM. The relationship between fusional vergence eye-movements and fixation disparity. Vision Res 1979; 19:1359–1367.

Sheedy JE, Saladin JJ. Association of symptoms with measures of oculomotor deficiencies. Am J Optom Physiol Opt 1978;55:670–676.

Sheedy JE, Saladin JJ. Phoria, vergence and fixation disparity in oculomotor problems. Am J Optom Physiol Opt 1977;54:474–478.

Sheedy JE. Fixation disparity analysis of oculomotor imbalance. Am J Optom Physiol Opt 1980;57:632–639.

# Richard London
# STRABISMUS 16

*The situation in which the line of sight of one fovea fails to intercept an object of regard under conditions of attempted binocular fixation is termed* strabismus. *Synonyms are tropia, squint, heterotropia.*

## BACKGROUND

Under normal viewing conditions, innervation to the extraocular muscles permits bifixation of objects of interest. Obstacles to accurate bifixation are largely overcome by fusional reflexes. When these reflexes are successful in allowing central fusion (within the central Panum's fusional area) with a deviation demonstrable only under dissociated conditions, a heterophoria or latent squint exists. If the reflexes are not successful in overcoming the obstacles, a manifest deviation or strabismus is present. In general, there are two fundamental etiologies of strabismus: a failure of the development of the fixation reflexes or disruption of existing reflexes from functional or structural causes. Therefore, reduced unilateral visual acuity in early life, hyper- or hypotonus of the horizontal or vertical extraocular muscles, an excessive near reflex, trauma, paresis, fibrosis, or faulty muscle insertion can all be causes of strabismus. Table 16.1 shows the general descriptors of strabismus by frequency and direction of deviation. Note that the direction of deviation is frequently a combination of the listed terms (e.g., exo-hypertrope).

Unilateral decrease in visual acuity in infancy may be due to anisometropia, sensory deprivation resulting from lid or media obstructions, congenital amblyopia, congenital strabismus, or pathology. Parents may notice that the child uses significant head turning when objects are presented to the poor side, in an effort to visualize the target with the good eye. If the good eye is occluded the child becomes disgruntled, a condition not apparent when the poorer seeing eye is covered. This difference in acuity does not allow central sensory fusion to develop, with the typical sequelae of the poorer eye drifting to a position where the two foveas are misaligned. In young children this is typically a nasal deviation. Ocular injury or traumatic cataract can result in disruption of binocular vision usually leading to esotropia in children under 5 years of age, and to exotropia in older children and adults. This suggests that tonic divergence dominates tonic convergence in the absence of binocular vision in adults and children above preschool age.

Alterations of the innervational pattern to the extraocular muscles results in

151

Table 16.1
Classifications of Strabismus

| Frequency | |
|---|---|
| *Type* | *Incidence (%)* * |
| Constant | 100 |
| Intermittent | 1–99 |
|   Periodic | |
|     direct (near point) | |
|     indirect (far point) | |
|     certain cases of | |
|       nonconcomitancy | |
|   Nonperiodic | Unpredictable |
| Nonstrabismic | 0 |
| Cyclic | Recurrent |
|   Heterophoria (always latent) | |
|   Orthophoria | |

| Direction | |
|---|---|
| *Deviation* | *Rotation of Deviating Eye with Fixating Eye in Primary Position* |
| Horizontal | |
|   Eso (convergent) | Inward |
|   Exo (divergent) | Outward |
| Vertical | |
|   Hyper | Upward |
|   Hypo | Downward |
| Torsional | |
|   Incyclo | Top of eye inward |
|   Excyclo | Top of eye outward |

| Additional Qualifiers | |
|---|---|
| *Type* | *Deviation* |
| Concomitant | Angle equal (within 5 prism diopters) in all directions of gaze with either eye fixating |
| Noncomitant | Angle varies more than 5 prism diopters in one or more positions of gaze or when fixating eye is changed |
| Consecutive | Change in direction of preexisting strabismus, usually following surgery |

**Table 16.1**
*(continued)*

| Duane-White | |
|---|---|
| *Deviation* | *Description* |
| Eso | |
| Convergence excess | At least 10 prism diopters (perhaps 15) greater at near than at distance fixation |
| Divergence insufficiency | At least 10 prism diopters (perhaps 15) greater at distance than at near fixation |
| Basic | Distance and near within 10 prism diopters of each other |
| Exo | |
| Convergence insufficiency | At least 10 prism diopters (perhaps 15) greater at near than at distance fixation |
| Divergence excess | At least 10 prism diopters (perhaps 15) greater at distance than at near fixation |
| Basic | Distance and near within 10 prism diopters of each other |

*Percentage of the time that deviation is manifest.

characteristic strabismus. For a complete review of the neural pathways and disorders see Chapter 19 on oculomotor assessment.

## Esotropia

Owing to its external course in the craninum, the sixth nerve is the most vulnerable to injury and increased intracranial pressure. The first opportunity for trauma to nerve VI occurs with forceps delivery at birth—look for a telltale indentation or scar, usually near the temple. Transient lateral rectus paresis in children may occur following nonspecific illness with resolution within 6 weeks.

Congenital strabismus is manifested between birth and 6 months of age. Most frequently, it is esotropia of large magnitude (over 50 prism diopters). Alternation of the fixating eye, slight refractive error, no amblyopia, dissociated vertical divergence, often latent nystagmus, and an equal angle of deviation at distance and near are commonly associated signs. Hypertonus of the medial rectus may be considered a suspect etiology. A cross fixation pattern, which simulates a bilateral abducens palsy, may develop. Occlusion of one eye for several days should loosen the abduction ability in cross fixators. If the pattern if not too strongly established, the doll's head maneuver or vestibular nystagmus may be adequate for differential diagnosis. Also to be considered are two congenital paralyses of the sixth nerve: Möbius' syndrome and Duane's retraction syndrome.

Möbius' syndrome is a complete bilateral paralysis of nerves VI and VII, plus a lateral gaze paresis. In addition, deafness, chest malformations, and head and feet deformities may be present.

Duane's retraction syndrome patients usually do not show an esotropia in the primary position, in fact, a slight exotropia may be present. A retraction of the globe on attempted adduction (probably owing to a cocontraction of the horizontal recti muscles) and a narrowing of the lid fissure are hallmarks; decreased abduction is also present.

Accommodative esotropia had previously been thought to develop around age 2 years, but recent studies suggest onset may be as early as 4 to 6 months. Thus, in the diagnosis of congenital strabismus, an accommodative component must be ruled out. Two separate etiologies for accommodative esotropia have been described. Refractive accommodative esotropia is found in patients with uncorrected hyperopia and insufficient base-in ranges. Nonrefractive accommodative esotropia is found in patients with a high AC/A ratio or high proximal convergence; that is, the convergent strabismus angle is greater at near than at distance. The abnormal A/AC synkinesis results in increased convergence tonus at near when accommodation is stimulated. Care must be taken to keep comparisons of distance and near deviations in the same position of gaze, otherwise a V-pattern esotropia could be mistaken for an accommodative strabismus. Note that with accommodative esotropia the near angle is always greater than at distance regardless of the position of gaze.

In cases of long standing, uncorrected accommodative esotropia, secondary changes may occur in the muscles precluding easy remediation by means of lenses. Partially accommodative esotropia presents as above; a residual convergent angle of deviation remains following full refractive and bifocal correction. Recheck the refraction taking care to eliminate barriers to fusion such as aniseikonia and astigmatism.

A "spasm of the near reflex" has been discussed by Cogan (1956). The patient shows an esotropia along with miosis. Attempted abduction results in further miosis. This is not a paresis, but a spasm, and usually clears with time. Some clinicians claim that this is more common in patients with an emotional overlay.

Increased intracranial pressure often first presents as an esophoria at distance. If a slightly blurred disk without spontaneous venous pulsation is observed on ophthalmoscopy, a very careful cover test must be done at 20 feet. Use a specific target like the meeting of the two lines in an L or T. The increase in eso at distance is usually quite rapid over a period of days. Although a posterior fossa tumor is often culpable, no true localizing significance is possible (see Chapters 31 and 32).

Sudden onset favors neurological lesions except in cases of trauma where the inferior muscles may be trapped between an orbital fracture. Forced duction testing will differentiate paretic from mechanical causes.

# Exotropia

Exotropia differs from esotropia in respect to the age of onset, effect of sensory adaptation, progression, and, as a result of these, prognosis. Congenital exotropia is considerably rarer than congenital esotropia. In fact, some authors have suggested that an intensive examination to rule out pathology should be performed on any constant exotropes under 6 months of age. Most exodeviations appear to begin as exophorias, which then progress to intermittent exotropia. The deviation may remain intermittent, be present constantly at one distance and not another, or progress to a constant exotropia. Because the deviation is absent or present only occasionally during the early years of many exotropes, binocular vision has a chance to develop to some extent. Even though the angle of deviation tends to increase with age in some exotropes (possibly as a sequel to decreasing tonic convergence), prognosis for the stimulation of single, binocular vision is better than for most nonaccommodative esotropes. The presence of anomalous correspondence is not as ominous to a favorable prognosis in exotropia.

Some children will show a change from esotropia to exotropia or vertical tropias that will vary in an irregular manner over time. Most commonly this is found in patients with cerebral palsy.

Insult to the third cranial nerve produces the most devastating picture of any of the innervators of the extraocular muscles. In the ipsilateral eye the medial and inferior recti, inferior oblique, levator, pupil, and accommodative ability may be affected, along with the contralateral superior rectus. The precise manifestations depend on whether the damage is nuclear, supranuclear, or fascicular. A full review of these various possibilities is covered in Chapter 19.

Particular concern should be shown for any transient third nerve problem that resolves with subtle residual signs. Signs of aberrant regeneration include: lid-gaze dyskinesis, Czarnekis' sign, pseudo-von Graefe's sign, pseudo Argyll-Robertson pupil, and adduction on attempted vertical gaze. They are ominous because the etiology of aberrant regeneration is frequently aneurysm, which, if left untreated, could rupture. Aberrant regeneration is not due to diabetes, so even in a diabetic who demonstrates a transient third nerve palsy with residual signs of aberrant regeneration, aneurysm must be strongly suspected.

An acquired exo deviation, poor adduction, irregular movements on conjugate gaze, and increased end-point nystagmus in a young, healthy adult warrants concern of an internuclear ophthalmoplegia. Rule out history that may suggest multiple sclerosis: paresthesias, transient unilateral decrease in color vision or acuity, Uhthoff's syndrome, and Lhermitte's sign.

# Vertical

Vertical misalignments may be a primary deviation or secondary to the horizontal component. Differential diagnosis is imperative to proper therapy. Establishment of a centration point (that place in real space where the visual axes cross) by means of vergence or lens additions elim-inates the horizontal component and allows for the measurement of the residual, primary vertical deviation. With small-angle esotropes, a centration point may be obtainable without need for additional lenses. If plus lenses are required, a useful starting point is found by the formula listed in the examination section. Prepresbyopic exotropes with an adequate AC/A can be brought to an ortho position by use of minus lenses. Interestingly, the primary vertical deviation may actually be in the opposite direction from that found when the horizontal component is manifest. Prismatic correction of the primary vertical deviation is recommended.

Congenital esotropes have a high incidence of double hyperdeviation (dissociated vertical divergence), often caused by an overaction of the inferior obliques. This deviation may remain latent until periods of visual inattention. If the hyperdeviation is large it may be cosmetically unpleasant. Large-angle exotropes may demonstrate secondary vertical deviations in either hyper- or hypo-directions. These deviations disappear during periods of convergence.

Primary vertical deviations are usually nonconcomitant. Concomitant primary vertical deviations are rare except in cases of orbital asymmetry. When the onset of a concomitant deviation is sudden (especially when accompanied by vertical diplopia), skew deviation must be considered in the differential diagnosis. This entity occurs in association with brain stem or cerebellar disease; testing should therefore include probes of these areas.

The trochlear nerve is the thinnest and has the longest course of any extra-ocular muscle innervator. It is also the only totally crossed motor cranial nerve; the right nucleus supplies the left superior oblique. Patients may manifest a congenital fourth nerve paresis, but a more common etiology is trauma in middle age. Rear end auto collisions may result in a fourth nerve palsy with immediate onset of diplopia; these usually clear in 3 to 6 months. The two fourth nerves cross each other en route to their contralateral end organs. Injury to the site of crossing at the anterior medullary velum can lead to bilateral paresis, manifesting with eso and torsion in down gaze. Patients may, therefore, present with a chief complaint of reading difficulties.

Third and fourth nerve palsies may occur concurrently. To test for fourth nerve involvement in patients with third nerve palsy, have the patient attempt to look down and in. Since the third nerve problem places the eye outside the normal action of the superior oblique (it can't adduct) the fellow eye is observed—it will move down and in. A small intorsion of the paretic eye may be noted if the conjunctival vessels are carefully watched, indicating an intact fourth nerve (mnemonic: "*inferior* people and *muscles extort*").

Head tilts, facial turns, and chin elevation or depression are commonly seen in pareses of the vertical muscles, particularly predictable with the obliques. It is commonly assumed that these actions are attempts to maintain fusion. When a patient is not quite able to fuse disparate images by these methods, however, the proximity of the diplopic images may be quite disconcerting. At this point, the patient may adopt an exact opposite posture to place the images as far away from each other as possible, allowing suspension of one of the images.

# HISTORY

Cosmetic concerns frequently are the presenting complaint from strabismic patients or their parents (Table 16.2). This is probably the chief reason for infants and young children being brought in for examinations. Questions must address age of onset and duration of the observed turn. Is the turn intermittent or constant? Equal visual acuities suggest either an intermittent or alternating strabismus. Has the frequency of the turn increased or remained stable? While parents may be fooled by factors resulting in pseudostrabismus, such as epicanthus, hypertelorism, orbital asymmetries, and large-angle lambdas, they are frequently very sensitive observers of their children and their input must be considered, especially in evaluating intermittent squint and visual behavior. Ask whether the child tends to close one eye in bright sunlight. This is often found in patients with intermittent exotropia. Interestingly, the closed eye may not be the one in the sun, as in common photophobia. Occlusion of the eye by the lid or hand, or turning the head may be observed in preschool and school-aged children during times of increased visual demand. Most likely, this indicates a fragile binocularity and a tendency toward

diplopia and asthenopia. Patients with alternating strabismus may report an actual jump of the target as fixation changes.

Preschool and early grade school children may be referred for strabismus evaluation because of amblyopia discovered during a school screening. Whenever a patient specifically requests an appointment for evaluation of a possible eye turn, they should be encouraged to bring with them old, unretouched photographs of the child

**Table 16.2**
**Anatomic Factors in Cosmesis of Strabismus**

| Favorable for Esotropia Unfavorable for Exotropia | Favorable for Exotropia Unfavorable for Esotropia |
|---|---|
| Positive angle kappa | Negative angle kappa |
| Narrow bridge of nose | Wide bridge of nose |
| Absence of epicanthus | Presence of epicanthus |
| Large interpupillary distance | Small interpupillary distance |
| Narrow face | Wide face |

at different ages. These may help clarify age of onset of turn and associated conditions of head tilts and turns.

Family history of strabismus should be explored. General health, history of trauma, and birth delivery information should be questioned. For example, injury from forceps delivery may lead to an apparent congenital esotropia from an injured sixth nerve.

Previous treatment of the squint or concurrent conditions, such as amblyopia, should be investigated fully. It is not sufficient to know that the child was patched for several months 4 years previously. Inquire about compliance, active exercises, whether the patch was alternated or kept unilaterally, and the best obtained acuity. Too often parents are discouraged because the acuity improved during the patching period only to regress when the patch was removed. The clinician should share his encouragement upon hearing this, realizing that the improvement is reclaimable if need be. In fact, if binocularity is obtainable, the acuity may be stabilized at the improved level. In summary, information regarding previous therapy is very important in developing a prognosis, and careful inquiry is necessary.

Adult onset of strabismus demands a special history. Refer to the chapters on oculomotor palsies and diplopia.

# EXAMINATION

Concern about cosmesis and ocular health is important in determining the management of strabismus. Inquire if functional or cosmetic cure is desired.

Examination of the strabismic patient must probe the same areas of other general examinations, evaluating acuity, refractive error, ocular and systemic health, binocular status, and with children, perceptual skills.

Visual acuity must be estimated in a matter that accounts for the crowding phenomenon demonstrated in amblyopia. Flom's psychometric chart (S-chart) is the most sensitive measure because it controls for contour interaction and provides many acuity test lines throughout the range from 20/277 to 20/9. Snellen chart acuity should be recorded as to chart, line, and letter acuities, with the latter considered the prognostic acuity following therapy. AO children's picture or tumbling E slides may be substituted for younger children. An inexpensive substitute is the tumbling E cards with contour interaction bars produced by the University of California. These cards allow single letter presentations at 10 feet but will adequately distinguish amblyopic responses. For very young children, STYCAR testing may suffice. A preferential looking apparatus will give a good acuity estimate in infants. This is particularly helpful in infants who have undergone strabismus surgery and appear to have straight eyes, but may have a residual amblyopia preventing the development of binocularity.

Visual behavior is particularly important to observe in young children. Squinting, head tilts or turns, fussing during occlusion of one but not the other eye are all indicators of potential visual problems.

Methods of refraction vary with the patient's age. Retinoscopy is the best clinical indicator of refractive error in young children from whom subjective responses are not possible. Mohindra's near retinoscopy helps control the infant's attention and reportedly gives results comparable to cycloplegia. Alternatively, cartoon loops, which are very successful in holding children's attention, may be purchased. Lens bars to neutralize the reflex in free space are preferable to placing the child behind the phoropter because it is easier to monitor attention and head position.

Cycloplegia with two drops of 1% cyclogel spaced 5 minutes apart provides adequate control of accommodation for most patients and may affect the angle of deviation. In addition, the accompanying mydriasis allows for more complete fundus evaluation. On the negative side, the mydriatic pupil produces a scissors movement that is difficult to neutralize. Children are also occasionally disturbed by fear or momentary discomfort from the instillation of the drops. When this happens, cooperation may be lost and the drug dosage affected by tearing or squeezing of the lids.

A thorough examination to rule out pathology is especially important with strabismic patients, since the ocular deviation may be secondary to various ocular or systemic diseases. Four main types of obstacles may prevent fusion: optical, sensory, motor, and psychological. Each factor must be ruled out or accounted for as completely as possible.

Pupils should be examined for size, shape, and responsiveness. An afferent pupillary defect should be carefully sought in cases of unexplained acuity loss. In young children, optic nerve gliomas may lead to reduction of acuity and subsequent squint without any other behavioral signs besides a positive Marcus Gunn pupil.

An evaluation of the anterior segment with loupe or slit lamp should focus on signs of optical or sensory obstacles such as displaced lens, corneal opacities, or cataracts. A Placido's disc may be helpful in determining corneal irregularities and astigmatism.

Fundus evaluation should concentrate on macular lesions, optic nerve atrophy or hypoplasia, and causes of sensory obstacles in children such as retrolental fibroplasia and retinoblastoma. Binocular indirect ophthalmoscopy is preferred because of its advantages in field of view and resolution. In infants and young children with poor fixation control, these advantages may determine whether an adequate view of the fundus is possible.

Sensory obstacles may be present anywhere along the retinocerebral pathway, so a careful study of visual fields is mandatory whenever possible. The Amsler grid provides a good measure of the central field, whereas tangent screen or perimeter is needed for detection of neurologic lesions. With amblyopia or central scotoma, a large cross placed on the screen provides an adequate fixation target. Motor obstacles are in the section on binocular evaluation. Psychogenic and hysterical conditions have occasionally been reported as an etiology of concomitant strabismus. In these cases, supportative therapy by psychologists or counselors is necessary.

Evaluation of a patient's binocular status consists of a diagnosis of the deviation, correspondence, and sensory and motor fusion. Any obstacles to sensory fusion, such as aniseikonia, amblyopia, and media opacities, should be noted during the general examination.

Diagnosis of the deviation consists primarily of an analysis of the frequency, magnitude, laterality, and direction of the deviation, concomitancy, and AC/A ratio. In general, testing should proceed from the most habitual state (natural or associated viewing condition—both eyes open and attempting to view a target of regard) to a less natural (dissociated) viewing condition.

Observation is the least obtrusive testing procedure, and the examiner should begin watching the patient's visual behavior from the moment of their introduction. Is there a head tilt or turn? Does the squint patient freely alternate fixation? Are there any gross restrictions in the field of gaze necessitating head movements into certain fields?

The Hirschberg test introduces a penlight fixation target held at 33 to 50 cm on the patient's midline. The examiner sights behind the light and compares the light reflex in each eye. Assuming that the foveas are located in corresponding locations in each eye, the displacement of the light reflex in the deviating eye will be equal to the true angle of strabismus. Displacement of 1 mm converts to 22 prism diopters of squint. Obviously, this is a rather gross technique, most useful with infants and uncooperative patients, for whom finer measures are unavailable. Confirmation of the Hirschberg estimate is made by placing compensating prisms before the deviating eye and judging when the reflexes appear equal (Krimsky technique). Care must be taken that no ocular movement occurs as a result of the introduction of the prism. Some authors suggest placing the prism before the fixating eye, presumably to introduce a known amount of versional movement (equal to the prism power). While this reduces the possibility of unknown amounts of movement, it is not as reliable in cases of nonconcomitancy.

Cover testing is a sensitive measure of the magnitude, direction, and laterality of the deviation. Targets should be chosen that are visible to each eye. When acuity allows, letters with sharp perpendicular lines are good targets at distance. Encourage the patient to look where the lines intersect. If acuity is poor, a muscle light is adequate. At near the target should demand accommodative accuracy. Small pictures with detail that the patient can be asked to describe are preferable to single letters since they maintain interest and, therefore, accommodative accuracy for a longer period.

Unilateral (cover-uncover) testing should be performed first since it is simply a probe of the patient's habitual binocular (associated) posture. Enough time must be given between probes to allow the patient to refixate the target in an associated condition. If squint is present, note if the eyes alternate freely to pick up fixation or whether a unilateral preference is evidenced.

Besides strabismus, several conditions can lead to movement on the unilateral cover test: eccentric fixation, uncorrected anisometropia, poor fixation maintenance, possibly large fixation disparities, and movement secondary to large

heterophorias that may pull the fixating eye off target because of yoked muscles (see Chapter 14).

Magnitude of the ocular deviation is most easily accomplished by the alternate cover test. In this test, one eye is always occluded so that the dissociation is complete and full deviation revealed. The actual magnitude must take into account eccentric fixation. Similar signs add to obtain the true deviation; that is, nasal eccentric fixation is added to esodeviation and subtracted from exodeviations.

Upon completion of the measure of magnitude, the occluder is removed and the recovery movement of the covered eye is assessed. This is particularly important in cases of intermittent squint. Ask the patient with a long latency prior to the recovery movement whether diplopia was noticed following the removal of the paddle. This is important information in developing a training program.

Remeasurement of the magnitude of the deviation with lenses before the eyes gives an indication of the AC/A ratio as well as the potential for passive therapy. This is particularly useful with esodeviations at near and with divergence excess exotropias. A good clinical starting point is a +3.00 add at near for esotropes and a −2.00 over manifest correction for distance measurements in divergence excess exotropes. Halberg clips are particularly helpful in this procedure since they allow both of the examiner's hands to be free to hold the occluder and neutralizing prism. Two formulas may be used to help determine more specific starting lenses in these measurements. The first formula is used to determine the AC/A ratio.

$$AC/A = PD + M (Hn - Hf),$$
where PD is in centimeters and
$M$ = fixation distance at near in meters (usually 0.4);
$Hn$ = objective angle of deviation at near;
$Hf$ = objective angle of deviation at far.

Eso deviations are positive.
Exo deviations are negative.

This calculated AC/A is usually higher than the gradient AC/A because of inclusion of proximal factors.

It can be seen that equal deviations at distance and near would cancel in the formula, leaving an AC/A equal to the *PD* (for example, a *PD* of 60 mm with 6-prism diopter esodeviation at distance and near would equal a 6/1 AC/A. When the eso is greater at near, or exo less at near, then at distance the AC/A is greater than the *PD*. Likewise, a lower eso at near, or higher exo at near indicates an AC/A of less than the *PD*.

Once the AC/A is calculated, an approximate neutralizing lens can be determined. For instance, if the patient has a 12-prism diopter exotropia at distance and AC/A of 4/1, by dividing the deviation by the AC/A (12/4), the overcorrection is found; in this example −3.00 DS is a distance addition. Remember when prescribing additional minus at distance that a bifocal may be required for comfort at near.

A second formula is useful for determining near additions. Simply by dividing the distance deviation by the *PD*, the near add is found. When a target is at the focal length of this lens, the eyes should be orthophoric. For example, an 18-prism diopter esotrope at distance with a 6-cm *PD* will be orthophoric with a +3.00 add when looking at 33 centimeters.

Concomitancy is a particularly important factor to investigate, especially in cases of recent onset of strabismus or diplopia. A change of 5 prism diopters or more in any position of gaze is considered nonconcomitant. Frequently, this may be observed during version testing. Be careful to note midline shifts of fixation, which may correspond to patient's reports of words jumping when reading. To make version testing more sensitive, it may be combined with the Hirschberg test. In this case, the observer either moves into the nine positions of gaze while sighting be-

hind a penlight, or, more conveniently, remains stable and moves the patient's head into the different positions while the patient maintains fixation on the penlight.

Alternate cover testing may be accomplished in the same manner as described above, the Hirschberg. Retain the neutralizing prism from primary gaze before the deviated eye and check for additional movement in the various diagnostic fields. Every patient with near-point complaints, even if never strabismic, should be given cover tests in upper and lower as well as primary positions of gaze checking for A or V patterns. These descriptive titles refer to the change of deviation in vertical gaze. A *V* pattern esotrope (exotrope) has more eso (less exo) in down gaze, while an *A* pattern esotrope has more eso (less exo) in up gaze. Patients with these problems may manifest chin elevations or depressions, which can cause neck discomfort.

Sensitive patients may be able to respond to subjective concomitancy tests such as red glass diplopia fields or the Hess-Lancaster screen. These tests allow greater refinement in measurement but are reliable only if normal correspondence is present. By a slight modification of these techniques, use of Maddox rod instead of red glass or lanterns with slit targets on Hess-Lancaster, cyclo components may be revealed.

When there is a significant vertical component, the Parks' three-step method can aid in determination of the paretic muscle: (1) Which eye is hyper in primary gaze? (2) Which direction of horizontal gaze shows an increase in the hyper deviation? (3) Upon tilting the head 30° toward the left and right shoulder, which yields an increase of hyper deviation? With very sensitive patients, a red glass may be used in each step, but usually the objective determination of the cover test is preferable. Remember, in step (3) the examiner must tilt his head to maintain a straight-on view of the patient's eyes to avoid confounding of torsial factors.

A simple method to interpret the three-step procedure is shown in Figure 16.1. The diagnostic action fields of each eye are shown. In primary gaze, the right eye is hyper, suggesting a problem with the depressors in that eye or the elevators of the left eye. Both of these groups are circled and labeled *number 1*. Next, place a vertical oval around the muscles involved in the direction of gaze showing an increase in hyper (number 2). Third, place a diagonal oval in the same direction as the patient's head tilt, which yields an increase in hyper (number 3). Only one muscle will have been circled three times: this is the paretic muscle.

Whenever there is evidence of recent nonconcomitancy, questions must address the "company it keeps." Ask about trauma, headache (especially if upon awakening or progressive), paresthesias, difficulty speaking, thyroid signs, and so forth. Presence of a spontaneous venous pulsation at the optic disc indicates an in-

tracranial pressure of less than 200 mm of water. While many normal patients do not manifest a spontaneous venous pulsation, its presence strongly suggests that increased intracranial pressure is not the cause of the current problem.

Once the deviation has been measured and health-threatening etiologies are ruled out, the remaining diagnostic variables, retinal correspondence, and sensory and motor fusion should be addressed.

Normal retinal correspondence refers to the fovea in each eye giving rise to a common visual direction. If the fovea of one eye is functionally linked to an extrafoveal point in the fellow eye, anomalous retinal correspondence is present. Three measurements are considered when discussing retinal correspondence: the objective angle of the deviation between the foveas of the two eyes, the subjective angle of directionalization, and the angle of anomaly, which is the difference between

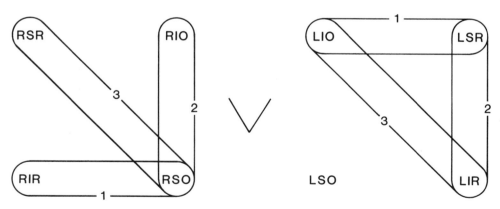

**FIGURE 16.1.**

Park's three-step method. A simple method to interpret the three-step procedure is shown. The diagnostic action fields of each eye are shown. In primary gaze, the right eye is hyper, suggesting a problem with the depressors in that eye or the elevators of the left eye. Both of these groups are circled and labeled number 1. Next, place a vertical oval around the muscles involved in the direction of gaze showing an increase in hyper (number 2). Third, place a diagonal oval in the same direction as the patient's head tilt, which yields an increase in hyper (number 3). Only one muscle will be circled three times; this is the paretic muscle. In this example, only the right superior oblique (RSO) is circled three times.

these two measures (Table 16.3). When the objective and subjective angles are equal, the angle of anomaly equals zero and normal correspondence is defined. If there is an objective angle while the subjective angle is zero, the angle of anomaly equals the objective angle. This is termed *harmonious anomalous retinal correspondence.* Any angle of anomaly not equal to the objective angle or to zero is referred to as *unharmonious anomalous retinal correspondence.*

Techniques for determination of correspondence may measure the objective and subjective angles, or directly measure the angle of anomaly. Most popular of the former techniques are the Bagolini striated lens combined with the unilateral cover test, and the major amblyoscope. After-image procedures permit direct assessment of the angle of anomaly, provided monocular fixation is central. If eccentric, compensation must be made as described previously for the cover test.

Manifest deviations of the visual axes create an obstacle to sensory fusion. Stereopsis, the highest level of sensory fusion, is reduced or absent in squint patients. Manley (1971) suggests a cutoff of 67 seconds of stereopsis to separate bifixation from monofixation. Linear disparity targets frequently used in practice (e.g., Titmus, AO circles, Bernell reindeer) may show better stereopsis than actually is present due to the monocular cues inherent in these tests. Random dot stereograms demand a higher order of stereoscopic processing and eliminate the monocular cues. Steropsis should be measured under the habitual conditions, with neutralizing prisms in place, and when possible, at the centration point.

When stereopsis is reduced, a measure of flat fusion should be made by means of targets such as the Worth 4 dot or the red glass technique.* Again it is important to

## Table 16.3
### Determination of Correspondence

Comparison of objective and subjective angles
  Bagolini striated lens
  Major amblyoscope
  Red glass/prism/cover test
  Vectographic methods for subjective
    measures
  Spontaneous diplopia in free space as a
    subjective measure

Direct measures of angle of anomaly
  Hering-Bielschowsky after-image
  Transferred after-image/Hadinger brush
  Hallden II
  Giesen
  Cüppers macula—macular test
  Binocular entopic phenomena

find out whether neutralizing prism or centration point can result in a fusional response. Attempts to establish fusion with prism may fail because of suppression of one of the targets.

In a natural environment, the recent-onset strabismic patient may see two different objects in the same place in space (confusion), or one object may be seen in two different places in space (diplopia). Suppression is probably the first mechanism employed (at least in young persons) to eliminate these annoyances. Suppression may be present with either normal or anomalous correspondence. Size of a suppression scotoma may be plotted on a Brock posture board, by adding prism to the suppressed eye until diplopia is first noticed in the horizontal and vertical dimensions, or by varying target size or distance to the suppressed eye until it is first seen.

Motor ranges around the objective angle are most easily determined in the major amblyoscope since many interesting targets of various sizes are available, and the

---

*  Strabismics, particularly divergent excess types, function well with stereoscopic targets, but break down under flat fusion. Flat fusion demands are present in common tasks like reading.

patient's eyes may be viewed to add objective confirmation to the patient's reports. Use of a prism bar in free space is an acceptable alternative procedure. Both base-in and base-out ranges should be determined. Intermittent exotropes may show decreases in base-out ranges as expected, but also deficient base-in ranges. Presumably, this is because as soon as the patient begins to turn the eyes out to meet the demand, control is lost and the tropia manifested.

# CLINICAL SIGNIFICANCE

## Conditions

### NONCONCOMITANT STRABISMUS

Most ominous of all the diagnostic variables are sudden onset and nonconcomitancy. Nonconcomitant deviations manifest a minimum change of 5 prism diopters in at least one field of gaze. Patients with nonconcomitant deviations are usually diplopic when looking into the affected muscle action field. While there are many etiologies of nonconcomitancy—anatomic, mechanical, and congenital—those caused by paresis are most threatening (Chapter 19).

Any patient suspected of having a nonconcomitancy deserves a specific diagnostic work-up (Table 19.4), which is attentive to all possible cases (Tables 19.1, 19.2, 19.3).

### CONCOMITANT STRABISMUS

Any strabismus that maintains an essentially equal diviation in all directions of gaze is considered concomitant. These deviations may be congenital, such as hypertonic medial rectus, or acquired, as in hypotonus of lateral rectus or disturbance of tonic vergence. Care must be taken, especially with infants and young children, to differentiate true from pseudostrabismus. Esotropia may be simulated by narrow interpupillary distance, epicanthal folds, and negative angle lambda, whereas an apparent exotropia may be due to hypertelorism. In many of these patients, the deviation may even appear to be nonconcomitant. If a case of pseudostrabismus later manifests an acquired strabismus, the history of onset and subsequent prognosis for functional care may be confounded.

Examiners must rely heavily on interview and clinical impression to gauge the psychologic impact of squint on the patient and family.

Primary vertical deviations usually are not concomitant. An exception is skew deviation, which may be concomitant or nonconcomitant. Skew deviation is associated with lesions of the brain stem, cerebellum, or labyrinth; therefore, any concomitant vertical deviation not secondary to surgery should alert the clinician to carefully seek associated signs or symptoms.

### MICROSTRABISMUS

Small-angle strabismics may present with almost no perceivable movement on cover testing but demonstrate amblyopia and reduced stereopsis. In any young patient with unexplained amblyopia, monofixation syndrome (microtropia, flick) should be suspected. A clue to this condition may be a slight flick movement during the unilateral cover test, followed by a much more pronounced movement on alternate cover testing, indicating that under normal viewing conditions a fusional movement is made that reduces the magnitude of deviation. More difficult to diagnose is the case where eccentric fixation is present in an amount equal to the objective angle of deviation, producing no movement on cover testing.

# Prognosis

Prognosis of a successful functional cure for strabismus, based on consideration of the variables of frequency, direction, magnitude, correspondence, and sensory fusion, was suggested by Flom (1958).

In general, congenital onset has a poor prognosis unless there is early intervention. Acquired nonaccommodative tropias have a fair prognosis, while accommodative onset has a good prognosis unless of long duration.

Anomalous correspondence is a strongly negative prognostic factor in esotropes, while not for most exotropes. This is because fusional vergence to the orthoposition is capable of changing retinal correspondence (covariation). Since it is much easier to converge than diverge the eyes, exotropes have a marked advantage in overcoming anomalous correspondence. In addition, exotropes frequently have had some early experience with binocular interaction and, therefore, a better prognosis for reestablishment of binocularity.

Concomitant squint is thought to have a better prognosis than nonconcomitant strabismus, although some authors believe variability of the angle of deviation may keep adaptations from becoming embedded, and is therefore favorable.

Intermittent strabismus has a more favorable prognosis than unilateral squint. Alternation appears to be as treatable as unilateral cases. In fact, since alternators normally are free of amblyopia they have one less obstacle to overcome.

Deep suppression, peripheral suppression, horror fusionis, and lack of correspondence are unfavorable factors.

In general, a strabismus manifest at distance is more difficult to treat than one at near.

Microtropia or monofixation syndrome usually has a poor prognosis for establishment of bifixation. If symptomatic, however, monofixators frequently respond well to standard orthoptic procedures with a goal of developing a more efficient monofixator.

# References

Cogan DG. Neurology of the ocular muscles. Springfield, Ill.; Charles C Thomas, 1956;2nd ed.;131.

Duke-Elder S. System of ophthalmology. VI. St. Louis: C.V. Mosby, 1973;

Flom MC. The prognosis in strabismus. Am J Optom 1958;35(10):509–514.

Griffin JR. Binocular anomalies procedures for vision therapy. Chicago: Professional Press, 1982;2nd ed.

Hugonnier R, Clayette-Hugonnier S. Strabismus, heterophoria, ocular motor paralysis. Véronneau-Troutman S, trans. St. Louis: C.V. Mosby, 1969.

Koch PS. An aid for the diagnosis of a vertical muscle paresis. J Ped Ophthal Strab 1980;17:272–276.

Manley DR. Symposium on horizontal ocular deviations. St. Louis: C.V. Mosby, 1971.

Parks MM. Ocular motility and strabismus. In: Duane TD ed. Clinical ophthalmology. Hagerstown, Md.: Harper & Row, 1979;1–20.

Roy, FH. Practical management of eye problems: glaucoma, strabismus, visual fields. Philadelphia: Lea & Febiger, 1975.

Von Noorden GK. Burian-von Noorden's binocular vision and ocular motility. St. Louis: C.V. Mosby, 1980;2nd ed.

# Michael W. Rouse
## Richard London
# DEVELOPMENT AND PERCEPTION 17

*Development is the process of progressive change in structure and properties of behavior that takes place in the course of an individual's lifetime.*

*Perception is the active process in which the individual searches for, selects, computes, compares, stores, and uses information that specifies objects or events.*

## BACKGROUND

Perception provides the individual with knowledge about the world and is more than simply what we see or how we respond. It involves an active interaction with the environment. It is the process by which information regarding the environment is gained through the senses in a direct and immediate way and, in turn, is acted upon by the individual.

There are several theories of perceptual development, but all tend to agree that the environment contains stimuli that must be received and acted on by the individual. If the individual does not attend to the stimulation, although sensory and perceptual capacity may exist, there is no effective acquisition of information.

The efficiency of the visual system is imperative if visual input is to be accurate. Any defects in the oculomotor, accommodative, or vergence systems may result in decreased attentional abilities. In addition, these systems are intimately involved in the basic development of perception.

There are many perceptual abilities that appear to be innate or develop early in life. Although many abilities appear to be present on a rudimentary level, the continued development of these skills requires an interaction between maturation and experience. In order to appreciate the interaction between perception and development, observe the developing infant.

Infants live virtually exclusively in a perceptual world. There are few memories to rely on, and the ability to anticipate the future is undeveloped. They are in a true sense stimulus bound. Any novel stimulus is likely to be sufficient to attract the infant's attention. Repetitive stimuli develop internal representations or schema of the stimulus, which allow quick and accurate perceptual matches. The infant is then able to block or turn off stimuli that match schema, permitting them to attend to new objects of interest. This process is known as habituation. Imagine the difficulty in the acquisition of new knowledge if habituation to common stimuli were absent.

The ability to attend selectively to stimuli is part of the normal development of all perceptual and motor systems. The infant's motor system responds in a very global manner initially. Stimulation of one part results in compensatory movements throughout the entire body. At about 4 months of age the child begins to control certain parts of the body, such as the arms, without moving other parts. Note that in the young child there is a need for redundant multisensory stimulation. Objects are seen, touched, heard, and tasted. Gradually, as schema and the knowledge base are increased, the perceptual systems become reciprocal; the need for redundancy is reduced. The child should be able to develop selective attention, either visually, auditorily, or tactilely, depending on the demands of the situation, and be able to match mentally the information coming through any single channel with its representation in other sensory systems. This ability to match visual, verbal, and kinesthetic information is imperative for efficient perceptual ability.

While the perceptual systems are beginning to reciprocate, a hierarchy is established, with the visual system assuming a dominant role. This permits a more efficient sampling system. Objects out of reach can now be visually explored and information gathered without the necessity of direct physical contact. The child learns to look and then act. Cognitive development continues away from sensorimotor dominance to the ability to visualize and abstract.

Developmental trends of the motor and perceptual systems emphasize the dependent relationship between these systems. By the time the child is of school age, it is assumed that development has proceeded normally. The teaching methods and learning environments are geared toward the child who has not only developed correctly, but has done so on a timetable dictated by the demands of the school system. Therefore, when developmental tests are performed on children with suspected lags,

it is recommended that the areas of motor skills, visual perception, visual-motor integration, and auditory perception be carefully explored.

The evaluation of perceptual abilities reflects the development of the child. Any deficits may prevent the child from receiving the full benefit of teacher instruction. As an example, perceptual motor problems may affect the timely development of perceptual and attention skills.

Furthermore, children who cannot sit still in school may have difficulty in attending to the teacher. Children who fail to develop reciprocity between their perceptual systems may show some of the same classroom behavior; that is, they are stimulus bound and highly distractable. Possibly even may be adversely affected, since he may be labeled derogatorily by peers and excluded from common athletic activities.

The role of the primary care practitioner/vision specialist in screening for perceptual skills is simply an extension of the testing for the patency of the sensory system. Intact sensation without the ability to form organized percepts may result in a number of problems. Receptive aphasia (loss of the faculty to receive ideas by language in any form) and alexia (loss of the power to grasp the meaning of written or printed words and sentences) are severe manifestations of this perceptual breakdown.

Less severe deficits in perceptual skills may result in a myriad of deficient skills that may impede performance, especially in school. The incidence of these deficiencies is significantly greater in the population of children labeled as having "learning disabilities." *Learning disabilities* is a generic term that refers to a heterogeneous group of disorders manifested by significant difficulties in the acquisition and use of listening, speaking, reading, writing, reasoning, or mathematical abilities. These disorders are intrinsic to the individual and are presumed to be due to CNS dysfunction. Even though a learning disability may occur concomitantly with other handicapping conditions (e.g., sensory impairment, mental retardation, social and emotional disturbance) or environmental influences (e.g., cultural differences, inefficient/inappropriate instruction, psychogenic factors), it is not the direct result of these conditions or influences.

Learning disabilities are estimated to affect as many as one of seven students, or almost 7 million children. By most definitions, these children have at least average IQ scores but are not performing as well as expected in certain areas. Many of these children may easily learn many everyday skills, but when placed in a stan-

dard classroom setting they are unable to process information dealing with symbols. Children with below average IQ scores may have deficient perceptual skills, but are not strictly classified as learning disabled, rather they are defined as mentally retarded or educationally handicapped. These children may even have difficulty learning everyday skills and may require special full-time educational assistance.

Since early intervention and remediation is often highly successful in developing efficient perceptual strategies, the establishment of an adequate screening regimen for visual and perceptual deficits is a critical patient care service.

# HISTORY

The optometric evaluation of children with suspected visually related learning problems starts with a complete case history. The school, in most cases, has already concluded that the child is having academic problems before the referral to the optometrist is made. The parent usually reports a main complaint of the child having difficulty in school, and the teacher or psychologist has referred the child to investigate whether problems with the child's eyes are contributing to the difficulties in school. Many parents may not volunteer this information and must be asked two questions: "Are you (the parent) satisfied with your child's school achievement?" and "Is the teacher satisfied with the child's school work and achievement?" If the parent did not initially volunteer that the child is having school difficulties and the answers to the two questions are yes, then it is relatively assured that the child is achieving up to the expectations of both parents and teachers. Many times the additional questioning elicits an outpouring of information from the parent, which might include a history of special classes, grade retention, or an impression that the child is a slow learner.

In addition to eliciting the main complaint, a developmental history should be completed. A developmental history is useful in identifying factors or events which may put a child "at risk." The developmental history can be divided into three periods: prenatal, neonatal, and postnatal. The prenatal history should center on whether the mother experienced a normal pregnancy. Any exposure of the mother to toxic agents or infectious diseases, especially during the first trimester, as well as any other abnormalities, should be noted. The neonatal history evaluates whether the child was full term and had a normal delivery and birth weight. The postnatal history includes questions about the child's medical, developmental growth, psychological/social, and school experiences. The child's medical history may reveal serious childhood diseases that may have resulted in high fevers or hospitalization. Extended periods of hospitalization may seriously interfere with the child's normally expected acquisition of perceptual skills. Chronic problems with allergies or ear infection should also be noted. Many children with academic problems may be on medication to control hyperactivity or other neurologic difficulties, such as epilepsy. Questions should address the type of medication, dosage, and changes in behavior noticed. Psychosocial development should address questions about adjustment to school and relationships with peers and family.

Question the parent also about the child's achievement of important early developmental milestones, especially ages at which the child crawled, walked, and spoke his first words (Table 17.1). Delayed acquisition of these milestones may indicate future difficulties with perceptual development and learning in general. A written developmental history chart may be completed by the parent before or during the examination for a more complete developmental history (Table 17.2).

A review of the child's school history is necessary. Important questions to ask are the age of the child when in kindergarten, whether the child was ever retained, what types of problems were especially noticed, and whether achievement in lower grades is comparable to the present level.

Some children will start out achieving adequately and then have difficulties when reaching the third and fourth grades. Difficulties at this stage implicate visual efficiency deficiency, or an inability to compensate for deficient perceptual skills. Problems can be triggered by the change from learning to read to reading to learn at approximately the third grade, requiring longer periods of concentration on material with smaller print size. Other children may do poorly from the beginning of their academic career, which may implicate more profound perceptual deficiencies. Many children enter kindergarten just under the age limit and may not be perceptually ready for the increasingly academic emphasis now present.

Parents are often unaware of the child's specific difficulties beyond readily observable problems with reading and/or arithmetic. Contact with the child's teacher is an excellent avenue to confirm the presence of behavioral signs and symptoms that correspond to diagnostic findings (for example, deficient saccadic eye-movement skills corresponding to teacher reports of the child skipping words or using a finger to keep the place). Contact with the teacher can be verbal or written. Table 17.3 is an example of a teacher's information form that has provided useful. In addition, a concerned phone call to the teacher may be an important contact for further referrals.

Table 17.1
Summary of Developmental Progress

| Age (months) | Gross Motor | Vision and Manipulation | Hearing and Vocalization | Social |
|---|---|---|---|---|
| 1 | Gradual development of head control. Movements coarse and jerky. | Begins to fixate on nearby familiar objects. Watches mother's face. Following with eyes. | Cries when hungry or uncomfortable. Freezes or quiets to sounds. | Sleeps and feeds. Evokes much affection and accepts this passively. |
| 2 | Dominance of primary reflexes on posture and movements. | Visually takes 'hold' of objects. | | Quiets in response to cooing and rocking. Regards nearby face. Smiles in response. |

**Table 17.1**
*(continued)*

| Age (months) | Gross Motor | Vision and Manipulation | Hearing and Vocalization | Social |
|---|---|---|---|---|
| 3 | Head lag, when pulled from supine to sitting, disappearing. | Holds objects placed in hands momentarily. | Response to sounds varies, e.g., dislikes loud harsh sounds, may excite to familiar sounds. | Reacts to familiar pleasant situations, e.g., feeding, bathing. |
| 4 | In prone, head and chest raised. Later, support taken on forearms. | Visually associated reaching develops. | Cry pattern more mature. Vocalizes in response to overtures. | Likes handling. Feeding now a social activity. |
| 5 | Feet to mouth, plays with toes. Rolls front to back, and usually later back to front. | Recognizes everyday objects, e.g., cup. Watches hands. | | |
| 6 | Held upright takes weight in legs. | Mature visual following and convergence. Eyes used together, no squint. | Turns to sounds. Wider range of vocalization. Chuckles. | Spontaneously responsive and smiling. |
| 7 | In sitting, head steady and back straight. | Transfers objects, e.g., cubes, hand to hand. | Beginning to imitate rhythms of sounds. | |
| 8 | Reciprocates with legs. Protective support reflexes of limbs appearing. | Looks for dropped objects. | Practices vocalization. | Beginning to be aware of strangers and to modify responsiveness. |
| 9 | Stable in sitting position. Sideways and forward support with arms. | Moves cover in order to see object. Index finger use appearing. | Babbles, uses voice purposefully. Vocal imitation. | Responds to adults; plays imitative games. |
| 10 | Attempts to move—creep, crawl, squirm, shuffle. Pulls to stand. | Visually very alert. Pincer grip for small objects. | Mature localization of sounds. | Reacts to encouragement and discouragement. |

**Table 17.1**
*(continued)*

| Age (months) | Gross Motor | Vision and Manipulation | Hearing and Vocalization | Social |
|---|---|---|---|---|
| 11 | Plays standing holding on. Cruises around furniture. | Glances around, makes quick visual appraisals. Beginning to look at pictures and may point with index finger. | Beginning to understand words and single simple commands. Beginning to vocalize recognizable words. | Shows affections. Plays pat-a-cake; waves bye-bye. |
| 12 | May take first steps. | | | |

| Age | Motor | Vision and Manipulation | Hearing and Language | Social |
|---|---|---|---|---|
| 12–18 months | Independent walking develops. Likes to push and pull wheeled toys. Often squats when playing. Climbs on to chairs. Goes up stairs usually with hand held and may attempt coming down, sometimes by bumping down on bottom. | Enjoys picture books, points with finger. Much practice of eye-hand coordination. Sees small objects and picks them up with thumb and index finger. Does not yet turn book pages individually. | Rapid development of vocabulary, especially of concrete nouns and verbs of action. Likes jingles. Understands single simple commands. | Becoming independent in feeding. Aware of and disapproves of wetness. Plays alone, but needs adult nearby. Vulnerable in unsuitable environment. |
| 18–24 months | Earlier motor skills more proficient. Beginning to attempt kicking and throwing ball. Shows better judgment of size and position of objects, e.g., chairs. | Likes to scribble with pencil, imitates vertical stroke. Turns book pages singly. | Beginning to join words. Echolalia often normally present. Carries out verbal requests. | Responds to adult guidance and control. Not yet cooperative with peers although may play alongside them. Domestic mimicry. |
| 2–3 years | Very mobile, using this ability for exploration. Likes nursery | Responds to Stycar single letter vision tests and good visual | Language well developed. May be expressed so quickly that | Clings to mother. Often has favorite toy or rag. May rebel |

**Table 17.1**
*(continued)*

| Age | Motor | Vision and Manipulation | Hearing and Language | Social |
|---|---|---|---|---|
| | climbing frame and large boxes to climb into and out of. Rides tricycle. Much more nimble. Walks sideways and backwards. | acuity is demonstrable. More mature hold of crayon. Copies circle. Beginning to thread beads and use scissors. | intelligibility is reduced. Uses language for questioning and to direct actions. Repeats and sings nursery rhymes. | over feeding. Beginning to help with undressing and dressing. Will help with tidying up. |
| 3–4 years | Now skillful in motor activities. Modifies speed and negotiates skillfully. Likes to try new skills, e.g., standing tiptoe, hopping. | Beginning to make recognizable two-dimensional line drawings, e.g., house, man. | Previous verbal skills and activities increased. Likes to hear and to relate long stories. | Imaginitive play in which everyday activities are imitated and children take adult roles. Tolerance of short separation and waiting developing. Beginning to share. Understanding good and bad. |
| 4–5 years | Walks on straight line. Stands on one leg. Hops and skips with alternating feet. Responds to rhythm and music and movement group activities enjoyed. | Hand skills developing rapidly. Colors pictures. Much neater and quicker. | Fluent speech free of infantile patterns. | More confident and independent. May like to be 'king of the castle.' Likes small groups but group identity not strong. Play influenced by sex of child and culture. |

| Age (years) | Area of Activity | Motor Abilities | Manipulation | Daily Activities | Personal–Social | Language |
|---|---|---|---|---|---|---|
| 5 | Home kindergarten. | Stands on one leg. Hops Jumps off step. | Draws with dynamic tripod. | Does simple errands. | Parents and adults held in awe; active imagination, fears and | Increasing ability to express thoughts and use language |

**Table 17.1**
*(continued)*

| Age (years) | Area of Activity | Motor Abilities | Manipulation | Daily Activities | Personal–Social | Language |
|---|---|---|---|---|---|---|
| | | | | | fantasies, exaggerations, tells tales. | directively. |
| 6 | | | | Manages own daily care, e.g., dressing, going to bed. | Increasing link to peer group, but still needs adult support and direction. | New concepts developing rapidly; greater understanding of size, shape, weight, distance, etc. |
| 7 | Elementary school. | Runs, climbs. | Prints large irregular letters. | May get self to school. | Ideals of right; God as punitive super-father. | |
| 8 | | | | | Needs acceptance by peers; resents social isolation. | Ability to hypothesize and solve problems beyond the here and now. |
| 9 | Increasing activity outdoors, parks, etc. | All skills performed more smoothly and efficiently; competitive games. | Joined up, neat writing; bat and ball games. | Beginning to help in household tasks, e.g., washing up, making light meals. Increasing reliability when doing tasks. | Tendency to brood; single-sex gangs. | |

# EXAMINATION

The examination of a child presenting with parental or teacher complaints of learning difficulties should include a complete evaluation of visual acuity, refractive status, ocular health, visual efficiency, and perceptual development. A thorough evaluation of the child's visual efficiency includes testing to probe ocular motilities, accommodative, vergence, and sensory systems. A screening to evaluate the child's perceptual development should include testing to investigate the developmental level of visual and auditory perceptual skills.

Visual acuity testing may have to be modified from the standard Snellen chart for these children. Many have poor recognition and knowledge of the alphabet, read from right to left, skip letters, and read letters out of order. Tumbling Es may also be difficult because of problems with directional concepts of right and left. This type of behavior should raise the clinician's level of suspicion concerning a perceptual difficulty. It may be necessary to give the child a cut-out E, which he can match to the test presentation to make the task easier. Picture cards, such as Lighthouse cards or AO children's slides that utilize familiar figures, may be helpful in getting repeatable and reliable findings. Having the child view cartoon loops or slides of animals helps greatly in keeping the child's attention during retinoscopy. The clinician should be sensitive to small hyperopic refractive errors, which may relate to deficient accommodation skills, such as high lags or infacility. A thorough evaluation of the child's external and internal eye health should be completed. Common childhood conditions, such as blepharitis, may be related to teacher reports of the child rubbing the eyes, suggesting a possible problem with visual efficiency.

The incidence of visual efficiency deficiencies has been reported to be significantly higher in children with learning problems. They may even affect the acquisition of some perceptual skills. A complete evaluation should be conducted to diagnose or rule out problems that may be contributing to the child's poor school performance. Visual efficiency diagnosis has been described extensively elsewhere in this text (Chapters 5, 13, and 14). Symptoms and clinical findings that support a diagnosis of difficulties in the ocular motor, accommodative, vergence, and sensory fusion systems are summarized in Tables 17.4 to 17.8.

An optometric evaluation of every child should include some minimal assessment of the child's visual perceptual skills. This assumes that every clinician should recognize the problems and make intelligent recommendations and referrals based on information obtained from the history and collated with diagnostic findings and observations.

Designing a visual perception screening evaluation is a complex problem. Evaluations range from observations to single and multitest developmental/perceptual test batteries, from batteries of tests requiring accurate observations with poorly standardized test norms to standardized tests, which seemingly ignore important observations of how the child accomplished the task. A blend of these two extremes will allow the clinician to make an intelligent assessment of the child's perceptual skills.

The history and observations made by the clinician during the previous testing may raise questions about visual-perceptual development. If a deficit is suspected, an appropriate test should be given.

**Table 17.2**
**Preexamination Developmental Questionnaire**

|  | mo. | day | year |
|---|---|---|---|

Child's name _____   Birthday _____/ _____/ _____
School _____   Teacher _____
School Address _____
Grade_____   Number of children in family _____

Mother's occupation _____   Father's occupation _____
Who referred you to this clinic? _____

I.  Please state the major reason you would like this child examined: _____
_____

II.  Visual Symptoms

| | Yes | No | Often | Occasionally |
|---|---|---|---|---|
| 1) headaches | ____ | ____ | ____ | ____ |
| 2) blurred distance vision | ____ | ____ | ____ | ____ |
| 3) blurred reading vision | ____ | ____ | ____ | ____ |
| 4) holds books closer than normal | ____ | ____ | ____ | ____ |
| 5) eyes hurt | ____ | ____ | ____ | ____ |
| 6) eyes tire | ____ | ____ | ____ | ____ |
| 7) double vision | ____ | ____ | ____ | ____ |
| 8) eye turn (crossed or wall-eyed) | ____ | ____ | ____ | ____ |
| 9) blinks excessively | ____ | ____ | ____ | ____ |

III.  School

| | Yes | No |
|---|---|---|
| 1) Does child like school? | ____ | ____ |
| 2) Does child like teacher? | ____ | ____ |
| 3) Is school satisfied with child's performance? | ____ | ____ |
| 4) Are you satisfied with child's school performance? | ____ | ____ |
| 5) Has a grade been repeated? | ____ | ____ |

IV.  Directions: Please rate this child on the following items. Place a number in the blank to the left of the item which describes the child's school or home behavior.

1—Always   2—Frequently   3—Occasionally   4—Rarely   5—Never   6—Unknown

_____ Hyperactive                     _____ Poor ability to organize work
_____ Short attention span            _____ Indistinct speech
_____ Easily frustrated               _____ Awkward or clumsy
_____ Easily fatigued                 _____ Behavior problems
_____ Emotional Problems
_____ Confusion following a series of verbal instructions
_____ Variable school performance (from hour to hour or day to day)
_____ Reverses letters, words or numbers in reading and/or writing

V.  At what age in years and months did the child:
speak words clearly _____ walk unaided _____
Which phrase describes the child's physical maturity (circle number)?
1—physically immature for age     2—average physical maturity     3—advanced physical maturity
                                          for age                    for age

**Table 17.2**
*(continued)*

VI. Rate the child's progress in the following subjects:

1—below average        2—average        3—advanced

\_\_\_\_\_ Reading     \_\_\_\_\_Spelling

\_\_\_\_\_ Writing     \_\_\_\_\_Arithmetic

VII. Is there a history of pregnancy or birth complications?     No _____Yes _____
If yes, please explain: _____
Has there been any severe childhood illness, high fever, injury or physical impairment? No \_\_\_\_
Yes _____ . If yes, please explain: _____

Has this child received a hearing test? No _____Yes _____Date _____
Has a hearing or speech deficiency been previously diagnosed? No _____Yes_____
If yes, please explain: _____
Has this child received a complete eye examination? No _____Yes _____
Date _____
Has a visual problem been diagnosed? No _____Yes _____
If yes, please explain: _____
Does the child have any allergies? No _____Yes _____
If yes, please explain: _____
Is the child currently taking any medications or pills? No _____Yes _____
List medication(s) and their purpose: _____

Has the child previously taken medication for hyperactivity?     No _____Yes _____

VIII. Has there been any therapy for a learning problem?     No _____Yes _____

| *Type of Therapy* | *Dates* | *Results* |
| --- | --- | --- |
| | | |
| | | |

If you wish a copy of our examination results sent to any individual or agency, please list the name and address below:

1) _____
2) _____
3) _____
Signature _____Date _____
Relation to child _____
Comments:

Thank you.

## Table 17.3
### Teacher's Report

TO THE TEACHER OF _____GRADE _____SCHOOL _____

The child named above is receiving vision care at our center. In order to more clearly assess the impact of vision problems on classroom performance, we request your observations of this child.

Please respond to the items pertinent to this child and return the report to us as soon as possible. Your cooperation will be greatly appreciated.

Sincerely,

Vision Therapy Service
Southern California College of Optometry
2001 Associated Road
Fullerton, CA 92631

OBSERVABLE CLASSROOM BEHAVIORS POSSIBLY RELATED TO VISION PROBLEMS:

1. APPEARANCE OF EYES:
   One eye turns in or out at any time _____
   Reddened eyes or lids _____
   Eyes tear excessively _____
   Encrusted eyelids _____
   Frequent styes on lids _____

2. COMPLAINTS WHEN USING EYES:
   Headaches in forehead or temples _____
   Burning or itching after reading or desk work _____
   Nausea or dizziness _____
   Print blurs after reading a short time _____
   Print "runs together" or jumps _____
   Blurred when looks up from reading _____

3. BEHAVIORAL SIGNS OF VISUAL PROBLEMS:

   A. *Eye Movement Abilities (Ocular Motility)*
   Head turns as reads across page _____
   Loses place often during reading _____
   Needs finger or marker to keep place _____
   Displays short attention span in reading or copying _____
   Too frequently omits words _____
   Repeatedly omits "small" words _____
   Writes up or down hill on paper _____
   Rereads or skips lines unknowingly _____
   Orients drawings poorly on page _____

   B. *Eye Teaming Abilities (Binocularity)*
   Complains of seeing double (diplopia) _____

Repeats letters within words _____
Omits letters, numbers or phrases _____
Misaligns digits in number columns _____
Returns to "drawing with fingers" to decide likes and difference _____
Squints, closes or covers one eye _____
Tilts head extremely while working at desk _____
Consistently shows gross postural deviations at all desk activities _____

C. *Eye-Hand Coordination Abilities*
Must feel of things to assist in any interpretation required _____
Eyes not used to "steer" hand movements (extreme lack of orientation, placement of words or drawings on page) _____
Writes crookedly, poorly spaced; cannot stay on ruled lines _____
Misaligns both horizontal and vertical series or numbers _____
Uses his hand or fingers to keep his place on the page _____
Uses other hand as "spacer" to control spacing and alignment on page _____
Repeatedly confuses left-right directions _____

D. *Visual Perception*
Mistakes words with same or similar beginnings _____
Fails to recognize same word in next sentence _____

**Table 17.3**
*(continued)*

Reverses letters and/or words in
  writing and copying ___

Confuses likenesses and minor
  differences ___

Confuses same word in
  same sentence ___

Repeatedly confuses similar
  beginnings and endings of words ___

Fails to visualize what is read either
  silently or orally ___

Whispers to self for reinforcement
  while reading silently ___

E. *Refractive Status (Nearsightedness,
    Farsightedness, Focus Problems, etc.)*

Comprehension reduces as reading
  continued; loses interest
  too quickly ___

Mispronounces similar words as
  continues reading ___

Blinks excessively at desk tasks
  and/or reading;
  not elsewhere ___

Holds book too closely; face
  too close to desk surface ___

Avoids all possible near-
  centered tasks ___

Complains of discomfort in tasks
  that demand visual
  interpretation ___

Closes or covers one eye when
  reading or doing desk work ___

Makes errors in copying from
  chalkboard to paper on desk ___

Makes errors in copying from
  reference book to notebook ___

Squints to see chalkboard, or
  requests to move nearer ___

Rubs eyes during or after short
  periods of visual activity ___

Fatigues easily; blinks to make
  chalkboard clear up
  after desk task ___

4. PEER RELATIONSHIPS:
   Gets along with classmates ___
   Others make fun of child ___
   Competes in games ___
   Chosen by other children for group
     activities ___
   Prefers older child as playmate ___
   Prefers younger child as playmate ___

5. CLASSROOM BEHAVIOR:
   Withdrawn ___
   Aggressive ___
   Behavior problem(s) ___
   Sits still ___
   Maintains interest in task at hand ___

PLEASE COMMENT ON THE FOLLOWING QUESTIONS:
1. Does this child have any major scholastic problems? Yes ___ No ___
   If so, please explain (e.g., subject material, behavior, etc.)
   _____

2. Is (s)he in the top third, middle third, lower third of his class? _____
3. How does achievement compare with potential? _____
   _____

4. Is (s)he reading below grade level? Yes ___ No ___
   If below grade level, at what level does (s)he read? _____
   Please check what seems to be any special areas of difficulty.
   Vocabulary ___          Word recognition ___          Oral reading ___
   Rate ___                Interpretation ___            Silent reading ___
   Attention ___           Comprehension ___             Memory ___
   If below grade level, what seem to be the factors that are interfering with learning to read? ___
   _____

YOUR OBSERVATIONS AND/OR COMMENTS:

**Table 17.4**
**Grading System for Evaluating Ocular Motor Abilities**

| | |
|---|---|
| 1. Pursuit ability for either eye<br> 4 + smooth/accurate<br> 3 + one fixation loss<br> 2 + two fixation losses<br> 1 + more than two fixation losses | 2. Saccadic ability for either eye<br> 4 + smooth/accurate<br> 3 + slight undershoot<br> 3 + gross undershooting or overshooting or<br>   increased latency<br> 1 + inability to do task or increased latency |

**Table 17.5**
**Ocular Motor System**

| Symptoms of Difficulties | Findings Indicating Difficulties |
|---|---|
| 1. Excessive head movement when reading<br>2. Frequent loss of place when reading or copying materials<br>3. Omission of words when reading or copying materials<br>4. Skipping of lines when reading<br>5. Use of the finger or a marker of some kind when reading in order to maintain place<br>6. Lack of comprehension when reading<br>7. A short attention span manifest when performing visual tasks | 1. Position maintenance<br>  a. Greater than $1\frac{1}{2}$ square deviation (eye trac) over 10 sec<br>  b. Less than $3^+$ on fixation observation<br>2. Saccades<br>  a. Less than $3^+$ on observation<br>  b. Greater than ISD or 1 year below on the Pierce Saccade Test<br>  c. 1 year below on King-Devich Saccade Test<br>  d. Poor performance on eye trac<br>    1. L–R (large) saccades<br>    2. 5 × 5 dots (small) saccades<br>    3. Reading paragraph<br>3. Pursuits<br>  a. Less than $3^+$ on observation<br>  b. Poor performance on eye trac<br>    1. Rotating drum<br>    2. Metronome |

## Table 17.6
### Accommodative System

| Symptoms of Difficulties | Findings Indicating Difficulties |
|---|---|
| 1. Asthenopia at near associated with excessive rubbing of eyes<br>2. Periodic blurring at distance after near-point activities on blurring at near<br>3. Reduced vision at distance<br>4. A working distance closer than expected when doing near-point tasks<br>5. Reports of headaches or nausea with near-point activities<br>6. Diplopia periodic at near<br>7. Excessive general fatigue toward the end of the day<br>8. Difficulty or inability to sustain near-point work | 1. NRA and PRA of lower than $+$ and $-1.75$.<br>2. $+$ and $-2.00$ flipper test monocularly and binocularly showing less than 12 cycles/minute with the patient viewing a 20/30 line at 16 inches, or a difference of more than 2 cycles/minute between the two eyes<br>3. M E M Retinoscopy—lag greater than 0.75 diopter<br>4. Net 14B greater than 0.75 diopter<br>5. Reduced amplitude of accommodate of more than 2 diopters below Donders' Age Expecteds, or greater than 0.50 diopter difference between the two eyes |

## Table 17.7
### Vergence System

| Symptoms of Difficulties | Findings Indicating Difficulties |
|---|---|
| 1. Asthenopia at distance and/or near<br>2. Intermittent diplopia at either distance or near<br>3. Patient confused about what is seen<br>4. Patient reports closing or covering one eye<br>5. Repetition of letters within words or difficulty aligning columns of numbers<br>6. Patient manifests a head tilt<br>7. Postural changes noted when working at a desk<br>8. Letters, words, or both appear to float or move around | 1. A near point of convergence manifesting a break-point greater than 5 cm and/or a recovery greater than 8 cm<br>2. Phoria at distance greater or less than 0.2 exophoria<br>3. Phoria at near greater or less than 0.6 exophoria<br>4. Distance vergence ranges:<br>Base-out to blur—less than 7 prism diopters<br>Break of less than 15 diopters<br>Recovery of less than 8 prism diopters<br>Recovery of less than 3 prism diopters<br>5. Near-vergence ranges<br>Base-out to blur less than 14 prism diopters<br>Break less than 18 prism diopters<br>Recovery less than 7 prism diopters<br>6. Opposing vergence blur should be twice the phoria<br>7. A manifest fixation disparity of any amount<br>8. Flipper prisms with 4 base-in and 8 base-out lenses at distance and 8 base-in and 12 base-out at near. The prisms are used as in the accommodative flipper test and the patient views a 20/30 line of print. 8–10 cycles/min expected. |

### Table 17.8
### Sensory System

| Symptoms of Difficulties | Findings Indicating Difficulties |
|---|---|
| 1. Report of the loss or absence of stereopsis<br>2. Report of the sensation that both eyes are "not working together"<br>3. Patient reporting that one eye is not seeing as clearly as the other<br>4. Report of turning his head away from the straight ahead position in order to get the clearest image | 1. Lack of second- or third-degree fusion as manifested on the Worth 4-dot or red lens test and tests for stereopsis, respectively.<br>2. The patient should manifest better than 60 seconds of arc on tests for stereopsis. (It is important that tests for the stereopsis be done at appropriate distances or be recalculated to give accurate results.)<br>3. The patient should be able to manifest far-point simultaneous binocular vision on the 20/30 line of the vectographic slide.<br>4. Any difference of greater than one line visual acuity after correction between the two eyes, or worse than 20/25 corrected acuity in both eyes. |

# Perceptual Areas

The areas of concern to optometry are loosely grouped below. The outline includes behavioral signs and symptoms and screening tests for the five perceptual areas.

I. Perceptual motor coordination: the ability to coordinate bilateral gross motor tasks with the effective use of visually guided movement
  A. Behavioral signs and symptoms
    1. Lack of coordination and balance between two sides of systems
    2. Excessive falling and banging into objects
    3. Poor athletic performance
    4. Tends to play with younger children
    5. Difficulty with rhythmic activities
    6. Difficulty sitting or standing still and generally controlling motor activities
    7. Tendency to work with one side of the body while other side doesn't participate
    8. Can't sit still
  B. Testing
    1. Southern California Perceptual Motor Survey
    2. Purdue Perceptual Motor Survey

II. Laterality/directionality: laterality relates to the internal awareness of the two sides of the body, directionality to projecting this internal awareness into external space
  A. Behavioral signs and symptoms
    1. Difficulty learning right and left
    2. Reverses letters and words when writing or copying
    3. May read either left to right or right to left
  B. Testing
    1. Piaget Right/Left Awareness test
    2. Jordan Reversal-frequency test (Gardner)

III. Visual perceptual discrimination and attention skills
  A. Form perception/discrimination: ability to discriminate dominant features in different objects; for example, the ability to discriminate position, shapes, forms, and also colors and letterlike forms

1. Behavioral signs and symptoms
   a. Confusion of likeness and minor differences
   b. Mistakes words with similar beginnings
   c. Tends to use other senses to make what should be visual discriminations (tactile, kinesthetic, and verbal).
   d. Difficulty recognizing the same word repeated on the same page
   e. May have difficulty recognizing letters or even simple forms
   f. Tends to overgeneralize when placing objects into classes
2. Testing
   a. Motor Free Visual Perceptual test
   b. Frostig Developmental Test of Visual Perception

B. Figure ground: ability to distinguish an object from its background
   1. Behavioral signs and symptoms
      a. Difficulty determining what is significant from what is insignificant
      b. Tends either to stop work before completion or perseveres on details when copying, writing, or drawing
      c. Tendency to have difficulty completing work
      d. Unaware of what should be attended to
      e. Performs slowly compared to peers
   2. Testing
      a. Motor Free Visual Perceptual test
      b. Southern California Figure Ground test
      c. Frostig Developmental Test of Visual Perception

C. Visual closure: ability to identify incomplete figures when only fragments are presented
   1. Behavioral signs and symptoms
      a. Ignores details when doing visual tasks
      b. May be able to perform several parts of task but cannot put them together
      c. Work incomplete
      d. Performs slowly compared to peers
      e. May manifest poor comprehension when doing visual tasks such as reading
   2. Testing
      a. Motor Free Visual Perceptual test
      b. Visual closure, subtest of Illinois Test of Psycholinguistic Abilities (ITPA)

D. Visual memory and sequencing: ability to recall dominant features of one stimulus item or to remember the sequence of several items
   1. Behavioral signs and symptoms
      a. Difficulty visualizing what is read
      b. Poor comprehension
      c. Difficulty learning new materials
      d. Difficulty anticipating next step in tasks presented
      e. Poor spelling
      f. Poor recall of visually presented materials
      g. Tends to whisper to himself when reading silently
      h. Uses other sensory support when doing visual tasks
      i. Difficulty with mathematical concepts
      j. Difficulty placing visual information into groups
      k. Difficulty with tasks that require more than one step
   2. Testing
      a. Motor Free Visual Perceptual test

      b. Visual Attention Span for Letters

      c. Monroe-Sherman Visual III

IV. Visual motor integration and organization abilities: ability to integrate visual discrimination with the eye-hand coordination system to motorically reproduce a pattern from a model

  A. Behavioral signs and symptoms

    1. Sloppy writing or drawing skills

    2. Poor spacing and inability to stay on lines

    3. Excessive erasures when doing written work

    4. Uses hands to keep place when writing or reading

    5. Poor performance of eye-hand coordination tasks

    6. Poor ability to properly place materials on page when drawing or writing

    7. Can respond orally but cannot get answers on paper

    8. Seems to know materials but does poorly when tested

  B. Testing

    1. Winterhaven Copy Forms

    2. Developmental Test of Visual Motor Integration (Berry)

    3. Bender-Gestalt Drawing test

    4. Rutger's Drawing test

V. Auditory perceptual discrimination: ability to discriminate between pairs of words different in a single phoneme or analyze single words into their separate parts (phonemes)

  A. Behavioral signs and symptoms

    1. Confuses similar words presented verbally

    2. Tendency to ignore auditorially presented materials

    3. Poor spelling

    4. Difficulty relating what is seen with what is heard

    5. Difficulty relating symbols to their sounds

    6. Difficulty with phonic method of learning to read

  B. Testing

    1. Wepman Auditory Discrimination test

    2. Rosner's Test of Auditory Analysis Skills

# Perceptual Screening

A screening battery can be developed to evaluate the areas of concern outlined above. An example might be:

1. Reversal-frequency test (Gardner) provides information about the child's acquisition of directionality skills by measuring letter and number reversals in children aged 5 through 12 years.

2. The Motor Free Visual Perception Test avoids motor involvement and assesses visual perception in five areas: spatial relationships, visual discrimination, figure-ground, visual closure, and visual memory.

3. Developmental Test of Visual Motor Integration (Berry), as the name implies, investigates visual-motor integration by assessing the child's ability to copy a series of increasingly difficult geometric forms.

4. Rosner's Test of Auditory Analysis Skills tests the child's ability to analyze words into their component parts (phonemes).

There are numerous tests that can be substituted, but the clinician must remember that objectivity is essential in diagnosis. Each of these standardized tests provides guidelines for administration and scoring. Results are then evaluated by comparison to normative scales to evaluate the child's developmental status. When the clinician selects testing instruments to evaluate a patient's perceptual skills, this issue of objectivity must be considered. Standard test results also facilitate communication between school personnel and the optometrist.

Although objectivity is essential, test scores are only part of the process of arriving at an accurate diagnosis. Observations must also be made of the patient's behavior. In addition to behavioral signs already listed, the clinician should be a sensitive observer during administration of the test. Some clues to developmental status are

1. Close working distance
2. Blinking or rubbing eyes
3. Inadequate pencil grip
4. Excessive pencil pressure
5. Excessive erasures
6. Need to trace figures with the fingers
7. Impulsive behavior
8. Low frustration level
9. Poor attentiveness
10. Needs instructions repeated frequently

If children younger than 5 years are evaluated, the Denver Developmental Screening Test (DDST) serves as an excellent screening instrument.

The DDST is made up of 105 items, with the examiner testing the child on only 20 or so simple tasks or items. These items are arranged on the test form in four sections.

1. Personal-social: tasks that indicate the child's ability to get along with people and to take care of himself
2. Fine-motor-adaptive: the child's ability to see and to use his hands to pick up objects and to draw
3. Language: the child's ability to hear, follow directions, and to speak
4. Gross motor: the child's ability to sit, walk, and jump

By interpreting the results, the examiner can evaluate whether the child shows normal, questionable, or abnormal development in each of these areas.

Since symptoms alone are not diagnostic, the number reported is unimportant, although they may reflect the severity of the problems. Their presence only serves to alert the clinician to the possibility of deficiencies in a particular area. These must be further evaluated by clinical testing and careful observation. On the other hand, aberrant clinical findings without symptoms would be considered suspect, initiating further questioning of patient and parent. Therefore, symptoms reported by the child or behavior signs reported by parents or teachers should correlate with clinical findings in order to achieve a final diagnosis.

# CLINICAL SIGNIFICANCE

The goal of the optometric evaluation of children with learning problems is to identify visual efficiency or perceptual development deficits that may be contributing to the child's problem of responding to educational teaching. An educational system expects that the child will have acquired the basic visual and perceptual skills necessary to facilitate learning. Unfortunately, only upon the child's failure to succeed is there an interest in investigating whether these skills are developed appropriately. It is likely that only a small percentage of children have learning problems caused solely by visual problems. On the other hand, there may be many more whose learning difficulties are exacerbated by visual and/or perceptual difficulties.

The incidence of significant refractive, visual acuity, or ocular health problems is reported to be no higher in children with learning problems than in children achieving normally. Nevertheless, the examiner should be sensitive to small hyperopic refractive errors, as they may be related to accommodative deficits discovered in the visual efficiency evaluation. There may not be any blurring or discomfort symptoms reported, but rather a decline in reading efficiency or an avoidance of close work.

Many children will be found to have difficulty with accommodative skills, especially facility and accommodative posture. Initially, difficulties in accommodation may not prevent a child from learning to read, since the print is large and attentional demands minimal. When prolonged reading is attempted, however, children may experience asthenopia or use the defense mechanism of avoidance to deal with the problem. Similarly, for the child with poor vergence skills, reading may become quite laborious and associated with fatigue or possible avoidance. Numerous studies have recently presented evidence that supports the contention that a primary eye movement abnormality may play a contributing role in reading problems. Most reports have stressed that inadequate readers tend to make frequent regressions, an increased number of fixations, longer pauses between saccades, and abnormalities in the return sweep. These visual efficiency problems may affect attention, which might result in the inability to perform or even to develop adequate visual perceptual skills.

Children found to have perceptual difficulties may be difficult to teach, failing to understand and grasp basic concepts and ideas. Perceptual motor integration problems result in poor gross motor skills, causing difficulty with peer and social adjustment. Significant difficulties may necessitate a referral to an occupational therapist or adaptive physical education teacher for further evaluation and special physical education considerations. Deficient development of bilateral integration may contribute to poor body awareness and an inability to visually guide the motor system and may lead then to difficulties with laterality and directionality concepts. This may result in significant problems with reversals, especially with letters such as b, d, p, and q, which are directional dependent. Form perception and discrimination may result in the child having difficulty with learning the alphabet, word recognition, and basic math concepts of size, magnitude, and position. Figure ground difficulties may result in poor selective attention skills, making it difficult for the child to attend to the important features of a visual display. Visual memory and visualization skills problems may contribute to poor comprehension, spelling, and sight vocabulary. Visual-motor integration difficulties may manifest in poor written work or unusually long periods of time to complete written work.

Auditory perceptual skills relate heavily to reading, especially in the decoding phase, when the phonetic approach to reading is being taught. Difficulties detected in this area necessitate a referral to the school or outside source for a speech and hearing evaluation. The evaluation should include not only testing for auditory acuity, but for auditory perceptual skills as well.

These types of problems often interfere with efficient learning and may seriously impair an individual's ability to respond to standard teaching. Efficient learning depends on accurate assimilation of printed symbols. Any factor that makes this process less efficient may serve to interfere, to some degree, with learning. Learning problems appear to arise when the negative factors tending to contribute to learning problems become too intense or numerous.

The child's problem may be complicated still further when adults decide to "wait and see" if "he will grow out of it." Rarely do children outgrow a problem before complications occur. Generally, the child falls even further behind during the period of "wait and see." Early intervention is essential to shortcut failure and possible associated emotional disturbances.

Clinicians will set their own levels of involvement. Some elect to diagnose problem areas and then refer to appropriate sources for their correction; others decide to treat the visual and perceptual deficits in their own office. It must be emphasized that school underachievement requires a multidisciplinary approach from education, psychology, medicine, and optometry for complete evaluation and successful remediation. The importance of the vision specialist in the diagnosis and treatment of these children is generally no greater than the participation of specialists from other disciplines, with each viewing the problem as primarily within their discipline. What must be recognized and emphasized is that there is no single known cause. Learning problems are brought about by a multiplicity of factors, many of which are interrelated.

Optometry must accept its responsibility, as a primary care vision provider, to identify those youngsters who can profit from appropriate visual and perceptual diagnosis and treatment. Since visual efficiency and perceptual problems are readily detected, and in most cases treatable, it would seem appropriate to be sure that these factors are not contributing to the child's learning problem.

# References

Bower TGR. Perceptual world of the child. Cambridge, Mass.: Harvard University Press, 1977.

Carter DB, ed. Interdisciplinary approaches to learning disorders. Philadelphia: Chilton Book Company, 1970.

Greenstein TN, ed. Vision and learning disability. St. Louis: American Optometric Association, 1976.

Hoffman LG. An optometric learning disability evaluation. Optom Monthly 1979;70(2):118–121;70(3);201–205; 70(4):279–283.

Hoffman LG, Rouse MW. Referral recommendations for binocular function and/or developmental perceptual deficiencies. J Am Optom Assoc 1980; 51(2):119–125.

Holt KS. Developmental pediatrics—perspectives and practice. Woburn, Mass.: Butterworth, 1977.

Rosinski R. The development of visual perception. Santa Monica, Calif.: Goodyear, 1977.

Solan HA, ed. The treatment and management of children with learning disabilities. Springfield: Charles C Thomas, 1982.

Wold RM, ed. Visual and perceptual aspects for the achieving and underachieving child. Seattle: Special Child Publications, 1969.

Wold RM, ed. Vision: its impact on learning. Seattle: Special Child Publications, 1978.

# III

# ASSESSMENT OF THE EYE AND VISION SYSTEM

# J. David Higgins
# PUPIL 18

*The pupil is the central aperture in the iris-diaphragm*
*responsible for controlling retinal illumination.*

## BACKGROUND

Pupil size is determined by the relative tonus in two sets of opposing smooth muscles: the radially oriented dilator, which is sympathetically innervated, and the circumferentially oriented sphincter, which is parasympathetically innervated. The sphincter has more influence in determining pupillary size. Dilator tonus acts more as an opposing spring, permitting rapid and full mydriasis when sphincter tone is released.

Lesions affecting the sphincter result in incomplete miosis in bright light. Thus, anisocoria greater in bright light implies a defect in the parasympathetic pathway on the side of the more mydriatic pupil. A sympathetic defect fails to produce much effect when the sphincters are active, with the hallmark being slow and somewhat incomplete dilation in darkness—that is, anisocoria in dim light, especially in the first few seconds, with the more miotic pupil being on the side of the sympathetic lesion.

Approximately 20% of the population show a perceptible amount of anisocoria (physiologic anisocoria), with the pupillary difference being equal or slightly more obvious in dim versus bright illumination. More marked anisocoria often shows a family tendency, and the extent of the defect may vary considerably from day to day.

A subset of retinal ganglion cells serve as the afferent arc for the light reflex. These pupillary fibers leave the tracts prior to the lateral geniculate body to reach their central pretectal synapse alongside the aqueduct near the posterior commissure. Slightly in excess of 50% of the pupillary fibers cross in the chiasm, and again after the central pretectal synapse on the way to the Edinger-Westphal components of the third nerve nuclei (Figure 18.1). These crossing biases account for sophisticated pupillometric recordings finding the direct response to be slightly in excess of the consensual, and for the pupillary escape that can sometimes be seen when a normal eye is obliquely stimulated to illuminate temporal retina while its partner receives nasal stimulation.

The manner in which the accommodation-related input reaches the third nerve nucleus is poorly understood; however, midbrain lesions affecting fibers just approaching or leaving the pretectal synapse often abolish the light reflex but spare the accommodative reflex.

The parasympathetic pupillary outflow of the Edinger-Westphal nucleus is via the third nerves, which emerge from the brain ventrally between the cerebral peduncles

189

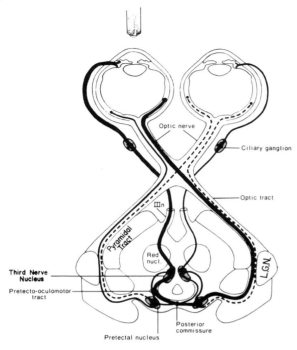

**FIGURE 18.1.**
Light reflex pathway showing partial decussation of pupillary afferents both in chiasm and tectum. Crossing fibers at both locations are drawn heavier to indicate their greater weight in producing pupillary drive.
Adapted from Thompson HS, ed. Topics in neuroophthalmology. Baltimore: Williams & Wilkins, 1979.

in the lateral gray of $T_1$ and $T_2$ (Figure 18.2). Preganglionic fibers exit at this level into the thorax and ascend the sympathetic chain to synapse in the superior cervical ganglion. From here, postganglionic fibers follow the carotid artery to reach the orbit by way of the superior orbital fissure and the long ciliary nerves. Fibers serving the sweat glands of the face leave those destined for the iris dilator and Müller's muscle of the lids at the level of the carotid bifurcation. This anatomic fact has clinical localizing significance.

A wide variety of influences affect the size of the pupils. Miotic pupils are the rule in infancy, senility, and sleep and are often observed in long-standing diabetes where they may be slightly irregular, difficult to dilate, and show a bit of pupillary atrophy to transillumination (pseudo-Argyll Robertson pupil). Direct and indirect cholinergic agents used in glaucoma commonly render the pupils miotic, as do organic phosphate insecticides and morphine derivatives. Miotic, but reactive, pupils are characteristic of comatose patients suffering from brain stem injuries. Miosis is also a hallmark of intraocular inflammation.

Mydriatic pupils are characteristic in youth, blonds, myopes, blue-eyed people, and in anxiety, but also of pheochromocytomas and hyperthyroidism. A wide variety of sympathomimetic and anticholingeric substances may render the pupils somewhat mydriatic, such as over-the-counter decongestants, antihistamines, gastric motility inhibitors, and others. The most important substances are lead, arsenic, and rarely, those associated with botulism and diphtheria toxins, where accommodation is usually affected as well.

When facing an apparently healthy patient with a fixed dilated pupil, it is always appropriate to consider the possibility that the patient accidentally placed a substance in the eye, especially if a hospital worker. In contrast to neurologic lesion, such pharmacologically blocked pupils will not constrict to a drop of pilocarpine 2%. This should not be attempted if there is

and then course forward alongside the posterior communicating arteries to pierce the wall of the cavernous sinus. The pupillary fibers travel superficially in the nerve, perhaps accounting for their relative sensitivity to compression. In the sinus, the third nerve is closely related to the first and second divisions of the fifth nerve before entering the orbit via the superior orbital fissure to synapse at the ciliary ganglion. Postganglionic fibers then reach the sphincter via the short ciliary nerves.

From its central origin in the posterior hypothalamus, sympathetic pupillary efferents traverse the brain stem to synapse

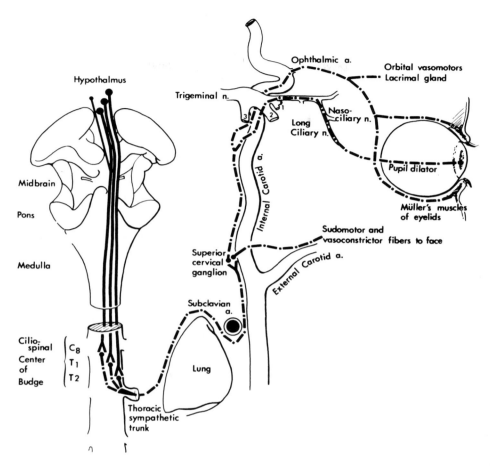

**FIGURE 18.2.**
**Sympathetic pathway to eye.**
Reprinted by permission of the publisher, from Glaser J. Neuro-
ophthalmology. Hagerstown, Md.: Harper & Row, 1978.

any strong suspicion of a neurologic disorder, as drug-induced miosis will render
the pupil untestable should the condition
rapidly evolve into an acute neurologic
syndrome.

Myoneural blockage by trauma often
produces sector or complete pupillary paresis and usually is not a clinical problem
to the examiner. Similarly, mydriasis
caused by reflex irritation, as from a foreign body or myoneural failure in acute
glaucoma, usually is well recognized and
does not pose a problem in interpretation.

# EXAMINATION

The afferent pupillary pathway is tested by
the "swinging flashlight test." Here the examiner directs the patient's fixation to a
distant object in a nearly darkened room.

A bright steady penlight is then shown *directly* into the pupil for a second or two until maximum miosis occurs and then abruptly switched to directly stimulate the contralateral eye. After a brief rest the procedure is reversed. In normal eyes both pupils will be seen to hold their size immediately after switching, the critical observation moment. When an optic nerve conduction defect exists the pupils will spring open a bit immediately upon switching the penlight to the suspect eye (pupillary escape or Marcus Gunn pupil) and usually reconstrict a little bit when the penlight is again switched to stimulate the good side. When in doubt, it is sometimes necessary to repeat the test several times to be sure of the response because of the effects of normal hippus and pupillary fatigue. It is important to stress that a maximum stimulus to miosis be used: dark room, distance fixation, and a bright steady light. Allowing accommodation to fluctuate, stimulating eccentrically, and waiting too long before switching will all diminish the power of the test and can produce false positives and false negatives.

The efferent pathway is tested by looking for pupillary inequality both under conditions of full illumination and under dim illumination. The shape of the pupil is best evaluated using the slit lamp. Comparing the size of the pupils in full room illumination presents no difficulty, but doing so in dim illumination is difficult if the irises are dark. It is often helpful to use oblique illumination from the penlight, such as prior to checking for the depth of the anterior chambers. Have the patient fixate in the distance and stimulate one eye with the penlight, and then move the penlight a foot or two away below the line of sight, still illuminating the pupils while observing redilation for anisocoria.

If anisocoria is observed to be about equal in extent in dim and bright illumination it is almost certainly physiologic. Nevertheless, lid position should still be checked for possible Horner's syndrome. If anisocoria is observed to be more notable in dim illumination, it represents a relative loss of sympathetic tone in the more miotic pupil. Always carefully observe lid position for signs of Horner's syndrome. A convenient shorthand for recording such a finding would be "anisocoria OD>OS (1 mm)>dark, lids equal." If the anisocoria is greater in bright illumination, this can never be recorded as physiologic and strongly suggests a third nerve defect on the side of the more mydriatic pupil if no obvious ocular cause of the defect exists (e.g., posterior synechiae). All cases of anisocoria should be pointed out to the patient and old pictures secured if the anisocoria gives any signs of not being of the physiologic variety.

Only when the pupils show almost no sign of a response to light (use slit lamp) is it necessary to evaluate the response to near. This is best accomplished by having the patient shift his gaze from distance to his own finger held a few inches in front of the face. If the response to near exceeds the response to light it is so recorded, and the examiner must now consider a variety of entities (tonic pupil, Argyll Robertson pupil, and Parinaud's syndrome).

# CLINICAL SIGNIFICANCE

## Marcus Gunn Pupil

Afferent pupillary defects strongly implicate a conduction defect in the neural pathways, even in the presence of normal or near normal visual acuity. Pupillary escape owing to retinal lesion or media opacity is distinctly uncommon and would be associated with obvious pathology of disastrous proportions. While this test should be done routinely, it should be done compulsively, or even repeated, in infants and young children and in any patient in whom refraction fails to produce equal visions and the cause is not apparent. By virtue of permitting a longer working distance, the indirect ophthalmoscope can be very valuable in assessing pupillary reactions in blepharospastic infants who would not tolerate instruments near the face. Patients with occult neurologic lesions affecting the conduction pathways often complain of dim vision, poor contrast, faded appearance to colors, and difficulty at night. Such complaints must be taken seriously even with 20/20 acuity; looking for an afferent pupillary defect is one simple and objective component of a battery of tests that should be run on all patients whose visual loss is unexplained (see Chapter 4).

A wide variety of optic nerve lesions will produce a Marcus Gunn pupil: inflammatory, neoplastic, demyelinating, nutritional, toxic, and so on. In the presence of homonymous hemianopia with undisturbed Snellen acuities, the observation of pupillary escape ipsilateral to the field defect strongly implicates a lesion in the contralateral optic tract. When tract lesions impinge on the chiasm the acuities may be affected, and a Marcus Gunn pupil will be manifest in the more severely involved eye, usually ipsilateral to the lesion.

## Anisocoria More Marked in Bright Light

The observation of increased pupillary inequality to stimulation by bright light always requires a search for an important third nerve lesion on the side of the larger pupil. Thus, ptosis and accommodation defects should be sought, as well as signs of inconcomitancy indicating involvement of the extraocular muscles served by the third nerve. Look for signs of aberrant regeneration where miosis may occur on up gaze or adduction. Periorbital sensation should be compared to wisps of cotton on both sides, and the corneal reflex should be tested to assess fifth nerve function. The orbit and retromastoid fossa should be auscultated for bruits suggesting a possible posterior communicating artery aneurysm, which may present with isolated internal third nerve involvement. In older patients, a history of antecedent head trauma in the preceding weeks should suggest that chronic subdural hematoma is beginning to herniate the cerebrum through the tentorium to impinge upon the brain stem (Figure 18.3). Such patients are likely to appear somewhat confused and are usually suffering from headache. The observation of a Hutchinson's pupil represents a true emergency.

A variety of other masses may occasionally present with isolated pupillary involvement, but when there is no company, one is usually dealing with Adie's tonic pupil. Affected patients are usually healthy young women who often present acutely noting either the anisocoria or blurred near vision in the eye because of simultaneous involvement of the accommodative fibers. This entity usually represents benign idiopathic lesion in the postganglionic fibers at or distal to the ciliary ganglion in the orbit. In 20% of the cases, the fellow eye may become fully involved. In an acute presentation, the diagnosis is usually made from the lack of company in a healthy patient and by the distinctive slit lamp appearance of sector paresis, where small arcs of the pupillary circumference will still show their normal radius compared to flatter unreactive segments (Figure 18.4). Interestingly, the sector paresis may be associated with sectors of corneal anesthesia and clinically measurable astigmatic accommodation, both of which tend to improve with time as contrasted with the pupil. In these intact areas, iris folds will be seen upon light stimulation with the typical vermiform attempts at contraction. In fresh cases, the pathognomonic tonicity may not be clearly manifest. This is sought by having the patient fixate the thumb a few inches away from the face in a bright room for several minutes; if the

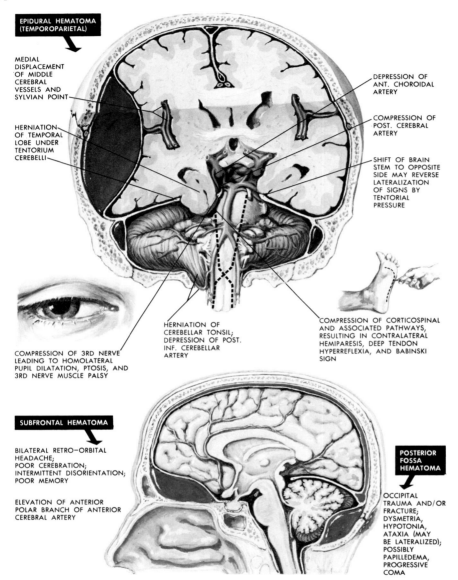

EPIDURAL HEMATOMA
(TEMPOROPARIETAL)

MEDIAL
DISPLACEMENT
OF MIDDLE
CEREBRAL
VESSELS AND
SYLVIAN POINT

HERNIATION
OF TEMPORAL
LOBE UNDER
TENTORIUM
CEREBELLI

DEPRESSION OF
ANT. CHOROIDAL
ARTERY

COMPRESSION OF
POST. CEREBRAL
ARTERY

SHIFT OF BRAIN
STEM TO OPPOSITE
SIDE MAY REVERSE
LATERALIZATION
OF SIGNS BY
TENTORIAL
PRESSURE

COMPRESSION OF 3RD NERVE
LEADING TO HOMOLATERAL
PUPIL DILATATION, PTOSIS, AND
3RD NERVE MUSCLE PALSY

HERNIATION OF
CEREBELLAR TONSIL;
DEPRESSION OF POST.
INF. CEREBELLAR
ARTERY

COMPRESSION OF CORTICOSPINAL
AND ASSOCIATED PATHWAYS,
RESULTING IN CONTRALATERAL
HEMIPARESIS, DEEP TENDON
HYPERREFLEXIA, AND BABINSKI
SIGN

SUBFRONTAL HEMATOMA

BILATERAL RETRO–ORBITAL
HEADACHE;
POOR CEREBRATION;
INTERMITTENT DISORIENTATION;
POOR MEMORY

ELEVATION OF ANTERIOR
POLAR BRANCH OF ANTERIOR
CEREBRAL ARTERY

POSTERIOR
FOSSA
HEMATOMA

OCCIPITAL
TRAUMA AND/OR
FRACTURE;
DYSMETRIA,
HYPOTONIA,
ATAXIA (MAY
BE LATERALIZED);
POSSIBLY
PAPILLEDEMA,
PROGRESSIVE
COMA

**FIGURE 18.3.**
Signs and symptoms in epidural and subdural hemorrhage. Ipsilateral
mydriasis may be the presenting sign of early tentorial herniation many
weeks after head trauma in a case of "chronic" subdural hematoma.

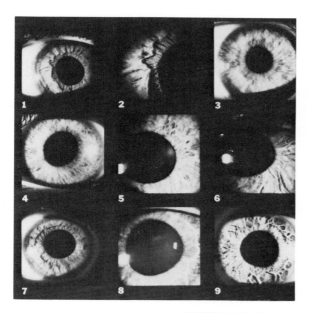

**FIGURE 18.4.**
Nine cases of Adie's syndrome emphasizing frequency of pupillary irregularity. Note sectors having intact "accordion folds" adjacent to flatter radius sections, which are denervated, e.g., at 11 o'clock in *photo 2,* and at 12 o'clock in *photo 8.*
Reprinted by permission of the publisher, from Thompson HS. Segmented palsy of the iris sphincter in Adie's syndrome. Arch Ophthalmol 1978;96:1615–1620. Copyright 1978, American Medical Association.

(knee and ankle jerks); a few patients may show more generalized autonomic involvement with segmental loss of sweating (Ross's syndrome), orthostatic hypotension, or migraine. Such patients are more likely to demonstrate bilateral pupil involvement.

When an Adie's pupil is of some duration, the sphincter muscle may become hypersensitive to cholinergic stimulation. Such denervation sensitivity is manifest by application of $\frac{1}{16}$% pilocarpine, which constricts the Adie's pupil but usually not the normal eye. A good slip lamp exam of the normal eye may also show slight flattening of small arcs in the pupillary margin, indicating bilateral but asymmetrical involvement, a helpful corroborating sign.

In all cases it is necessary to look for signs of orbital involvement (engorged conjunctival veins, proptosis), as even a postganglionic lesion may occasionally represent a mass (e.g., lymphoma, sarcoidosis). As both tonicity and hypersensitivity may not be present in the more important cases of recent onset, the slit lamp exam of both eyes, history, and general neuroophthalmologic exam are paramount to diagnosis. The significance of Adie's pupil is to distinguish it from serious causes of an internal third nerve paresis.

pupil seems to have gotten slightly smaller one then looks for tonic redilation as the patient shifts fixation to a distant object, where several minutes may be required for the pupil to open up when viewed against its partner in dim light. The observation of tonic redilation virtually makes the diagnosis. Interestingly, if an Adie's pupil is first noted in the dim light of the exam room it often appears smaller than its partner until tonic redilation occurs. This should not confuse the astute examiner.

Many patients with Adie's pupil show associated defects in the deep tendon reflexes, especially in the lower extremities

## Midbrain Pupils

When both pupils show little or no response to light one must consider the presence of a toxic substance, bilateral Adie's syndrome, myopathy/neuropathy, or a midbrain lesion affecting the input/output of the pretectal synapse. The hallmark of midbrain pupils is that the response to near-point stimulation is usually normal, or even enhanced, such that it exceeds a greatly diminished or absent response to light. This point usually serves to distinguish it from other causes of diminished pupillary responses (toxins, chronic alcoholism, multiple sclerosis, diabetes, and occasionally myotonic dystrophy or severe hypothyroidism).

The Argyll Robertson variety of the midbrain pupil is nearly pathognomonic for neurosyphilis. Besides its almost universal bilaterality and predominance of the near response over the light response (Figure 18.5), these pupils are typically miotic, somewhat irregular, show a bit of pupillary iris atrophy to slit lamp iris transillumination, and are difficult to dilate. These signs are similar to the pupils in long-standing diabetes, except for the paradoxical near response, which is only rarely present in diabetes. Even in the absence of a positive history of syphilis, the pupil may be the sole presenting sign prior to onset of general paresis or tabes. Securing a VDRL and especially an FTA-ABS is essential in these cases.

The other major variant of the midbrain pupil is that accompanying the sylvian aqueduct (Parinaud's syndrome). Here the pupils are also fixed to light, but often respond to near; however, these pupils tend to be semidilated rather than miotic. Other parts of the syndrome that may be present are accommodative and convergence paresis, lid retraction, and an incomplete vertical gaze apraxia usually more notable in up gaze. Bell's reflex is usually normal, and even upward refixations or pursuits may be intact; however, voluntary up gaze is usually absent (say "Look up, please!"). Convergent/retraction nystagmus is pathognomonic for the condition and is observed by rotating an optokinetic target downward, whereupon jerky convergence or retraction of the eyes is seen in place of the normal upbeat nystagmus. In some cases, vertical gaze may be asymmetrically affected, producing diplopia in up gaze. Because of the staring appearance (posterior fossa stare) and lack of up gaze, thyroid myopathy may be wrongly suspected if other aspects of the syndrome are not looked for. The more prominent causes of Parinaud's syndrome are occlusion of the deep penetrating twigs of the posterior cerebral artery in the el-

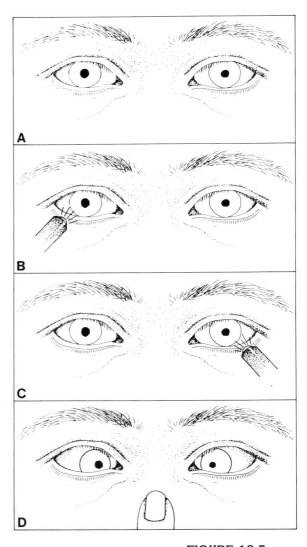

**FIGURE 18.5.**
*A.* Typical miotic and irregular appearance of pupils in neurosyphilis. *B,C.* Neither pupil reacts well to light, but a definite response is seen to a near stimulus (*D*).

derly and racemose AV malformations, and especially pinealomas in younger patients in whom increased intracranial pressure may also be manifest early in the clinical course.

While unilateral light-near disassociation can occur, it is rare. Always consider anomalous regeneration of the third nerve. Here fibers destined for the medial rectus may regrow to serve the iris sphincter, and miosis will occur on adduction as well as convergence. While such anomalous innervation may be congenital, it also follows third nerve palsies, especially those caused by mass lesions.

## Horner's Syndrome

Sympathetic denervation of the Horner's pupil produces slow incomplete redilation in dim light. Anisocoria will be observed to be more marked in darkness, implicating the more miotic pupil as part of a Horner's syndrome. In most cases, small (less than 1 mm) amounts of anisocoria, observed to be slightly more apparent in dim light, are benign. The more miotic eye must always be scrutinized for mild ptosis, however, owing to concomitant loss of sympathetic tone in Müller's muscles.

It must be emphasized that both the relative miosis and the ptosis need not be marked in a Horner's syndrome. The smaller pupil may give nearly an equal measurement between the top of the pupils and upper lid margins, masking the ptosis; so it is important to search for "upside-down ptosis" or lack of sympathetic retraction of the lower lid as well (Figure 18.6). This is not invariably present, but is best viewed by sighting over a fixation light in the midline while depressing the patient's chin and noting whether the limbus is first exposed in the contralateral eye. Other confirmatory signs of sympathetic pupillary paresis are in noting maximal anisocoria several seconds after removing the light stimulus (slow redilation) and a relative hypotony on the involved side. Central sympathetic stimulation may serve to enhance the anisocoria as well as startling the patient by dropping a book or pinching the nape of the neck. Occasionally, a patient with Horner's syndrome may notice relative accommodative inertia in looking near to far, but

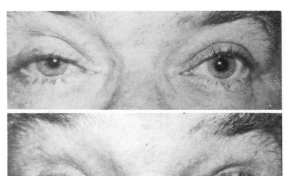

**FIGURE 18.6.**
Horner's syndrome with pupillary miosis and ptosis of both upper and lower lids evident in right eye (*top*). Lack of response to 4% cocaine further confirms the clinical diagnosis (*bottom*).
Reprinted by permission of the publisher, from Glaser JS. Case presentation D: anomalies of the pupil—Raeder's paratrigeminal syndrome. New Orleans Academy of Ophthalmology, Symposium on Neuro-ophthalmology. St. Louis: C.V. Mosby, 1976.

this is usually not manifest as a clinical symptom. Finally, on rare occasions the distinctive appearance of an irritative Horner's syndrome may present, wherein mydriasis and lid retraction may precede sympathetic failure.

Horner's syndrome is a significant finding, as approximately one-third of fresh cases without obvious cause are due to neoplasms. Since the most important lesions occur prior to the superior cervical ganglion (preganglionic), the clinical appearance is paramount, as these pupils show no reliable distinguishing attributes to any sort of pharmacologic testing. If the lesions occur proximal to the carotid bifurcation, the clinician may search for facial anhidrosis on the involved side. In most offices electrodermal impedance or iodine-starch testing is not done, and one may grossly assess this feature by tightly taping down a piece of plastic over talcum powder on each side of the face and observing whether sweating is induced to cake the powder.

The onset of the syndrome can often be dated if it is either very recent or congenital/infantile. In a fresh Horner's syndrome, the eye may show transient erythema and tearing. Hypotony is much more characteristic of a fresh case as well. When onset is congenital, the iris on the involved side is often lighter in color under daylight or fluorescent lighting, and there may be some facial asymmetry/hemiatrophy owing to loss of trophic innervation in the involved hemiface. In most cases without obvious causes, it is necessary to secure old photographs to document whether the lesion is important in the sense of being of relatively recent onset.

In patients without obvious causes (e.g., endarterectory, thyroidectomy, etc.) and in whom the onset may be recent, it is helpful to know whether the postganglionic fibers remain intact in the dilator. If so, use of the indirect sympathomimetic 1% hydroxyamphetamine (Paredrine) will cause release of norepinephrine, producing mydriasis similar to the good eye. If the lesion is postganglionic, however, the relative miosis will remain and become even more marked after the drops are instilled. It is important to try to obtain equal penetration of the drops. The test should not be done after tonometry; full drops should be placed in the cul-de-sacs in quick succession to avoid the diluting effect of tearing. Lack of stinging on the affected side always suggests simultaneous involvement of nerve V; here, test the corneal reflexes.

Most Horner's pupils show relatively poor dilation to 4% cocaine; however, it is difficult to obtain and keep fresh solutions and the response cannot be relied upon to distinguish among central, preganglionic, and postganglionic lesions. The use of weak epinephrine solutions to identify and localize a Horner's syndrome is no longer considered to have merit. In most offices, therefore, the diagnosis is made by the clinical appearance, and localization is attempted by using hydroxyamphetamine and considering associated signs and symptoms.

Postganglionic Horner's pupils are the most likely to be benign, especially if accompanied by a history of cluster headaches, with which they are often associated. Since the sympathetics follow the carotid artery and are closely related to the first division of the fifth nerve, Paredrine-unreactive Horner's pupils always demand auscultation of the neck and eye and testing of corneal and facial area sensitivity. Cranial nerves III, IV, and VI should, of course, be evaluated and a search for symptoms of nasopharyngioma made (epistaxis, swallowing difficulty, ear/maxillary pain, nasosinus obstruction, blocking and popping of the eustachian tubes, dysarthria, oral paresthesias, etc.).

Prominent causes of Horner's syndrome are many (Table 18.1). The one that must never be forgotten is that of apical lung tumor; all patients with hydroxyamphetamine-responsive pupils should be asked about a recent history of dyspnea, coughing, and shoulder pain.

In general, Horner's pupils that dilate equally to hydroxyamphetamine should be referred to the internist when there is no neurologic company. Paredrine-unresponsive syndromes usually can be safely followed if there is no company, especially when a history of cluster headache exists.

## Table 18.1
### Selected Causes of Horner's Syndrome

| Benign, Cause Suggested via History/Physical Exam | Associated with Potentially Serious and Progressive Disease |
|---|---|
| Congenital (iris heterochromia and facial hemiatrophy may accompany) | 1st neuron (Paredrine reactive) |
| | cervical spurs, dislocated disc, ankylosing spondylitis |
| Cervical/thoracic surgery (radical neck, thyroidectomy, endarterectomy) | syringomyelia/syringobulbia |
| Trauma (pneumothorax, congenital brachial plexus palsy, broken collar bone, from toting skiis on shoulder) | posterior inferior cerebellar artery infarct |
| | cerebellar angioblastoma |
| | tabes |
| Other (congenital cervical rib, prominent cervical nodes, cluster headaches, mandibular tooth abscess) | tumors of the hypothalamus, brain stem, and cervical cord |
| | 2nd neuron (Paredrine reactive) |
| | mediastinal lymphadenopathy (e.g., TB, lymphomas) |
| | aortic aneurysm |
| | masses (chiefly apical lung cancer or granuloma) |
| | 3rd neuron (Paredrine unreactive) |
| | paratrigeminal mass (e.g., meningioma) or nasopharyngioma |
| | atherosclerotic carotid artery dissecting aneurysm |
| | goiter/thyroid cancer |

# References

Adie WJ. Argyll Robertson pupils true and false. Br Med J 1931;2:136–138.

Bell R, Thompson RS. Relative afferent pupillary defect in optic tract hemianopias. Am J Ophthalmol 1978; 85:538–540.

Giles CL, Henderson JW. Horner's syndrome: an analysis of 216 cases. Am J Ophthalmol 1958;46:289–296.

Grimson BS, Thompson HS. Drug testing in Horner's syndrome. In: Glaser JS, Smith JL, eds. Neuro-ophthalmology symposium. St. Louis: C.V. Mosby, 1975;VIII;13:265–270.

McNealy DE, Plum F. Brainstem dysfunction with supratentorial mass lesions. Arch Neurol 1962;7:10–32.

Miller S, Thompson HS. Pupil cycle time in optic neuritis. Am J Ophthalmol 1978;85:635–642.

Seybold ME, et al. Pupillary abnormalities associated with tumors of the pineal region. Neurology 1971;21:232–237.

Thompson HS, Corbett JJ, Cox TA. How to measure the relative afferent pupillary defect. Surv Ophthalmol 1981; 26:39–42.

J. David Higgins
# OCULOMOTOR SYSTEM 19

*Disorders of the oculomotor system can be any departure from normal performance in the quality of fixation, pursuits, saccades, or convergence. Clinical conditions result from lesions in the final common pathway (nerves III, IV, or VI), or in higher "supranuclear" control centers responsible for coordinating precise dynamic bifoveal fixation of the object of regard.*

## BACKGROUND

Cranial nerve lesions may occur at the level of their nuclei, fasciculi within the substance of the brain stem, or in the nerve trunks (see Figures 19.1 and 19.2). Nuclear and fascicular lesions are likely to produce related brain stem neurologic defects, whereas trunk lesions more commonly present with isolated involvement of cranial nerve function. Disease in the extraocular muscles may mimic a neurologic lesion. Regardless of the etiology, the chief symptom of nuclear and infranuclear oculomotor pathology is the acute onset of diplopia.

Acute oculomotor palsy is a noteworthy event, as about one-third of the patients with this condition fail to survive 5 years because of processes related to the CNS lesion itself or to coexisting systemic disease. Even patients with persistent stable palsies of a year's duration or more must be examined regularly, despite apparently normal neurologic status.

The hallmark of supranuclear disease often is the lack of patient symptomatology, and many such disorders are overlooked by both patient and doctor. Proper interpretation of nondiplopia-producing anomalies often is the cornerstone of early neurologic diagnosis. Unlike the relative simplicity of infranuclear pathways, the pathways for supranuclear control are complex, often ill-defined, and involve almost all parts of the brain.

## EXAMINATION

The following discussion highlights the appearance of anomalous oculomotor patterns. Discussions are elaborated in succeeding sections of this chapter.

### Stability of Fixation

Instrument-oriented practitioners may fail to fully assess the gross appearance of the

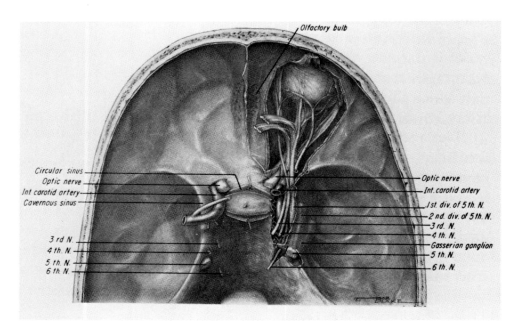

**FIGURE 19.1.**
**View of base of skull from above with orbit and cavernous sinus**
**unroofed on right to show relationships of cranial nerves.**
Reprinted by permission of the publisher, from Odom GL. Ophthalmic involvement in neurologic vascular lesions. In: Smith JL, ed. Neuro-ophthalmology symposium. Springfield, Ill.: Charles C Thomas, 1964.

eyes at rest at the outset of the exam. Unless the patient is directed initially to fixate an object held by the examiner in good room illumination, asymmetry of lid and orbit position, iris color, pupillary size, and fixational stability may be overlooked entirely. All patients, except the very young, anxious, hyperactive, or inattentive, should be able to sustain precise fixation for 10 seconds or more.

In observing fixation, a *peripheral micronystagmus,* such as that associated with vestibular disease, might be manifest. These rhythmic oscillations of the eyes are usually horizontal or horizontally rotary and independent of the position of gaze. With central nystagmus the amplitude usually varies with gaze. *Quiver* is evident as intermittent spring-like oscil-

lations of the eyes during fixation and suggests myasthenia. *Ocular flutter* looks much the same and is likely to occur just before a saccade, but reflects cerebellar disease. Flutter often includes a succession of overshooting and undershooting dysmetric movements at the end of a saccade. *Opsoclonus* is chaotic disassociated movements of both eyes, which often pass through a stage of flutter and then dysmetric movements with recovery.

*Square wave jerks* differ from other nystagmoid movements and exhibit a just perceptible latency between involuntary saccadic oscillations away from fixation and back again. These movements may occur spontaneously to either side of fixation, with amplitudes of from a few degrees to even 15 or 20 degrees. Square wave jerks

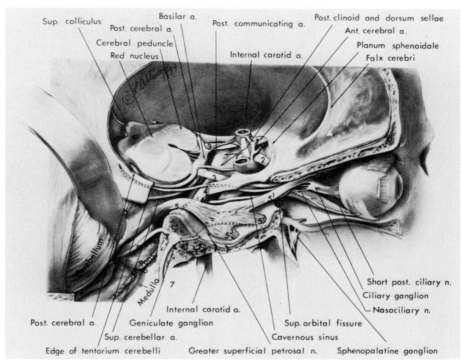

**FIGURE 19.2.**
**Lateral view of the brain showing course of cranial nerves II–VIII from brain stem to orbit.**
Reprinted by permission of the publisher, from Glaser JS. Neuro-ophthalmology. Hagerstown, Md.: Harper & Row, 1978.

give the patient a shifty-eyed or noncooperative appearance and are clearly abnormal. They occur in progressive supranuclear palsy, but are otherwise hallmarks of cerebellar disease, such as ataxic telangiectasia.

Patients with significant brain stem disease, such as basilar artery stroke, may exhibit *ocular myoclonus,* a rapid nystagmoid movement almost always accompanied by similar clonic spasms of the oropharyngeal or even diaphragmatic bulbar musculature. *Ocular bobbing* is also seen in significant brain stem disease and usually accompanies major palsies of gaze. Here the eyes shoot downward and return to the primary position so slowly as to make differentiation from downbeat nystagmus

unmistakable. Bobbing usually is worst when the patient attempts to move the eyes.

Episodic attacks of torsional flicks in one eye represent superior oblique myokymia, typically a benign condition. Other seizure-like movements, called *oculogyric crises,* are seen in chorea (poststreptococcal, Huntington's, postencephalitic parkinsonism, and occasionally with birth control pills). Here the eyes undergo spasmotic sustained eccentric deviations, usually upward. These should be distinguished from lateral deviations seen during a generalized seizure, which suggest a contralateral frontal lobe focus, or from more brief, subtle, and frequent petit mal occurrences in children. These partial seizures may be accompanied by apnea, fluttering of the lids, a cry, and mental absence.

# Position of the Eyes

Occasionally a patient will demonstrate a resting bias of both eyes to one side of midline fixation. This is not an obvious face turn to gain fusion with a horizontal rectus palsy, nor an attempt to quiet gaze nystagmus. The most common cause for such an observation would be lateral gaze palsy caused by brain stem or frontal lobe lesions. A second cause is lateral-pulsion, in which the patient often lists to the side of the eye bias and on attempted saccades will tend to overshoot to the side of the bias and undershoot to the other. This disorder reflects ipsilateral cerebellar disease and is often part of a Wallenberg syndrome, a potential neurologic emergency.

By far the most common cause of anomalous eye position is strabismus (see Chapter 16). This chapter, however, is concerned with nonconcomitant or acute paralytic strabismus, which is always heralded by diplopia unless one eye is severely amblyopic to begin with, or the patient is an infant or toddler.

While characteristics of specific cranial nerves are discussed in the following sections, certain general principles apply. First, unlike decompensating phorias, the onset of a neurologically significant diplopia is never vague, and the patient can usually name the exact time when the symptom began. Second, the extent of the deviation depends on position of gaze always being worst when the eye in question moves into the field of action of the affected nerve or muscle. This may be obvious from simple inspection or by examining symmetry of the pupillary reflexes on version. Quantitative subjective or objective measurements using the prism bars and cover test, Maddox rod, red glass, or Hess screen may be necessary. These tests usually isolate the nature of the palsy in fresh cases. In older lesions, the deviation is likely more concomitant but is almost always larger when the affected eye is fixing (secondary deviation). For example, consider an apparent right hypotropia of equal extent in up and down gaze. If the deviation increases in right gaze then the differentiation is between a right superior rectus palsy (partial third nerve lesion) and a left fourth nerve lesion. Here, if the cover test shows a greater angle when the left versus right eye is fixing (i.e., cover moved OD to OS), then a paralysis of the left superior oblique is suggested.

In general, there are few problems with horizontal disconjugations; for example, a right third nerve lesion will show weakness of all muscles save the lateral rectus and superior oblique. The eye will be in a down and out position. In addition, the exotropia will be worse in left versus right gaze and in near versus distance fixation because of the need for medial rectus action in these positions. Ptosis, poorly reactive pupils, and sluggish accommodation always suggest third nerve disease but are not always present.

A right sixth nerve paresis affecting the abducens will present with an esotropia worse in right gaze, worse with the right eye fixing (secondary deviation), and worse in distance versus near. As with any palsy, severe muscle paretic nystagmus may be seen on attempted right gaze. The patient may turn the head into the field of action of the affected muscle if this gains fusion (e.g., to the right in the above example). Patients usually will fix with the good eye, as this avoids the misreaching and ocular vertigo that occurs when the paralytic eye is used. This is a helpful tendency, but occasionally patients will fix with the bad eye to increase the magnitude of the diplopia to lessen perceptual confusion.

Sometimes a preexisting large horizontal phoria exists and will mask the nature of the lesion. If the horizontal deviation is roughly concomitant, a small vertical imbalance may be the culprit. Here it is best to focus only on the vertical component using the Maddox rod. Although eight vertically acting muscles exist, isolated neurologic involvement of the inferior recti and obliques is a truly rare expression of partial third nerve palsy. It is always a problem to differentiate involvement of the superior rectus (third nerve) of the hypo eye from a superior oblique (fourth nerve) lesion in the contralateral hyper eye. If the deviation does not change radically in up versus down gaze and it is roughly the same with each eye fixing, then use the Bielschowsky head tilt test (Figure 19.3). The rule for elevators/depressors is simply that the vertical deviation will be greatest when the head is tilted toward the involved superior muscle (SR/SO), and greater when tilted away from the involved inferior muscle (IR/IO). Thus a patient with a right hypertropia greater in the left gaze could have a right fourth nerve lesion (RSO) or a partial left third nerve lesion (LSR). If there is no left ptosis or internal ophthalmoplegia and the deviation is otherwise concomitant, then an increase of the deviation in tilt toward the right shoulder suggests RSO, while an increase on left tilt suggests LSR. In general, this test is definitive when it supports an SO palsy, confirmatory when it supports an SR palsy, and not of great value when dealing with inferior muscles.

In general, partial third nerve palsies are rare. Always consider a myopathy in isolated pure exotropias or in isolated upgaze weakness when the pupil is not involved.

Finally, attention should be paid to acute onset of vertical diplopia that is not affected by head tilt. Such an event might be a supranuclear defect such as occurs occasionally with Parinaud's syndrome or, more commonly, in skew deviation. Both of these entities are discussed in following sections.

## Convergence

The assessment of convergence is only occasionally of neurologic importance. Convergence insufficiency is common and is

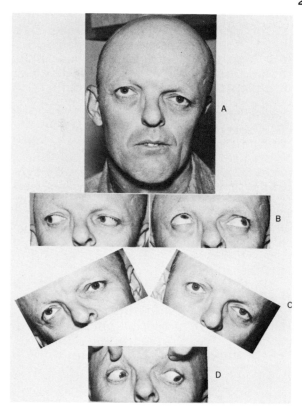

**FIGURE 19.3.**
*A.* Right hyper deviation. *B.* More apparent in left gaze with inferior oblique overaction. *C.* More apparent in right, versus left, head tilt. *D.* Poor depression in adduction. Diagnosis: right superior oblique palsy.
Reprinted by permission of the publisher, from von Noorden, GK. Maumenee's atlas of strabismus. St. Louis: C.V. Mosby, 1977; 3rd ed.

discussed in Chapter 14. It is occasionally complete and refractory to treatment as a congenital syndrome; a weakness of accommodation usually is evident.

A partial third nerve palsy might be most evident during reading because of the increased action of the medial recti in convergence. This usually would be obvious, but myasthenia gravis must be considered in cases of recent afternoon diplopia during reading when the examination of the rested patient shows little deficit. Lateral rectus involvement in infiltrative thyroid eye disease will also make reading difficult. In assessing recent onset of diplopia at near with apparently good convergence, do not overlook the small vertical or torsional imbalance of oblique disease, especially after head trauma.

Significant acute neurologic impairment of convergence and (sometimes) accommodation suggests Parinaud's syndrome or even Wilson's disease (see section on vertical gaze). It is also occasionally seen with internuclear ophthalmoplegia, wherein an absence or slowness of adduction is seen on quick saccades; in most cases, however, convergence is spared in this disorder.

Finally, a functional malady, spasm of the near reflex, may present with rigidly converged eyes simulating bilateral sixth nerve palsies. The typical profile of accommodative spasm, small pupils, and a recent history of intense near-point work in a healthy patient, and quick response to binasal spectacle occlusion and homatropine, differentiates this disorder from an acute midbrain lesion.

## Pursuit Defects

It is common experience to note lack of smooth-following movements in children under 6 years, in older hyperactive children, in mentally distraught or otherwise very nervous patients, and in patients taking tranquilizers. Except for these cases, the examiner should always expect smooth and accurate pursuit movements in all positions of gaze. Nystagmoid movements are only normal at the extreme limits of gaze; otherwise, nystagmus signifies a posterior fossa gaze nystagmus, a brain stem gaze paretic nystagmus, a muscle paretic nystagmus, or an abduction nystagmus (internuclear ophthalmoplegia). Myasthenic muscle weakness may stimulate any of these disorders.

In general, the most common neuro-logic affliction of pursuit is *cogwheeling*, or steplike pursuits that are used in place of smooth pursuit to follow the target. Here the usual problem is to decide whether this reflects basal ganglia disease, such as parkinsonism or cerebellar disease. Cogwheeling may be asymmetrical, perhaps occurring on right, but not leftward, pursuit. This usually reflects parietal lobe disease. It is often observed that patients unable to voluntarily pursue will hold fixation nicely when the head itself is passively rotated by the examiner (doll's head maneuver). This attests to the complex supranuclear basis of the disorder and can be helpful in topical diagnosis. If doll's head movements are absent, then sparing of more reflexive movements, such as holding the upper lids open while the patient attempts to close the eyes (Bell's reflex) or by irrigating the ears with ice water (caloric testing), can be sought.

## Saccadic Dysfunction and Gaze Palsy

In the general assessment of pursuit it may become obvious that there is a marked limitation of conjugate gaze to one or both sides. In this event, no movement will usually be seen to attempted saccades as well ("look at my pen, please"). While this could represent a case of chronic progressive external ophthalmoplegia, it usually represents some form of major gaze palsy.

Usually gaze disturbances are far from this complete, and the latency, velocity, accuracy, and ability to maintain eccentric gaze must be assessed. In testing gaze, hold the patient's head while asking for large refixations, as from the examiner's nose to an eccentrically held penlight. Patients with oculomotor apraxias often are unable to initiate a saccade unless the head is free to move to lead the eyes (head thrusting). While this is often a congenital anomaly, it sometimes reflects progressive neurologic deterioration. In very young children who appear to show a paucity of optically elicited eye movements, it is often helpful to hold the child up and spin him around to see if this combination of optokinetic and vestibular stimulation produces nystagmoid eye movements.

Hesitant, long latency, hypometric, and ill-sustained saccades are common in a variety of CNS degenerations. Often they are also detectibly slow, as in Alzheimer's disease or most of the basal ganglia degenerations. Hypometric and ill-sustained saccades are also characteristic of cerebellar disease, but here the velocities are normal. Partial brain stem gaze palsies are characterized by slow drift away from an eccentrically fixated object followed by refixating saccades (gaze paretic nystagmus). *Dysmetria* is characterized by a series of small homing-in saccades necessary to attain eccentric fixation owing to a tendency to either overshoot or undershoot. Rarely, one may note that small sac-

cades seem too quick for their amplitude. Such darting movements are termed *glissades* and are characteristic of myasthenia.

Occasionally there are disconjugate saccades in the absence of strabismus. Here, when the patient is requested to produce a large saccade to one side or the other, the adducting eye will not follow the leading eye or will lag behind in latency (Figure 19.4). Such an internuclear ophthalmoplegia reflects a lesion in the median longitudinal fasciculus of the brain stem and may be either unilateral or bilateral (see section on lateral gaze disorders).

In addition to examining random saccades and optically elicited movements, it sometimes is important to check specifically for the integrity of voluntary saccades. Patients with frontal lobe apraxias

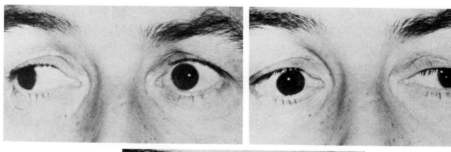

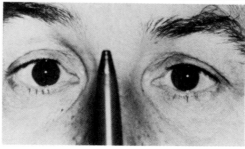

**FIGURE 19.4.**
**Bilateral weakness of adduction despite retention of convergence in internuclear ophthalmoplegia.**
Reprinted by permission of the publisher, from Huber A. Eye signs and symptoms in brain tumors. Blodi FC, ed. and trans. St. Louis: C.V. Mosby, 1976; 3rd ed.

of gaze to one side will often show reasonably good refixations and pursuits but will be unable to move the eyes on command ("look to your left, please"). This partial disassociation often appears in presenile dementia and is common in vertical gaze palsies from an aqueductal tectum lesion in the midbrain as part of Parinaud's syndrome.

Use of the optokinetic tape is especially helpful in unmasking subtle saccadic and pursuit defects: 2″ × 2″ red squares are sewn 2 inches apart on a 2″ by 4′ strip of white cloth. The tape is then drawn past the patient's eyes with the simple instruction to watch the tape. In the normal patient, brisk symmetrical nystagmoid movements will result in all directions. The fast phase is opposite the motion of the tape. Besides demonstrating that vision is grossly intact, this test is helpful in unmasking internuclear ophthalmoplegias in brain stem disease and unilateral pursuit defects in parietal lobe disease. Passing the tape downward before the eyes leads to diagnosis of a Parinaud's syndrome if convergent-retraction nystagmus is elicited. Finally, patients with aberrant regeneration of the third nerve may produce conjugate following movements but often will show obvious disconjugations to an optokinetic challenge, such as the adducting eye manifesting an up gaze component on the fast phase.

Some patients require reflexive attempts to elicit a fast phase. For example, the eyes will rarely move to caloric vestibular stimulation in a brain stem gaze palsy, whereas they will in frontal lobe gaze palsy. A patient with lid retraction, an up gaze palsy, but good elevation via Bell's reflex, has a supranuclear lesion and is suffering from midbrain disease—and not thyroid ophthalmoplegia.

Eliciting a Bell's reflex is also useful as a screen for lateralized cerebral involvement in suspicious patients who do not exhibit localizing CNS signs; for example, a patient suspected of early dementia. On attempted closure of the lids, the great majority (98%) of normal patients will show either an upward or downward excursion, which may also be disconjugate. Patients with hemispheric disease, however, sometimes show a conjugate Bell's, where the eyes will both move to the left or right as well. This suggests a lesion in the hemisphere contralateral to the deviation.

# CLINICAL SIGNIFICANCE

Oculomotor abnormalities can reflect disease anywhere in the central nervous system. The sections that follow alert the reader to the more subtle defects and assessment of their clinical significance. Unfortunately, many eye practitioners have relegated this complex area to the neurologist and the neurologist has shifted it back to the eye practitioner. It is the eye practitioner, however, who is more likely to observe these anomalies. Increased awareness is crucial. Simply performing a cover test and casually observing the duction is not sufficient. It is necessary to carefully observe the eyes at rest and to precisely assess all aspects of the quality of pursuit and saccadic movements.

# Third Nerve Disorders

*The third cranial nerve innervates the superior, inferior, and medial recti, the inferior oblique, iris sphincter, ciliary body, and levator muscles.*

## BACKGROUND

The third cranial nerve derives from paired nuclei in the floor of the aqueduct of silvius at the pons-midbrain junction. Fibers run anterior-ventrally near the midline, in close proximity to the substantia nigra and red nucleus, to emerge between the cerebral peduncles before piercing the dura (Figure 19.5). From here, fibers course forward under the junction of the posterior communicating and posterior cerebral arteries, under and alongside the tracts and then chiasm near the posterior communicating artery, through the cavernous sinus, and enter the orbit through the superior orbital fissure (Figures 19.1 and 19.2). At the fissure the superior division separates to innervate the superior rectus and levator. In the cavernous sinus and superior orbital fissure area, important associated structures include the sympathetics to the eye, the intracavernous carotid artery, cranial nerves IV and VI, and the first division of nerve V.

## HISTORY AND EXAMINATION

The appearance of a complete third nerve palsy is unmistakable. The eye is down and out with a severe ptosis, dilated and unreactive pupil, and paresis of accommodation. Whenever any of these are even minimally affected, it is crucial to check all other third nerve functions completely. Pupillary involvement is most consistently associated with mass lesions. In subtle pupil involvement, assess whether the relative mydriasis is more apparent in bright light—the hallmark of third nerve involvement.

Outside of pure internal ophthalmoplegia, the other major variants of partial third nerve palsy are ptosis and superior rectus weakness. Here, the Bielchowsky test may be valuable. Also examine the pupil; levator weakness may mask a Horner's syndrome. Relative miosis on the affected side more apparent several seconds after dimming room illumination suggests Horner's syndrome. Such a pupil will not dilate to hydroxyamphetamine and indicates multiple nerve involvement in the carotid sinus. While isolated involvement of inferior oblique or inferior or superior rectus can occur with a neurologic lesion,

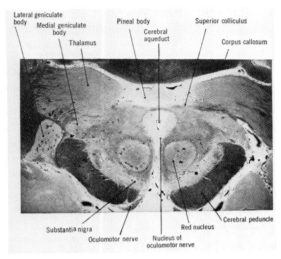

Lateral geniculate body
Medial geniculate body
Thalamus
Pineal body
Cerebral aqueduct
Superior colliculus
Corpus callosum
Substantia nigra
Oculomotor nerve
Nucleus of oculomotor nerve
Red nucleus
Cerebral peduncle

**FIGURE 19.5.**

**Cross section of midbrain showing oculomotor nucleus in floor of aqueduct. Note proximity of red nucleus, substantia nigra, and cerebral peduncle to fascicular portion of the third nerve.**

Reprinted by permission of the publisher, from Gardner E. Fundamentals of neurology. Philadelphia: W.B. Saunders, 1963; 4th ed.

such partial presentations are rare, and the cause is more likely orbital disease or myopathy.

Nuclear disorders are truly rare and usually show bilateral involvement along with other midbrain signs. Divergent eyes with poor adduction bilaterally, along with bilateral ptosis and occasional pupillary involvement, is suggestive of a midline nuclear lesion. With progressive bilateral third nerve weakness in an alert patient, suspect bilateral nerve trunk involvement from an interpeduncular mass. Compression in this area is more likely to affect the pupil early on, and aneurysm must be ruled out.

Fascicular lesions within the substance of the brain stem almost always will present with other company (Figure 19.5). Lesions of the pyramidal fibers present as Weber's syndrome, with crossed signs of hemiparesis (cerebral peduncle lesion); Benedict's syndrome with contralateral resting tremor or chorioathetosis (red nucleus lesion); or Nothnagel's syndrome, with contralateral ataxia (brachium conjunctivum lesion).

Patients with nuclear and fascicular disorders more likely present to the neurologist. But some patients are surprisingly tolerant of progressing subacute neurologic defects. Part of the workup of patients with third nerve disorders therefore is a search for company in this area of the brain. For example, with a ventral lesion affecting the peduncle, look for a little leg swing on the opposite side; check for flexor rigidity in the arm and extensor rigidity of the leg accompanied by hyperactive reflexes; perhaps a positive Babinski reflex may be all that is observed. Lesions with this sort of company can never be considered neuritic and serious causes should be ruled out.

Nerve trunk lesions are the most common cause of third nerve palsies. These lesions can occur at the base of the brain as the nerves emerge or as they course forward into the cavernous sinus along with nerves IV, V, and VI, and through the superior orbital fissure into the orbit. Lesions producing trunk damage are unlikely to have signs of altered cerebral function unless the palsy presents very late in the course of the disease, or is part of a devastating picture of trauma or a subarachnoid hemorrhage. The one major exception is where an expanding hemispheric mass results in herniation of the uncus, hippocampus, or temporal lobe through the tentorium to impinge upon the brain stem (Figure 19.6). In such cases, third nerve signs are an early warning of impending disaster, and ipsilateral pupillary involvement is a very consistent omen (Hutchinson's pupil). The major cause that must be remembered in office practice is the chronic subdural hemorrhage of the el-

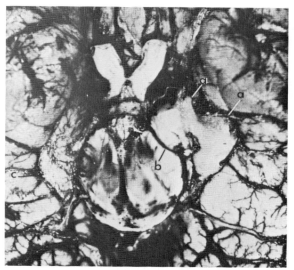

**FIGURE 19.6.**
Tentorial herniation in temporal lobe glioblastoma. Note herniated uncus (*a*) indenting cerebral peduncle (*b*). Brain-stem compression also evident via congestion and petechiae. Ipsilateral mydriasis may be an early sign of this serious complication of enlarging supratentorial masses, especially hematoma.
Reprinted by permission of the publisher, from Wood EH, Taveras JS, and Tenner MS. The brain and the eye. Chicago: Yearbook Medical Publishers, 1975. Copyright 1975, American College of Radiology.

derly, where rebleeding and expansion of the clot may result in this sign even several months after minor head trauma. Such patients may present only with an internal or partial third nerve palsy with the minimal company of headache and mild confusion. Always inquire as to an antecedent trauma.

With apparently isolated third nerve palsy, always look for a simultaneous fourth nerve palsy evidenced by lack of intorsion at the slit lamp on attempted down-and-in gaze (Figure 19.7). Again, a neuritic lesion can never be accepted with such evidence of dysfunction in two adjacent cranial nerves.

In a relatively intact patient presenting with seemingly isolated third nerve trunk disease, the search for company also involves the nearby cranial nerves, including brow and corneal sensation; the ventral brain stem and pyramidal tracts; the pituitary-endocrine system; the cavernous sinus-superior orbital fissure/orbital area (e.g., proptosis, venous congestion, bruits); and, of course, systemic disease (e.g., myasthenia, sarcoid). Exophthalmometer readings must always be taken in any case of acute diplopia, but it is well to remember that 2 or 3 mm of proptosis is expected with any complete third nerve palsy.

# CLINICAL SIGNIFICANCE

The most common causes of isolated third nerve palsies (Table 19.1) are aneurysm (20%) and vascular disease (20%, most commonly diabetes); about 15% of the cases represent trauma, and 10% to 12% represent tumors. Perhaps 30% are neuritic, in which no definite cause is found but that often follow a viral illness.

Of particular interest is the entity of the painful third nerve palsy of relatively acute onset. Here the major diagnostic dilemma is differentiating an infarct secondary to microvascular disease (chiefly diabetes, but also syphilis, lupus, hypertension) from aneurysm (chiefly a posterior communicating artery aneurysm) (Figure 19.8). In a cavernous sinus infarct, pain is present in about half the cases and usually spares the pupil (80%). These palsies are often preceded by a day or more of smoldering orbital or retro-orbital ischemic aching, which resolves abruptly when the actual infarct and palsy occur. The pupillomotor fibers are thought to be frequently spared because of their superficial location in the nerve trunk in the

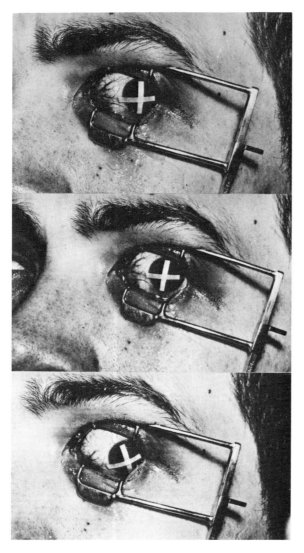

**FIGURE 19.7.**
Third nerve palsy with patient attempting to look up (*top*), straight ahead (*middle*), and down (*bottom*). Retention of intorsion in depression signifies sparing of the fourth nerve. Reprinted by permission of the publisher, from Cogan D. Neurology of the ocular muscles. Springfield, Ill.: Charles C Thomas, 1956; 2nd ed.

**Table 19.1**
**Common or Important Causes of Apparently Isolated Third Nerve Palsy**

Occult diabetes mellitus in patient past 40
Aneurysm of posterior communicating artery
Other masses:
    Parasella/cavernous sinus (e.g., carotid aneurysm/fistula, adenoma)
    Superior orbital fissure (e.g., meningiomas, granulomas)
    Orbital apex (sarcoma, lymphomas, thyroid, pseudotumor)
Myasthenia gravis/thyroid eye disease
Arteritis (collagen vascular and giant cell)
Granulomatous disease (syphilis, sarcoid, tuberculosis)
Chronic subdural hematoma (elderly and substance abusers)
Recurrent migrainous palsy in children
Idiopathic (presumed vascular, etc.)

cavernous sinus. Interestingly, in many diabetic palsies the patient is unaware of the preexistence of occult adult-onset diabetes, which again stresses the importance of diabetic screening.

Truly abrupt onset of severe pain at actual onset of the palsy is characteristic of aneurysm (nearly 100% are painful). Pupillary loss is also highly characteristic and occurs in 95% of the patients. In contrast to diabetes, where cessation of the ache often accompanies the onset of diplopia, aneurysms may progress with persistence or worsening of the pain, the palsy, or even the patient's general condition (e.g., hemiparesis, nucchal rigidity, or even obtundation). Also in contrast to diabetes, the pain tends to be sharper and often localized to the brow. Check for loss of facial sensation to light touch and/or a decreased corneal reflex in suspicious cases. The examiner may also hear an orbital or retromastoid bruit with the bell stethoscope.

Carotid-posterior communicating artery junction aneurysms often rupture without any warning. Because of their importance and prevalence (accounting for

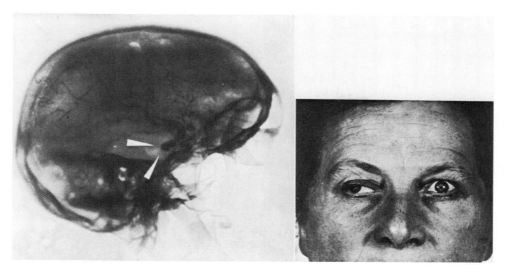

**FIGURE 19.8.**
**Middle-aged woman with right oculomotor paresis and partial ptosis.**
**Angiography demonstrates a right carotid-posterior communicating**
**artery aneurysm.**
Reprinted by permission of the publisher, from Huber A. Eye signs and
symptoms in brain tumors. Blodi FC, ed. and trans. St. Louis: C.V.
Mosby, 1976; 3rd ed.

one-third of all intracranial aneurysms), however, they must be suspected even with an incomplete syndrome (internal ophthalmoplegia, facial numbness, abrupt onset of orbital pain, intermittent diplopia/ptosis). Four-vessel angiography may be needed. Persistent relative mydriasis in bright light, and especially aberrant regeneration point to a mass lesion, such as aneurysm, regardless of the initial diagnosis. Most frequently, aberrant regeneration is manifested by pupillary contraction on adduction (use slit lamp), lid retraction on down gaze (pseudo-Graefe sign) (Figure 19.9), or adduction on attempted up gaze (Figure 19.10). The latter two extraocular anomalies are best seen with a challenge using the optokinetic tape to induce repetitive down or upbeating nystagmus. Symptomatic aneurysms are almost nonexistent in childhood and are most common in middle-aged women.

Painful ophthalmoplegia, with more obvious signs of multiple palsies such as fifth nerve involvement, loss of vision, proptosis, and congestion, suggests more anterior disease, such as anterior cavernous sinus, superior orbital fissure, or of the orbit itself. Thyroid disease, cellulitis, orbital masses, pseudotumors, lymphomas, sphenoid meningiomas, cavernous sinus masses, and fistulas lead the list along with the relatively benign Tolosa Hunt syndrome. A slow progression of cranial nerve involvement in a middle-aged woman suggests a meningioma (Figure 19.11).

Some authors use the term Tolosa Hunt syndrome to refer to any inflammatory orbital disease accompanied by diplopia and that is steroid responsive; however, the syndrome classically refers to a recurrent granulomatous inflammation of the dura adjacent to the carotid artery in the cavernous sinus, which typically affects older males. It is characterized by recur-

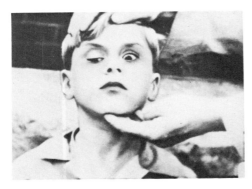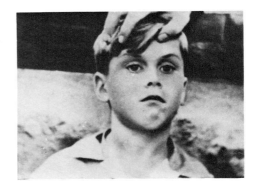

**FIGURE 19.9.**
Retraction of lid on down gaze in a case of aberrant regeneration of the third nerve (pseudo-Graefe sign, *left*). Compare with normal lid position in primary position (*right*).
Reprinted by permission of the publisher, from Cogan D. Neurology of the ocular muscles. Springfield, Ill.: Charles C Thomas, 1956; 2nd ed.

rent painful third nerve palsies, often with first division fifth nerve anesthesia and orbital congestion. The patients may have some malaise, the ESR is elevated in half the cases, and the inflammatory mass may be outlined by a dent in the intracavernous carotid artery on angiography, or by orbital venography (positive in 60% to 70% of the cases). Almost without exception, the pain and then the palsy resolve rapidly with high-dose steroid therapy. A note of caution: many diseases, including edema related to tumors, may improve with steroids. Thus, transient improvement of a palsy with steroids does not prove inflammation.

A frequently misdiagnosed disorder is that of a low-flow dural artery-cavernous sinus fistula. Practitioners are familiar with the explosive symptoms of a high-flow carotid-cavernous fistula with proptosis, congestion, pain, motility restriction, pulsation of the globe, and a bruit. This usually occurs after trauma, but may occur spontaneously in the elderly. The low-flow variety is more likely to occur spontaneously, and often episcleral dilation and mild proptosis are the only signs; patients usually present because of the red eye or

headache. Usually no bruit is heard, but intraocular pressure (IOP) is elevated and blood is seen in Schlemm's canal, indicating high episcleral venous pressure. The significance of this disorder is to recognize it as a cause of diplopia and to save the patient unnecessary treatment save for the management of the glaucoma itself.

While "migrainous ophthalmoplegia" affecting the third nerve is a well-known entity, a better pseudonym would be "benign idiopathic headache followed by transient third nerve palsy dominated by ptosis." It usually occurs in young boys and is exceedingly rare. This diagnosis can never be proved, but is a diagnosis of exclusion to be accepted only after a complete neuroophthalmologic workup. Signs of aberrant regeneration are totally inconsistent with this diagnosis.

The reader is referred to standard neuroophthalmologic texts for a full discussion of oculomotor palsy. Management of these disorders naturally depends on the preliminary diagnosis. Brain stem signs, multiple cranial nerve, or early pupillary involvement suggest a referral to neurology, on an emergency basis if an aneurysm or brain stem herniation is suspected. Iso-

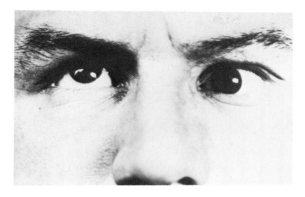

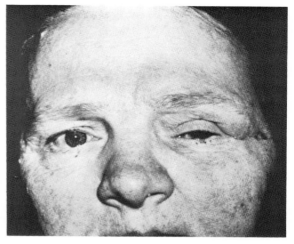

**FIGURE 19.11.**
Meningioma (en plaque) filling in the left temporal fossa in a case of sphenoid wing tumor. Patient was a 40-year-old woman with a congested eye, blurred vision, and proptosis. Reprinted by permission of the publisher, from Cogan D. Neurology of the visual system. Springfield, Ill.: Charles C Thomas, 1966.

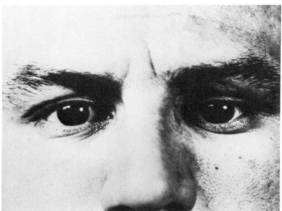

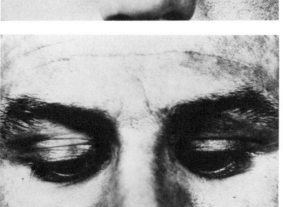

**FIGURE 19.10.**
Anomalous adduction of left eye in attempted up gaze with eyes straight in primary position.
Reprinted by permission of the publisher, from Cogan D. Neurology of the ocular muscles. Springfield, Ill.: Charles C Thomas, 1956; 2nd ed.

lated signs of orbital disease suggest an ophthalmologic referral. A pupillary-sparing third nerve palsy in a known diabetic is little cause for concern, but an emergency referral to the internist after a stat ESR is indicated when company suggesting temporal arteritis is present.

A complete neurologic workup can be both expensive and risky. The provisional diagnosis at presentation must include a full inquiry into how the patient has been feeling recently. To overlook weight loss, thyroid hyperplasia, and palpitations in a middle-aged woman with diplopia in up gaze may mean that such symptoms are never volunteered again to a tertiary specialist to whom you have incorrectly referred the patient, and the true diagnosis of Graves' disease is likely to be delayed. Consider the mode of presentation of the disorders listed in Table 19.1.

# Sixth Nerve Disorders

*The sixth nerve (abducens) innervates the lateral rectus muscle
and is responsible for abduction.*

## BACKGROUND

The sixth nerve emerges at the lower border of the pons near the junction of the basilar and anterior inferior cerebellar arteries. It runs forward in the subarachnoid space of the pontine cistern up the clivus to pierce the dura about 2 cm below and lateral to the posterior clinoid process. Here the sixth nerve, in close proximity to nerve V, passes up over the petrous apex in a groove to then bend sharply forward to enter the cavernous sinus and then passes through the superior orbital fissure into the orbit (Figures 19.1 and 19.2). Perhaps because of its long course or its fixation over the petrous, the sixth nerve is the most vulnerable to trauma and to downward movement of the brain with increased intracranial pressure or expanding hemispheric masses. The sixth nerve also is the most commonly affected from presumed postviral demyelination, which usually follows a childhood illness. In the brain stem proper, the sixth nerve nucleus is closely associated with rootlets of the seventh nerve and nucleus para-abducens, which controls ipsilateral conjugate gaze.

## HISTORY AND EXAMINATION

The appearance of a full sixth nerve palsy is unmistakable, with evident esotropia greater at distance, greater in ipsilateral lateral gaze, and greater with the involved eye fixing. Besides a general ocular exam and inquiry for systemic complaints, the examination for lateral rectus palsy follows that of third nerve disease—looking for neurologic company in the lower brain stem and cranial nerves, cavernous sinus/superior orbital fissure area, and the orbit itself. More than with any other cranial nerve, however, it is vital to search for signs and symptoms of increased intracranial pressure, including peripapillary retinal edema, loss of venous pulse, morning headache, irritability, lethargy, and vegetative signs. In young children, measure head circumference and listen for a "cracked-pot" sound to a sharp rap on the skull by the tip of the fingers.

Several entities may simulate an acquired sixth nerve paresis. In congenital esotropia, for example, one often sees a failure to abduct the affected eye, but this disappears after patching the good eye for several days. Duane's retraction syndrome, with abducens aplasia, is rarely associated with diplopia and is recognized by the anomalous innervation pattern causing the fissure to narrow (or even globe retraction) on attempted adduction. Thyroid fibrosis of the medial rectus is suspected in middle-aged women with progressive symptoms; here the forced duction will be positive.

Lastly, convergence spasm is not rare and will present with distance diplopia and blurred vision owing to pseudomyopia. Here, further miosis on attempted abduction in a nervous patient who does intense close work suggests the diagnosis. The symptoms should remit over several days with homatropine and binasal occlusion. This is mainly a disorder of young people.

Finally, one should always measure the extent of the deviation on initial presentation to gauge the clinical course. Neuritic palsies should start improving in 6 to 8 weeks, while progression always suggests a mass.

# CLINICAL SIGNIFICANCE

The causes of sixth nerve palsy are legion; some of the more common and/or important ones are presented in Table 19.2.

Nuclear and fascicular lesions, by virtue of their brain stem location, are almost always associated with significant company. Damage must also occur to nucleus para-abducens producing an associated palsy of gaze ipsilaterally and usually other company, such as an ipsilateral seventh nerve. Isolated sixth nerve weakness and gaze palsy in a relatively healthy patient suggests an extremely localized lesion such as a demyelinating plaque in younger patients, brain stem twig infarct or lacuna in older hypertensives, or Wernicke's encephalopathy in debilitated alcoholics. In general, sixth nerve weakness is the only oculomotor palsy that can be considered compatible with a diagnosis of Wernicke's syndrome, no matter how much the patient drinks.

In fascicular lesions, contralateral motor weakness owing to pyramidal involvement might be expected, along with an ipsilateral seventh nerve palsy (Millard-Gubler syndrome), and perhaps an ipsilateral gaze palsy as well (Foville's syndrome). In the preantibiotic era, the spread of an otitis into the petrous bone with involvement of the sixth and seventh nerves and referred pain to the orbit was termed Gradenigo's syndrome. At present, metastatic tumors and nasopharyngiomas have replaced osteomyelitis as the most common cause of this rare syndrome.

In the pontine subarachnoid space, meningitis and basal skull fractures are likely to affect nerves V to VIII. Always inquire as to malaise and stiff neck. Because cerebello-pontine angle tumors in this location may affect the sixth nerve, one should always compare corneal and facial sensation on both sides, and be alert for asymmetry of the facial muscles, loss of hearing, and ipsilateral gaze nystagmus.

More anteriorly, disorders of the cavernous sinus and superior orbital fissure are likely to present with the multiple cranial nerve signs and orbital symptoms discussed for the third nerve.

Most often, however, a sixth nerve paresis occurs as an isolated event without brain stem or other company, and a precise cause is never proved. In older patients, therefore, most physicians are reluctant to order higher risk procedures, such as air studies or angiography, unless there is company or signs of progression.

In children without history of trauma

**Table 19.2**
**Common or Important Causes of Apparently Isolated Sixth**
**Nerve Palsy (Weakness of Abduction)**

| Unilateral | Bilateral |
|---|---|
| Diabetes mellitus in patient past 40 | Congenital brain-stem aplasia (Möbius' syndrome) |
| Postviral demyelination: | Bilateral abducens aplasia (Duane's syndrome) |
|   Acute exanthems in children | Trauma (always consider battered child) |
|   Mono and URIs in young adults | Neurosyphilis |
|   Zoster in elderly | Wernicke's encephalopathy |
| Nonlocalizing sign in mass lesions | Divergence insufficiency in increased intracranial pressure |
| Masses: | Convergence excess with anticholinergic medicines |
|   Parasella, cavernous sinus, superior orbital fissure and orbit | Spasm of the near reflex |
|   Aneurysm a rare cause of truly isolated palsy | |
|   Cerebellar-pontine angle masses and nasopharyngioma | |
|   Petrous invasion in metastatic disease and otitis | |
| Collagen/giant cell vasculitis | |
| Multiple sclerosis in young adults | |
| Wernicke's encephalopathy | |
| Lacunar stroke in elderly hypertensives | |
| Myasthenia/thyroid eye disease | |
| Following lumbar puncture, spinal anesthesia, myelogram | |
| Idiopathic palsy common with sixth nerve | |

or recent flu, however, even isolated palsy of sixth (or third or fourth) nerve must always be considered as being due to a mass unless proved otherwise. Although tumors are relatively common causes of sixth nerve paresis, it again should be recalled that if signs and symptoms of hydrocephalus exist, a sixth nerve defect alone cannot be considered to have localizing significance.

In older patients with isolated sixth nerve paresis, diabetes and involutional disease are most common, but temporal arteritis should always be ruled out. Sixth nerve paresis also represents the most common ocular presentation of nasopharyngioma, a highly aggressive malignancy. These growths are most common in elderly males and may also cause a Paredrine-unreactive Horner's pupil and/or periorbital pain and paresthesia. Pain is more common in the maxillary or ear region, however. Other company includes fullness and popping of the ears, serous otitis, nosebleeds, oropharyngeal paresthesias and congestion, dysarthria, and dysphagia. A reassuring point concerning the sixth nerve is that an intracavernous aneurysm as a cause of isolated palsy is quite rare.

While acute sixth nerve palsy is unmistakable, a partial and variable palsy may occasionally occur with raised intracranial pressure and thus may present a difficulty in differentiating from decompensating phoria or myasthenia. In patients with morning predilection of diplopia on distance viewing, rule out sixth nerve palsy and search for signs of inconcomitancy and raised intracranial pressure.

Finally, isolated sixth nerve palsy in a previously healthy young adult always raises the possibility of multiple sclerosis. Inquire about other short-lasting defects with special note of previous diplopia, episodic distal paresthesias, leg weakness, sphincter control problems, vertigo, optic neuritis, and neuralgialike facial pain. Patients with isolated sixth nerve palsies are unlikely to show elevated myelin-basic proteins but may show an increased cerebrospinal fluid (CSF) gamma globulin fraction. Even asymptomatic patients may show delayed nerve conduction with the visual-evoked potential, brain stem auditory-evoked potential, or peripheral nerve conduction studies. In the eye, look for minimal subjective signs of optic nerve conduction failure, retinal ganglion cell defects, arcuate field defects, and subclinical internuclear ophthalmoplegias.

While sixth nerve palsies are common and often have no identifiable cause, one must always conduct a diligent search for other neurologic accompaniments as well as a general review of the patient's health.

# Fourth Nerve Disorders

*The fourth (trochlear) nerve innervates the superior oblique muscle and is primarily responsible for down gaze when the eye is in the adducted position.*

## BACKGROUND

The fourth nerve originates lateral and ventral to the aqueduct of silvius at the level of the inferior colliculus. Fibers of the fourth nerve are unique in that they both cross almost completely in the anterior medullary velum and are the only cranial nerves to emerge from the dorsal part of the brain. After a somewhat lengthy and circuitous course, the fourth nerve passes laterally to the dorsum sella, pierces the dura, passes through the lateral wall of the cavernous sinus and through the superior orbital fissure into the orbit (see Figures 19.1 and 19.2).

## HISTORY AND EXAMINATION

Acute onset of a fourth nerve palsy is associated with a diplopia with a measurable hyper component (4 to 10 prism diopters) that increases in adduction and more so on down-and-in gaze. The deviation is greater with the affected eye fixing and increases on head tilt to the affected side.

Bilateral fourth nerve palsies reflect the lack of support in the anterior medullary velum, where the nerves decussate. Such palsies occur most commonly after vertex head trauma or abrupt deceleration, as from falls and with whiplash injuries. The patient may have little complaint at distance, but complain of "focusing" problems reading, as they rarely recognize the torsional nature of the diplopic impedi-ment—this is similar to the misnaming of diplopic symptoms in convergency insufficiency. In these patients there may be no vertical deviation in the primary position, but a hyperdeviation will be bilaterally present in adduction and the Bielchowsky will show hyperdeviations on whichever side is tilted towards the shoulder. The patient may recognize torsional diplopia if a fine-drawn line held at the reading position is illuminated by a penlight in an otherwise darkened room. Often the complaint goes unrecognized.

Increasing hyperdeviation on adduction is also common in V-pattern esotropia. This is contrasted with the alternate hyperdeviation in abduction, which usually represents a supranuclear skew deviation from cerebellar disease or Arnold-Chiari malformation.

Otherwise, the approach to fourth nerve palsies is similar to that already outlined for third and sixth nerve palsies.

# CLINICAL SIGNIFICANCE

The fourth nerve is commonly involved in congenital paresis in the young and vascular accidents in the elderly. Trauma is the major cause of these palsies in the middle years (Table 19.3). Typically, frontal trauma is associated with single sphenooccipital (SO) palsy, where bilateral palsies often follow blows to the vertex or whiplash injury.

Aneurysms are rare causes, and tumors account for only 10% to 15% of incidence. Aside from congenital defects, small-vessel disease is by far the most common cause (e.g., senile, with diabetes, hypertension, collagen disease, sickle cell, etc.). In an older healthy patient, therefore, if blood pressure, glucose tolerance test, ESR, skull films, and a neuroscreen are normal, one can practically assure full recovery in 4 to 6 weeks of a so-called cryptogenic or presumed vascular palsy. In children, however, as with sixth nerve palsies of uncertain origin, rigorous investi-gations must be carried out, as tumors are common causes. Sometimes, with apparent onset of diplopia in childhood, a tell-tale long history of head tilt toward the opposite eye may be elucidated. Careful inquiry in these patients usually determines that in the past these children upon adopting unusual postures have been vaguely aware of "a second TV set in the doorway," to quote an example of one child. In such patients a congenital palsy is suggested, especially when the deviation is relatively concomitant, except to a head tilt. Decompensation of these deviations to produce a relatively vague and intermittent diplopia in later life probably is more common than generally believed.

The list below is a sample first stage workup useful in the initial approach to unexplained isolated oculomotor palsies of any sort.

1. BP, formal glucose tolerance test, and general medical, neurologic and toxic screen as indicated
2. CBC, differential, and heterophile
3. Skull and sinus series
4. FTA-ABS for neurosyphilis; other serology as indicated
5. $T_3$, $T_4$, FTI and TRH if orbital congestion, middle-aged woman, etc.
6. Collagen vascular screen in young and middle-aged women
7. Stat ESR if over 55 and giant cell arteritis suspected
8. Muscle and tensilon testing
9. LP for pressure; red, white, and malignant cells; and protein fraction
10. Nerve conduction studies if multiple sclerosis suspected

#### Table 19.3
#### Common or Important Causes of Apparently Isolated Fourth Nerve Palsy

Trauma to orbit, vertex; after whiplash injury or frontal sinus surgery
Decompensating congenital palsy
Occult diabetes mellitus in patient past 40
Masses (rare, but must be considered in childhood)
Aneurysms (rare)
Collagen vascular disease
Multiple sclerosis (rare, in young adults)
Myasthenia
Paget's disease in elderly
With zoster in elderly
Idiopathic onset (most common cause in elderly)

11. Metastatic cancer screen if pain, progression, or pupillary involvement in middle-age or later

12. Four-vessel angiography if unexplained pain or pupillary involvement

13. Other tests based upon clinical suspicion (e.g., CAT scan, ultrasound, tomograms, venograms, etc.)

# Myopathic Disorders

*Anomalous oculomotor function caused by primary disease at
the myoneural junction or in muscle cell itself.*

## BACKGROUND

While significant neurologic causes of diplopia remain paramount, such patients often have other symptoms that place them in the hands of the neurologist. Relatively speaking, myopathic disease thus presents much more commonly in the eye practitioner's office than would be expected, given its low prevalence in the general population.

The prevalence of ocular symptoms in myopathic disease probably reflects several factors. First, the extraocular muscles themselves are histologically unique and subject to isolated involvement, as in the chronic progressive external ophthalmoplegias. Second, Hering's law of equal innervation makes them exquisitely sensitive to symptomatic malfunction at a stage when other muscle involvement would still be occult. Third, the extraocular muscles are innervated by bulbar structures and share their predisposition to early involvement in several myopathic diseases. Finally, a specific facilitating immunologic pathway may exist for these muscles in Graves' disease, accounting for the preeminence of ocular muscle symptomatology in this illness.

## HISTORY AND EXAMINATION

Specific points of history and clinical testing depend on suspicion of a particular myopathy; however, several general points can be made. First, Graves' disease is always highly suspect simply because it is the single most common cause of diplopia. Second, family history of a generalized muscular disorder or motility problem always implicates a myopathic basis. Third, be especially suspicious of muscle disease when the motility exam fails to show the clear-cut field-of-action characteristics expected of specific cranial nerve weakness. This is especially true with the concomitant presence of a ptosis or orbicularis weakness. The most common presentation of myopathies usually is weakness on up gaze, while pupillary involvement virtually rules out muscle disease. Fourth, look especially closely at the remaining bulbar musculature, and also inquire and test for proximal (limb-girdle) weakness; listen for nasalization as a sign of vagus weakness; inquire as to trouble swallowing, enunciating, and chewing; inquire as to symptoms while holding the arms up as in brushing the hair, and test for weakness in shoulder shrugs and head turning (accessory nerve); note any tongue wasting or difficulty in lateral strength against resistance (hypoglossal nerve); note any lower extremity proximal weakness suggested by difficulty getting out of chairs and walking up stairs and hills.

Myasthenia may simulate any oculo-motor syndrome from gaze nystagmus to an internuclear ophthalmoplegia. If the cause of an apparent neurological motility disorder is at all elusive, then IV tensilon testing is mandatory to rule out myasthenia.

# CLINICAL SIGNIFICANCE

The myotonic dystrophies are the only major muscular dystrophies that commonly affect the eye muscles. Significant dysfunction occurs only late in the disease. The levator and orbicularis muscles are typically affected earlier and more severely than the extraocular muscles. The pupil may occasionally be sluggish, a finding never observed in the chronic progressive external ophthalmoplegias (CPEOs). Light/near disassociation has even been observed with myotonic disease. The disease complex is suggested by its familiar nature (autosomal dominant) and by progressing weakness, muscle atrophy, and accompanying myotonia. The inability to relax muscles once contracted is often characterized by the oft-quoted inability to relax a handshake, but also by sustained blepharospasm after forced closure or lid lag on quick down gaze. Typically the symptoms are worse in cold weather. Faces are characteristic with loss of fullness especially marked in temporalis, paper thin orbiculari, loss of expressiveness, and often premature frontal balding (Figure 19.12). It is also the only ocular myopathy associated with distal muscle weakness, exemplified by dropping objects or tripping on rugs. With significant extraocular muscle weakness, hypotony may be noted, but in general, eye muscle signs are a late accompaniment. Iridescent and/or cortical snowflake cataracts are not late signs, however, and may be seen early in the disease.

The CPEOs represent a diffuse group of poorly defined abiotrophies with severe dystrophic changes limited mainly to the eye muscles. All forms of inheritance have been identified, the worse cases usually being sex linked or those beginning in childhood. At onset, ptosis is usually the most obvious symptom, although orbicularis weakness is just as evident when specifically tested for (Figure 19.13). Ptosis repair may result in a total inability to close the eyes, resulting in visual catastrophe from exposure. Diplopia and limitation of gaze, usually up gaze first (as with all myopathies), may follow. The final picture of fixed exotropic eyes takes years to evolve. Patients are usually surprisingly tolerant of the motility disorder.

Unlike myotonia, the proximal and bulbar muscles are the most common non-ocular muscles affected, although this usually is not severe. Characteristically, these patients have weak neck flexors and cannot overcome even moderate force against the forehead in strength testing. Other eye signs may include optic atrophy, gyrate atrophy, and pigmentary degeneration. Systemic accompaniments may include short stature, early gonadal atrophy, cerebellar ataxia, and heart block.

Since heart block poses by far the most significant and only treatable problem associated with CPEOs, it is important to realize that this complication tends to occur most commonly in the Kearns-Sayres triad (CPEO, heart block, and retinal pigmentary degeneration). It is important to note that the retinal disorder is not bone-spicule in character, but more granulated, as seen in rubella. Although most evident in the macula, central vision is usually quite good, and the ERG is near normal.

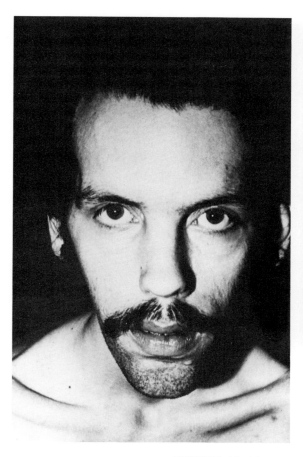

**FIGURE 19.12.**
Advanced myotonic dystrophy with temporalis
wasting, expressionless "hatchet" face, loss of
folds and orbicularis weakness evident as
lagophthalmos. Tensions were 10 mm OU,
and punctate lens opacities were present.
Reprinted by permission of the publisher,
from Donin JF and Keane JR. Diagnostic
problems in neuro-ophthalmology. New York:
Famous Teachings in Modern Medicine,
Medcom, Inc., 1973.

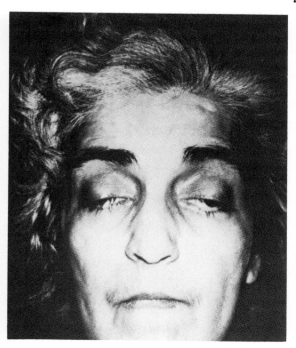

**FIGURE 19.13.**
Face in CPEO is flaccid and expressionless
with marked ptosis, paper-thin orbiculari,
lagophthalmos, and fixed exotropic eyes.
Reprinted by permission of the publisher,
from Lessel S. Chronic progressive external
ophthalmoplegia. In: Glaser JS and Smith JL,
eds. Neuro-ophthalmology, vol. VIII. St. Louis:
C.V. Mosby, 1975.

While occasionally autosomal dominant, Kearns-Sayres triad usually appears
sporadically and tends to begin in early
adolescence with prominent ptosis and facial weakness (Figure 19.14); the children
are often short in stature and by their
twenties may show a bit of ataxia and
hearing loss; laboratory testing often dis-
closes abnormal glucose tolerance, EEG
slowing, and increased CSF protein. It is
important never to overlook the potentially
fatal heart block in patients who tend to
fall into this class. Always take the pulse
and refer the patient for ECG if there is
any doubt.

The oculopharyngeal variety of CPEO
appears dominant, with a consistent
penetrance; usually it is limited to mid-life
onset of ptosis, dysphagia, and sometimes
mild dysphonia. A great many of those
affected are of French Canadian descent.

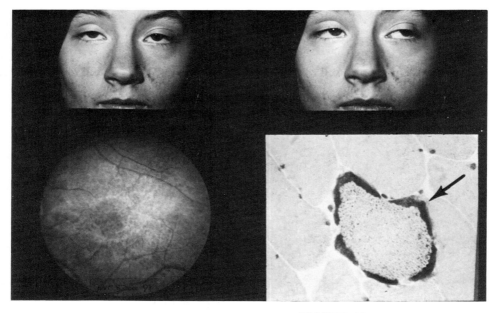

**FIGURE 19.14.**
Fifteen-year-old girl with complaints of failing night vision and ptosis (*upper left*). Extraocular weakness moderately evident in left lateral gaze (*upper right*). Atypical pigmentary retinopathy also evident (*lower left*). Biopsy of extraocular muscle demonstrates "ragged red" fibers (*lower right*). Diagnosis: Kearns-Sayre's syndrome.
Reprinted by permission of the publisher, from Miller NR and Fine SL. The ocular fundus in neuro-ophthalmologic diagnosis. In: Sights and sounds in ophthalmology, vol. III. St. Louis: C.V. Mosby, 1975.

Regurgitation is the most significant problem, and a barium swallow test is used for definitive diagnosis and to ascertain whether the swallowing difficulty can be improved with surgery. These patients often retain a Bell's reflex and good orbicularis function, making them potential candidates for cosmetic ptosis surgery. These patients can name at least one close relative with the same disorder. Although sporadic cases are said to occur, these tend to have some degree of limb-girdle dystrophy and may not represent the same disease as familial cases.

Myasthenia gravis as a cause of myoneural failure is rare (1/25,000, with a 3:2 female preference, generally nonfamilial) but must be entertained in any unexplained ptosis, diplopia, or other gaze disturbance. Ocular motor disturbances are the presenting signs in some 50% to 60% of patients, and for this reason alone myasthenia deserves consideration.

Myasthenia is especially to be considered when symptoms are variable, occur more at the end of the day, and are not associated with a clear-cut nerve palsy. Diplopia often occurs in up gaze; a partial third nerve palsy may appear to exist with an intact pupil; saccades are quick and flicklike, but slow up as they reach extremes of gaze (glissades); asymmetric or monocular quiver may be seen after refixations.

Early findings tend to present in the limb-girdle or bulbar muscles, such as with dysphonia upon prolonged conversing or having the patient count rapidly, or inability to continue chewing. Muscle failure need not be accompanied by subjective feelings of fatigue, but simply by an inability to push the body up another step or to proceed in other simple repetitious efforts.

When myasthenia is suspected, the clinical approach revolves around demonstrating deterioration of function with continued effort. Thus, a worsening of a ptosis after sustained up gaze or effort to open the eyes against resistance is confirmatory. In like manner, lagophthalmos that develops several seconds after eye closure would represent orbicularis fatigue (Figure 19.15). A gaze nystagmus present only after several seconds of side gaze would represent myasthenia-consistent muscle paretic nystagmus, as would an apparent internuclear ophthalmoplegia where adduction begins normally and then fails on further side gaze. In some cases, the onset of fatigue phenomenon is so rapid that one looks for the reverse, that is, a brief restoration of function after a rest. This is the basis of Cogan's lid twitch test, in which the patient looks down for a minute or so then looks suddenly upward. If the ptotic lid briefly raises to nearly equal its partner then droops again, a positive lid-twitch test for myasthenia would be recorded.

While the IV tensilon test is usually diagnostic if it restores function, lack of response in fresh cases does not rule out myasthenia. Also, improvement of a complicated and variable extraocular muscle anomaly may not be easy to document; for this reason an increase in IOP using concurrent tonography is sometimes useful in assessing restoration of overall muscle tone via Tensilon.

Although a rare cause of significant morbidity and occasionally even mortality, the significance of myasthenia for the optometrist is that it presents in the office much more often than its prevalence in the general population would indicate.

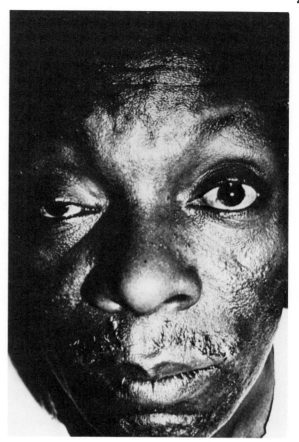

**FIGURE 19.15.**
Apparent right third nerve paresis in patient with nasalized speech and leg weakness originally thought to have Wernicke's encephalopathy. Exotropia was greater in right gaze, indicating left medial rectus palsy in combination with right ptosis. Multiple myopathic symptoms eventually proved to be myasthenia.
Reprinted by permission of the publisher, from Donin JF and Keane JR. Diagnostic problems in neuro-ophthalmology. New York: Famous Teachings in Modern Medicine, Medcom, Inc., 1973.

Myasthenia must always be kept in mind since it can mimic almost any ocular motor disorder and may be diagnosed later in a patient thought to be a chronic complainer if no abnormality is seen at the time of the exam.

Lastly, relatively sudden onset of widespread myasthenialike symptoms may reflect remote carcinoma (Eaton-Lambert syndrome). Treatment of myasthenia has changed radically over the last few years and is best carried out through a neurologic center. Although a serious disease still, if symptoms remain only ocular for 2 years or so, the patient's prognosis is favorable.

Thyroid myopathy (Graves' disease) represents the single most common cause of diplopia and should always be suspected in symptomatic females, even when they seem in good health (Table 19.4). Along with thyroid hyperplasia and its systemic and ocular signs indicating increased sympathetic tone, some patients with hyperthyroidism also show inflammatory signs of an autoimmune nature, chiefly involving muscles, especially extraocular.

Thyroid myopathy usually is associated with or may precede idiopathic goiter, but not nodules, subacute or chronic thyroiditis, nor malignancies. Often the worse cases follow surgical or radioactive normalization of clinical hyperthyroidism. Patients with ocular signs may be euthyroid initially, but the eye practitioner's suspicions are usually borne out when clinical and laboratory evidence follow. $T_3$ and $T_4$ in fact are more often normal than not at presentation. A free thyroxine index should be obtained by radioimmune assay, not by calculation from resin uptake. Special testing is more likely to show faulty regulation, and here the Werner suppression test has been largely supplanted by the safer and more sensitive thyroid releasing hormone test.

Thyroid myopathy usually presents with proptosis of one or both eyes; only rarely can diplopia exist in its absence. Proptotic asymmetry seldom is greater than 4 mm. Barely measurable asymmetry often will be more obvious by simply comparing prominence of the eyes by looking down over the brows. Other diagnostic signs include resistance against digital ballottement of the eyes backward into the orbit and signs of congestion, such as enlarged veins over the horizontal recti and

#### Table 19.4
#### Signs and Symptoms in Graves' Disease

| General | Eye |
|---|---|
| Palpable diffuse thyroid hyperplasia | Lid retraction |
| Hoarseness/sensation on swallowing | Staring appearance/infrequent blinking |
| Nervousness/insomnia | Lid lag on quick down gaze |
| Fine tremor in outstretched hands | Signs of orbital infiltration: |
| Rapid speech |    Venous congestion over horizontal recti |
| Thinning of hair |    Fingerlike edema of upper lid |
| Weight loss despite increased appetite |    Proptosis |
| Palpitations/tachycardia with little response to digitalis |    Diplopia |
| Systolic hypertension/cervicle venous hum/possible orbital bruit |    If severe chemosis, disc edema, exposure keratitis, retinal folds, glaucoma, and optic atrophy may occur |
| Heat intolerance/warm, moist hands/increased perspiration | Dysthyroid ophthalmopathy rarely may occur with Cushing's syndrome, cirrhosis, Crohn's disease, patients taking thyroid extract for weight loss, and secondary to remote carcinoma. |
| Fatigue, muscle wasting, pretibial myxedema | |

of fingerlike edema of the upper outer lids (Figure 19.16). In addition, orbital congestion usually results in no decrease of the exophthalmometer reading when the patient is reclining versus the usual drop of 2 to 3 mm observed in normal eyes. Always consider carotid-cavernous fistula when this type of presentation is unilateral.

One must remember that diplopia in dysthyroid myopathy (which usually is worse in up gaze, as in other myopathies)

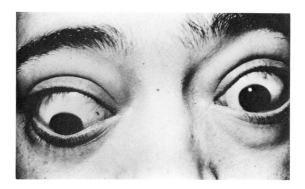

**FIGURE 19.16.**
**Tethering of the eyes in attempted up gaze in a case of dysthyroid ophthalmoplegia. Note marked lid retraction and characteristic fingerlike edema of the upper lids.**
Reprinted by permission of the publisher, from Abrahamson IA, Jr. Ophthalmic manifestations of medical and neurological diseases. New York: Famous Teachings in Modern Medicine, Medcom, Inc., 1972.

reflects not a paresis, but a mechanical restriction to motion from the inflammatory process in opposing muscles: lymphocytic infiltration, edema, and fibrosis. This supplies the *raison d'être* for the forced duction test; an enlarged and fibrotic inferior rectus simply will not allow good passive motion when it is grasped in an attempt to rotate the eye upward with forceps. Equally diagnostic would be the observing of a marked rise in Schiøtz tensions when the patient attempts to move the eyes into the field of action of maximum diplopia. Although forceps with cocaine anesthesia is the classic method of doing a forced duction, the eye with a simple neurogenic palsy is exceedingly easy to push into the impaired field of action by using a Q-tip at the limbus and proparacaine anesthesia. Of course, ask the patient to attempt to move the eyes to relax the antagonists; if the eye does not move freely, suspect a mechanical restriction as from an orbital fracture entrapment or Graves' disease.

In general, thyroid disease resolves over 1 to 2 years, and most patients escape with little but the need to lubricate the eyes at night plus some permanent residual proptosis and lid retraction. One is reluctant, therefore, to suggest muscle surgery. Patients with major disease threatening sight from increased tension, severe exposure, or optic nerve compression are candidates for systemic steroid treatment, orbital radiation, or orbital decompression.

# Anomalies of Lid Position

*Any deviation from the normal relative position of the lids with respect to the vertical limbi can be caused by anomalies in levator/orbicularis function, or by an abnormal forward/aft position of the globe in the socket.*

## BACKGROUND

Defects in eyelid position should not be forgotten in routine examination in preference to the extraocular muscles. Subtle defects often are not recognized by the patient and can be critical neurologic observations. For example, the slight widening of the fissure representing seventh nerve weakness has been the first sign of many a brain tumor.

Although there is wide variation, the usual position of the upper lid is that which covers the limbus by a millimeter or two; the lower lid usually rests near the limbus or slightly below. This position is subject to some variability due to factors such as age, race, and refractive error; for example, the eyes are somewhat larger and thus more forwardly positioned in high myopia, producing a wider fissure, while the upper and lower lids are both somewhat slacker and lower in position with senility.

The levator muscle controls the posi-tion of the upper lid and is innervated by the third nerve. Ptosis owing to third nerve disorder usually is readily suggested by disorders of motility or anisocoria.

The smooth retractor muscle of the lids (Müller's muscle) is controlled by sympathetic fibers, and here the ptosis is usually less marked and may also include some degree of lower lid ptosis. Spastic orbicularis function, as after recovery from Bell's palsy, may also produce a pseudo-ptosis, but this is usually obvious in surrounding periorbital facial muscles.

More often seen is orbicularis weakness manifest as lagophthalmos. When myopathic, the levator and other facial muscles are often bilaterally affected. When of neurologic import, the chief concerns are ipsilateral seventh nerve function, ipsilateral brain stem and associated cranial nerve function, or contralateral hemisphere disease (supranuclear palsy).

## HISTORY AND EXAMINATION

Observe the gross appearance of the eyes before the detailed eye exam so as not to overlook an asymmetry in the size of the palpebral fissures. When noted, it is not always evident whether a mild asymmetry is due to a ptosis on the smaller side or lid retraction, proptosis, or orbicularis weakness on the larger side. Levator weakness generally is evident by an abnormally low position of the upper lid relative to the pupil, in one or both eyes. Obviously, the effects of anisocoria or a vertical tropia will have to be taken into account when present. Nonemergency causes of ptosis commonly are bilateral but may be asymmetrical.

Proptosis and orbicularis weakness usually result in a widening of the fissure by exposing more sclera below (Figure 19.17). Lid retraction usually is bilateral but may be asymmetrical and always widens the fissure by exposing sclera above. It may vary considerably with the state of mind, being more obvious when the patient is nervous or attentive.

It is always necessary when confronted with a palpebral fissure asymmetry to use a good parallax exophthalmometer; what appears to be a ptosis may turn out to be a contralateral proptosis, and what appears to be proptosis may turn out to be a slack lower lid caused by orbicularis weakness. Fissure differences often accompany orbital/facial asymmetry, and the more forward-positioned globe simply reflects a more shallow orbit. In these patients, look for facial asymmetry, such as

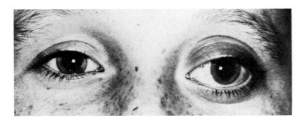

**FIGURE 19.17.**
Widening of the fissure exposing more sclera below as is characteristic of proptosis—in this case, caused by childhood glioma of the optic nerve.
Reprinted by permission of the publisher, from Lloyd LA. Gliomas of the optic nerve and chiasms in childhood. In: Smith JL, ed. Neuro-ophthalmology update. New York: Masson Publishing USA, 1977.

a hypo-orbit, to interpret properly the exophthalmometry readings. Although norms vary with race and refractive error, a good rule of thumb is that 21 mm represents the upper limit of normal, with 3 mm of asymmetry or more needing explanation. The full discussion of proptosis appears in Chapter 20.

Excluding a congenital ptosis, which is usually marked and denoted by absence of the upper lid fold, common causes of ptosis are bilateral and mild. These include senility, familial tendency, and chronic hard contact lens wear. Blepharochalasis may obscure lid margin position and simulate ptosis; the redundant skin has to be gently retracted to ascertain the true state of affairs. Myopathies were discussed in the preceding section and are suspected when a ptosis is bilateral, progressive in midlife or before, subject to significant day/night variation as in myasthenia, or accompanied by facial, bulbar, proximal limb-girdle or extraocular weakness, with or without a familial tendency.

Always look for a mechanical cause of ptosis and palpate the orbit for a mass. Simple lid edema from chronic allergies, giant pappillary conjunctivitis, hypothyroidism, and a water-retention tendency in middle-aged women may produce a thickening of the lids and mild ptosis that is most evident on arising. If ptosis and swelling show a purplish cast, look for enlargement of the tongue, which suggests amyloidosis or myeloma; if there also is weakness and soreness of other muscles, consider an inflammatory cause such as trichinosis or dermatomyositis.

Slack orbicularis function is common in senility and often is part of the presentation of myopathies. It is most evident in its exposure of the lower sclera and may produce morning irritation from lagophthalmos, poor tear pumping with epiphora, or even ectropion. It often is not noted until bifocal heights are measured, and the novice examiner may mistakenly order unequal bifocal heights and miss a neurologically important sign. It is crucial here to look for other signs of facial muscle asymmetry, such as loss of wrinkles or the nasolabial fold or a drooping of the corner of the mouth. Inspect symmetry of function while the patient wrinkles the brow, frowns, smiles, and grimaces spontaneously and on command. Test orbicularis power by holding the upper lids while the patient attempts forcibly to close the eyes. Also note lower lid tone by pulling the lids away from the globe and watching for a tendency for one lid to take longer to return to apposition. See if the patient can retain air when puffing out the cheeks.

Finally, it is surprising how often patients will suddenly become aware of a preexisting fissure asymmetry. If there is a concomitant complaint such as headache, the patient may even present as an emergency. Always ask for old pictures to be sure that the sign is one of true emergency.

# CLINICAL SIGNIFICANCE

## Lid Retraction

The appearance of unilateral lid retraction occasionally reflects excessive levator tonus being employed to aid a contralateral ptosis; have the patient close the other eye to see if the retraction disappears to make this diagnosis. Furthermore, since about 5% of myasthenia cases are associated with Graves' disease, one may indeed encounter ptosis on one side with a bonafide lid retraction on the other. Here, if one mechanically elevates the ptotic lid, the other lid suddenly droops, producing a most distinctive sign of myasthenia: "seesaw ptosis."

The most common cause of lid retraction is thyroid disease, and although usually bilateral, it may present asymmetrically. Lid retraction, on occasion, is the only eye sign of Graves' disease, and usually the patient is euthyroid, but the thyrotroprin-releasing hormone (TRH) test is often positive. If there are no midbrain signs, and lid lag is observed on quick down gaze, the diagnosis is almost certain, especially in young and middle-aged women. Assuming no treatable thyroid anomaly, lid retraction that persists for more than a year represents fibrosis and will be permanent in most cases. An experienced cosmetic surgeon will usually obtain a good result in these cases.

Fibrotic scarring from lid lacerations also produces lid retraction but is little problem in the differential. Not uncommonly, there is a markedly variable lid retraction in neurotic patients who commonly complain of symptoms suggesting hyperthyroidism. Here the lid position will tend to normalize in casual conversation toward the end of the exam, and no lid lag is observed. Finally, it is possible to see unilateral sympathetic irritation and lid retraction as a paradoxical presentation of a Horner's syndrome. The pupil may be enlarged, and this entity seems more common in thoracic lesions such as aortic aneurysm.

The most important neurologic cause of bilateral lid retraction is a midbrain lesion in the tectum near the aquaduct— Collier's sign or "posterior fossa stare." Look for other components of a Parinaud's syndrome (see section on vertical gaze anomalies), as these patients may simulate thyroid eye disease with large pupils and deficient up gaze; there is no lid lag, however (Figure 19.18). In infants, always rule out hydrocephalus (setting-sun sign) by measuring the head circumference and percussing the skull for a cracked pot resonance (Figure 19.19). In children and young adults consider pinealoma or midbrain AV malformation. In somewhat older patients masses are most common. The most common cause, however, occurs in the elderly: basilar artery stenosis.

While lid retraction often is not a part of parkinsonism, it is occasionally seen in

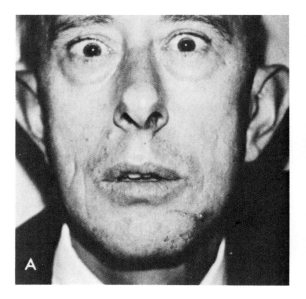

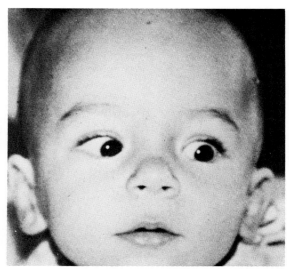

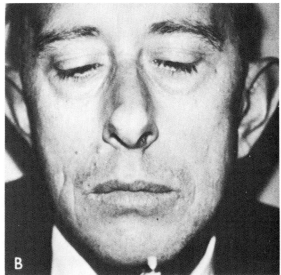

**FIGURE 19.18.**
**Posterior fossa stare in Parinaud's syndrome.**
Note lack of lid hangup in quick down gaze, unlike the lid retraction seen in thyroid disease. Pupils were mid-dilated and fixed in this patient suffering from a pinealoma.

these patients, along with other autonomic involvement such as profuse sweating. Refer to the section on pursuit pathology for a discussion of parkinsonism.

## Ptosis

Aside from myopathic disease already discussed, there are several important neurologic causes of ptosis to consider. Preeminent among these are oculosympathetic paresis and third nerve disease. While these have already been discussed (Chapter 18), it is worth reiterating that in any case of a fresh ptosis, the ipsilateral pupil is the key to diagnosis. If it is relatively miotic a moderate ptosis may be easy to miss, but one must strongly suspect a Horner's syndrome. If it is relatively mydriatic, one must carefully assess third nerve function.

Aside from these two key entities, ptosis is sometimes a component of Wernicke's encephalopathy and may be rather sudden in onset. Inquire about drinking and eating habits and look for signs of ataxia, gaze weakness, nystagmus, dysmetria, and diplopia. Assess the patient for general debilitation and look for evidence of rosacea. Check to see if distal vibratory sensitivity is intact.

In younger patients it is possible to see an isolated ptosis as a component of multiple sclerosis. Here, as always, the history of other typical symptoms will indicate a neurologic diagnosis. One cannot underestimate the importance of a good eye exam to detect subacute conduction and oculomotor defects in such patients.

## Orbicularis Dysfunction

Orbicularis weakness as a component of general bulbar muscle weakness has been discussed in the section on myopathies. Here the diagnosis is suggested by thin, recessed, ptotic, slightly purplish lids in an expressionless face. Unlike this type of bilateral involvement, neurologically important causes are always unilateral.

Facial and orbicularis weakness on one side most commonly reflects Bell's palsy (in five of six patients, often young males). This sudden loss of function is the result of an unknown inflammatory process, often in the petrous bone aspect of the nerve. This condition may reflect a postviral demyelination, perhaps caused by herpes simplex. Occasionally, a specific diagnosis may be herpes zoster, Paget's disease, or sarcoid. It is best to get a glucose tolerance if the patient is over 40, as the incidence of diabetes in this group will approach 20%.

The palsy generally is complete, involving the upper and lower halves of the face on the same side. Depending on the proximity of the lesion, it may also affect taste (anterior two-thirds of the tongue), decrease salivation and lacrimal output, and occasionally may affect the stapedus nerve to produce hyperacusis. The picture is typical (see Chapter 21), with a slight pseudolid retraction and ectropion on the involved side, the mouth pulled over toward the unaffected side, and loss of wrinkles and folds on the involved side. Some physicians prescribe steroids when the patient is seen soon after onset and the lesion is proximal (e.g., loss of taste), but usually Bell's palsy shows early signs of recovery on its own in several weeks or so. Delayed recovery (past 2–3 months) is more likely to mean incomplete recovery, often with anomalous reinnervation (e.g., jaw winking).

An old Bell's palsy may present as a persisting cause of lagophthalmos. Here the examiner should be alert to distinguish the orbicularis atonicity from apparent exophthalmos.

Mild orbicularis weakness tends to show up as a touch of lagophthalmos with tremor in gentle eye lid closure; look for this with morning irritation complaints or lower corneal stippling. In most severe dysfunction, the involved eye may even open sharply on attempted closure, owing to superior rectus/levator cocontraction via Bell's reflex. One may also test strength by holding the eyelids during attempted forced closure, or have the patient gently close his eyes while looking up. The side with the weaker orbicularis is less likely to close fully.

Brain stem facial weakness may simulate a Bell's palsy when of acute onset, such as that caused by stroke. There are likely to be other pontine cranial nerve signs (nerves V, VI, and VIII) as well as crossed sensorimotor ones. An ipsilateral gaze palsy is common. With lagophthalmos, keep in mind cerebellopontine angle mass—usually acoustic neuroma. Check the corneal reflexes and facial sensation, as well as hearing and ipsilateral cerebellar function (listing, gaze nystagmus, dysmetria). This entity often is progressive over the years, the symptoms are rarely noted early, and it is a common tumor in von Recklinghausen's disease. Many patients have noted decreased hearing for 15 years or more before more ominous signs present. A reduced corneal reflex usually is present in such patients.

Supranuclear facial palsy is a different entity altogether. Descending hemispheric fibers reaching the final common path in the seventh nucleus are mostly crossed, except for those subserving the upper half of the face, of which about half are crossed. Thus, a patient with lower face weakness on the right, perhaps a little orbicularis weakness but equal brow wrinkling on both sides, almost certainly has a supranuclear palsy, which is more serious than Bell's as it represents cerebral disease, in this case on the left side. These patients sometimes retain emotional input to the nucleus and might show spontaneous expressions that seem impossible with the inability to reproduce voluntary movements. Often, neither patient nor family note the change in facial appearance when it is subtle. Pyramidal tract function should be evaluated in such patients and the examiner should be alert for subtle parietal lobe signs of a middle cerebral artery hemorrhage. Elderly patients with lower facial weakness always deserve auscultation of the contralateral carotid bifurcations.

The presence of hyperactive orbicularis function, blepharospasm, is quite common. To some degree, episodic appearance of transient spasms in children is normal under stress. Occasionally, the spasms become progressively worse and may become a strong habit, which is difficult to treat by any means.

Other cases of "essential" blepharospasm develop for no apparent reason in seemingly normal patients. This bilateral progressive disorder can become so severe as to make even walking dangerous. The disorder occasionally reflects a more generalized parkinsonianlike dyskinesia. Always inquire as to whether the patient is a habitual decongestant user, as this is a recognized cause of the disease.

The most common presentation, however, is that of myokymia, a rapid mild episodic twitching of the lids. Often patients claim that the eye itself "jumps." Especially if confined to the lower lid and occasionally alternating eyes, myokymia is both common and harmless. Some authors feel that it may be related to stress, eye strain, fatigue, or neuroticism. One should ask if there are any other spastic muscles to rule out a general condition, such as hypoparathyroidism or electrolyte imbalance. Quinine or vitamin E are sometimes helpful. Although most cases are functional, progressive unilateral involvement of both upper and lower lids and periorbital facial musculature in a more sustained blepharospasm or facial tic is cause for concern. If testing denotes lateralized signs of facial muscle weakness concomitant with the spastic tendency, there is a significant possibility of pontine glioma and a stem neurologic screen and follow-up visit, at the very least, are required. Multiple sclerosis has also been known to cause an irritative partial facial weakness as well; inquire as to historical evidence of other suggestive problems in young adults.

Bilateral hyperreflexive blepharospasm is common in the neurotic, the elderly, and is most marked in parkinsonism and the Steele-Richardson-Olchevsky syndrome, where the patient may have considerable trouble opening the eyes. Blepharospasm occurs episodically in a variety of stroke syndromes, and such patients often cry inexplicably at these moments. Such patients usually cannot refrain from blinking to repeated glabella taps, a useful sign in considering a diagnosis of parkinsonism.

In children, pathologically increased startle with blepharospasm has been noted as an early sign of subacute sclerosing panencephalitis (SSPE), which is a uniformly fatal disease associated with an increased measles titer. Like other habit spasms, persistent squinting is often seen in myopes and albinos, even after remediation of the condition is made with lenses.

Finally, fluttering of the lids may cause parents to bring in a child and should be recognized as a common sign of petit mal in children. It may be accompanied by a cry, apnea, staring expression, mental absence, conjugate deviation of the eyes, or more obvious fleeting signs.

In summary, the significance of disorders of lid function can be far ranging. The optometrist must not forget that two cranial nerves innervate these structures—an indication of their value as windows to the integrity of the nervous system.

# Pursuit Disorders

*Absence of smooth pursuit in one or more directions in the presence of normal or near normal saccades indicates a pursuit disorder.*

## BACKGROUND

Smooth pursuit movements are incapable of being voluntarily produced in the absence of relative motion of the object of regard. Pursuit movements probably derive from the extrapyramidal control systems responsible for so many other involuntary "postural" adjustments.

One of the chief functions of the vestibular systems is to stabilize the eyes and aid retention of fixation during head and body movement (doll's head pursuits). Optically elicited pursuit such as that produced by large optokinetic targets probably serves to aid in the vestibular system in maintaining sustained fixation. A quite different ability is to smoothly track moving objects independently of vestibular input. To do this accurately when the head is also turning to aid in tracking the object of regard actually requires extrapyramidal suppression of vestibular input, or else the eyes would contravert.

Retention of vestibularly generated pursuit requires the integrity of a three-neuron arc from sensory vestibular apparatus to brain stem control, from brain stem control to oculomotor nuclei, and from oculomotor nuclei to extraocular muscles. Retention of optically elicited pursuit and vestibular suppression, however, requires extrapyramidal integrity: the basal ganglia and cerebellum. Optically elicited pursuit also requires cortical integrity of vision and descending influences. Although this pathway is not worked out, it is clear the focal point in the descending hemispheric control for lateral smooth pursuit is the ipsilateral deep parietal lobe near the occipital junction. It is not surprising, therefore, that isolated pursuit defects nearly always reflect lesions in the cerebellum, basal ganglia, or parietal lobe.

## HISTORY AND EXAMINATION

Occasionally, there may be complete absence of optically elicited tracking in the presence of normal saccadic movements. Much more common, however, is cogwheeling, or a series of small saccades employed in place of pursuit to follow the examiner's penlight. Mildly jumpy pursuits are commonly seen in young children, in patients with cerebral palsy, the developmentally disabled, the inattentive, very nervous patients, and those on tranquilizers. The complete absence of smooth pursuit to a slowly moving target in patients past the age of 5 years is always pathologic, however, and requires explanation. When there is doubt as to the integrity of these movements in one or more directions, the defect will usually become more obvious with use of the optokinetic tape, on which little or no nystagmus will be evident when the tape is moved in the suspect direction(s).

With major brain stem gaze palsies, slow pursuit movements are not retained even with doll's head or caloric stimulation. In non-brain-stem apraxias of saccadic gaze, however, one may see retention of optically directed pursuit and, almost always, preservation of doll's head movement. Indeed, even in the absence of smooth pursuit, these movements are usually intact with vestibular augmentation.

In cerebellar disease and the more severe basal ganglia degenerations, testing for integrity of vestibular suppression may be considered. This is done by having the patient seated in the chair and fixing his finger in front of his face while the chair is rotated. In cerebellar disease, vestibular stimulation often will contravert the eyes away from the object of regard. There will be, therefore, a series of misaligning drifts followed by corrective saccades, or nystagmus. While most characteristic of cerebellar disease, lack of vestibular suppression may also occur in progressive supranuclear palsy, where lack of the saccadic redress usually occurs—that is, the eyes amazingly just drift to the end point when the chair is rotated in deference to the patient's fixational wishes.

# CLINICAL SIGNIFICANCE

A major absence of pursuit is often seen in lipid storage diseases, where it may accompany a total oculomotor apraxia. This should be remembered in children with failing vision, macular opacification, dysmyelinating symptoms, psychomotor failure, and hepatosplenomegaly. Even here, smooth doll's head pursuits are usually retained. Whether this defect reflects basal ganglia deposition is unknown. Certainly the most common causes reflect basal ganglia disease (Table 19.5).

Using parkinsonism as the prototype, general signs and symptoms of degenerative diseases are

1. Bradykinesia: masklike face; paucity of spontaneous movements, including saccades and blinking, small steps, failure to swing arms, tiny handwriting, etc.

2. Poor reflex suppression: increased startle, inability to suppress blink to glabella taps, lack of vestibular suppression, blepharospastic tendency.

3. Resting tremor and mild ataxia: "pill-rolling" fingers, head nodding, shuffling, swaying, stooping, and widening of stance in gait.

4. Rigidity: Difficulty initiating action, neck rigidity with tendency to turn whole torso; rigidity may be of cogwheel type on passive motion versus the "lead-pipe" rigidity seen upon arm extension in pyramidal disease.

5. Autonomic defects: Seborrheic blepharitis, sweating, tearing, drooling, postural hypotension.

6. Mild dementia and depression: "Look sad, feel sad."

7. Other oculomotor disturbances: Poor vertical gaze, convergence and accommodation; long latency, slow, hypometric, and ill-sustained saccades.

8. Choreoathetoid movements: spasmodic sudden twitches of extremities and writhing, twisting movements that include spasmodic episodic upward eye deviation (oculogyric crises).

### Table 19.5
### Causes of Basal Ganglia Syndromes

Parkinsonism
Parkinsonism plus degenerations (e.g.,
    progressive supranuclear palsy)
Long-term high-dose phenothiazines
Carbon monoxide poisoning, asphyxia, shock
Wilson's disease
Part of the spectrum of presenile dementias
Part of the spectrum in hereditary lipid storage
    disease (e.g., Niemann-Pick)
Huntington's chorea
Poststreptococcal (Syndenham's) chorea
Lenticulostriate artery hemorrhage
Mass lesions (rarely)
Low-tension hydrocephalus

While the usual picture of Parkinson's disease is unmistakable (Figure 19.20), always consider the other entities in Table 19.5, especially in patients younger than 55 or 60 years. With sudden onset of a parkinsonianlike motor disorder plus mental confusion, always consider low-tension hydrocephalus—a treatable cause of dementia in the elderly in which the computed axial tomographic (CAT) scan shows dilated ventricles, but intracranial pressure is found to be normal.

Because dementia is often so apparent in conducting an eye exam, Table 19.6 lists the most prominent causes roughly by frequency to encourage the optometrist always to suspect one of the treatable entities, so great is their tendency to be overlooked. As can be seen, the majority of the diseases listed are either treatable or preventable, and many have prominent eye signs.

Two particular disorders deserve special attention. Progressive supranuclear palsy (PSP or the Steele-Richardson-Olchevsky syndrome) is the prototype of the "parkinsonism-plus" basal ganglia degenerations. It typically presents in late middle age, most frequently in males, and often with early mental deterioration. The rigidity, especially cervical, usually is more apparent than tremor at disease onset. In addition to cogwheel pursuits, these patients are extremely likely to show deficient saccades, especially voluntary ("look down, please"). While mild up-gaze insufficiency is characteristic of parkinsonism, patients with PSP have marked difficulty in looking down, despite retention of doll's head movement. They may require base-down prism in both lenses to walk safely and to read. At the late stage the patient may have a total pseudoophthalmoplegia, save the lack of ptosis.

PSP is the only noncerebellar extrapyramidal disorder in which square-wave jerks are common—that is, the patient appears to look away randomly from the object of regard and back again quickly, despite instruction to fix. Rigidity may be manifest in the inability to reopen the eyes after forced closure or even in lid lag on quick down gaze. Finally, these patients often show an interesting lack of vestibular suppression as mentioned earlier. PSP is uniformly progressive over the years, with a high incidence of some degree of dementia and often premature death. There is no treatment and the disorder is not familial, but it should be recognized to spare unnecessary trips to medical centers and excessive testing.

Wilson's disease (hepatolenticular degeneration) is perhaps the best example of a disease not to be missed by the optometrist. Despite its rarity, this autosomal recessive metabolic disease progresses with liver (hepato-) and basal ganglia (lentiform) signs owing to increased copper deposition in these tissues. Signs and symptoms of the disease may bring the patient (usually an adolescent or young adult) to the doctor at a stage where the pathognomonic corneal copper deposition may not be obvious (Kayser-Fleischer rings) (Figure 19.21). The liver disease may be overlooked or misdiagnosed, and thus a knowledge of the extrapyramidal signs may be crucial in making the diagnosis. In addition to the eye signs already discussed in this section, accommodative pa-

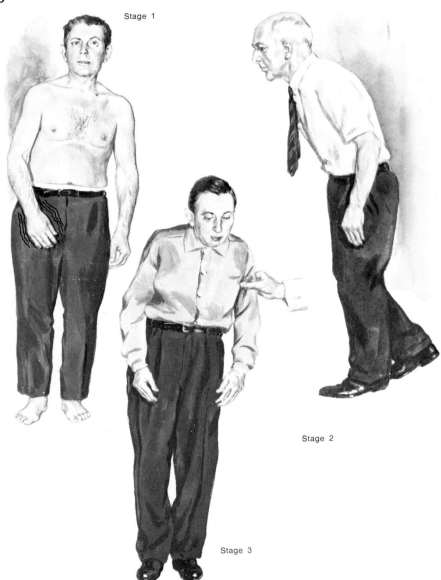

Stage 1

Stage 2

Stage 3

**FIGURE 19.20.**
**Stages in parkinsonism.** *Top left,* blank staring face with mild flexion of
right arm and finger tremor at rest. *Top right,* more generalized ataxia
with stooping and slow shuffling gait. *Bottom* indicates progression to
marked postural instability with tendency to fall.

## Table 19.6
### Most Common Causes of Dementia Roughly by Frequency

Diffuse CNS degenerations
   Alzheimer's disease
   Pick's disease
Vascular disease
   Multiinfarct arteriolar disease in hypertension
   Atheromatous disease
   Collagen vasculitis
   Temporal arteritis
Toxins
   Alcoholism
   Heavy metals
   Hydrocarbons
   Hypoxia/carbon monoxide
   Chronic drug toxicity
Normal pressure hydrocephalus
Intracranial masses
Other degenerative diseases
   Parkinsonism
   Progressive supranuclear palsy
   Spinocerebellar degenerations
   Huntington's chorea
   Recurrent seizures
Infections/inflammatory diseases
   Neurosyphilis
   Encephalitis/meningitis/abscess
   Multiple sclerosis
   Creutzfeldt-Jakob disease
   Dysmyelinating syndromes
   Behcet's disease
   Whipple's disease
Posttraumatic/including chronic subdural
   hemorrhage
Metabolic
   Hypothyroidism/hypopituitarism
   Vitamin deficiency
   Hepatic disease
   Parathyroid disease
   Hypoglycemia
   Uremia
   Remote carcinoma

sion, mutism, and dementia following with the more obvious motor signs of ataxia, tremor, and choreoathetosis (including the eye movements); note staring face sign in Wilson's disease versus facial rigidity with Huntington's chorea (Figures 19.21, 19.22). Untreated, Wilson's disease is fatal. The diagnosis is made by noting increased urinary copper and decreased serum copper and ceruloplasm in assays.

Unaffected heterozygotes may show positive laboratory evidence, necessitating a liver biopsy. It is essential to suspect this disease early, as penicillamine stops further progression in most cases, but does not return CNS function already lost. Thus an uncoordinated, drooly 10-year-old with a peculiar facial rigidity, spider angiomas, and jerky pursuits, who is brought in by his mother because of an episode where

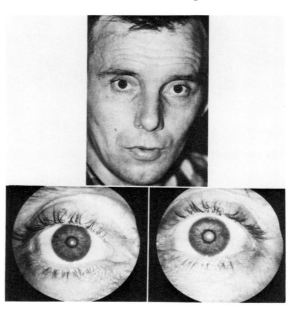

**FIGURE 19.21.**
**Fixed staring face in Wilson's disease, with peripheral iris detail masked by copper deposition in corneas.**
Reprinted by permission of the publisher, from Goodman RM and Gorlin RJ. Atlas of the face in genetic disorders. St. Louis: C.V. Mosby, 1974; 2nd ed.

resis may be present while other early findings may be still subtle, such as poor fine coordination expressed in bad penmanship. Drooling, dysphagia, and slurred speech are characteristic, with depres-

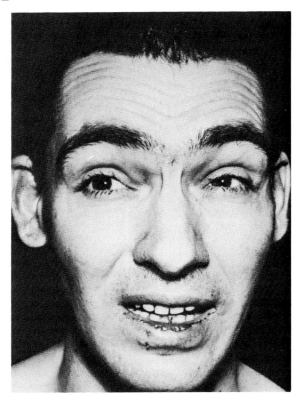

**FIGURE 19.22.**
Marked facial rigidity evident in a patient with Huntington's chorea attempting to open mouth.
Reprinted by permission of the publisher, from Perrine GA Jr and Goodman RM. A family study of Huntington's chorea with unusual manifestations. Ann Intern Med 1966; 64:570–574.

lesions and is a very valuable localizing sign seen even in patients with intact visual fields. Such patients may show an absence of smooth pursuit *only toward* the side of the lesion, that is, targets going away from a field or visual inattention defect if present. The defect may be subtle, however, and is best viewed using an optokinetic challenge, in which case a lack of brisk optokinetic nystagmus (OKN) will be seen when the stripes are moved only toward the side of the lesion (asymmetrical optokinetic nystagmus). This test should be carried out in all patients with homonymous field defects, as a negative OKN test almost rules out parietal lobe disease, which is second in frequency only to occipital lobe disease in causing such field defects but much more commonly is associated with masses.

The third type of pursuit pathology is the cogwheeling seen in cerebellar disease that is virtually identical to that seen in basal ganglia disease. Although familial spinocerebellar degenerations are common, cerebellar signs often herald acute significant disease. Here one makes the distinction by noting the relative absence of basal ganglia signs versus the existence of the distinct company of cerebellar signs discussed in a succeeding section. For example, tremor in cerebellar lesions is usually of the intention rather than resting type seen in parkinsonism.

The significance of pursuit defects of course depends on their cause. This subtle abnormality may be the only ocular finding suggesting further observations, tests, and history leading to the discovery of serious treatable illnesses such as Wilson's disease, parietal lobe glioma, or cerebellar hemiangioblastoma.

the eyes jerked into right up gaze, has Wilson's disease until proved otherwise.

The second important type of selective pursuit pathology occurs with parietal lobe

# Vertical Gaze Apraxias

*Vertical gaze apraxia is the loss of the ability to elevate or depress the eyes despite intact oculomotor nuclei, nerves, and muscles.*

## BACKGROUND

A localized cortical area responsible for vertical gaze does not seem to exist. In some animals both the substantia nigra and tectum possess receptotopic motor maps, which when stimulated produce directed eye movements to the appropriate area of the field. Neither area sends fibers directly to the oculomotor nuclei, however, and their significance is not known in humans. Unilateral substantia nigra lesions seem to have no effect on human eye movements, while the bilateral degenerations discussed in the pursuit section seem to have only a modest effect on vertical gaze. Tectal lesions, however, have a marked effect on vertical gaze but little on horizontal. Clinically speaking then, the more voluntary aspects of vertical gaze seem to be centered in the pretectal periaqueductal gray of the midbrain near the red nuclei.

## HISTORY AND EXAMINATION

Simply asking the patient to pursue the examiner's penlight in up and down gaze often is sufficient to disclose a vertical gaze apraxia. When a midbrain syndrome is suspected, however, it is necessary also to require voluntary saccades ("look up, please; look down, please"). Furthermore, if a deficiency of vertical gaze of any sort is suspected, or if other components of a possible midbrain syndrome are evident, it is also necessary to pass the optokinetic flag up and down before the patient's eyes. Absence of even voluntary up gaze strongly suggests a midbrain lesion, and observation of convergent-retraction nystagmus to an OKN challenge is even more suggestive.

Nonneurological causes of deficient upgaze include extreme old age, myasthenia, the progressive external ophthalmoplegias, thyroid ophthalmoplegia, and traumatic entrapment syndromes involving the inferior muscles. These have already been discussed.

While some loss of up gaze is common in the elderly, especially those with Parkinson's disease and other basal ganglia degenerations, the company with a midbrain lesion is usually distinctive. The vertical gaze paresis usually is of up gaze. A complete Parinaud's syndrome would also include lid retraction (posterior fossa stare), poor convergence and perhaps accommodation, and often mid-dilated pupils with little response to near effort. An incomplete presentation may not be so obvious and may even mimic thyroid disease with its lid retraction and poor up gaze, especially if up gaze is asymmetrical and diplopia ensues, since Parinaud's syndrome is one of the few supranuclear syndromes where diplopia can occur (Figure 19.23). Similarly, the occasional existence of up-beat nystagmus on attempted up gaze might bias the examiner toward a cerebellar lesion if the remainder of the syndrome is not sought.

Often the vertical gaze paresis is minimal and should best be called an apraxia, as the patient may show good up pursuit, or even refixating saccades, but be totally unable to demonstrate voluntary up gaze: to look up on command. Even when all of these are abnormal, doll's head maneuver or forced closure may show intact function of the cranial nerves, thus pointing to the supranuclear nature of the defect. An important test when a midbrain syndrome is suspected is to challenge up gaze with the OKN tape, passing it downward before the patient's eyes; instead of the normal up-beating nystagmus, one may see *convergent/retraction nystagmus*, where the eyes repeatedly jerk inward or even retract into the orbit. This finding strongly suggests midbrain lesion. Some patients may not present with the full-blown syndrome, so it is advisable to check for all components when any one or two are manifest.

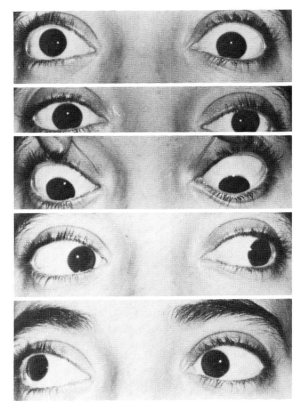

**FIGURE 19.23.**
Inability to elevate the eyes with left hypotropia in Parinaud's syndrome (*top*); lid retraction evident in primary gaze (*second photograph*). Versions were otherwise full. Parinaud's syndrome is one of the few supranuclear lesions that may produce diplopia and may simulate dysthyroid ophthalmoplegia. Patient suffered from a midbrain arteriovenous malformation.
Reprinted by permission of the publisher, from Huber A. Eye signs and symptoms in brain tumors. Blodi FC, ed. and trans. St. Louis: C.V. Mosby, 1976; 3rd ed.

# CLINICAL SIGNIFICANCE

The clinical significance of Parinaud's syndrome is the integrity of the subthalamic midbrain. While pinealoma is the classic cause (said to account for 50% of the cases, especially in younger people), other tumors, lues, multiple sclerosis, thalamic AV malformation (Figure 19.24), and posterior cerebral artery occlusions are all occasional causes. In infants, obstructive hydrocephalus often produces Collier's, or the "setting sun," sign. In private practice, however, it would seem that basilar artery insufficiency in the elderly represents by far the most common cause and may underlie the patient's complaint of not seeing well when relatives move up near the head of the bed.

A final clinical note is that while spasm of the near reflex (miosis, esotropia, pseudomyopia) is usually a functional disorder, it may on occasion represent an irritative Parinaud's syndrome, and a midbrain cause must be ruled out if it doesn't quickly remit with binasal occlusion and cycloplegics. Masses in this area are prone to closing off the aqueduct of Silvius, and thus signs and symptoms of increased intracranial pressure make a Parinaud-like syndrome all the more ominous. For example, a headachy 13-year-old with Parinaud's syndrome and disc edema almost certainly has a pinealoma.

Although not clearly a related pathology, seesaw nystagmus is often associated with diencephalic disease and is mentioned here. The entity of one eye elevating and intorting while the other is depressing (and extorting), and then vice versa, occurs most often in children and suggests a lesion in the area of the floor of the anterior third ventricle, which may affect hypothalamic or chiasmal function. Thus, a field if possible and a review of vegetative function (appetite, sleeping, etc.) is in order. When the referral to the optometrist for this oculomotor disorder is made in an infant whose failure to thrive is painfully

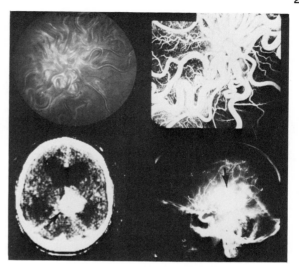

**FIGURE 19.24.**
Retinal arteriovenous malformation (*top left*) that was competent to fluorescein (*top right*). Enhanced CAT scan shows a large midbrain mass and dilated lateral ventricles (*bottom left*). Angiography shows the mass to be a large vascular malformation. Diagnosis: racemose AV malformation of the midbrain and retina (Wyburn-Mason syndrome).
Reprinted by permission of the publisher, from Miller NR, Fine SL. The ocular fundus in neuro-ophthalmologic diagnosis. In: Sights and sounds in ophthalmology, vol. VIII. St. Louis: C.V. Mosby, 1975.

obvious to all concerned, a glioma can be almost guaranteed; radiation may produce remarkable long-term improvement. Even the existence of uniocular vertical bobbing or spasmus nutans should be suggestive of a diencephalic mass in emaciated children.

# Lateral Gaze Disorders

*Disorder of lateral gaze is any deviation from the normal in the latency, velocity, amplitude, and conjugacy of the horizontal excursions of the eyes, given intact oculomotor nerve and muscle function.*

## BACKGROUND

Based upon stroke and tumor data, the origin of the horizontal saccadic system is in a diffusly represented in the contralateral frontal lobe. Descending influences cross near the level of the midbrain to become associated with uncrossed "pursuit fibers" originating near the parietal-occipital junction. These horizontal gaze fibers continue caudally through the paramedian pontine reticular formation to the nucleus of the para-abducens. Output of this nucleus goes to the adjacent sixth nerve nucleus to produce abduction of the ipsilateral eye, and across to the contralateral medial longitudinal fasciculus (MLF) to ascend to nerve III to produce adduction of the contralateral eye as necessary for conjugate gaze. Obviously, lesions in the MLF may lead to disconnection syndromes, where it may appear that the right eye truly does not know what the left eye is doing.

## HISTORY AND EXAMINATION

When a gaze weakness is suspected, it is necessary to study carefully the excursions to a variety of stimuli—pursuit, doll's head maneuver, optically elicited saccades, voluntary saccades, and the optokinetic tape; when all else fails, the ear on the gaze deficient side can be irrigated with ice water. Hold the patient's head to more fully manifest disorders of gaze.

Patients with gaze weakness are usually ignorant of the exact nature of the defect. One memorable patient complained only of not seeing oncoming cars well, leading one to suspect a myopic shift or field defect; a complete left gaze palsy was evident, however.

The search for associated signs and symptoms depends on the site of the lesion. Generally speaking, if the patient is relatively intact neurologically, the office exam focuses on several possibilities. These include myopathies, diffuse cerebral degenerations, acute frontal lobe disease, bilateral parietal lobe disease, and cerebellar disease; the most severe and obvious presentations, however, involve the brain stem. As discussed in the next section, each of these disease classes presents somewhat characteristically.

# CLINICAL SIGNIFICANCE

A complete *lateral gaze palsy* usually presents no difficulty in diagnosis. Some patients are not so obliging, however, and are likely to present with incomplete or bilateral syndromes that appear to be apractic. For example, bilateral, delayed onset, hypometric but normal velocity saccades occur in diffuse cerebellar lesions, such as the familial spinocerebellar degenerations or Louis-Bar syndrome. Other cerebellar signs, such as ataxia, are usually prominent and are described in the next section.

Bilaterally infrequent, *slow*, and ill-sustained saccades are also common in diffuse cerebral degenerations such as Alzheimer's disease and basal ganglia disease (see section on pursuit for the distinctive company of these diseases). Here the apractic nature of the defect is exhibited by little or no movement on command, but there are full rotations during fixation when the examiner passively rotates the patient's head. In these apraxias the paucity of gaze is usually more obvious when the patient's head is held rigid. Children with congenital oculomotor apraxia characteristically use rapid head thrusts to break fixation to allow saccadic initiation. In some of these children the initiation of a voluntary saccade is totally impossible (spasm of fixation), and the head thrust serves to totally contravert the eyes to the end points. Further face turning then serves to break fixation mechanically and allow a shift of gaze (Figure 19.25). Infants with this disorder may appear blind to the examiner if head thrusting has not yet developed; however, oculomotor apraxia presents with normal pupillary responses, normal eye movement when the baby is rotated en bloc, and normal visual evoked response (VER). Congenital oculomotor apraxia improves with age and is rarely associated with progressive disease although such children often have strabismus, mild retardation, and are clumsy. Always consider a lipid storage disease if the child is not developing normally and especially if smooth pursuit defects or apraxias of vertical gaze co-exist.

The progressive *external ophthalmoplegias* will present with a paucity of gaze, but the ptosis, other muscular involvement, family history, and impairment of gaze to all stimuli usually suggest the diagnosis. Myasthenia can cause confusion as well, but here the saccade starts abruptly with normal speed and then slows (glissades): enhanced end-point, muscle-paretic nystagmus and/or diplopia may also result, especially with sustained eccentric gaze (myasthenic gaze fatigue).

Finally, infrequent, ill-sustained, and markedly inaccurate saccades are seen occasionally in bilateral parietal lobe damage as part of Balint's syndrome (see Chapter 32).

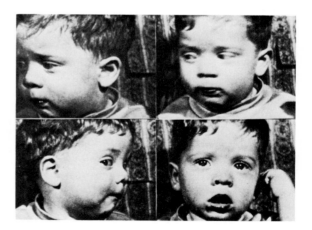

**FIGURE 19.25.**
Oculomotor apraxia: child initiates a change in fixation (*top left*) by thrusting the head (*top right*) while eyes remain contraverted at the end point. When fixation is finally attained (*bottom left*), head returns to primary position (*bottom right*).
Reprinted by permission of the publisher, from Felker GV, Ide CH, and Hart WM. Congenital ocular motor approxia. *EENT Monthly* 1973;52:104. Copyright Insight Publishing Co.

A contralateral *gaze apraxia* lasting 2 to 3 weeks is most commonly seen after a major frontal lobe stroke in elderly patients. Here, a resting bias toward the side of the lesion is also usually seen, and the patient may complain of inability to see to the other side, suggesting a field defect. Conversely, an irritative frontal lobe lesion may present with a history of episodic spasms of contralateral gaze. In office practice, always consider subdural hemorrhage.

Finally, the term *spasticity of conjugate gaze* is sometimes applied to the observance of a conjugate Bell's reflex seen on attempted forced lid closure with the examiner's fingers holding the upper lids. While normal eyes may not always drift upward, a conjugate deviation to one side or the other occurs in only 2% of the population; the observation of a conjugate Bell's reflex has little localizing significance but is useful to help confirm a hemispheric lesion somewhere on the side opposite the lateralized eye movement.

The major characteristic of *brain-stem gaze palsies* is that they are complete to all stimuli, including vestibular. Stroke is the most common cause. Other signs of brain-stem pathology, such as hemiparesis, will be obvious. As opposed to signs of frontal lobe lesions, the eye will drift *toward* the hemiparetic side, as the gaze palsy is ipsilateral to the stem lesion, and the descending pyramidal motor fibers have not yet decussated. Often there will be cranial nerve defects, especially of nerves VI and VII. A seemingly isolated true gaze paresis in an otherwise intact patient visiting the office suggests a microlesion, such as lacunar infarct in hypertension, a demyelinating plaque, lues, and, especially, Wernicke's encephalopathy with an accompanying sixth nerve palsy (Figure 19.26).

Brain-stem gaze paresis does not recover as well as that seen in frontal lobe disease. If incomplete, it is often associated with very slow drifts away from the eccentrically fixated object of regard, fol-

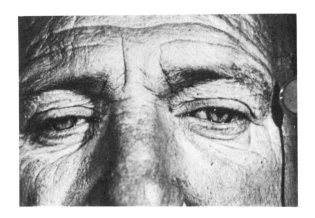

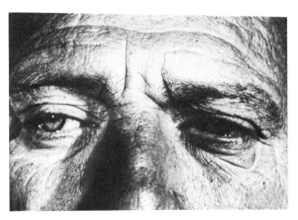

**FIGURE 19.26.**
**Bilateral paresis of conjugate gaze in Wernicke's encephalopathy. Patient had a history of chronic alcoholism as evidenced by furrowed orange peellike skin and nasal sebaceous hypertrophy.**
Reprinted by permission of the publisher, from Donin JF and Keane JR. Diagnostic problems in neuro-ophthalmology. New York: Famous Teachings in Modern Medicine, Medcom, Inc., 1973.

lowed by attempted refixations. Such gaze-paretic nystagmus beats are evident only on the involved side and will not be seen in other positions of gaze.

A particularly interesting brain-stem variant is that of a dissociated gaze palsy, *internuclear ophthalmoplegia* (INO) (Figure 19.27). Here the command for ipsilateral gaze may leave the right nucleus para-abducens to produce ipsilateral abduction via the right sixth nerve, but crossing fibers ascending the left MLF are interrupted. Thus, the left third nerve never receives the message; that is, the eye ipsilateral to the MLF lesion fails to adduct, with the good eye often showing abduction nystagmus.

Such an INO is clearly not a left medial rectus (MR) palsy, as the eyes are usually straight in the primary position, and adduction is usually evident on convergence. While often a part of major brain-stem syndromes, isolated INO in the office tends to reflect a microlesion. Bilateral INO in an intact patient (especially a young adult) is virtually pathognomonic for multiple sclerosis, although this sign is not nearly as common as paresthesias, leg weakness, and optic neuritis. Brain-stem lesions can produce both an ipsilateral gaze palsy and

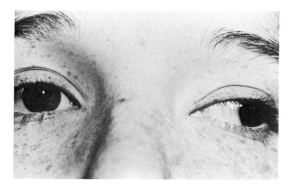

**FIGURE 19.27.**
Right internuclear ophthalmoplegia evident by failure of right eye to adduct in left conjugate gaze despite normal third nerve function. Patient has suffered from bilateral leg weakness and recurrent optic neuritis. Diagnosis: multiple sclerosis.
Reprinted by permission of the publisher, from Donin JF and Keane JR. Diagnostic problems in neuro-ophthalmology. New York: Famous Teachings in Modern Medicine, Medcom, Inc., 1973.

an INO (one-and-one-half syndrome); here no movement toward the side of the lesion takes place and only abduction occurs contralaterally.

INO may present subclinically in multiple sclerosis, since conduction along the MLF may be impaired. Such patients may present with apparently normal extraocular muscle movements (EOM), except for abduction nystagmus in one or both eyes. While pursuits may be normal, watching the patient make large saccades produces the unsettling feeling that the adducting eye attains the end point slightly behind its partner.

The full integrity of the MLF may then be challenged using the OKN tape as follows: move the tape to the patient's left; the right eye will show a brisk, right-beating OKN. If the left eye shows a diminished fast adduction phase, one has demonstrated asymmetrical optokinetic nystagmus. This is not to be confused with the asymmetrical responses of parietal lobe lesions that pertain to rightward versus leftward moving tapes.

Examining rapid large saccades or using the OKN tape is required for patients in whom brain-stem lesions or multiple sclerosis is suggested by other signs of history. Obviously, any case of unilateral INO should also be challenged to the opposite side, since the observing of a subclinical INO on the other side then makes the case a bilateral one with very different implications. Myasthenia (as in so many eye movement pathologies), may also occasionally mimic an INO, and brain-stem pathology may be all the more suspect, with pseudobulbar weakness caused by the characteristic distribution of transmission failure (shoulder girdle, dysarthria, dysphonia, dysphagia, facial weakness). If myasthenia is suspected, Tensilon will usually settle the matter. Lastly, tricyclic antidepressants and phenothiazines have been reported to be associated with the development of INO.

Two additional syndromes associated with major lesions in the brain stem (such as basilar artery strokes) deserve attention. *Ocular myoclonus* is an extremely disconcerting syndrome in which constant, extremely rapid myokymialike flutter of the eyes usually accompanies a similar myoclonus in much of the bulbar musculature (facial, lingual, palatal, pharyngeal, and diaphragmatic). Little improvement is to be expected.

*Ocular bobbing* can be mistaken for down-beat nystagmus, as it is characterized by a quick downward phase followed by an extremely slow return; it usually accompanies major restrictions of gaze and generally is more active when the patient attempts to move the eyes in any direction. Down-beat nystagmus characteristically is not associated with gaze restrictions and is most evident in down and eccentric gaze. A number of other oculomotor anomalies associated with brain-stem cerebellar disease are discussed in other sections (see sections on nystagmus and skew deviation).

In summary, there are numerous explanations for a patient's inability to produce timely, quick, full saccades on command, and the clinical significance may be complicated and extensive. The major areas of interest are the brain stem, cerebellum, basal ganglia, and frontal lobe, and each exhibits distinctive characteristics.

# Oculomotor Disorders and Cerebellar Disease

*A variety of fine tuning and postural defects affecting the stability and precision of dynamic fixation are indicative of cerebellar disease contributing to oculomotor disorders.*

## BACKGROUND

Perhaps nowhere is the contribution of the cerebellum to the extrapyramidal motor control system more evident than in oculomotor function. Although not involved in the initiation of eye movements, it can be said that the cerebellum possesses the detailed cybernetic programs and plasticity that move the eyes smoothly and accurately from point A to point B once this is "willed"—regardless of such obstacles as head position, body motion, acquired vestibular imbalances, and the altered magnification of new glasses. Animal studies show the flocculus of the cerebellum to be capable of actually reversing the direction of the doll's head reflex in just 2 weeks after reversing prisms are instituted. Perhaps elderly patients taking longer than this to adjust to new glasses can indeed be said to have lost cerebellar plasticity with age. The lack of improvement of an oscillopsia/nystagmus after several weeks is thus itself evidence of cerebellar localization.

## HISTORY AND EXAMINATION

Excluding nystagmus, which is discussed in the following section, other instabilities of the eyes at rest may be evident in cerebellar disease. These include the dysmetria-flutter-opsoclonus triad and square-wave jerks.

Ocular dysmetria refers to a dampening defect in which a series of unusually large correctional oscillations are seen on refixations. It occasionally may be asymmetrical and on right gaze a series of to and fro overshooting saccades eventually will attain fixation; whereas on left gaze a step-series of hypometric saccades is required to reach the target. In such asymmetry, there is usually a bias of both gaze and gait to the overshooting side as well, and the tendency is then called *lateropulsion*. A common cause is infarct of the lateral medullary plate, where brain-stem signs are also evident.

Ocular flutter is a burst of springlike, decreasing horizontal oscillations, which may accompany small fixations or even appear to occur spontaneously during fixation. The ultimate in underdampening is opsoclonus (saccadomania), where one sees a more pronounced, almost constant, chaotic series of semiconjugate movements (underdampening of microsaccades?). While serious lesions may be at fault, the progressive improvement from opsoclonia to flutter to dysmetria to normal is a relatively common sequel to postviral encephalitis in children.

Another interesting disorder is that of square-wave jerks, in which at random intervals a saccade (2°–20°) interrupts fixation, and after a barely perceptible delay, the patient again attains fixation. Such patients may have no insight into the defect and may look "shifty-eyed" or inattentive. Such an inability to sustain gaze with concentrated effort, however, is clearly abnormal. The exception to its usual cerebellar origin is in progressive supranuclear palsy, in which it usually is found if carefully sought.

In addition to square-wave jerks, patients with cerebellar disease may otherwise seem unduly inattentive or uncooperative. Additional signs are cogwheel pursuits, probably the most common sign in cerebellar disease, and delayed onset and hypometric saccades, which are also characteristic and may be seen on request to refixate. Such saccades have normal velocities as opposed to those in a patient with myasthenia or PSP, for example. Although an eye movement recording may be necessary to show this, retention of normal saccadic velocity is extremely helpful in distinguishing cerebellar cogwheeling from that seen in basal ganglia degenerations. Delayed, hypometric saccades are most characteristic of diffuse cerebellar damage, as in ataxia telangiectasia or the familial spinocerebellar degenerations.

Gaze nystagmus also may indicate cerebellar disease. While characteristic of stem disease, horizontal and, especially, up-beat nystagmus commonly occur in cerebellar disease. Usually other signs point to the cerebellum, but the observation of rebound is characteristic: for example, in a patient with spontaneous right-beating nystagmus that is worse in right gaze, the examiner may ask the patient to maintain fixation to the right for a minute or two. If, on return to the primary position, a left-beating nystagmus is now evident, rebound is demonstrated.

Acquired pendular nystagmus (usually late multiple sclerosis) is also thought to represent cerebellar damage and may convert to gaze nystagmus on vertical gaze, as opposed to the benign ocular variety.

Finally, isolated skew deviations usually reflect vascular accidents (70%) in the posterior fossa in general, not just the cerebellum. These vertical deviations are often perfectly concomitant but occasionally change in magnitude, or even direction, with right or left gaze. The supranuclear nature of the defect is seen in that no change in the measured imbalance occurs in up or down gaze or with head tilt. Several patients with diplopia seen by the author during a migraine attack have demonstrated just this sort of deviation.

Besides typical oculomotor accompaniments, patients with cerebellar disease usually demonstrate other posterior fossa signs (hypotonia, ataxia, intention tremor, listing, dysdiadochokinesia, dysarthria, long tract signs, cranial nerve dysfunction, signs of increased intracranial pressure, etc.). A basic screen of cerebellar function includes observing the stability of the patient with eyes closed and feet together (Romberg test), tandem walking for ataxia, finger-nose testing and heel-shin testing for dysmetria, and testing quick alternating movements such as an alternate pronation/supination of the hands for undue "stickiness" (dysdiadochokinesia). Very helpful in the differentiation from basal ganglia extrapyramidal disease is that tremor is less when the patient is at rest, with increasing oscillation observed as the patient reaches for objects.

Finally, one may look for lack of vestibular suppression in suspected cerebellar dysfunction. Here, the patient attempts to fixate his own finger while his whole body is rotated in the chair. If fixation drifts contralaterally to the direction of motion and back to the finger again, then lack of vestibular suppression has been demonstrated. While not always present in cerebellar disease, it is distinctive, being only present in one other condition—PSP, where usually only the slow drift, which pins the eyes to the end point, is observed.

# CLINICAL SIGNIFICANCE

Observation of a cerebellar sign may reflect all classes of disease—trauma, congenital, neoplastic, infectious/inflammatory, vascular, metabolic/degenerative. Although cerebellar signs in major head trauma and congenital spastic disorders are common, they are not of major significance in office eye practice.

Neoplasia probably is the most important disease category and is suggested by steady progression. A cerebellar pontine angle tumor (e.g., an acoustic neuroma in neurofibromatosis) may proceed so insidiously that ipsilateral loss of hearing, facial power, and corneal reflex may all go unnoticed. Vestibular function may be extinguished so slowly that cerebellar plasticity may constantly "reset the gain" such that there is no vertigo. In such cases, listing to the side of the tumor and an ipsilateral gaze nystagmus may be the presenting signs.

While gliomas probably are the most common masses in children, consider a medulloblastoma if progression is rapid. In these unfortunate cases, up-beat nystagmus and truncal ataxia may be the presenting signs. The most important tumor, however, is the hemangioblastoma (Fig. 19.28). These tumors may be hereditary as part of the Hippel-Lindau disease and account for about 20% of posterior fossa tumors in adults. They are often eminently treatable by surgery and, untreated, almost always produce life-threatening symptoms of compression or leakage by midlife. Therefore, in any patient with cerebellar signs, inquire as to family history, onset of cervical headache or stiff neck,

listen for bruits, and always dilate the eyes to look for associated retinal tumors. Conversely, in any patient with retinal angiomas, look for cerebellar signs *before* referring for argon laser therapy.

Infection and inflammation etiologies are not common, but remember that postviral opsoclonus in children and collagen vascular disease in adults may produce

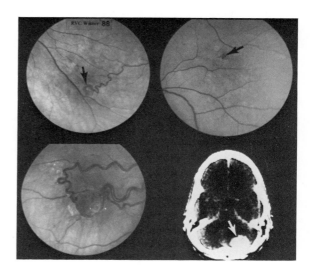

**FIGURE 19.28.**
**Three retinal angiomas in a patient with right-sided cerebellar hemangioblastoma evident on enhanced CAT scan. Diagnosis: Hippel-Lindau syndrome.**
Reprinted by permission of the publisher, from Miller NR, Fine SL. The ocular fundus in neuro-ophthalmologic diagnosis. In: Sights and sounds in ophthalmology, vol. VIII. St. Louis: C.V. Mosby, 1975.

ischemic symptoms any place in the nervous system.

A vascular etiology of cerebellar disease is suggested by sudden onset in an older patient with risk signs. Elderly patients with acute onset of lateropulsion often will also show one or more symptoms of a complete Wallenberg syndrome: lateropulsion of the eyes and body to the side of the lesion, perhaps a skew deviation with the hypo-eye on the same side, perhaps an ipsilateral Horner's syndrome with referred facial ache and hypoesthesia, and sometimes a perceived tilt to the world. A crossed loss of pain and temperature sensation is common in the extremities. Such a presentation should suggest an acute cerebellar hemorrhage or posterior-inferior cerebellar artery infarct. Here brain-stem compression can result in a dizzy patient presenting in the office and expiring in relatively short order; it represents a true emergency. Anterior-inferior cerebellar artery infarct will present with similar features, but usually with an ipsilateral hearing loss and sixth nerve paresis plus crossed pyramidal tract signs in the extremities.

Metabolic degenerative disorders are the most common cause of insidious onset of cerebellar signs and symptoms. The most common of these are the familial spinocerebellar degenerations. Dominant forms usually present in the third or fourth decade, while recessive forms tend to present in the first or second. Skew deviations and nystagmus may precede generalized ataxia. These disorders often cause down-beating nystagmus.

Ataxia-telangiectasia is rare and recessive; affected children are often thought to be simply clumsy. They also suffer a form of immunologic incompetence that makes them prone to frequent colds, ear infections, and at risk for lymphomas. By mid-childhood the telangiectatic vessels generally become obvious on the palpebral, then bulbar conjuctiva, as well as the malar regions and ears (Figure 19.29). Although any signs may occur, these children invariably demonstrate square-wave jerks and distinctly long latency saccades that are poorly sustained and hypometric.

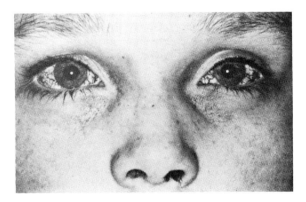

**FIGURE 19.29.**
**Conjunctival telangiectases in a child with ataxia telangiectasia (Louis-Bar syndrome).**
Courtesy Dr. G. Gaull. Reprinted by permission of the publisher, from Merritt, HH. A textbook of neurology. Philadelphia: Lea & Febiger, 1973; 5th ed.

# Overview of Nystagmus and the Dizzy Patient

*Nystagmus is a rhythmic, involuntary oscillation of the eyes characterized by slow drifts in one direction, followed immediately by saccadic redresses in the opposite direction.*

## BACKGROUND

Aside from congenital varieties, nystagmus usually reflects vestibular pathology from a destructive lesion in the sensory pathway on one side (labyrinth or eighth nerve). Alternatively, a lesion may occur in the central brain-stem/cerebellar comparator mechanism responsible for assessing vestibular information. Nystagmus may also result from central lesions affecting the eccentric gaze-holding mechanism (leaky integrator or gaze-paretic nystagmus in brain-stem disease).

Whatever the cause, misinformation sent to the extraocular muscles produces a pursuit to compensate for nonexisting head motion, after which the resulting error in fixation is detected and a saccadic redress is made. Convention dictates that the direction of the fast redress defines the direction of the nystagmus rather than the pursuit.

Nystagmus can be characterized as being coarse or fine, but more accurately, the terms first degree ($< 5°$), second degree ($5°-15°$), and third degree ($> 15°$) should be used. Electronystagmography best defines these and other parameters in various positions of gaze with eyes both closed and open. Clinically, however, terms like *right-fine-jerk* nystagmus are used.

Because of the fine tuning of the vestibular mechanism, if it were not for CNS plasticity, unequal sensory wear and tear would result in the detection of an imbalance in the central comparator and produce constant lifelong vertigo. Fortunately, the CNS is capable of resetting the gain between the ears when imbalances do occur. This is all the more incredible as vestibular-ocular movements are mediated by only a three-neuron arc. While the cerebellar flocculus seems to be critically involved in modulating sensory input, there is also good evidence for cortical suppression via inhibitory efferents at the level of the hair cell as well as at the interneuron. A good example of the deleterious effects of losing inhibition is after the use of depressants, such as alcohol or barbiturates, where dizziness is universal. Cortical atrophy in the elderly may also make manifest, in the form of dizziness, acquired imbalances between the ears, which previously had been well compensated. Stimulants (such as Ritalin), are often effective in relieving this common symptom of aging.

# HISTORY AND EXAMINATION

More often than not, patients seek the optometrist's counsel or are inappropriately referred by other physicians, not because of the jumpy eyes, but because they complain of dizziness. When a history of periodic dizziness may be secondary to vestibular or CNS disease, it is crucial to determine whether the patient is suffering from true vertigo versus light-headedness versus ataxia (Figure 19.30).

Vertigo is a specific symptom of vestibular disease; actual motion/spinning/swimming, with a definite time of onset, is usually perceived by the patient, often with some degree of nausea. Oscillopsia is also a sensation of rotation, but rather than creating an overpowering global whirling feeling, the patient is more likely to describe a restricted clearly visual phenomenon, similar to the rolling of a television picture that is out of vertical synchronization; oscillopsia of this kind is much more likely to represent CNS disease.

When the patient cannot volunteer any sense of motion, it usually is very difficult to obtain a clear picture of what "dizzy" means without obtaining a series of equally vague eponyms: "like walking on eggs," "woozy," "nothing seems real," "high," to describe the clouding of consciousness. Such feelings may represent a whole host of processes that indirectly affect CNS function: peripheral neuropathies, neurotic depression, fatigue, postural hypotension, hypoglycemia, polycythemia, viremia, anemia, presyncope, TIAs, cardiac block, arrhythmias, hyperventilation, anxiety. Also, never underestimate the effect of a wide range of medications in underlying this type of complaint.

Patients suffering from ataxia will also often complain of dizziness. Attention must be paid to questions and tests directed toward dysequilibrium signs of swaying, listing to one side, and falling. Consider here tests for cerebellar function (heel-shin, finger-pointing, EOM abnormalities, dysdiadochokinesis, tandem walking) and for posterior column disease (Romberg sign, two-point discrimination, tingling/burning of the feet, bandlike sensations, decreased distal vibratory sensitivity). Often patients with peripheral neuropathies may be suffering from disease that will have additional eye manifestations (e.g., diabetes, multiple sclerosis, the elderly, spinocerebellar degenerations, Wernicke's encephalopathy, myxedema, pernicious anemia, tabes, and a variety of drugs toxic to the second and/or eighth cranial nerves). Use the 250 CPS tuning fork in evaluating vibratory sensory loss over bony prominences in the lower extremities when a "dizzy" patient may be ataxic. Patients with a sensory ataxia have most trouble in the dark, as when going to the bathroom at night and especially when walking on uneven ground in the dark.

# CLINICAL SIGNIFICANCE

Patients whose history and examination suggest a cerebellar or sensory ataxia always deserve a neurologic exam when the cause is not evident; otherwise, refer them to the specialist suggested by the findings. For example, refer to the internist a case of peripheral neuropathy in a postgastrectemy patient with fatigue, conjunctival pallor, and a beefy red tongue since these symptoms strongly suggest pernicious anemia. Likewise, unexplained true vertigo is best worked up by the otolaryngologist, except when the diagnosis seems obvious and treatment can properly be rendered by the family physician, as in Meniere's disease.

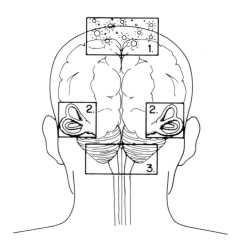

or seventh nerve dysfunction, and worsening with quick head movements or closure of eyes.

*Consider:*
 Labyrinthitis
 Viral vestibularitis
 Meniere's disease
 Benign positional vertigo
 Demyelinating disease
 Vertebro-basilar-acoustic artery stenosis
 Posterior fossa masses

## 3. CEREBELLAR/POSTERIOR COLUMN

*Characterized by:* balance difficulty, swaying, listing, difficulty walking on uneven ground or in dark, distal paresthesias.

*Check for:*
Tingling, numbness, neuralgia, bandlike constrictions, distal vibratory sensitivity, Romberg's sign, Lhermittes' sign.
Cerebellar signs: quick alternating movements, finger-nose, heel-shin, heel-toe, hypotonia, dysarthria.

*Consider:*
Metabolic states; chiefly pernicious anemia and diabetes
Vitamin deficiency; in alcoholics, depressed elderly widows
Hereditary disorders; Refsum's disease, spinocerebellar degenerations, Louie Bar, Bassen-Kornzweig syndrome, etc.
Primary CNS disease; spinocerebellar degenerations, extrapyramidal syndromes, cerebellar hemorrhage, infarct, angioblastoma, glioma, medulloblastoma, neuroma, Arnold-Chiari malformations
Infectious; tabes, Guillain-Barre, postviral ataxia in childhood
Toxic; heavy metals, drugs such as aspirin, INH, Dilantin, barbiturates, etc.
Multisensory impairment in disorientation of elderly
Miscellaneous; amyloidosis, collagen disease, remote effect of cancer especially lung, hypothyroidism
Demyelinating diseases

## 1. GLOBAL CNS DYSFUNCTION

*Characterized by:* a lack of clear vertigo or dysequilibrium and difficulty in describing the exact nature of the disorientation or clouding of consciousness.

*Consider:*
Anoxia; congestive heart failure, emphysema, the anemias, etc.
Ischemia; artheromatous disease, heart block, arrythmias, etc.
Medications; tranquilizers, Digitalis, Diuretics, antidepressants, etc.
Presyncope; postural, autonomic neuropathy, antihypertensive, etc.
Functional; neurotic depression, hyperventilation with anxiety
Toxic states; viremia, occult fever, hypoglycemia, hepatic failure, hypothyroidism, vasculopathies, electrolyte disturbances, etc.
Primary CNS disease; seizures, masses, low tension hydrocephalus, Alzheimer's disease, etc.

## 2. VESTIBULAR DISEASE

*Characterized by:* sensation of apparent motion, oscillopsia, swimming, etc.

*Check for:* hearing defect, tinnitus, nystagmus, fifth

**FIGURE 19.30.**
**Diagnostic categories to consider in approach to dizzy patient.**

"Fuzzy-headed" patients certainly deserve a thorough eye exam and careful history. Often the cause will remain unclear even after checking the pulse, blood pressure, listening for carotid bruits, and a neurologic screen. Such patients are best referred back to the managing physician for a thorough workup.

In some cases, however, there will be distinctive signs and symptoms that will be best interpreted by the eye practitioner. Some of these presentations are of the greatest significance and are reviewed in the following sections.

# Acquired Peripheral Nystagmus

*Certain nystagmoid movements of the eyes have the defined characteristics and associated symptomatology expected of disease in the peripheral vestibular-sensory apparatus.*

## BACKGROUND

Vestibularly generated eye movements are best understood as a mechanism that aids in maintaining fixation under conditions of head and body movement. Thus, rotating the head causes relative stimulation of the hair cells in the leading ear, and the eyes contravert as if to maintain fixation. Similarly, irrigating the left ear with warm water (thermally increasing baseline hair-cell discharge) will produce a rightward rotation interrupted by a leftward refixation saccade. A series of such nystagmoid movements is produced and, of course, vertigo results as the brain perceives the head to move when, in fact, it is still (Figure 19.31). Cold water or a destructive peripheral lesion in the right ear decreases baseline hair-cell discharge and will also produce repetitive rightward drifts and leftward saccades. Since convention depends on naming the direction of the fast phase, results of caloric testing can be remembered by the acronym COWS (cold—opposite, warm—same). A peripheral destructive lesion reacts similarly to cold water and, therefore, produces a nystagmus toward the good ear. The opposite is true in brain-stem/cerebellar lesions. Thus, while hearing loss or tinnitus in a dizzy patient with nystagmus favors a peripheral lesion, the observation of a right-beating nystagmus in a patient with right-sided hearing loss who lists to the right would not be consistent with a right-sided labyrinthian disease; it points instead to a right-sided CNS lesion such as acoustic neuroma.

## HISTORY AND EXAMINATION

The cardinal feature of vestibular disease is not mere dizziness, but a clear-cut major league vertigo with a definite time of onset. This being ascertained, the examination strategy is threefold: first, look for the characteristic signs and symptoms signifying a peripheral vestibular lesion; second, rule out the presence of features that suggest a CNS origin of the vertigo and nystagmus (next section); and third, if at this stage a peripheral sensory lesion is still suggested, carry out specific inquiry and tests to help suggest the specific vestibular pathology at hand.

The word peripheral does not necessarily mean benign. The same presenta-

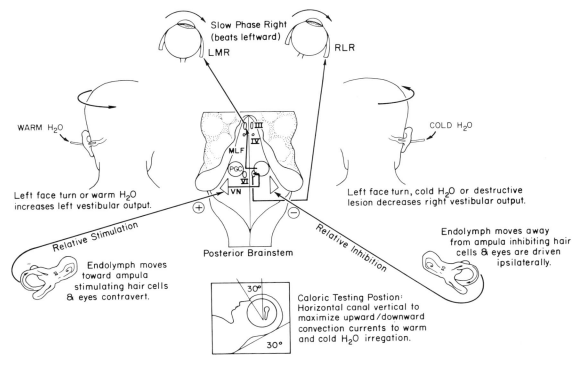

Slow Phase Right
(beats leftward)
LMR

RLR

WARM H₂O

COLD H₂O

III

IV

MLF

PGC

VN

VI

Left face turn or warm H₂O
increases left vestibular output.

Left face turn, cold H₂O or destructive
lesion decreases right vestibular output.

(+)

(−)

Relative Stimulation

Relative Inhibition

Posterior Brainstem

Endolymph moves
toward ampula
stimulating hair cells
& eyes contravert.

Endolymph moves away
from ampula inhibiting hair
cells & eyes are driven
ipsilaterally.

30°

30°

Caloric Testing Postion:
Horizontal canal vertical to
maximize upward/downward
convection currents to warm
and cold H₂O irregation.

**FIGURE 19.31.**
**Vestibular gaze mechanisms. Exitatory input from left eighth nerve reaches ipsilateral vestibular nuclei (*VN*) in brain stem. Second order afferents cross to synapse in contralateral pontine gaze center (*PGC*). From here, efferents travel to adjacent sixth nerve nucleus and also to contralateral third nerve nucleus by way of the median longitudinal fasciculus (*MLF*). Coordinated output of these nuclei produces rightward pursuit.**
Adapted with permission of the publisher from Gay AJ, Newman NM, Keltner JL and Stroud MH. Eye movement disorders. St. Louis: C.V. Mosby, 1974.

tion can result from end-stage organ failure as with otitis, senile arteriosclerosis, labyrinthitis, Meniere's disease, trauma, or from the effects of a destructive lesion in the vestibular portion of nerve VIII or its first order brain-stem connections, as with neoplasms, vascular insufficiency from stroke, TIAs, and occasionally migraine, demyelinating disease, postviral vestibularitis, and many medicines.

Evidence of hearing loss, earache, sensation of fullness, or tinnitus on the side opposite the direction of nystagmus is strong evidence of a peripheral etiology. Even though peripheral nystagmus is very symptomatic, the eye movements themselves must be examined. They are invariably perfectly symmetrical, horizontal or horizontal/rotary, and usually fast and of fine degree. Both the vertigo and the nystagmus itself are worse with the eyes closed or in the dark, and better with sustained fixation of reference points in the room. Here, one can obstruct fixation with high plus lenses to look for worsening. It is also very important that the nystagmus beats remain the same regardless of position of gaze.

Almost invariably, the symptoms are worse with quick head movements. Most patients are painfully aware of this, but one can have the patient stand with the feet close together and eyes closed while the head is turned from side to side; usually patients will tend to fall forward or backward depending on the direction of turn.

No matter how severe a vestibular lesion may be, the integrity of central plastic repair mechanisms provides another important clinical rule: in peripheral nystagmus, both the vertigo and eye movements should be improved in several days and cured in 2 weeks. The only exceptions are viral vestibularitis, where minor symptoms may occasionally occur on quick head movements for months or years, and recurrent episodic disorders such as TIAs or Meniere's disease.

Occasionally, a brain-stem disorder will present with a few features suggesting peripheral nystagmus. This underlies the importance of the second rule in approaching these disorders: rule out the presence of features characteristic of central nystagmus as discussed in the next section, or an important mixed presentation could be missed. This being done, a consideration of the more common presentations can then be entertained.

# CLINICAL SIGNIFICANCE

In a middle-aged patient, especially female, recurrent vertigo of 10 minutes to hours in duration, usually with concurrent fullness, tinnitus, and progressive hearing loss on the involved side, generally is attributed to Meniere's disease or "benign vestibular hydrops." The probable pathology is defective subarachnoid resorption of endolymph. Here, history and findings are consistent with peripheral nystagmus: severe vertigo better with fixation, for example. The condition improves with treatment with diuretics, brain-stem suppressants such as antihistamines or tranquilizers, and restriction of salt and water intake. Some severe causes require surgery.

Vertigo and hearing loss in the elderly are common, as in nonspecific dizziness and sensory ataxia owing to loss of dorsal column input from the extremities. In these patients, symptoms are often too quickly attributed to arteriosclerosis. While benign positional nystagmus is common in this age group, a history of short episodes of severe vertigo, especially on arising, should suggest a vertebrobasilar TIA. Such episodes may be monosymptomatic, as with a plaque at the origin of the acoustic artery. Question thoroughly for other spells indicative of posterior fossa ischemia, such as bilateral paresthesias, weakness, cervical headache, ataxia, drop attacks, dysarthria, perioral paresthesias, diplopia, and transient field defects. Blood pressure should be checked in both arms of such patients to rule out a treatable subclavian steal syndrome, and the carotid arteries should be auscultated for evidence of generalized artheromatous disease. Some consideration of cardiac emboli and arrhythmias should be entertained as well.

In the absence of labyrinthian inflammation (visible otitis, pain, and fever), acute onset of severe vertigo in young people with a motionless nauseated patient is often attributable to a postviral demyelinating lesion (viral vestibularitis) and usually clears up over a period of a week despite its severity. Obviously, previous focal neurologic episodes in other systems calls for considering the possibility of multiple sclerosis as well. Occasionally, a long history of episodic vertigo and vertical diplopia (skew deviation) will represent a stereotypical aura preceding migraine in young people.

In any acute presentation suggesting

a posterior inferior cerebellar artery hemorrhage or infarct, immediate hospitalization is advised because of the very real possibility of early brain-stem compression and death. Such symptoms are often treatable if the cause is suspected at the onset. Symptoms are dizziness, vertical diplopia, ipsilateral lateropulsion, and swaying, headache, and numbness radiating to the ipsilateral eye and, perhaps, ipsilateral Horner's syndrome.

Finally, all seemingly healthy patients presenting with vertigo to the optometrist should have the function of nerves V, VII, and VIII checked, as well as a brief screen of motor and cerebellar function. To be remiss may mean that the neurologist will

later find a cerebellar-angle tumor based on a reduced corneal reflex. Because of their slow, steady growth these tumors often produce few vestibular symptoms, even with total eighth nerve destruction (i.e., central compensation is able to occur); a mildly symptomatic central-gaze nystagmus toward the side of the tumor (indicating cerebellar compression) is, therefore, much more common than a contralaterally beating peripheral nystagmus (Figure 19.32).

There are many other causes of peripheral nystagmus. When the cause is not clear, referral usually is to the otolaryngologist.

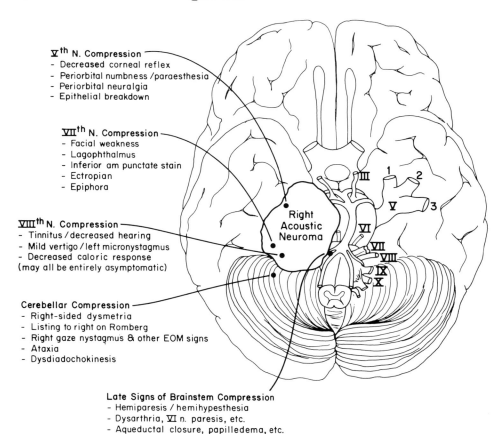

V<sup>th</sup> N. Compression
- Decreased corneal reflex
- Periorbital numbness /paraesthesia
- Periorbital neuralgia
- Epithelial breakdown

VII<sup>th</sup> N. Compression
- Facial weakness
- Lagophthalmus
- Inferior am punctate stain
- Ectropian
- Epiphora

VIII<sup>th</sup> N. Compression
- Tinnitus /decreased hearing
- Mild vertigo /left micronystagmus
- Decreased caloric response
(may all be entirely asymptomatic)

Cerebellar Compression
- Right-sided dysmetria
- Listing to right on Romberg
- Right gaze nystagmus & other EOM signs
- Ataxia
- Dysdiadochokinesis

Right Acoustic Neuroma

Late Signs of Brainstem Compression
- Hemiparesis / hemihypesthesia
- Dysarthria, VI n. paresis, etc.
- Aqueductal closure, papilledema, etc.

FIGURE 19.32.
Signs and symptoms with cerebellar pontine angle tumors.

# Central (Gaze) Nystagmus

*Central (gaze) nystagmus is secondary to posterior fossa disease and usually has a prominent gaze component.*

## BACKGROUND

Sensory information from the semicircular canals of both ears is processed in the brain stem and modulated by a wide variety of influences, which seem to be chiefly integrated in the cerebellum. Lesions in these structures can produce central vestibular pathology that results in nystagmus. Additionally, subtotal brain-stem conjugate-gaze palsies commonly are associated with gaze-paretic nystagmus.

The cerebellum is also concerned with both the ballistic and fine-tuning aspects of eye movements, and lesions affecting these mechanisms or their brain-stem connections may produce gaze nystagmus and other nystagmoid instabilities. The reader should therefore consult sections of this chapter dealing with lateral-gaze palsies and cerebellar disease.

## HISTORY AND EXAMINATION

Most often, central nystagmus will be readily apparent when the patient is asked to look in various positions of gaze as it is usually coarse, often of second or third degree. A cardinal diagnostic point is that patients with CNS lesions and nystagmus often have little vertigo, may suffer some degree of oscillopsia, *or be entirely asymptomatic.* Furthermore, central nystagmus almost always has a prominent gaze component where the magnitude or even direction of nystagmus will vary with changes in eye position. Thus a patient with a barely observable right fine-jerk nystagmus in the primary position may, for example, show an obvious course right-beating nystagmus in right gaze, and even a moderate left-beating nystagmus in left gaze as well. While horizontal gaze nystagmus is sometimes benign and/or congenital, the observation of vertical gaze nystagmus almost always implies a significant lesion.

In brain-stem disease there might also be a partial paresis of conjugate gaze. Here, attempted gaze in the direction of the palsy produces a series of slow, very coarse, negatively accelerated drifts away from eccentric fixation followed by refixing saccades—so-called gaze-paretic or leaky-integrator nystagmus. The pathology reflects normal ballistic saccade initiation (the pulse) superimposed on a brain-stem error in the eccentric holding component (the step).

Some patients occasionally will show a mixture of signs and symptoms of both central and peripheral nystagmus, central vestibular nystagmus (Table 19.7). For example, a patient may present with a fine horizontal rotary nystagmus with minimal vertigo. Except for perhaps the lack of tinnitus or hearing loss, such a patient might be thought to be suffering a vestibular lesion. Nevertheless, further workup might reveal that the nystagmus has persisted for 4 weeks, that it increases in amplitude in right gaze, and that symptoms are better with the eyes closed and no worse with quick head movement. Such a mixed presentation obviously becomes a cause for greater concern. In intracranial lesions, however, one does not usually expect to find the signs and symptoms seen in peripheral vestibular disease. Their absence always argues strongly for considering a central lesion.

# CLINICAL SIGNIFICANCE

The clinical significance of central nystagmus lies in its potential for representing progressive posterior fossa disease. If not congenital, a thorough search for company must ensue. Again, a wide variety of lesions throughout the brain stem and cerebellum may be responsible. Thus, the observation of distal ataxia with an intention tremor on pointing and loss of quick alternating movements would strongly suggest an ipsilateral hemispheric cerebellar lesion. The direction of nystagmus and the tendency to fall will be on the same side as the lesion (as opposed to peripheral nystagmus): for example, a mild ataxia with tendency to swerve to the right and a positive Romberg sign might be noted in a patient with right gaze nystagmus and dysmetria upon slow pointing movements with the right hand. Refer to the section on cerebellar disease for a full discussion of associated signs and symptoms and the approach to the examination.

In children, especially, the new observation of up-beat nystagmus, in the absence of other signs of a Parinaud's syndrome unfortunately often turns out to represent a medulloblastoma. In young children with progressive nystagmus and ataxia, the observation of conjunctival tel-

Table 19.7
Differential of Peripheral versus Central Nystagmus

| Peripheral | Central |
|---|---|
| Vertigo usually marked | Vertigo minimal or absent; oscillopsia sometimes present |
| Definite onset | Onset usually vaguer |
| Worse with head movement | Head turn has no effect |
| Worse when eyes closed | If anything, better with eyes closed |
| Hearing loss, fullness, pain, tinnitus often present | Hearing symptoms usually absent |
| Nystagmus usually fine, fast and primarily horizontal/rotary | Course nystagmus that is purely horizontal or vertical depending on gaze |
| Gaze has no effect | Direction and amplitude of nystagmus usually gaze dependent |
| Beats to side opposite lesion | Beats to side of lesion |
| Improves rapidly | May persist or worsen |
| Little CNS company | May have posterior fossa signs |

angiectases would essentially make the diagnosis of Louis-Bar syndrome. Affected children are likely also to show delayed hypometric EOMs, square-wave jerks, and tend to die young because of immunodeficiency associated with recurrent infections and/or lymphomatous disease.

In adults, hereditary hemiangioblastomas must especially be considered by the optometrist, and part of the workup of any posterior fossa sign should include a dilated retinal exam looking for angiomas. The observation of an angioma in an asymptomatic patient with gaze nystagmus is potentially life-saving, as the early diagnosis of Hippel-Lindau syndrome may save the patient from a disastrous cerebellar hemorrhage later in life.

As with any posterior fossa lesion, cerebellar masses often are accompanied by symptoms and eye signs of increased intracranial pressure. Along with specific cerebellar signs, persisting nystagmus without improvement is more likely to represent cerebellar rather than brain-stem disease, especially if it is accompanied by *rebound* nystagmus. This is noted on continued side gaze where the degree of nystagmus is observed to gradually diminish and then to actually reverse in direction on return to the primary position. Although gaze (often vertical) nystagmus is associated with a variety of medicines, only phenytoin (Dilantin) can produce it with therapeutic levels, while it represents overdosage when seen with CNS depressants, especially barbiturates. In the absence of significant mass lesions, trauma, or obvious stroke, the onset of central nystagmus is seen most commonly in Wernicke's encephalopathy, in the familial spinocerebellar degenerations, and in late demyelinating disease.

When isolated brain-stem lesions are associated with gaze nystagmus, the presentation may be the same as in cerebellar disease, except that one is more likely to see long tract signs (e.g., a positive Babinski) and gaze and cranial nerve palsies. In a patient with *down-beating* nystagmus (most evident in eccentric down gaze), however, special attention must be given the lower brain stem. These patients often note oscillopsia similar to a rolling TV picture. Even with adult development of symptoms, rule out congenital malformations, platybasia, and Arnold-Chiari syndrome when the cause is not already clear, as with established multiple sclerosis or spinocerebellar degeneration. While such patients may have a predisposing history of infantile hydrocephalus or spina bifida, the presentation can also occur in a healthy adult, and suspicion of the cause can prevent a fatal herniation of the brain. *Periodic alternating* nystagmus, a condition where the nystagmus cyclically slowly quiets, then reverses direction over a course of minutes, also is often associated with lower brain-stem disease. If the examiner is not astute, he or she may simply think that the nystagmus varies somewhat in amplitude and miss the key point of alternation.

Finally, it is common in eye practice to see patients complaining of a very distinct nystagmoid syndrome known as *benign positional* nystagmus. The complaint of episodic vertigo that reliably occurs only upon changing from one posture to another is common in older patients. Usually occurring on reclining and arising, the dizziness sometimes occurs only upon attaining a precise head position on the pillow. The pathology is the resettling of loose otoliths in the vestibules or their rolling into the semicircular canals to stimulate hair cells. Therefore, it is a peripheral nystagmus and typically produces major vertigo such as bed spinning that is worse in the dark and better with sustained fixation. It is important to inquire as to the latency of onset since the benign variety takes several seconds to develop. Furthermore, it shows rapid adaptation so that if the patient sits up abruptly, a second recline is much less symptomatic. Finally, it tends to show rebound, such as recurrence when the patient arises in the morning. Patients otherwise in good health with history of such stereotypical episodes can be assured of the benign nature of their disorders.

Positional nystagmus also occurs after head trauma, whiplash, and with a variety of depressants such as ethyl alcohol. The relatively common accompaniments of the posttraumatic syndrome also include chronic headache, blepharospasm/photophobia, accommodative instabilities, and, occasionally, partial bilateral fourth nerve weakness, which may also produce reading complaints.

The clinical significance of benign positional nystagmus is to distinguish it from a look-alike variety of central positional nystagmus, which has been the sole presenting symptom in a number of posterior fossa tumors. Generally, these presentations are those that tend to involve younger patients without antecedent trauma and in whom symptoms are progressing over a brief time span. More specifically, a posterior fossa lesion is to be strongly suspected when vertigo is mild, when it occurs immediately upon changing position without a latency, when it doesn't adapt or show rebound, and when symptoms are better with the eyes closed than with fixation. Even in the absence of suspicious company, these patients deserve a prompt neurologic referral.

In summary, central nystagmus can be the first presenting sign of posterior fossa lesions in a totally asymptomatic patient. Suspicious company should always lead the examiner to look specifically for gaze nystagmus (e.g., dysarthria, balance difficulty, blurred optic discs, retinal angiomas, facial asymmetry, and so forth). Therefore, always closely observe the patient's conjugate movements and distinguish them from physiologic nystagmus, which is only permissible at the very end points of gaze.

# Nystagmus of Early Onset

*Nystagmoid oscillations of the eyes may be noted at birth or in infancy.*

## BACKGROUND

Several types of nystagmus are commonly seen in childhood. For the most part, they do not have neurologic import; however, they are often very disturbing to both parents and pediatricians, and such children usually have their eyes examined.

## HISTORY AND EXAMINATION

Outside of the usual prenatal, birth, and developmental histories, the most important initial aspect of examination is in simply studying random eye movements and those that occur on optically elicited eccentric gaze. Careful inspection will usually reveal one of four major patterns to be discussed. It is important for the eye practitioner to be thoroughly versed in the typical appearance and characteristics of each form, as occasionally a neurologically significant entity may present masquerading as one of them.

*Pendular nystagmus* is manifest as slow, predominantly lateral oscillations without a fast component and may be partially disassociated. Pendular nystagmus occasionally is a familial condition but usually reflects a fairly severe reduction in overall vision or faulty macula development, such as occurs with congenital cataracts, aniridia, albinism, Leber's retinal dystrophy, and achromotopsia. If the cause is not seen, all such infants deserve an ERG. Pendular nystagmus caused by purely ocular disease never occurs in adults.

The benign ocular variety often converts to jerky nystagmus on lateral gaze, but never on vertical gaze. Acquired pendular nystagmus reflects brain-stem or cerebellar damage, may convert to jerky nystagmus on vertical gaze, and is seen most commonly in late multiple sclerosis. It may produce oscillopsia, while the ocular variety does not. The significance of pendular nystagmus is in finding the cause of visual loss when it is congenital and in taking steps toward uncovering a neurologic lesion when the symptom is acquired or when a jerky nystagmus is manifest.

*Latent nystagmus* is a jerky nystagmus manifest in each eye only upon covering its partner and almost always occurs in association with congenital esotropia. When a congenital esotropia is accompanied by latent nystagmus, it is likely to show double hyperphoria and may be accompanied by episodic torsional twitching as well. If the nystagmus is small enough to be evident only upon using the ophthalmoscope, which occludes one eye, it is helpful to remember that the slow movement is always toward the occluded eye. As with all forms of congenital nystagmus, neither vertigo or oscillopsia accompany the movement, although the monocular visions may be reduced somewhat. This is a totally benign entity, but a little knowledge can be dangerous.

Note that many forms of nystagmus get worse when one interferes with fixation, and the observation with the ophthalmoscope of a micronystagmus is not necessarily harmless; it *must* differ in direction depending on the eye occluded. Many of these patients actually show a micronystagmus with both eyes open, such as that seen with the slit lamp; the symptom is simply more obvious when occluding an eye—a manifest latent nystagmus. The significance of latent nystagmus is simply to recognize the condition and its common associations and to not confuse with acquired nystagmus.

*Spasmus nutans* is an acquired nystagmus, usually beginning in the second year of life and generally a horizontal, fast, low-amplitude nystagmus accompanied by head turning or nodding; the nystagmus may be much greater in one eye (partially disassociated). Fortunately, the disorder clears spontaneously, usually by the third year of life, with no known cause of residua. X-ray films of the sella are still indicated because of an infrequent coexistence with diencephalic/chiasmal lesions. If vertical, seesaw, or monocular nystagmus develops in a failure-to-thrive infant, a full neurologic workup is definitely indicated, even in the presence of head nodding. These symptoms more likely reflect an anterior third ventricle glioma then simple spasmus nutans. With this exception, the

chief significance of the disorder is in providing adequate reassurance to the parents that it will pass.

*Congenital jerk nystagmus* is a form of horizontal-gaze nystagmus present right after birth; sometimes it is familial. It generally improves somewhat with age, being worse when the child is nervous. Vision is decreased somewhat, although this is not usually a severe problem owing to the magnification the young eye can obtain by close viewing during the learning process. In most cases there is a null point, or a position of gaze, wherein the nystagmus is much reduced. On either side of the point, nystagmus is in the direction of gaze and increases in coarseness with eccentricity. As with pendular nystagmus, any vertical conversion in up or down gaze must be taken as a potential sign of a posterior fossa lesion, even in a child. Most cases also show a decrease in amplitude upon convergence; however, trying base-out prism to improve stability and hence the vision does not elicit a full "near reflex" and generally is a total failure. Nevertheless, when the patient has a definite face turn to use a good null point, a cosmetic improvement can sometimes be made with press on prisms or surgery. Biofeedback has been tried with some success as well. An interesting characteristic distinguishing the congenital variety from acquired gaze nystagmus is inversion with OKN; for example, in a right-beating nystagmus passing the stripes to the patient's left actually diminishes the nystagmus, although it would induce a right-beating nystagmus in normal eyes. This is a useful test in an older patient who is uncertain as to whether the eyes have always been jumpy. Except for the cosmetic and visual factors, this disorder has little significance for the patient's health.

# CLINICAL SIGNIFICANCE

The clinical significance of nystagmus of early onset is discussed separately for each form in the preceding paragraphs. Although each type is usually easily recognized and has its unique implications, perhaps the chief significance of these entities lies in overlooking a simulating neurologic presentation. Always look for vertical conversion in pendular and congenital jerk nystagmus, lack of reversal in apparent latent nystagmus, and diencephalic/chiasmal signs in atypical spasmus nutans.

# References

Cogan DG. Neurology of the ocular muscles. Springfield, Ill.: Charles C Thomas, 1956; 2nd ed.

Daroff RB, Troost BT. Supranuclear disorders of eye movements. In: Glaser JS, ed. Neuro-ophthalmology. Hagerstown, Md.: Harper & Row, 1978;201–218.

Gay, AJ, ed. Eye movement disorders. St. Louis: C.V. Mosby, 1974.

Lennerstrand G, Bach-y-Rita P. Basic mechanisms of ocular motility and their clinical implications. New York: Pergamon Press, 1975.

## Nerve Palsies

Bajandas BJ. The six syndromes of the sixth nerve. In: Smith JL, ed. Neuro-ophthalmology update. New York: Masson, 1977;49–69.

Burde R, Karp J. The efferent visual system and the orbit. Int Ophthalmol Clin 1978;18(1):1–186.

Burger LJ, Kalvin NH, Smith JL. Acquired lesions of the fourth cranial nerve. Brain 1970;93:567–574.

Coppeto JM, Lessel S. Cryptogenic unilateral paralysis of the superior oblique muscle. Arch Ophthalmol 1978; 96:275–277.

Dell'osso LP, Daroff RB. Eye movement characteristics and recording techniques. In: Glaser JS, ed. Neuro-ophthalmology. Hagerstown, Md.: Harper & Row, 1978;185–199.

Gay AJ, ed. Eye movement disorders. St. Louis: C.V. Mosby, 1974.

Glaser JS. Infranuclear disorders of eye movement. In: Glaser JS, ed. Neuro-ophthalmology. Hagerstown, Md.: Harper & Row, 1978;245–284.

Helper RS, Cantu RC. Aneurysms and third nerve palsies. Arch Ophthalmol 1967;77:604–608.

Hoyt WF, Keane JR. Superior oblique myokymia. Arch Ophthalmol 1970; 84:461–467.

Hunt WE, et al. Painful ophthalmoplegia: its relation to indolent inflammation of the cavernous sinus. Neurology 1961;11:56–62.

Leigh RJ, Zee DS. The neurology of eye movements. Philadelphia: F.A. Davis, 1983.

Lennerstrand G, Bach-y-Rita P. Symposium on basic mechanisms of ocular motility and their clinical implications. New York: Pergamon Press, 1975.

Phelps CD, Thompson HS, Ossoinig KC. Atypical carotid-cavernous fistula. Am J Opthalmol 1982;93:424–436.

Victor M. Neuro-ophthalmic disorders due to alcoholism and malnutrition. In: Smith JL, ed. Neuro-ophthalmology, focus 1980. New York: Masson, 1979;37:357–378.

Weber RB, Daroff RB, Mackey EA. Pathology of oculomotor nerve palsy in diabetics. Neurology 1970;20:835–838.

## Myopathies

Daroff RB. Chronic progressive external ophthalmoplegia. Arch Ophthalmol 1969;82:845–850.

Drachman DA. Ophthalmoplegia plus: the neurodegenerative disorders associated with progressive ophthalmoplegia. Arch Neurol 1968;18:655–674.

Eaton LM, Lambert EH. Electromyography and electric stimulation of nerves in diseases of motor unit: observations on myasthenic syndrome associated with malignant tumor. JAMA 1957; 163:1117–1124.

Glaser JS. Infranuclear disorders of eye movement. In: Glaser JS, ed. Neuro-opthalmology. Hagerstown, MD.: Harper & Row 1975;245–284.

Keans TP, Sayre GP. Retinitis pigmentosa, external ophthalmoplegia and complete heart block. Arch Ophthalmol 1958;60:280–289.

Leveille AS, Newell FW. Autosomal dominant Kearns-Sayre syndrome. Ophthalmology 1980;87:99–108.

Osher R, Glaser JS. Myasthenic sustained gaze fatigue. Am J Ophthalmol 1980;89:443–445.

Osher R, Griggs R. Orbicularis fatigue (the "peek" sign) of myasthenic gravis. Arch Ophthalmol 1979;97:677–697.

Shaivits JS. Timolol and myasthenia gravis. JAMA 1979;242:1611–1612. (Letter)

Victor M, Haynes R, Adams RD. Oculopharyngeal muscular dystrophy. N Engl J Med 1962;207:1267–1272.

# Lid Position

Cogan DG. Myasthenia gravis: a review of the disease and a description of lid twitch as a characteristic sign. Arch Ophthalmol 1965;74:217–221.

Collier J. Nuclear ophthalmoplegia, with especial reference to retraction of lids and ptosis and to lesions of the posterior commissure. Brain 1927;50: 488–498.

Epstein G, Putterman AM. Aquired blepharoptosis secondary to contact lens wear. Am J Ophthalmol 1981;91:634–639.

Forster RK, Shatz NJ, Smith JL. A subtle eyelid sign in aberrant regeneration of the third nerve. Am J Opthalmol 1969;67:696–698.

Powers JM. Decongestant-induced blepharospasm and orofacial dystonia. JAMA 1982;247:3244–3245.

Revilla AG. Neurinomas of the cerebellopontine recess: a clinical study of one hundred and sixty cases including operative mortality and end results. Bulletin of the Johns Hopkins Hospital 1947;80:254.

Smith JL. Pathological lid retraction and lid position in neurology. In: Smith JL, ed. Neuro-opthalmology update. New York: Masson, 1977;9–16.

Teaser RB. Myokymia and facial contraction in multiple sclerosis. Arch Intern Med 1976;136:81.

Teaser RB, Corbett JJ. Myokymia and facial contraction in brain stem glioma: an electromyographic study. Arch Neurol 1974;30:425.

Williamson PD. Facial nerve paralysis. In: Walsh TJ, ed. Neuro-ophthalmology: clinical signs and symptoms. Philadelphia: Lea & Febiger, 1978;183–194.

# Pursuit

Cartwright GE. Current concepts: the diagnosis of treatable Wilson's disease. N Engl J Med 1978;298:1347–1350.

Cogan DG. Congenital ocular motor apraxia. Can J Ophthalmol 1966; 1:253–260.

Curran RE, Hedges TR III, Boger WP. Loss of accommodation and the near response in Wilson's disease. J Pediatr Opthalmol Strabismus 1982;19:157–160.

Smith JL. Ocular signs of parkinsonism. J Neurosurg 1966; 24(suppl.):284–285.

Starr A. A disorder of rapid eye movements in Huntington's chorea. Brain 1967; 90:545–564.

Steele JC, Richardson JC, Olszewski J. Progressive supranuclear palsy. Arch Neurol 1964;10:333–359.

Tyler HR. Abnormalities of perception with defective eye movements (Balint's syndrome). Cortex 1968;4:154–171.

## Vertical Gaze

Chamberlin W. Restriction in upward gaze with advancing age. Am J Ophthalmol 1971;71:341–346.

Christoff N. A clinicopathologic study of vertical eye movements. Arch Neurol 1971;31:1–8.

Daroff RB, Troost BT. Supranuclear disorders of eye movements. In: Glaser JS, ed. Neuro-ophthalmology. Hagerstown, Md.: Harper & Row, 1978;201–218.

Smith JL, et al. Nystagmus retractorius. Arch Ophthalmol 1959;62:864–867.

## Lateral Gaze

Daroff RB. Ocular motor manifestation of brainstem and cerebellar dysfunction. In: Smith JL, ed. Neuro-ophthalmology. Hallandale: Huffman, 1970;5:104.

Smith JL, Cogan DG. Internuclear ophthalmoplegia. Arch Ophthalmol 1959;61:687–694.

Smith JL, Gay AJ, Cogan DG. The spasticity of conjugate gaze phenomenon. Arch Ophthalmol 1959;62:694–696.

Waltz AG. Dyspraxias of gaze. Arch Neurol 1961;5:638–647.

## Cerebellar Disease

Cogan DG. Ocular dysmetria: flutter-like oscillations of the eyes and opsoclonus. Arch Ophthalmol 1954;51:318–335.

Cogan DG, Chu FC, Reingold DB. Ocular signs of cerebellar disease. Arch Ophthalmol 1982;100:755–760.

Dell'osso LF, Troost BT, Daroff RB. Macro square wave jerks. Neurology 1975;25:975–979.

Levin DB, Boynton JR, Smith JL. Down beating nystagmus and hereditary cerebellar degeneration. In: Smith JL, ed. Neuro-ophthalmology update. New York: Masson, 1977;337–338.

Meyer KT, Baloh RW, Krohel GB. Ocular lateropulsion. Arch Ophthalmol 1980;98:1614–1616.

Miles FA, Fuller JH. Visual tracking and the primate flocculus. Science 1975;198:1000–1002.

Precht W. Cerebellar influences on eye movement. In: Lennerstrand G, Bach-y-Rita P, eds. Basic mechanisms of ocular motility and their clinical implications. New York: Pergamon Press, 1975;261–280.

Sandok BA, Kranz H. Opsoclonus as the initial manifestation of occult neuroblastoma. Arch Ophthalmol 1971;97:235–236.

## Nystagmus

Daroff RB, Troost BT, Dell'osso LF. Nystagmus and related ocular oscillations. In: Smith JL, ed. Neuro-ophthalmology. Hagerstown, Md.: Harper & Row, 1978;219–240.

Donin JF. Acquired monocular nystagmus in children. Can J Ophthalmol 1967;2:212–215.

Drachman DA, Hart CW. An approach to the dizzy patient. Neurology 1972;22:323–334.

Gay AJ, et al., eds. Eye movement disorders. St. Louis: C.V. Mosby, 1974.

Harbert F. Benign paroxysmal positional nystagmus. Arch Ophthalmol 1970;84:298–302.

Rubin W, Norris CH. Electronystagmography. What is ENG? Springfield, Ill.: Charles C Thomas, 1974.

# Barry J. Barresi
# ORBIT 20

*The orbit is the funnel-shaped opening in the skull. The globe occupies one-quarter of the orbital space, with the remaining space occupied mostly by adipose connective tissue, but also by the lacrimal gland, optic nerve, extraocular muscles, nerves, and blood vessels.*

## BACKGROUND

The contents of the orbit are well packed into small confines. An increase in orbital mass or contraction of orbital walls causes anterior displacement of the globe and widening of the palpebral fissure. Likewise, loss of orbital fat or increase in space, as with an orbital floor fracture, may cause enophthalmos.

The apparent position of the globe in a nondiseased orbit is subject to some variation. Facial asymmetry can raise suspicions of exophthalmos. Myopic, glaucomatous, and normal eyes, particularly in blacks, may appear unduly prominent. Cranial dysostosis with associated abnormal ossification and reduced orbital volume is rare, but when present may confuse the unwary observer. Crouzon's disease is the most notable cause of tower skull, but the full spectrum of anomalies of skull contour, tower skull, and shallow orbit are beyond the scope of this book.

The most common orbital disease is Graves' ophthalmopathy. The association of thyroid disease with exophthalmos, lid retraction, and lid lag has long been recognized. The etiology of thyroid ophthal-mopathy still is somewhat of an enigma. Autoimmunity appears to be the pathogenic mechanism for extraocular involvement, but autoimmunity does not explain the swelling of orbital fat.

Confusion in terms and classifications has plagued many clinicians trying to interpret clinical reports on thyroid eye disease. It seems best to refrain from linking the cause or state of thyroid function with the diagnosis and simply to state the physical signs. The Werner classification (Lyle 1978) was adopted by the American Thyroid Association. This classification defines seven classes of eye changes, with the first letter of each definition forming the pneumonic NO SPECS. The seven classes include:

0. No signs or symptoms

1. Only signs, no symptoms (upper lid retraction, stare, and lid lag)

2. Soft tissue involvement signs and symptoms

3. Proptosis

4. Extraocular muscle involvement
5. Corneal involvement
6. Sight loss (optic nerve involvement)

After Graves' disease, less frequently occurring orbital disease includes tumors, inflammation, and vascular disorders. Injuries can result in orbital foreign bodies, hemorrhage, or floor fractures.

Primary and secondary neoplasms of the orbit are of various types and may have some distinguishing clinical features, but in most cases can be differentiated only by biopsy. Inflammation, notably orbital cel- lulitis, is associated with injury or septi- cemia. Ethmoidal sinusitis, particularly in children, may lead to orbital involvement.

Vascular disorders can have a direct effect on increasing orbital mass or a re- mote effect of orbital passive congestion. Varices or other venous anomalies can in- volve the orbit and may show prominence of the superficial veins of the globe. Arte- riovenous fistulas arise from injury or as a consequence of rupture of an arterial aneurysm. Cavernous sinus thrombosis is an uncommon complication of orbital in- flammation or septicemia in the debili- tated patient.

# HISTORY

Proptosis is the cardinal sign of orbital disease. Other presenting features of or- bital disease include vision loss, diplopia, swelling, tearing, ptosis, and pain. Each feature should be qualified as to onset, se- verity, and course.

Orbital pain must be carefully differ- entiated from other local ocular conditions (Chapter 5). Also, sources of pain referred to the orbit from sinus disease, intracran- ial masses, and headache syndromes should be ruled out (Chapter 9). The most common cause of referred pain to the orbit is the muscle tension headache. Moderate to severe pain with orbital swelling sug- gests against an orbital neoplasm and in favor of orbital inflammation. With vas- cular orbital disorders, usually orbital var- ices, the valsalva maneuver (stooping or physical straining) typically exacerbates orbital pain. Discomfort in conjunction with a swishing orbital sound suggests an orbital bruit caused by vascular intercom- munication, such as with carotid cavern- ous sinus fistulas.

In the eye history be alert to ocular trauma and any previous treatment for proptosis or other orbital signs. While se- rial exophthalmometry readings may be of some value, a good facial photograph is even more helpful in gauging the extent of periorbital signs and eye prominence.

A medical history should consider signs and symptoms of thyroid disease (Table 19.4). Of course, the absence of current thyroid problems does not rule out Graves' disease. Carefully investigate any seem- ingly remote history of past surgical or radioisotope treatment for thyroid disease.

History of previous surgery can be helpful. A history of operations for carci- noma raises the possibility of orbital metastases.

# EXAMINATION

The investigation for orbital disease be- gins with inspection of the face and po- sition of the globe. Observe the con- figuration of the head and depth of the orbits from different viewpoints. Minor de- grees of exophthalmos can be easily re- vealed if the examiner, standing behind and above the patient, looks over the patient's brow. Misalignment of the optic axis and any vertical displacement of the eye should be noted.

Any suspected exophthalmos can be recorded by photography or the exophthalmometer. Use of the Hertel instrument is quite simple; a measurement of greater than 24 mm from corneal surface to lateral orbital rim is often noted as a cut-off point. Differences between the two eyes, and comparison of repeated measurement over time, usually is more valuable than the absolute measurements. Any noted vertical or horizontal displacement can be easily measured by use of a clear ruler placed across the bridge of the nose. Typically, if facial asymmetry is ruled out, the globe is displaced opposite to the position of any orbital mass lesion.

Anteriorly placed tumors may exhibit lid swelling and, particularly if in the upper quadrant, may be palpable by use of the tip of the little finger. One pitfall is to mistake a lobe of the lacrimal gland for a tumor. Recognition of orbital pulsation suggests AV malformations or a defect in the orbital roof, as in neurofibromatosis.

Inspection of the eyelids may reveal local swelling. A distinctly localized swelling probably is a chalazion. Other associations should be considered: upper-lid lateral swelling and lacrimal gland tumor or inflammation, upper-lid nasal swelling and mucocele, and lower-lid swelling and lymphoma of inferior fornix. Intense swelling and rubor is associated with orbital inflammation of cellulitis or pseudotumor. The puffy, itchy lids of atopic dermatitis or more localized inflammation of hordeolum or dacryocystitis should not be overlooked.

The position of the eyelids to the anterior landmarks of the limbus, pupil, and superior palpebral sulcus should be noted. Normally, the upper lid margin lies at a position halfway between the limbus and the pupil. Lid retraction, suggesting Graves' disease, usually pulls the upper lid to the limbus, and even in the absence of proptosis may expose more sclera. Henderson and Farrow (1980) make a distinction between the lid retraction of Graves' disease and the lid elevation of proptosis with orbital tumors (test of superior palpebral fold ratio). The distinction is evident by measurement of the distance between the upper lid margin and the superior palpebral sulcus. Normally this distance in adults is 3 mm. Henderson and Farrow report that the migrain-fissure distance shortens with Graves' lid retraction but is unaltered if the palpebral fissure is widened by ocular tumor proptosis.

Orbital mass lesions and inflammation can limit eye movement, but so can mechanical factors such as myopathies and nerve palsies. Bilateral limitation of motion, particularly on up gaze, and positive forced duction tests all suggest Graves' disease. The differential diagnosis of motility problems is quite extensive and is reviewed in some depth in Chapter 19.

Reduction in visual acuity can precede other signs. The loss in vision may be alleviated by a new, more hyperopic correction. A retrobulbar tumor, with compression of the posterior globe, may be to blame. In any case, the vision loss may be neural, owing to optic nerve compression, or ischemic and present with classic signs of optic nerve conduction defects. The first cause of reduced visual acuity to consider, however, is exposure keratitis.

Careful slit lamp study with flourecein and rose bengol staining should be performed to detect any tear-film abnormalities or exposure keratitis caused by incomplete blinking or lid closure. During the examination of the external eye, notes should be made of any "sentinel" vessels. A single, dilated episcleral vessel above the lateral rectus suggests thyroid eye disease. More diffuse dilated episcleral vessels may be sentinels for orbital AV malformations.

Orbital mass lesions may be manifested by fundus signs of passive venous congestion, compression of the globe, or damage to the optic nerve. Extensive retinal venous dilation can be a sign of orbital AV malformations. Choroidal folds, a nonspecific sign, and swollen disc in the presence of exophthalmos are indicative of orbital tumors. Optic atrophy can represent a late stage sequel of Graves' disease or result from tumor compressing the optic nerve.

Definitive diagnosis of orbital mass lesions invariably requires the use of sophisticated testing not available in office practice. Computerized axial tomography and ultrasonic methods have become almost indispensable. Fluorescein angiography, venograms, and biochemical investigation may in some cases offer adjunctive information.

# CLINICAL SIGNIFICANCE

A thorough review of the clinical features of orbital disease is beyond the scope of this book. Two conditions, however, are investigated here: Graves' ophthalmopathy, a common cause of orbital signs and symptoms, and orbital cellulitis, a life-threatening condition that requires prompt recognition and treatment. In addition, a brief discussion of orbital tumors reviews the classification and incidence of tumors.

## Graves' Ophthalmopathy

A wide spectrum of clinical manifestations are associated with Graves' ophthalmopathy. Diagnosis may be elusive when only minor lid or periorbital signs are present. On the other side of the spectrum, the more serious manifestations of proptosis and optic neuropathy may herald progressive vision loss. The role of thyroid disease and these manifestations of Graves' disease is equivocal, with about half of the hyperthyroid patients presenting clinically notable ocular signs (Figure 20.1).

The Werner classification provides a helpful schema for clinical diagnosis. The sites for ocular manifestations include eyelids, periorbital soft tissue, proptosis, extraocular muscle impairment, corneal exposure, and compressive optic neuropathy.

Eyelid signs are the most common clinical manifestation of Graves' disease. Lid retraction, stare, and lid lag may be unilateral or bilateral. Dry eye symptoms with pronounced lid retraction, the acute sign of exposure keratitis, may be reported by these patients.

These lid signs are quite suggestive, but not pathognomonic of Graves' disease. Dorsal midbrain lesions (Parinaud's syndrome) can present with bilateral lid retraction in the absence of lid lag. Typically, vertical gaze impairment, convergence retraction nystagmus with attempted up gaze, and pupil light-near dissociation are also present with midbrain syndrome (Figure 19.23).

Impaired venous return from the orbit is manifested by soft tissue swelling of the periorbital region, lids, and conjunctiva.

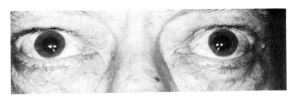
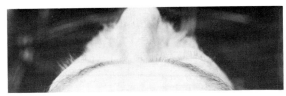

FIGURE 20.1.
Exophthalmos in Graves' disease. Note the slightly greater protrusion of the left eye verified by the superior frontal view. Exophthalmometry readings are OD 22 mm, OS 23 mm.

This mild edema can cause tearing or gritty sensations of a varying nature.

Muscle weakness, or actual fibrosis, can restrict the range of motion of extraocular muscles. Upward rotation is first restricted, then abduction. Rarely are other gaze directions restricted. Patients may note an achy, pulling sensation on attempted up gaze. If diplopia is present the complaint is intermittent and elicited with gaze above the horizon. In these patients a compensatory backward head tilt may ensue with consequent neck ache and stiffness. Another curious consequence of the inferior rectus fibrosis is an increase in intraocular pressure of 3 to 4 mm Hg on attempted up gaze.

Definitive diagnosis of extraocular muscle involvements with Graves' disease requires the use of the forced duction test and, in some cases, ultrasonography and high resolution, computerized tomographic scanning.

Proptosis, which in most series is noted in one of five patients with Graves' disease, is typically associated with restrictive myopathy and lid retraction. Old photographs are the most sensitive method of detecting subtle presentations of proptosis and lid retraction. Exophthalmometry is most useful for sequential examination to follow the course of the disease.

Postural changes in exophthalmometry measurements is an additional clinical sign. With "settling" of the orbital contents, the supine position reading in the normal eye may be up to 3 mm less than the seated position reading. Findings of bilateral orbital resistance (equal supine and seated readings) suggest Graves' ophthalmopathy, while unilateral orbital resistance suggests a retrobulbar tumor. Asymmetric proptosis greater than 6 mm also suggests retrobulbar tumor.

Corneal integrity is threatened by exposure from lid retraction, proptosis, and limitation of upward gaze. Prolonged exposure, if not treated, can cause progression from superficial erosions to corneal keratitis and ulceration.

While corneal exposure can lead to vision loss, the possibility of optic nerve compression must be ruled out. The optic neuropathy of Graves' disease typically results in curtain scotomas, inferior arcuate nerve fiber bundle deficits, and exhibits expected afferent defect pupillary signs.

## Orbital Tumors

One of the largest surveys of orbital tumor cases is the Mayo Clinic Series. Henderson and Farrow (1980) reported the distribution of orbital tumor in 764 consecutive cases.

The five most common primary orbital tumors in their series were as follows:

| | |
|---|---|
| Hemangiomas | 55 |
| Malignant lymphoma | 38 |
| Lymphocyte inflammatory pseudotumors | 35 |
| Meningioma | 23 |
| Optic nerve glioma | 19 |

The five most common secondary orbital tumors in their series were:

| | |
|---|---|
| Mucocele | 65 |
| Squamous cell carcinoma | 58 |
| Meningioma | 45 |
| Vascular malformations | 40 |
| Malignant melanoma | 27 |

Definitive diagnosis of orbital tumors invariably requires consultation. While precise pathologic evaluation ultimately requires biopsy, nonsurgical evaluations, particularly the use of computerized tomographic scanning and ultrasonography, are of considerable assistance.

## Orbital Cellulitis

This is a life-threatening condition. Orbital cellulitis demands immediate consultation and prompt referral for treatment. In acute cases, the infection can quickly proceed backward and cause cavernous sinus thrombosis and death. A high index of suspicion is most important with debilitated, alcoholic, or immunosuppressed patients.

Usually trauma or local inflammation of the lids or paranasal sinusitis precede orbital involvement. Therefore, it is important to look for evidence of hordeolum, conjunctivitis, dacryocystitis, and dacryoadenitis. Signs of sinusitis, however, can be difficult to distinguish from orbital cellulitis. Frontal sinusitis, more common in adults, and ethmoidal sinusitis, more common in children, can present with periorbital swelling and local pain. It is best to be cautious and proceed to rule out orbital cellulitis in any case of periorbital inflammation signs and pain.

Ocular clinical features of orbital cellulitis include proptosis, conjunctival injection and chemosis, pain, and lid edema and erythema. Systemic features may include upper respiratory infection, fever, nausea, and leukocytosis. The additional association of vision loss and ophthalmoplegia is ominous and suggests cavernous sinus thrombosis. Differential diagnosis should consider primary eyelid inflammation, particularly acute meibomianitis, and periorbital swelling caused by allergy.

Prompt recognition and treatment of orbital cellulitis can save a patient's life. In particular, take care to rule out orbital cellulitis if history reveals antecedent trauma or poor health.

# References

Greenberg DA. Basic evaluation of exophthalmos. J Am Optom Assoc 1977; 48(11):1431–1433.

Henderson JW, Farrow GM. Orbital tumors. New York: Brian C. Decker, 1980;2nd ed.

Krohel GB, Stewart WB, Chavis RM. Orbital disease, a practical approach. New York: Grune & Stratton, 1981.

Lyle WM. Werner's classification of ocular changes in Graves' disease. Am J Optom Physiol Opt 1978;55(2):119–127.

# Lyman C. Norden
# EYELIDS 21

*The eyelid region extends from the brow above to the inferior sulcus on the cheek below. Inflammations and anomalies of this area are common, and their clinical characteristics result from the unique anatomic features of this region (Figure 21.1).*

## BACKGROUND

The outer skin covering the eyelids is quite thin and loosely attached by areolar connective tissue. Within the skin are numerous sebaceous glands. These features allow for the necessary stretching and folding of the outer skin during eyelid movements.

Enclosed within the tarsal plates are the meibomian glands, which secrete a lipid component to the preocular tear film. The other important glands in the eyelids are located at the margins in close association with the eyelash follicles. These are the glands of Zeis and Moll.

Eyelid motility and tonus are provided by three separate muscle groups: (1) the levator muscle, (2) Müller's muscle, and (3) the orbicularis muscle. The levator muscle originates at the top of the orbital apex and attaches to the anterior aspect of the superior tarsal plate. Innervation of the levator is supplied by a branch of cranial nerve III, the oculomotor nerve. Components of this nerve also supply the pupillary sphincter muscle and four of the six extraocular muscles. A single nucleus for the levator fibers of the two oculomotor nerves is located on the dorsal aspect of the oculomotor nucleus group in the mesencephalon.

Tonus of the elevated upper lid is maintained by Müller's muscle, which originates on the underside of the levator muscle and attaches to the upper border of the superior tarsal plate. This muscle is innervated by a branch of the cervical sympathetic nervous system. These nerve fibers originate in the diencephalon and follow a lengthy path down the spinal column to the thoracic region, past the superior aspect of the lung and back up the superior sympathetic chain to synapse in the superior cervical ganglion. Postganglionic fibers continue along the external carotid artery to sweat glands of the face and along the internal carotid to the pupillary dilator muscle and Müller's muscle. A small branch of this sympathetic system also supplies a smooth muscle group, the inferior division of Müller's muscle, located beneath the orbicularis muscle of the lower lid. Its function is to add tonus to the opened lower eyelid.

The orbicularis muscle is a thin sheet of striated muscle that encircles the palpebral fissure. Its contraction causes clo-

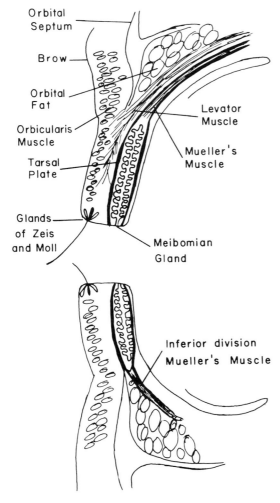

Orbital
Septum

Brow

Orbital
Fat

Orbicularis
Muscle

Tarsal
Plate

Levator
Muscle

Mueller's
Muscle

Glands
of Zeis
and Moll

Meibomian
Gland

Inferior division
Mueller's Muscle

**FIGURE 21.1.**
Eyelid cross section.

reaching the orbicularis and facial muscles. The sensory supply to the eyelids is by cranial nerve V.

Parts of the lacrimal drainage system are important components of the eyelids. The nasal superior and inferior puncta serve as entryways to the drainage system, which must remain in close apposition to the globe in order to function normally.

Certain structural and physiologic features predispose the eyelids to rather common inflammations. For example, the local environment mediated by sebaceous gland output favors bacterial proliferation, which causes exudative and ulcerative blepharitis.

The loosely attached, thin skin of the eyelids can swell remarkably with edema in the absence of inflammation in surrounding tissue. For example, relatively mild allergies can cause considerable eyelid edema and symptoms of itching in persons with no other signs of allergy. The eyes are said to be 10 times more clinically sensitive to allergens than other parts of the body.

Diffuse lid swelling and hyperemia can also occur with small insect or spider bite. Such a bite had little effect elsewhere on the body, but at the lids it can cause notable tissue swelling.

Dramatic eyelid swelling is also common in acute hordeolum. Although the primary inflammation in acute hordeolum occurs within a single meibomian gland, the surrounding tissue becomes secondarily inflamed and grossly chemotic. The resulting condition appears a lot worse than it really is to the patient and sometimes to the examiner (Figure 21.2).

Hordeolum (or stye) is an inflammation caused by bacterial proliferation within one of the glands of the eyelid. The causative organism usually is *Staphylococcus*, which is commonly found in the normal bacterial flora of the skin. If the microbe infects a gland of Zeis or Moll, the result is an external hordeolum. When it forms a head and drains, it does so toward the outer lid surface. A meibomian gland

sure of the eyelids, either forcibly under voluntary control or involuntarily as a blink. The orbicularis muscle is attached by the medial and lateral palpebral ligaments to the nasal and lateral aspects of the orbit. Innervation of the orbicularis muscle is by cranial nerve VII, the facial nerve. The facial nerve nucleus is located in the pons, and its fibers pass through a long canal in the petrous bone before

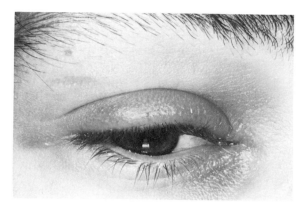

**FIGURE 21.2.**
Acute internal hordeolum. Note the diffuse lid swelling with localized inflammation midtemporally.

infection, however, causes an internal hordeolum which seldom points to the outer lid surface. A hordeolum usually has a rapid onset, and the swollen eyelid is moderately to severely painful, particularly to touch.

A meibomian gland can also become inflamed chronically and nonpainfully as a chalazion. This presents as a localized swelling without secondary lid edema. The etiology of chalazion is not clearly established.

Normally, the meibomian glands secrete a clear viscous fluid that forms a partial barrier against skin oils at the lid margins. Meibomian secretion also forms a lipid layer on the tear film to slow its evaporation. Light finger pressure usually is sufficient to bring a small amount of the secretion to the lid margin surface. For unknown reasons, particularly in elderly individuals, the meibomian secretion becomes abnormal or may be absent, even on forced expression. This often leads to formation of dry spots in the tear film and symptoms of intermittent, sharp, or stinging eye pains owing to corneal exposure. These pains may cause reflex tearing and resultant epiphora. Meibomian gland dys-

function is thought to be a complicating factor in contact lens wear.

Eyelid movements and positioning serve to protect the globe and maintain its optical integrity. They enable the lids to form a mechanical barrier to outside influences when necessary and to distribute the preocular tear film evenly over the cornea. Eyelid movements (i.e., blinking and forced closure) are mediated by the levator and orbicularis muscles. Positioning of the lids is controlled by Müller's muscle superiorly and inferiorly. Eyelid movement and positioning are directly affected by certain cranial and sympathetic nerve anomalies and by individual eyelid muscle disorders; they are indirectly affected by tarsal plate ligament tonus, eyelid tissue mass, and tissue scarring.

Dysfunction of the levator muscle causes ptosis. Ptosis can be mechanical, resulting from an accumulation of too much weight or mass within the lid tissue, thereby restricting levator function. A large chalazion is a good example of this condition.

Ptosis can also be myogenic, caused by impaired muscle function. An example of this is senile ptosis, in which age-related deterioration of the levator muscle occurs. Another example is myasthenia gravis, in which there is insufficient acetylcholine present at the myoneural junction for normal muscular function.

A third type of ptosis is neurogenic, caused by lesions of either the oculomotor nerve or of the cervical sympathetic nervous system (see Chapter 19).

Another important type of neurogenic ptosis involves the sympathetic supply to Müller's muscle. This occurs in Horner's syndrome. The classic features of Horner's syndrome are ptosis, miosis, and anhidrosis; it is possible, however, to have a partial Horner's syndrome that exhibits only one or two of the above signs. The causative lesion may occur at one of numerous locations along the cervical sympathetic pathway. Several examples are injury of the cervical spinal column, tumor of the superior lobe of the lung, and damage to the external carotid plexus (see Chapter 19).

The orbicularis oculi muscle plays an important role: first, it closes the eyelids when necessary, and second, it maintains close apposition of the lacrimal drainage apparatus against the globe. A lesion of the facial nerve results in paresis or paralysis of the orbicularis muscle as well as muscles of the cheek and mouth. Facial nerve palsy, therefore, causes a loss of facial expression and an inability to close the eyelids on one side of the face. The cause may be at the nuclear level, but usually it occurs in peripheral portions of the nerve. A common type of facial nerve palsy is Bell's palsy, the cause of which is unknown. In peripheral facial nerve palsy there usually is an intact Bell's phenomenon. This mechanism helps to protect the cornea from prolonged exposure by turning the eye and cornea upward under the upper eyelid during attempted forced blinking. This phenomenon is lost if the facial nerve lesion is nuclear (see Chapter 19).

A common problem in aging is loss of tonus of the orbicularis muscle and its ligaments. When this occurs, the lacrimal punctum falls away from the globe, thereby inactivating the lacrimal pump mechanism. When tears no longer drain normally, the pool fills excessively and eventually spills over onto the cheek. A typical patient response to epiphora is continual wiping of the eye and lower lid with a handkerchief. Over a long period of time, this further weakens the muscle and ligaments and can lead to an ectropion. The sequence of events listed above is believed to occur partially as a result of orbital fat accumulation with aging, which also decreases the tonus of the lower lid against the globe.

The same aging changes that cause ectropion can also lead to an entropion. This often occurs with a forced lid closure in an elderly person following an irritative stimulus to the external eye. If there is insufficient tonus in the lower aspect of the orbital muscle, the lid may remain turned inward, causing more corneal irritation and possible injury.

Loss of orbicularis muscle tonus can also cause lagophthalmos. This is an incomplete closure of the lids, usually during sleep, which leads to partial corneal exposure and epithelial erosion.

A fifth anomaly of orbicularis muscle function, myokymia, occurs most often in young and middle-aged adults. This is an episodic, involuntary twitching of the orbicularis muscle. Its cause is unknown, but the condition may be associated with stress, fatigue, or minor ocular irritation.

# HISTORY

The case history is a relatively straightforward element in the assessment of eyelid anomalies. These anomalies usually are so obvious that either the patient, or those around him, are able to give valuable information quite easily.

The duration of the abnormality is one of the most important diagnostic features. For example, a hordeolum usually develops rapidly, while a chalazion develops slowly. A ptosis that develops suddenly almost invariably will require a medical consultation, while a long-standing ptosis does not—unless surgical correction is being considered. Whatever the anomaly, the examiner should attempt to determine its duration.

The clinical course of the condition helps to establish its preferred mode of management. For example, a hordeolum that reportedly is still worsening when first seen by the doctor should be followed more closely than one improving by the time the patient presents. A chalazion or meibomitis that appears to recur more than once in the same location should alert the doctor to the possibility of a carcinoma.

In some cases, the patient may offer an explanation or probable cause for the eyelid anomaly observed. A patient with diffuse eyelid edema may be able to say that its onset was associated with chronic fatigue or recent exposure to a possible allergen, such as pet hairs. If the cause is not already apparent, it is often worthwhile to ask, "Do you have any idea what may have caused this?"

Related problems or symptoms are also worth investigating. A patient with recent onset of ptosis and subjective diplopia most likely has an oculomotor nerve lesion. If the patient has a history of diabetes mellitus, there is a good chance the cause will be diabetic neuropathy. If the patient with ptosis reports unusual fatigue, also of recent onset, myasthenia gravis should be considered.

Several aspects of the patient's past history also are of potential value. A history of previous occurrences of acute, painful lid swelling with spontaneous resolution supports a diagnosis of hordeolum. Previous occurrences of chalazia raise the possibility of rosacea, which often is medically treatable.

The patient's medical history can be useful when evaluating certain eyelid anomalies. Ptosis is a common problem following cataract surgery, resulting from the use of lid retractors. Horner's syndrome has been known to result from carotid angiography procedures.

In some cases, the family history becomes quite important. Xanthelasma, for example, has a familial tendency. Knowledge of the family history enables the doctor to predict more accurately whether a given patient will be similarly affected, whether there is likely to be an associated hematologic or metabolic anomaly, and whether surgical treatment is recommended. Family history is also valuable in the examination of ptosis, since this condition is sometimes hereditary. In some cases, a close examination of old family photographs will reveal in one of the parents a previously undiagnosed ptosis identical to that of the patient.

# EXAMINATION

The examination of eyelid anomalies consists of various techniques of gross observation, evaluation of lid position and function, and biomicroscopy. Most individual test procedures are highly specific for the particular disorder presented to the doctor. They will, therefore, be detailed with consideration given to presenting signs and symptoms.

## Gross Observation

In blepharitis the initial observation usually is hyperemia at the lid margins. There also may be diffuse conjunctival hyperemia caused by bacterial toxins produced at the lid margins. Often the person with blepharitis has oily appearing eyelid skin.

On the other hand, many who do not show this characteristic have scalp dandruff instead. Making this initial distinction aids in the differential diagnosis between staphylococcal and seborrheic blepharitis.

The initial evalution of eyelid swelling, or edema, should include a search for focal hyperemia, along with fingertip palpation. Palpation is done in an attempt to find a localized area of hardness within the swollen lid. If such an area is located, there usually is considerable pain or tenderness reported by the patient when it is touched. This is a sure sign of acute hordeolum.

If lid edema is unilateral and not obviously due to hordeolum, look for ipsilateral preauricular lymph node swelling. This would be readily apparent by gross observation in a case of Parinaud's ocu-loglandular syndrome.

If preauricular lymphadenopathy is not present, the lid swelling may be associated with a sinusitis. This may be unilateral or bilateral.

Bilateral lid edema also raises the prospect of local allergy. This characteristically appears as predominantly clear tissue swelling with relatively little hyperemia. The lid surface texture should be examined. In local, contact allergy it usually appears quite dry and cracked.

Lid swelling that is localized and non-painful as determined by palpation will almost invariably be a chalazion. If a lesion is not well localized by palpation, it could be a carcinoma and its size should be documented for future follow-up.

In a case of ptosis the first observation should be of the ipsilateral pupil. If it is dilated, there probably is an oculomotor nerve lesion such as aneurysm or tumor. If the pupil is constricted, the ptosis probably is a part of Horner's syndrome. If the pupil is unaffected, the probable cause is either myasthenia gravis or peripheral neuropathy in diabetes mellitus.

In suspected lid retraction, it is possible to rule out exophthalmos by observing ocular protrusion while standing behind the partially reclined patient. The relative protrusion of one eye can be compared to the other by using the frontal ridge as a baseline for this observation. A true exophthalmos should be quite obvious by this technique (see Chapter 20).

A pseudo-lid retraction can also appear secondary to a ptosis in the fellow eye. A patient with either mechanical or myasthenic ptosis may attempt to elevate forcibly the affected lid. Since there is equal innervation from a single nucleus to both lids, the opposite lid may elevate excessively. In some cases, a patient attempts to overcome ptosis by elevating both lids with the frontalis muscle. This usually will appear grossly as a furrowed brow on the patient.

The typical appearance of basal cell carcinoma is a darkly discolored, raised lesion with an eroded looking central crater with pearly, rolled edges (Figure 21.3). They are most likely to occur on the nasal aspect of the lower eyelid, and there often will be similar lesions behind the ear or along the rear scalp line. This feature may help to positively identify a questionable lesion.

Xanthelasma appears grossly as a yellowish, slightly raised plaque just beneath the eyelid skin surface. It is important to note the number and size of these lesions.

Many older patients complain of excess tearing; however, those with true epiphora usually have overflowing tears visible on the cheek at the time of examination. Also, they are usually seen to be continually wiping their lids and lid margins with a handkerchief (see Chapter 22).

# Lid Position and Function

Evaluation of lid position and function can provide additional valuable information in

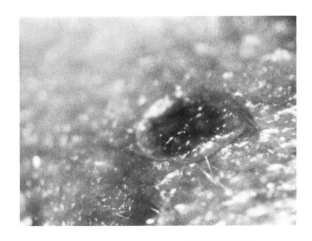

**FIGURE 21.3.**
Early basal cell carcinoma. Note the eroded central crater surrounded by a slightly rolled border.

the assessment of ptosis, lid retraction, facial palsy, and epiphora.

In Horner's syndrome, the lower eyelid on the affected side will be positioned slightly higher than on the fellow eye because of impaired smooth muscle function (Figure 21.4). The upper eyelid, although positioned lower than on the fellow eye, will have the same range of motion between down gaze and up gaze. This occurs because the levator muscle is unaffected.

The amount of declination in down gaze helps to establish whether the ptosis is congenital or acquired. In congenital ptosis, the affected lid does not depress as low as the lid of the fellow eye. In acquired ptosis, it usually drops to a lower position than its fellow.

Several noninvasive tests can be run for signs of myasthenia gravis in cases of acquired ptosis. One of these is known as Cogan's twitch sign. This phenomenon is a slight hyperelevation followed by a settling of the affected lid occurring with a voluntary eye movement from down gaze to primary gaze. Another dynamic feature

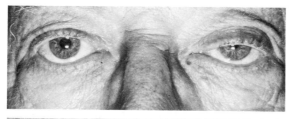
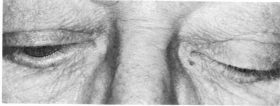

**FIGURE 21.4.**
Ptosis in Horner's syndrome. Note the miosis and the slightly elevated lower lid margin, *OS.* Also note the greater declination of the left superior lid in down gaze, indicative of acquired ptosis.

in myasthenia is fatigue of the upper lid after a series of repeated up- and down-gaze movements. A similar test involves a sustained voluntary up gaze. In myasthenia, the upper lid will begin to fatigue within a few seconds, while the normal will not. Definitive diagnosis usually is made by observing normal lid elevation following administration of edrophonium (see Chapter 19).

In differentiating true lid retraction from pseudo-lid retraction, as occurs in exophthalmos, it is sometimes useful to test elasticity of the levator muscle. This is done by grasping both superior eyelids at the lashes and pulling downward. In true lid retraction there will be noticeably more resistance on the affected side.

Facial palsy usually is not obvious by gross observation unless the examiner specifically watches the patient's facial expressions and movements. For example, if the patient is asked to smile, the affected side of the face will be unable to form this expression around the eye and at the corner of the mouth (Figure 21.5). Usually there will appear to be an overly exaggerated blink on the opposite side, as if the patient were attempting to compensate for the inactive side. If orbicularis dysfunction is not obvious, its tonus can be tested by placing thumb and fingers on the upper brow and lower lid and attempting to prevent orbicularis contraction while the patient performs a forced blink. The affected muscle will be noticeably weaker in this comparison.

If a facial palsy is diagnosed, check for Bell's phenomenon. When the eye does not rotate upward during attempted forced closure, there is not only a possibility of a nuclear lesion of the facial nerve but also a greater chance of ocular damage from exposure.

In cases of epiphora, it is possible to evaluate lower lid tonus by noting how far the lower lid margin can be pulled away from the globe. A distance greater than 6 mm indicates a significant loss of tonus.

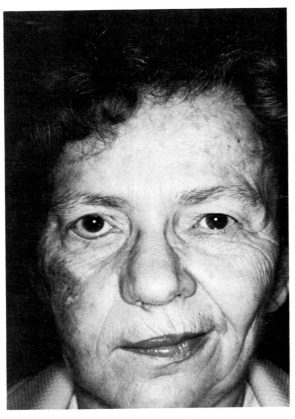

**FIGURE 21.5.**
Right facial palsy. Patient was asked to smile;
note right ectropian.

## Biomicroscopy

Biomicroscopy is especially useful in the evaluation of blepharitis, lid edema, meibomitis, epiphora, and myokymia.

Blepharitis scales may be classified as either dry or exudative. Dry scales look essentially like dandruff scales, while exudative scales have a waxy appearance and often are seen as collarettes around individual cilia. In more severe cases of exudative blepharitis, the lid margins may appear ulcerated.

The conjunctiva and cornea should also be examined biomicroscopically for signs of secondary inflammation in blepharitis. If the conjunctiva is only secondarily inflamed by staphylococcal toxins, there will be little more than diffuse conjunctival hyperemia with discharge and possible marginal keratitis.

In meibomitis, the meibomian secretion should be examined first, if it is present. Normally, it will appear as an almost clear dome of fluid over the meibomian gland orifice. In some cases, it may appear frothy if abnormal in quality. If the secretion is not readily visible, an attempt should be made to express the glands of the lower lid by finger pressure against the lid and globe. If there is secretion from no more than two or three glands, meibomian gland function can be considered to be abnormal. In such cases, forced expression of the glands with firm pressure against a solid object, such as a glass rod held behind the lid, will yield either no secretion or a semisolid discharge similar to toothpaste squeezed out of the tube.

Epiphora not caused by insufficient drainage, but rather by excess tearing, is frequently associated with an inadequate tear film. Therefore, a biomicroscopic tear film evaluation should be included in the assessment of epiphora when the cause is not an obvious loss of lower lid tonus or punctal stenosis.

Biomicroscopy is also useful in the evaluation of myokymia. Involuntary lid twitching sometimes may be caused by tear deficiency or local foreign body irritation.

# CLINICAL SIGNIFICANCE

In practice, many eyelid disorders and anomalies fail to present all of the expected diagnostic characteristics as outlined. In some cases, a tentative diagnosis may be based on the presence of one or two diagnostic features that can be elicited and the obvious absence of features related to other conditions. Appropriate follow-up includes a search for developing signs or symptoms that would alter the diagnosis and management.

When blepharitis is seen, it should first be classified as either dry or exudative. Dry blepharitis looks essentially like scalp dandruff.

Exudative blepharitis has a yellowish white, waxy appearance. This material often binds several cilia together as it hardens. Often it will appear as a collarette near the base of a single cilia, as if the cilia had grown directly through the scale. This material is a combination of sebum originating from skin glands and bacterial by-products produced by staphylococci. The bacteria are able to proliferate remarkably within this oily, warm environment, thus producing even more toxins that become harmful to the skin. This leads to local hyperemia and skin irritation. Susceptible individuals may develop small ulcerations of the skin surface (ulcerative blepharitis).

The bacteria are protected by the crusts of hardened exudative material, thereby rendering topical antibiotics relatively ineffective. The most important aspect of treatment is lid scrubs.

Eyelid edema not associated with hordeolum, chalazion, or infectious conjunctivitis is caused most often by allergy. A comprehensive allergy history often will isolate the cause. Contact allergens usually cause dry, cracked skin. Other allergens such as dust, pollen, and animal hairs usually cause little more than mild tissue swelling and itching, but they are also harder to isolate by history.

Lid edema caused by insect bite differs from allergy mostly in that it is unilateral. The absence of preauricular lymphadenopathy differentiates the condition from Parinaud's oculoglandular syndrome. The swelling and irritation can be expected to resolve within a few days. If lid swelling is of recent onset and does not improve within a few days, the possibility of sinusitis should be considered.

Chalazia are clinically very similar to subacute hordeola. The major difference is an absence of diffuse tissue swelling and resultant pain.

It is noteworthy, however, that persons with recurrent chalazia are more likely to have rosacea. Therefore, it is advisable to look for signs of increased flush of the nose, cheeks, chin, and forehead. If rosacea is suspected, referral to a dermatologist may benefit the patient. If chalazia appear to recur at a single location, the possibility of a squamous cell carcinoma should be considered. Fingertip palpation of a carcinoma is not likely to feel well localized, as with a chalazion.

Carcinoma should also be suspected if there is apparent recurring, unilateral, ulcerative blepharitis or chronic, unilateral lid swelling. The eyelids should be palpated to check for possible diffuse thickening and hardening of the affected lid as compared to the opposite lid.

Meibomian gland dysfunctions unfortunately are not well understood at present, but they are thought to be the cause for certain tear film deficiencies and contact lens complications. The problem is believed to develop in some individuals over a period of years in which there is inadequate eyelid hygiene and/or infection within the glands. During this stage, the meibomian secretion may appear either somewhat frothy or purulent.

Congenital or long-standing ptosis usually requires no special follow-up care once the diagnosis is established. A referral for surgical repositioning of the lid may be considered if the patient is sufficiently bothered by the ptosis.

Recently acquired ptosis should have some type of medical follow-up in virtually every case. The most common types of acquired ptosis without pupillary involvement are caused either by diabetic neuropathy or by myasthenia gravis, both requiring general medical care. Acquired ptosis accompanied by pupillary anomaly (either dilation or constriction) should be evaluated by a neurologist.

Facial palsy should also be referred to

a neurologist. Acute facial palsy of unknown cause is known as Bell's palsy. In most cases of Bell's palsy there is nearly complete recovery of facial muscle function over a period of several months.

Patients with lid retraction should be referred either to an internal medicine specialist for evaluation for possible thyroid disease or to an ophthalmologist, or to both.

The patient with suspected carcinoma should be referred to a dermatologist or to an ophthalmologist. A growth or pigmented lesion on the skin that obviously is not a carcinoma can be followed initially by either photographing it or by documenting its size and appearance and reexamining the lesion over a period of several months.

There are four common types of growths that do not require surgical treatment unless the patient wants a cosmetic improvement or there is unusual enlargement: (1) sebaceous cyst, (2) keratosis, (3) verruca, and (4) papilloma. Sebaceous cyst results from a plugged sebaceous gland (Figure 21.6).

Keratosis is a proliferation of the keratinized surface epithelium (Figure 21.7). It may appear as an extension of keratin, known as cutaneous horn, or as a discolored proliferation of cells, known as se-

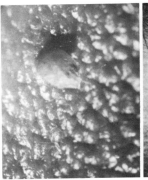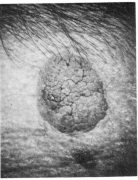

**FIGURE 21.7.**
Keratosis, an irritative, noninfectious proliferation of keratinized epithelial cells. A cutaneous horn. Seborrheic keratosis *(left)*. Seborrheic keratosis has distinctive surface structure unlike the eroded appearance of basal cell carcinoma *(right)*.
Photo courtesy of Dr. Gerald G. Melore.

borrheic keratosis. Either condition could be a precursor to basal cell carcinoma.

Seborrheic keratoses are frequently called verrucae. True verrucae, however, are typical warts caused by the papovavirus (Figure 21.8). As with seborrheic keratosis, most cases are only cosmetically objectionable, but some may cause chronic, low-grade conjunctivitis from leakage of metabolic by-products into the cul-de-sac. Either type of growth can be easily removed dermatologically.

Papilloma is a wartlike knob of epithelial proliferation connected to the skin surface by a thin stalk. This, too, is usually a benign lesion easily removed dermatologically if necessary. Ideally, any growth that has been excised should be examined by a pathologist for possible cancer, particularly if there has been documented enlargement.

Another infectious type of eyelid skin growth that should be specially managed is molluscum contagiosum (Figure 21.9). As its name implies, this is a highly contagious infection by the molluscum virus. Clinically, it appears as multiple, smooth

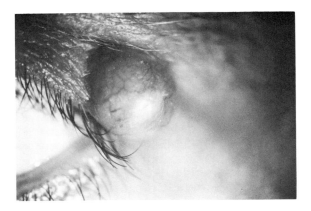

**FIGURE 21.6.**
Sebaceous cyst. This is a plugged, but not infected, sebaceous gland.

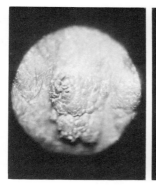 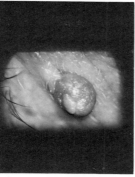

**FIGURE 21.8.**
*A.* Verruca, a common wart. *B.* Papilloma, a pedunculated wart. Both are caused by papovavirus infection.

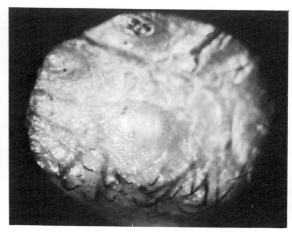

**FIGURE 21.9.**
Molluscum contagiosum with associated dermatitis.

elevations with slight central depressions. The toxins produced by the virus may cause an associated dermatitis and/or conjunctivitis. Because of these complications and possible contagion, molluscum lesions should be removed as soon as possible.

A patient with xanthelasma should be sent for blood lipid analysis, particularly if under age 40. The xanthelasma plaques often can be surgically removed, but there is a good chance of recurrence, especially if more than one eyelid is affected.

# References

Beard C. Ptosis. St. Louis: C.V. Mosby, 1980;3rd ed.

Duane TD, ed. Clinical ophthalmology. Hagerstown, Md.: Harper & Row, 1981.

Fitzpatrick TB, et al. Dermatology in general medicine. New York: McGraw-Hill, 1979;2nd ed.

Hurwitz JJ. Investigation and treatment of epiphora due to lid laxity. Trans Ophthalmol Soc UK 1978;98(1):69–70.

Jones WL. Basal cell carcinoma. A case of long standing neglect and a case of early detection. J Am Optom Assoc 1982; 53:999–1003.

Korb DR, Henriquez AS. Meibomian gland dysfunction and contact lens intolerance. J Am Optom Assoc 1980; 51(3):243–251.

# Barry J. Barresi
# LACRIMAL SYSTEM 22

*The lacrimal system secretes and drains tears. Structures
include the main and accessory lacrimal gland, conjunctival
secreting structures, and the drainage passages of the puncta,
canaliculi, lacrimal sac, and nasolacrimal duct.*

## BACKGROUND

The layered preocular tear film lubricates
and protects the external eye. Lubrication
of the corneal epithelium maintains a
smooth optical surface and prevents corneal dessication and subsequent erosion.
Lysozyme, a bacteriostatic tear constitu-
ent, helps prevent infection. Some foreign
bodies and irritants are washed out by the
tears.

### Secretion

Aqueous secretors are the main lacrimal
gland and the accessory lacrimal glands of
Krause and Wolfring. The main lacrimal
gland is situated in the lacrimal fossa under the upper temporal orbital rim. The
lateral extension of the aponeurosis of the
levator muscle divides the gland into an
orbital and a palpebral lobe. The glands of
Krause and Wolfring also produce watery
secretions. Located subconjunctivally,
these small glands are more numerous
above the upper tarsus.

Oily secretors are situated at the lid
margin and include the meibomian gland,
accessory sebaceous, and the glands of Zeis
and Moll. The meibomians are the oily secretors of principal importance in supplying the superficial lipid layer of the tear
film. The oil secretion is composed mostly
of cholesterol and cholesterol esters.

Mucin secretions are produced by the
conjunctival goblet cells, located mostly in
the interpalpebral bulbar area. The basal
secretion of mucin converts the corneal
epithelium into a hydrophilic aqueous
layer of the tear film.

Aqueous, lipid, and mucin secretions
combine to form the tear film. This dynamic, three-layered structure is contin-
uously renewed by the basic secretions and
blinking of the eyelids. The outermost superficial lipid layer consists mainly of waxy
and cholesterol esters and polar lipids and
is approximately 0.1 $\mu$m thick. The middle
aqueous tear layer comprises about 98%
of the total thickness of the tear film. It is
composed of water with dissolved inor-
ganic salts, glucose, urea, surface active
biopolymers, proteins, and glycoproteins.
Finally, the innermost mucin layer is a very
thin, less than 0.5% of tear film thickness,
coating of hydrated mucoproteins that

clings to the anterior microvilled surface of the corneal epithelium.

Dry spots form on the cornea when the continuity of the tear film is disrupted. Dry spots appear as randomly distributed, small, crater-like holes in the tear film. These breaks in the tear film are clinically observed in the test of tear-film breakup time.

Holly (1981) has presented three corollaries to support the clinical value of the tear-film breakup time as a measure of relative tear-film stability (Table 22.1). The tear-film breakup time is that interval between a blink and the appearance of the first random dry spot. Holly suggests that lipid contamination of the cornea-tear film interface leads to instability and subsequent dry spot formation. Recurrent dry spots can in turn lead to epithelial damage, as evidenced by superficial punctate staining.

An unstable tear film does not necessarily lead to harmful effects. More frequent, full blinking or increased tear secretion can compensate for premature tear-film breakup.

Causes of rapid tear-film breakup time identified by Holly (1981) include: (1) low tear volume, (2) poorly functioning mucus layer, (3) highly polar lipid contaminants (meibomianitis, skin conditions, cosmetics), (4) inadequate blinking pattern or poor lid-globe congruity, and (5) excessive debris or transient contaminants from the environment.

## Distribution

Tears are distributed by the movement of the eyelids and the globe. The blinking action of the eyelids, and on occasion the underlying motion of the globe, distributes the tear film constituents and reforms the three-layer tear film. Usually the blinking action occurs before or very shortly after dry spots form. Abnormal blinking patterns, such as infrequent or incomplete blinking, provide inadequate

Table 22.1
Aspects of Tear-Film Breakup

| | |
|---|---|
| Corollary I. | A continuous film 10 microns thick can only exist on a hydrophilic surface (low interfacial tension), since thickness is much lower than the critical thickness of rupture for films or hydrophobic surface. |
| Corollary II. | An increase in interfacial tension (conversion from hydrophilic to hydrophobic) will result in the immediate rupture of the film. Hence, such a rupture (dry spot formation) *must* indicate that the solid surface has locally become hydrophobic. |
| Corollary III. | Since the surface is initially hydrophilic, and since the original film thickness is much smaller than the critical thickness of rupture, and since the surface changes its character in time; *the time interval required for film rupture,* rather than the film thickness at rupture, becomes the relevant parameter. |

resurfacing of the tear film and lead to premature tear-film breakup. Lid surfacing of tear film can also be defective in cases of inflammation or structural alterations of the lid margins.

## Excretion

Tears are eliminated by evaporation and drainage. Except with low secretors, evaporation does not lead to drying because of inadequate tear volume. Rather, evaporation can lead to aqueous layer thinning, which in turn fosters migration of superficial lipids to the epithelium and causes tear-film breakup.

Drainage proceeds through the puncta, canaliculi, lacrimal sac, and nasolacrimal duct. The pumping effects of the blink and movement of the canaliculi and lacrimal sac aid in tear outflow. Tears are propelled nasally by the blink, with the largest volume exiting via the lower puncta and canaliculi. With a normal blink and pumping motion, the lower puncta can be seen to move several millimeters toward the nose.

Impairment of the drainage system can occur from failure of the pumping mechanism due to ectropic punctum, lid notching from past inflammation or trauma, and weak orbicularis muscle contraction associated with aging or a seventhnerve palsy. Lacrimal drainage may be blocked by obstructions in the puncta, canaliculus, lacrimal sac, and nasolacrimal duct.

# HISTORY

The strategy in history and examination is to: (1) identify patients with lacrimal disorder, (2) locate the part of the system involved (secretion, distribution, excretion), (3) assess the functional impact on corneal integrity and health of external eye, and (4) determine the etiology. Keep in mind that the initial history may not provide sufficient information. Often after clinical signs are noted and qualified during the exam, a return to interviewing the patient can provide needed insights for diagnosis.

Determine if vision or comfort is affected. Note any transient disturbances of blurring or lines in vision associated with ocular discomfort or tearing. Qualify any discomfort, such as a sandy, gritty, or tearing feeling, actual epiphora, or an achy eye. How does each eye compare and is there any pattern in the associations or progression of discomfort symptoms?

Determine how severe and frequent is the complaint. Does the patient suffer chronic symptoms or episodic symptoms associated with reading, time of day, or outdoor activity? Ask how the patient resolved the discomfort. Does the patient dab the eyes, use ocular decongestants, irrigate the eyes, or apply home remedies? To gauge severity of hyposecretion, ask the patient if tears are absent even when crying.

Investigate symptoms of current and past history of external eye inflammation. Ask about conjunctival redness, discharge, and matted lashes. In particular, be alert to a history of upper temporal or lower nasal lid swelling. Note if patient is aware of any structural or positional problem of the eyelids. Ask about history of exposure to airborne toxic or physical ocular irritants. Does the patient have any history of trauma or surgery to the nose or external eye?

Investigate the patient's medical history for the association of rheumatoid arthritis or other collagen-vascular disease. Note if the patient uses diuretics, antihypertensives, and antihistamines, and if the medication use precipitates symptoms of lacrimal dysfunction. Also, be alert to vitamin A deficiency caused by malabsorption syndrome, intestinal bypass surgery, or malnutrition.

# EXAMINATION

Assessment of the lacrimal system includes evaluation of the secretion, stability, distribution, and drainage. Techniques of assessment include external inspection of the lids and globe, biomicroscopy of the external eye, and functional testing of tear production and drainage.

External inspection can reveal signs of inflammation and eye lid position or movement abnormalities (Figure 22.1). Note any lacrimal gland (upper temporal quadrant) or lacrimal sac (nasal inferior quadrant) swelling. Inspection of lashes and conjunctiva should rule out signs of blepharitis conjunctivitis, or structural changes such as scarring, loss of lashes, trichiasis, and tumors (Figure 22.2).

Observe lid movements and assess lid closure. Noting the frequency and correctness of blink is quite relative. The blink rate should be noted in the external examination, although it really can not be interpreted by measurement; for a given eye, however, a desirable blink rate is one in which the typical blink interval is shorter than the tear-film breakup time. Assessing lid closure is done simply by in-

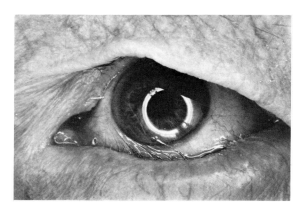

**FIGURE 22.2.**
Spastic entropion and trichiasis. Rule out abnormal lid position as a cause of epiphora. This patient complained of epiphora in evening.

structing the patient to gently close the eyes. With a penlight then look for incomplete closure with exposure of the conjunctiva and the cornea. Also look for any maceration of skin at canthi and at the cheek from tears spilling over.

The biomicroscope is useful for inspection of lid position, signs of inflammation, tear-film stability, and corneal integrity. Care should be taken to rule out an ectropion, entropion, or trichiasis, which may contribute to ocular irritation or epiphora. The lid margins should be carefully examined for exudates, edema, erythema, scaling, cilia loss, and neovascularization. The presence of blepharitis may inhibit proper blinking, but more important, it may result in dysfunction of meibomian glands. Abnormal lipid production and bacterial toxins may have an adverse effect on the cornea by precipitating dry spot formation, or they may disturb the corneal epithelium.

Assessing nasal lacrimal patency begins with examination of puncta patency, position, and movement with the blink. The puncta must be open and point into the tear lake. Orbicularis tone and the lac-

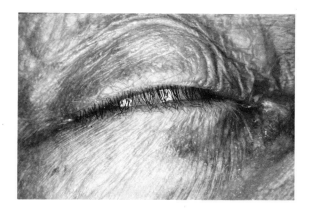

**FIGURE 22.1.**
Nocturnal lagophthalmos. Patient was asked to close eyes gently. Patient presented with a complaint of a "dry, achey" eye upon awakening in the morning.

rimal pump can be assessed by asking the patient to attempt lid closure while the examiner holds the upper lid. With attempted closure the inferior puncta should continue to point into the tear lake and move 3 to 4 mm nasally.

Palpation is helpful in assessing drainage of the lacrimal system. Mildly press on the inferior orbital rim and slowly move medially, feeling the tear sac. With chronic infections, mucopus can be expressed. With a palpable mass and a history of "bloody tears," suspect a lacrimal sac tumor.

Examination of the conjunctiva should rule out signs of dry eye such as symblepharon, Bitot's spots, tissue shrinkage, and interpalpebral injection. Signs of nonspecific conjunctivitis such as diffuse redness and papillary hyperplasia should also be looked for, since, as with any positive external finding, comparison of appearance between the two eyes is most helpful. A unilateral presentation more likely represents inflammation rather than the dry eye of senility or Sjögren's syndrome. Other causes of dry eye are listed in Table 22.2.

The goal of evaluating tear film is to gauge the volume, consistency, and stability of the corneal film. Observation of the marginal tear strip along the inferior lid margin can provide a relative measure of tear volume. A convex 1-mm-wide strip should be expected. With each blink the cornea should be resurfaced with a resulting smooth and uniform tear film. The pressure of ropy mucus strands, increased tear debris, and corneal filiments all suggest inadequate hydration. The debris and mucus strands in the inferior cul-de-sac can contribute to a foreign-body sensation. The technique for measurement of tear-film breakup time is described by the following steps:

1. Wet a fluorescein strip with preserved saline or (ideally) distilled water.

2. Instill drop from strip into lower cul-de-sac, being careful to minimize squeezing of eye lids.

**Table 22.2**
**Selected Causes of Dry Eye**

Hyposecretion
  Congenital absence lacrimal gland
  Riley-Day syndrome
  Senile hyposecretion
  Sjögren's syndrome
  Inflammation (e.g., sarcoid)
Exposure
  Proptosis
  Nocturnal lagophthalmos
  Facial palsy
  Ectropion
Disease mucous membranes
  Stevens-Johnson syndrome (erythema multiforme)
  Ocular pemphigoid
  Avitaminosis A
  Chemical or radiation burns
Drug side effects
  Parasympatholytic drugs
  Antihistimines
  Nasal decongestants
  Diuretics
  Tranquilizers
  Birth control pills

3. Observe the tear film using a low illumination on level, broad beam (3 mm or so) and the cobalt blue filter.

4. After three gentle complete blinks, then time the interval between the last blink and the first sign of a dry spot. Look for early spots by scanning the cornea from side to side.

5. Look for mucus strands, tear debris, lid-cornea incongruity, and epithelial staining.

Reduced volume of tears can cause premature tear-film breakup, but so can surface contamination. Excess oily secretions and production of free fatty acids are often associated with chronic blepharitis and meibomitis. Also, surface-active contaminants may be introduced by facial creams and eye cosmetics.

With the biomicroscope, look for colored interference surface phenomena. When light is reflected from a thin lipid layer the reflection from the anterior and posterior surface becomes phase-displaced, giving rise to a rainbow effect. This phenomenon occurs if the lipid layer is greater than 0.1 mm thick. The interference pattern is best seen in the reflection of the slit lamp mirror (specular reflection technique).

The tear film, made visible with fluorescein dye, is thickest immediately after a blink. The tear film generally thins due to evaporation and migration to the lacrimal lake. The film eventually ruptures into dry spots, noted as dark blue spots against the green of fluorescein. The most clinically useful test of tear-film stability is the tear breakup time (BUT). The appearance of dry spots in less than 10 seconds after a blink is considered a rapid BUT. Tear-film instability shown by a rapid BUT suggests reduced tear volume, deficient mucus layer, lipid contaminants from inflammation or cosmetics, or environmental irritants.

Comparison of the normal blink interval and the BUT is most important. Note if the formation of dry spot stimulates a blink. For example, a patient with a 15-second BUT may be symptomatic because of infrequent blinks, greater than 20-second BUT intervals, or because of incomplete blinks. In contrast, a patient with a rapid BUT may be compensating by more rapid blinking. Keep in mind that blink rates noted by gross inspection may differ from biomicroscopic observation. Also blink rates typically reduce with general fatigue or prolonged near-point tasks.

The purpose of biomicroscopy of the cornea in a lacrimal workup is twofold: to detect primary corneal disease that causes tear-film abnormality and to detect secondary corneal abnormalities, which are sequelae of dry eye. Distinguishing between primary and secondary corneal abnormality may be elusive in some cases, but the distinction is critical to selecting proper management. Look for such signs as areas of consistent nonwetting, local elevation of superficial epithelium, corneal filaments, erosions, dellen, ulcers, neovascularization, epithelial microcysts, and edema.

Biomicroscopic assessment of corneal integrity is greatly augmented by use of rose bengal and fluorescein dyes. Fluorescein is more helpful in assessing tear-film stability and corneal wetting. The dye will also pool in areas of dellen and epithelial disruption. Rose bengal, not as commonly used, is a vital dye that stains devitalized cells and mucin. Fluorescein and rose bengal staining, if associated with keratitis sicca, typically exhibit an interpalpebral or, more specifically, an inferior corneal pattern.

During the course of the remaining assessment of ocular health, if dry eye is present, keep in mind the manifestations of systemic causes. For example, the patient with rheumatoid arthritis along with dry eye is at risk for ocular inflammation, most notably iritis.

## Secretory Tests

Secretory tests are valuable if interpreted on the basis of their intent. These tests are just one in the battery of tests of tear-film stability, tear volume, and corneal integrity. In suspected cases of dry eye, repeated application of these tests can help qualify the severity and the natural history of the lacrimal disorder. Measurement of tear lysozyme ratio (Mackie 1981) offers consideration and promise as a supplement to Schirmer's tests.

### SCHIRMER #1

Tear production can be quantified by means of a filter paper absorbing tear fluid from the conjunctival sac. The #1 test is performed without instillation of local anesthetics. The folded short end of a Schirmer strip (Whatman #41 filter paper) is placed over the lateral lower lid at a point one-third away from the lateral canthus. The patient is instructed to look slightly above a direct line of gaze. The strips are left in place for five minutes and the amount of wetting is then measured on a mm scale.

Wetting less than 10 mm is considered suspect, while wetting less than 5 mm in 5 minutes is a positive finding of hyposecretion. Wetting greater than 10 mm or even more rapid wetting may be normal or represent a pseudoepiphora with the reflex secretors compensating for decreased basic secretion. Thus if the test is negative and dry eye is still suspect, one can proceed to the basic secretion Schirmer's test.

### BASIC SECRETION SCHIRMER'S TEST

Here the Schirmer's test is repeated after instillation of one drop of a suitable local anesthetic in the lower culs-de-sac. Wait two to three minutes, then proceed with application of the Schirmer's strip. Again, with this test, 10 mm of wetting is the guidepost. Greater than 10 mm is negative, less than 10 mm is suspicious, and less than 5 mm is a fairly reliable indicator of hyposecretion.

## Excretory Test

The Jones No. 1 and No. 2 are considered the standards of assessing patency of the lacrimal drainage system. Dye retrieval in Jones No. 1 can pose a problem. Hecht (1978) advocates a modification of the Jones No. 1 test. The test differs from the

**Table 22.3**
**Hecht Modification of Jones No. 1 Test**

1. Instill one drop of 2% fluorescein dye in each conjunctival cul-de-sac.
2. After 15 seconds, instill second drop; after 15 seconds, instill third drop.
3. Patient's head remains in erect position for 1 minute.
4. Patient's head placed down at 45° angle from erect position for 10 minutes.
5. With one nostril occluded, patient blows his nose 10 times into white tissue paper. Copious dye will commonly appear.

Source: Hecht 1978.

standard procedure in quantity of dye used, head position during testing, and length of time allowed for dye transit to nose (Table 22.3).

In an office screening of lacrimal drainage, the following sequence is suggested. First, assess the lids, puncta, and lid movement and rule out lid notching, ectropic puncta, or weak orbicularis muscle contraction. Next, perform the Schirmer #1 test to rule out dry eye as a cause of epiphora due to excessive reflex tearing. And, last, perform the modified Jones No. 1 fluorescein dye test. Beyond the three-step office screening procedure, some other diagnostic procedures to consider are standard lacrimal irrigation (Clompus 1983) and dacryocystography.

# CLINICAL SIGNIFICANCE

The most common presentation of lacrimal disorder is tear film instability and mild dry eye. The patient with a wet-feeling eye or with epiphora more likely has reflex tearing from keratosis sicca than hypersecretion or drainage block. While hypersecretions and drainage blocks are less common than dry eye, their consequences for patient discomfort can be quite nota-

ble, and they may be harbingers of neoplasm or inflammation of the lacrimal gland or drainage system. Care must always be taken to assess thoroughly the lacrimal secretion, distribution, and drainage, and initially to distinguish between diagnostic categories of dry eye, hypersecretion, and drainage block.

# Dry Eye

The range in severity of dry eye is quite broad. Accurately gauging that level of severity is the key to appropriate management. While distinguishing between the mucus-deficient versus the aqueous-deficient eye may be of interest to some clinicians, the initial diagnostic task is to qualify the severity, the current consequences to the patient's ocular comfort and corneal integrity, and the risk of harmful sequelae. An additional task is to be alert to dry eye as a manifestation of systemic disease or as a side effect of medication (Table 22.4).

With all cases of dry eye, care should be taken to rule out Sjögren's syndrome and the serious mucus deficiency of Stevens-Johnson syndrome, pemphigoid, and avitaminosis A.

When dry eye is associated with larger systemic involvement, it is referred to as *Sjögren's syndrome.* The syndrome includes the presence of dry eyes, dry mouth, and usually is accompanied by a connective tissue disease, typically rheumatoid arthritis. Other connective tissue diseases reported to be associated with Sjögren's are systemic lupus erythematosus, polyarteritis nodosa, and scleroderma. Patients should be asked about symptoms of dry mouth (xerostoma) and dryness of other mucous membrane organs such as the nose, vagina, and throat. Dry mouth may be reported as decreased saliva, oral dryness, food sticking to the mouth, and increased fluid intake with meals. Although Sjögren's syndrome may affect males and children, it has a striking preponderance in middle-aged women. The etiology is in doubt, but an autoimmune mechanism is strongly suspected. The clinical significance of Sjögren's syndrome goes beyond the importance of treatment of the dry eye and other symptoms. These patients deserve a thorough rheumatologic workup to investigate underlying connective tissue disease and should receive most appropriate treatment.

# Hypersecretion

When epiphora is caused by hypersecretion, the problem is more an annoyance than a condition as potentially serious as

Table 22.4
Notable Systemic Causes of Dry Eye

| Disorder | Characteristics |
| --- | --- |
| Sjögren's syndrome | Chronic dry mouth, usually connective tissue disease; middle-aged women |
| Stevens-Johnson syndrome | Acute bullous disease, mild to severe dry eye, onset usually <10 years old. |
| Pemphigoid | Chronic blistering disease, conjunctival vesiculae with eventual shrinkage of conjunctiva, average age over 60 years. |
| Avitaminosis A | Nutritional deficiency, usually preceded by night blindness. |
| Sarcoid | Granulomata in many organs possible, including lacrimal gland. |

impaired lacrimal drainage. A variety of conditions have been reported as being associated with hypersecretion. The most common causes are probably reflex tearing from environmental irritation and external inflammation. Also, for a period of time a patient with dry eye may actually complain of epiphora because of periodic reflex tearing. Of the other reported causes of hypersecretion, primary disease, either inflammation or neoplasm of the lacrimal gland, is the most important to rule out.

## Lacrimal Drainage

Inadequacy of block of lacrimal drainage with consequent epiphora can be caused by congenital and acquired disorders. Office screening of patients with suspected drainage impairment can be done by examination of lids, orbicularis function and patency, and excretory tests.

Congenital anomalies include absent or unformed puncta and absent or unformed canaliculi. Obstruction of the nasolacrimal duct is a common cause of epiphora in the newborn, although spontaneous correction occurs in most cases. Continued impairment can lead to conjunctivitis and dacryocystitis.

Eversion of the lower punctum, with or without ectropion, is an acquired disorder of the aged that often leads to epiphora. The elderly are also prone to orbicularis weakness and failure of the puncta to move nasally with the blink.

The punctum may become occluded as a complication of pemphigus and Stevens-Johnson syndrome. Canaliculi stenosis may also ensue. The concretion of fungus infection and primary tumors may block lacrimal drainage.

Dacryocystitis, when acute, presents a distinctive clinical picture of swelling below the medial canthal tendon, redness, and discomfort. Epiphora usually is overshadowed by the associated signs and symptoms of inflammation. Chronic dacryocystitis usually seen in adults, particularly women, presents with less dramatic inflammatory signs. Epiphora often is the presenting symptom, with or without lacrimal sac swelling.

Palpation may reveal tenderness and express pus. For dacryocystitis, prompt recognition and treatment can minimize the chance of secondary structural change and the risk of permanently impaired drainage.

# References

Clompus R. When the patient complains of excessive tearing. Rev Optom 1983; 120(3):51–56.

Hecht SD. Evaluation of the lacrimal drainage system. Ophthalmol 1978; 85:1250–1258.

Holly FJ. Tear film physiology and contact lens wear I,II. Amer J Optom Physiol Opt 1981;58:324–341.

Korb DR, Henriquez AS. Meibomian gland dysfunction and contact lens intolerance. J Am Optom Assoc 1980; 51:243–251.

Mackie IA, Seal DV. The questionably dry eye. Br J Ophthalmol 1981;65:2–9.

Veir ER. Lacrimal disorders: diagnosis and treatment. St. Louis: C.V. Mosby, 1976.

# Lyman C. Norden
# CONJUNCTIVA 23

*The conjunctiva lines the inner lids and the outer eyeball by means of a continuous tissue sheath. The excess tissue folds inward to form the conjunctival sac. Thus, there are three major conjunctival regions: palpebral, bulbar, and fornix.*

## BACKGROUND

The conjunctiva is so named because in effect it joins the eyeball to the lids. Since the conjunctiva and its contiguous structures are essentially the exposed parts of the eye, inflammations are common. Its high visibility enhanced by its white scleral background often leads to questions concerning mild inflammations, degenerations, and neoplasms. The differential diagnosis of these anomalies is based upon the conjunctiva's specific anatomic and physiologic characteristics.

The conjunctival mucosal surface is tightly adherent to the tarsal plate in the upper lid, while it is somewhat less firmly attached in the lower lid. The fornix and bulbar surfaces are least adherent because of their areolar submucosal structure. The mucous membrane epithelium is continuous with eyelid skin at the lid margins and with corneal epithelium at the limbus. Within the conjunctival epithelium are melanocytes, which usually are pigmented only in dark skinned individuals. When visible, they are often seen at the limbus, fornix, plica, caruncle, and the site where the anterior ciliary artery penetrates the sclera. Also, within the epithelium are nu-

merous goblet cells. These cells secrete mucin, which serves as a lubricant and as a corneal wetting agent for tears. Goblet cells increase in number during conjunctival inflammation.

Beneath the epithelial layer lies the submucosal lymphoid layer. This is a fine connective tissue meshwork containing numerous lymphocytes. During inflammation this tissue may proliferate, causing irregularities in the mucous membrane surface.

The conjunctiva has a rich vascular supply, which serves as a route for inflammatory cells during inflammation. It is the dilation and subsequent engorgement of these normally small vessels that causes the readily visible hyperemia seen even in mild inflammation. The pericorneal plexus of vessels contains two layers of diagnostic significance: the superficial conjunctival layer and the deep episcleral layer. The superficial layer becomes injected in corneal epithelial inflammation, while the episcleral layer does so in deep corneal, iris, and ciliary-body inflammation.

The conjunctiva has a lymphatic system that drains toward the lympatic ves-

301

sels emerging from the lids. Drainage from the lateral side is to the preauricular lymph nodes, and drainage from the medial side is to the submaxillary lymph nodes.

The sensory nerve supply of the conjunctiva consists of bare nerve endings for touch and pain and modified nerve endings for temperature sensation. Bare nerve endings are by far the most numerous.

Signs and symptoms of conjunctivitis include hyperemia, irritation (itching, burning, pain), tearing, and discharge. Conjunctival hyperemia is a common complaint, even in the absence of infection or serious insult, because it involves a readily visible, vascularized, and transparent tissue backed by white sclera. A similarly minor inflammation of other mucous membrane tissue in the body, as may be caused by ordinary environmental irritants, often will go unnoticed because they are not so visible.

The degree of irritation experienced by the patient is highly variable because of the bare nerve endings involved. Mild stimulation causes an itching sensation, while stronger stimulation yields pain. The variability in clinical presentation occurs because of individual variations in inflammatory response and interpretation of the sensation. Generally, however, the mild pressure associated with allergic tissue swelling yields nothing more than an itching sensation, while the inflammation with infection usually yields a mild painful foreign-body sensation.

Loose areolar structure and ready visibility predisposes the conjunctiva to visible swelling with inflammation. In allergy, the associated serum leakage causes a predominant sign of conjunctival chemosis, which with the abundance of bare nerve endings provides an explanation for the conjunctiva's relative sensitivity to allergens. Because of the conjunctiva's great allergic sensitivity, conjunctival allergies often occur in persons with an otherwise negative allergy history.

The submucosal lymphoid tissue often proliferates during inflammation to form, in essence, miniature lymph nodes. The newly formed germinal centers in this tissue yield primarily mononuclear inflammatory cells (lymphocytes) to combat the invading agent. As these germinal centers grow, they create elevations or bumps on the mucous membrane surface and are called *follicles* (Figure 23.1). Follicles usually are about one-half to several millimeters in size and show a slightly gray white discoloration. Because of the conjunctiva's loose attachment to the tarsal plate, follicles usually appear only in the everted lower lid. In more severe inflammation, the follicles increase in size and some may become visible in the upper lid. The superior lid is the main conjunctival site for polymorphonuclear cell production. This takes place within slightly elevated areas, much smaller than follicles, known as *papillae*. Papillae usually signify more severe inflammation than follicles.

Conjunctival irritation typically results in increased mucin production by the goblet cells. In relatively mild inflammation, the result is an accumulation of gray white mucoid discharge floating in the tears.

The conjunctival vasculature supplies inflammatory white blood cells in response to toxic stimuli. The white blood cells are actively drawn out of these vessels into the mucous membrane and tear film when there is either an allergic or infective stimulus. In more severe inflammation, there is increased accumulation of fibrinogen, which leads to fibrin formation at the mucous membrane surface (Figure 23.2). This yields the pseudomembrane sometimes seen on the superior palpebral conjunctival surface in more severe inflammation (Figure 23.3). It also adds substance to the purulent discharge seen in severe inflammation.

Because the conjunctival epithelium is continuous with the corneal epithelium, there is a tendency for primary conjunctival inflammation to develop into a secondary corneal inflammation (Figure 23.4). For example, bacterial conjunctivitis often

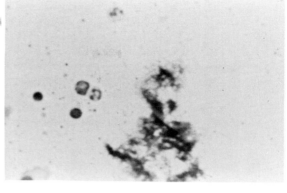

**FIGURE 23.2.**
Inflammatory cells in acute bacterial conjuctivitis. Shown are one cuboidal epithelial cell, one eosinophil, two mononuclear cells, three polymorphonuclear cells, and a large fibrinous mass (200 ×).

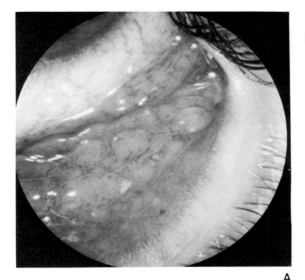

A

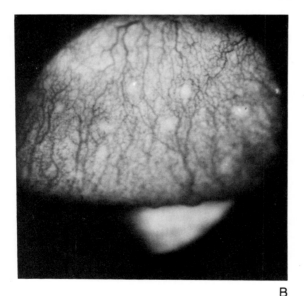

B

**FIGURE 23.1.**
Follicles in interior (*A*) and superior (*B*) palpebral conjunctiva.

results in a pooling of bacterial toxins and inflammatory cells in the lower tear meniscus. In mild cases this results in a characteristic form of epithelial erosion in the lower quadrant of the cornea. In more se-

vere cases it can lead to a marginal corneal ulcer.

The mechanism of sign and symptom production in conjunctivitis can be somewhat variable depending on the strength of the stimulus itself and on the individual sensitivity of the host. For example, an adenoviral infection and subsequent inflammation may be so severe as to resemble bacterial infection by producing considerable hyperemia, papillae, polymorphonuclear cells, and pseudomembrane. On the other hand, a bacterial infection may cause only a low-grade, subacute inflammatory response with little hyperemia, follicle formation, lymphocyte production, or mucoid discharge. In certain individuals, however, bacterial infection can cause unusually severe inflammation with considerable pain, hyperemia, and tearing. An example of this is phlyctenular conjunctivitis (Figure 23.5). If the inflammation is severe enough to cause corneal infiltrate or ulceration at the limbus, this condition may be called marginal keratitis.

Idiopathic inflammation of the superficial sclera can resemble a primary conjunctivitis with clinical presentation of

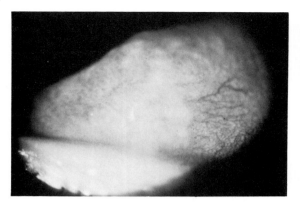

**FIGURE 23.3.**
Pseudomembrane on superior palpebral conjunctiva in acute bacterial infection.

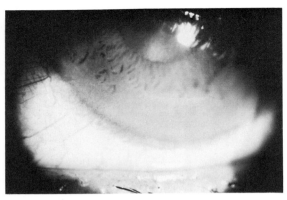

**FIGURE 23.4.**
Inferior corneal staining along lower lid line in bacterial conjunctivitis.

pain, hyperemia, and chemosis. The condition known as episcleritis (Figure 23.6) may be either diffuse or nodular. There is typically little or no corneal involvement, no sign of allergy or infection, and no related ocular complication, but it is often recurrent.

Vascular changes in the conjunctiva include hemorrhage, aneurysm, and telangiectasia. Spontaneous hemorrhaging occurs in the conjunctiva just as it does in other parts of the body. On the arms or legs it looks like a random bruise; in the conjunctiva it appears as a dark red accumulation of blood beneath its surface. Conjunctival aneurysms are said to occur in diabetes mellitus and other vascular diseases, but their appearance generally is not consistent enough to be of much clinical value. Small aneurysmlike areas are common in the normal eye. Large aneurysms are uncommon and may be of pathologic significance.

Telangiectasia is an irreversible dilation of preexisting vessels and may occur with local irritation or prolonged inflammation. Dilation of vessels near the rectus muscle insertions may be a sign of thyroid disease. Congested, dilated vessels may also be associated with a local anomaly, such as ciliary-body melanoma, or with a distant anomaly, such as carotid cavernous fistula.

Conjunctival pigmentary anomalies such as melanosis and nevi are common, particularly in nonwhite races. Nevertheless, the documented appearance of a newly pigmented area should be viewed with suspicion of possible malignancy.

Subconjunctival buildup of small individual yellowish deposits are signs of conjunctival amyloidosis. This abnormal glycoprotein is of pathologic significance when found elsewhere in the body, but not when seen only in the conjunctiva.

Degenerative changes of the conjunctiva include pinguecula, pterygium, and symblepharon. *Pinguecula* is a yellowish accumulation of connective tissue in the angular conjunctiva. Often this is accompanied by localized hyperemia, but there is no pathologic significance. *Pterygium* is a proliferation of vascularized fibrotic material that invades the cornea from the angular conjunctiva. Its growth appears to accelerate with chronic exposure to wind, dust, and ultraviolet radiation. Left untreated it could lead to blindness by covering the central cornea.

*Symblepharon* is a degenerative fusion of the palpebral and bulbar conjunctiva, which gradually eliminates the cul-

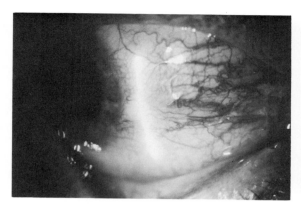

**FIGURE 23.5.**
Phlyctenule. Nodular swelling and localized hyperemia near the limbus are characteristic of this condition.

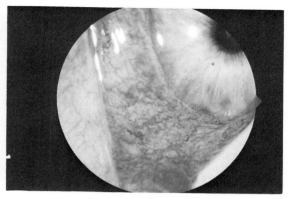

**FIGURE 23.6.**
Episcleritis. Note the marked, generalized conjunctival hyperemia and chemosis with no discharge.

de-sac. This is followed by shrinkage of the bulbar conjunctiva, loss of ocular motility, and finally loss of corneal integrity. Symblepharon and conjunctival shrinkage may be caused by chemical burn, severe infection, certain topical and systemic drugs, and disorders of the skin and mucous membranes, such as pemphigoid.

# HISTORY

The case history often yields valuable information useful in the diagnosis and primary management of conjunctival anomalies. For example, it is well known that bacterial conjunctival infections generally have a fairly rapid onset of several hours, while adenoviral infections appear gradually over a period of several days. Allergic conjunctivitis may have either a rapid or a gradual onset depending on the type of allergy. Tear deficiency conjunctivitis typically has a very gradual onset. With these characteristics in mind, it is important initially to classify conjunctival inflammations as either acute, subacute, or chronic. In acute conjunctivitis, the patient can usually relate which day and often what time of day the inflammation began. In subacute conjunctivitis, the onset can usually be related only to a given week or part of the week. In chronic conjunctivitis, the patient can hardly say which month the inflammation began.

The course of a conjunctival inflammation is also important to consider. Ask the patient if at the time of examination the condition seems better or worse than the day before. If the condition is still worsening, it is obviously potentially more serious and requires more vigorous initial treatment and closer follow-up than if the condition has already started to improve. In acute conjunctivitis, it is worthwhile to ask the patient if there has been recent exposure to a similarly affected individual. Although the reply is usually negative, when a positive reply is obtained, the conjunctivitis in question can usually be expected to run a similar course.

The type of irritation experienced by the patient with conjunctivitis often helps to identify the cause, particularly in mild conjunctivitis. As discussed earlier, allergic conjunctivitis usually presents with symptoms of itching, while infectious conjunctivitis usually presents with a foreign-body type of pain. Tear-deficiency conjunctivitis usually presents with symptoms of intermittent sharp or stabbing eye pains, often followed by reflex tearing.

There are two related problem areas involving mucous membrane tissue worth investigating in cases of mild to moderate conjunctivitis. The first of these is upper respiratory infection. A history of cold or sore throat just prior to the onset of conjunctivitis symptoms implies that the conjunctivitis is due either to secondary infection by the microbe or to residual inflammation of the underlying lymphatic tissue. In either case, the conjunctivitis will probably run the same clinical course as the upper respiratory inflammation. The second related area of concern is the urethra. Urethritis is a frequently associated symptom that helps to identify chlamydial infection of the conjunctiva.

Usually there is no history of previous occurrence in infectious conjunctivitis, but there may be in cases of phlyctenular conjunctivitis, marginal keratitis, and episcleritis. In such cases, the inflammation can reasonably be expected to run a clinical course similar to the previous episodes.

Previous occurrences sometimes are reported in cases of allergic conjunctivitis. The patient may know what the allergen is or under what circumstances to expect the inflammation (e.g., seasonal allergy). In some cases, however, it may be necessary to question the patient about specific environmental factors such as house dust, animal hair, cosmetics, and so forth. As noted, the clinician cannot count on there being a general allergy history because other areas of the body are much less sensitive than the conjunctiva.

The case history is relatively straightforward in other types of conjunctival anomalies, such as neoplasia and degeneration, because the patient usually recalls the onset of any significant changes. If the case history is noncontributory the clinician can rely on follow-up examinations. A form useful for conjunctival evaluation is displayed in Table 23.1.

# EXAMINATION

Examination of the conjunctiva should include a preliminary gross observation followed by biomicroscopy. Additional procedures to consider in conjunctivitis are smear analysis and culture studies. Although smear analysis usually is not worth the necessary additional time and effort for the experienced examiner, it is often helpful for those who wish to gain experience in this area and for occasional cases of questionable etiology. By the same token, culture studies are generally impractical for common conjunctivitis unless one is in the process of building clinical experience, or if the inflammation is unresponsive to initial therapy.

In the preliminary gross examination, carefully observe the patient's facial appearance, particularly in the orbital area. The allergy-prone individual often has a deep, slightly bluish skin tone and a diffuse edematous appearance in the orbital area. In adenovial conjunctivitis, there usually is mild diffuse hyperemia and chemosis of the eyelids (Figure 23.7). In blepharoconjunctivitis, there is typically a marked hyperemia at the lid margin.

With conjunctivitis, always check for lymphadenopathy by palpating the preauricular areas. A swollen lymph node characteristically feels like a small knot just below the skin surface. Sometimes the patient will report that the area is or has been tender to touch. Lymphadenopathy occurs in about 50% of patients with viral conjunctivitis and almost never in bacterial infection.

The patient's visual acuity should be routinely recorded in ocular inflammation, partially for medical-legal reasons and partially as an adjunct to ophthalmoscopy to rule out possible internal ocular involve-

**Table 23.1**
**Red Eye Evaluation Outline**

Patient's Name: _____ Age: _____ Telephone: _____

HISTORY
    Type of irritation: Pain? Burning? Itching? Foreign body? Other? _____
    Type of irritation: Constant? Intermittent?
    Onset: When? _____How rapid? _____
    Present course: Better/Worse/Same today compared to yesterday
    Effect on vision? _____
    Previous occurrence? _____
    Recent cold or sore throat? _____
    Taking any eyedrops? _____Response? _____

GROSS OBSERVATION
    Visual acuity: _____ Photophobia? _____
    Pupils: _____ Digital tensions: _____
    Lymphadenopathy? _____
    Eyelid hyperemia? _____ Swelling? _____
    Discharge: Sticky? Stringy? Purulent? Mucoid? Tearing?
    Hyperemia: Diffuse? Localized? Limbal?

BIOMICROSCOPY
    Lid margins: Crusting? Flakes? Collarettes? Ulceration?
    Cornea: Foreign body? Ulceration? Dendrite? Infiltrates, central?
        Infiltrates, marginal? Keratitis? Other? _____
    Anterior chamber: Cells? Flare? Grade: _____
    Conjunctiva: Follicles? Papillae? Chemosis? Other? _____
    Tear film: BUT _____Other? _____

OTHER
    Conjunctival smear: Polys? Monos? Epis? Other: _____
    Culture? _____
    Intraocular pressure: _____
    Ophthalmoscopy: Disc, CDR _____ Macula, foveal reflex _____

MANAGEMENT
    Drug allergies: Sulfa? _____Other? _____
    Treatment plan: _____
    Follow-up: Three-day? One-week? Other? _____
    Follow-up subjective: _____
    Follow-up objective findings: _____

ment. For patients with mild chronic symptoms suggestive of tear deficiency, it is sometimes worthwhile to note the normal blink interval while the patient is reading the near-point card. Many persons with complaints of sharp stabbing eye pains have a tendency to not blink normally while reading, driving, or performing other concentrated visual tasks. The blink interval can be noted without calling the patient's attention to it during near-point acuity testing. This interval can later be correlated with the tear-film breakup time.

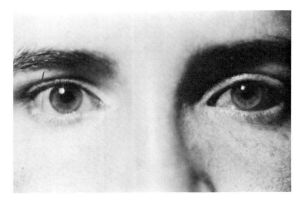

**FIGURE 23.7.**
Subacute adenoviral keratoconjunctivitis. Note the slightly swollen left superior eyelid. Appearance of equal pupils quickly rules out acute iritis and angle closure.

Routinely check pupils in all cases of ocular inflammation to screen for possible iritis or angle-closure glaucoma. In iritis, the affected pupil will usually be miotic, while in angle closure it will be middilated. These disorders are likely to become apparent in later testing, but it is best to recognize such problems as early as possible.

Digital tension estimates are another simple technique for detecting angle-closure glaucoma and acute iritis. If the intraocular pressure in the angle-closure eye is approximately 40 mm Hg or greater, the eye will definitely feel hard compared to the opposite eye. In some cases of ocular inflammation, digital tensions are preferable to applanation recordings because the applanation probe can actually pass an infectious agent on to subsequent patients (e.g., epidemic keratoconjunctivitis).

In biomicroscopy, pay individual attention to each of the following structures: eyelids, lashes, lower tear meniscus, tear film, palpebral conjunctiva, bulbar conjunctiva, cornea, and anterior chamber. Examine the lids and lashes for signs of scaling or exudation as occurs in blepharitis. Blepharitis can cause an associated conjunctivitis either by secondary infection or simply by discharge of bacterial toxins into the conjunctival sac. Attempts at treating the conjunctivitis without first eliminating the blepharitis usually are unsuccessful.

Examine the lower tear meniscus next. This appears as a bead of tear fluid between the tear margin and the globe. Observing the tear meniscus does not discreetly quantify lacrimal output, but it does give a helpful impression of lacrimal secretion without the introduction of an unusual stimulus (i.e., Schirmer's test). Narrowing the slit beam to an optic section allows observation of the mucinous content of the tear film. Bits of mucin and strands of gray white cellular debris seen flowing along the lower tear meniscus are signs of chronic low-grade inflammation (i.e., tear deficiency).

After evaluating the tear meniscus and before palpating the lids, look directly at the tear film over the cornea. Movement of the tear film itself, with its lipidlike surface texture, should be visible when the patient blinks. When this is absent because of meibomian dysfunction, the tear film is practically invisible. These patients are more likely to have other signs and/or symptoms of tear deficiency. Fluorescein breakup time (BUT) usually is reduced in these patients, but this test should be reserved until later in the examination. The addition of fluorescein will make anterior chamber evaluation for cells and flare and conjunctival smear analysis more difficult. Fluorescein studies should be done only after completion of all the nonintrusive tests but before the instillation of any eyedrops.

With diffuse illumination, examine the palpebral conjunctiva for proliferation of follicles and papillae. Follicles are characteristic of the subacute, mild-to-moderate inflammation resulting from adenoviral infection. Papillae appear in the more acute, moderate inflammation seen with bacterial infection and acute allergies. Papillae are also seen frequently in asymptomatic eyes and therefore should not be relied upon too greatly for differential diagnosis. While examining the superior palpebral conjunctiva, look for a pseudomembrane. This signifies a moderately severe inflammation. A pseudomembrane looks like a gray white, diffusely discolored area on the mucous membrane surface. It can be easily removed with a cotton-tipped applicator as a long, stringy, and sticky discharge. A similar type of structure, which cannot be removed without causing localized bleeding, is a true membrane. This would be a sign of even more severe inflammation.

An S-shaped fibrotic scar sometimes is seen in the superior tarsal conjunctiva in cases of recurrent chlamydial conjunctivitis (Figure 23.8). This sign is considered to be practically diagnostic when present in recurrent conjunctivitis. Next, examine the bulbar conjunctiva for chemosis and/or phlyctenule formation. Both are allergic phenomena. The evaluation of chemosis is mostly a qualitative judgment based on experience. Simply stated, the chemotic conjunctiva looks thick and water-logged compared to the normal structure.

Deep circumcorneal hyperemia char-

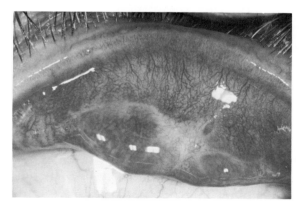

**FIGURE 23.8.**
S-shaped scarring of superior tarsal conjunctiva in recurrent chlamydial conjunctivitis.

acteristic of iritis sometimes is difficult to distinguish from the hyperemia of conjunctivitis. For this reason, examination time is often better spent in evaluating the pupil for miosis and the anterior chamber for cells and flare.

Another conjunctival feature that often is difficult to evaluate is the reported fluorescein staining pattern associated with keratoconjunctivitis sicca. Most patients with significant tear-deficiency problems do not show the characteristic conjunctival staining pattern, while many asymptomatic patients show fluorescein pooling and retention that resembles the reported sicca staining. Again, the time necessary for this evaluation is often better spent in evaluating the corneal epithelium for possible desiccation and in instituting a therapeutic trial with tear substitutes for the symptomatic patient.

Biomicroscopy of the cornea can yield important diagnostic information in conjunctivitis. The cornea is continuous with conjunctival epithelium, hence there frequently is a parallel or secondary involvement of the corneal epithelium. In bacterial conjunctivitis, there often is a characteristic fluorescein staining pattern in the inferior quadrant, where the lower lid margin normally rests. In adenoviral conjunctivitis, there is usually a concomitant diffuse epithelial staining pattern caused by the microorganism itself. In more severe inflammation, there may be scattered gray white subepithelial infiltrates of inflammatory cells. Diffuse corneal involvement usually indicates adenoviral infection. Marginal corneal infiltrates of gray white material are signs of phlyctenule marginal keratitis and sometimes diffuse episcleritis.

Be sure to rule out corneal ulceration away from the limbus. Central corneal ulcers usually are caused by direct invasion of a pathogen, which of course demands urgent and specific antimicrobial treatment.

Finally, examine the anterior chamber with the biomicroscope. Fine details such as cells and flares are most visible if all room lights are turned off. Direct a narrow beam of light obliquely across the pupillary zone, avoiding reflected glare from the cornea and iris. Flare looks like finely smoke-laden air while illuminated with a bright light beam. Grade I flare is just detectable, while Grade IV nearly obscures iris details. Cells look like dust particles floating in air while viewed in a bright light beam. Grade I cells are just detectable, while Grade IV are too many to count. If there is any question about either appearance, simply look at the other eye for comparison. Iritis is almost always unilateral (see Chapter 26).

The conjunctival smear technique provides a view of the cellular response in conjunctivitis. The specimen is from the mucous membrane surface of the lower cul-de-sac and is taken with a cotton-tipped applicator and transferred to a microscope slide. The simplest staining procedure is the Diff-Quick™ method (made by Harleco), which can be done in the office.

The noninflamed conjunctiva usually will yield only a few cuboidal epithelial cells. Presence of more than a few random white blood cells indicates that some type of inflammatory stimulus is present in the conjunctiva. A predominance of neutrophils usually indicates an acute bacterial infection. Eosinophils appear in acute or immediate type allergies. A predominance of mononuclear cells (lymphocytes and monocytes) usually occurs in subacute adenoviral infections; however, lymphocytes only may appear in a delayed type of allergy. Relatively equal numbers of neutrophils and mononuclear cells may occur in subacute bacterial infection, moderately severe adenoviral infection, and in chlamydial infection. In such cases it is helpful to evaluate the epithelial cells (Figures 23.9–23.11).

In bacterial infections, there usually are relatively few epithelial cells in the smear, and they often contain a large volume of cytoplasm compared to the size of the nu-

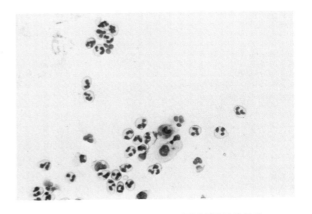

**FIGURE 23.9.**
Conjunctival smear showing predominantly polymorphonuclear cells (neutrophils) in acute bacterial conjunctivitis. Note the single epithelial cell with small, uniformly staining nucleus (200×).

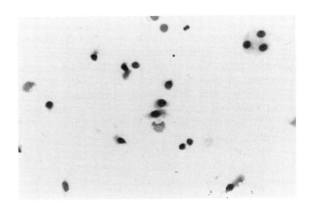

**FIGURE 23.10.**
Conjunctival smear showing predominantly mononuclear cells (lymphocytes) in subacute adenoviral conjunctivitis (100×).

cleus. In adenoviral infection, the epithelial cells usually show signs of direct invasion by the microbe. The epithelial cells usually are quite numerous and contain relatively large and distorted nuclei resulting from the damage caused by the virus. Chlamydial infections sometimes show intraepithelial inclusion bodies in the

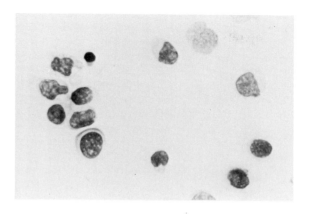

**FIGURE 23.11.**
Conjunctival smear showing karyolytic, vacuolated epithelial cell nuclei in subacute adenoviral conjunctivitis (400×).

smear (Figure 23.12), but this feature is not consistent enough to be diagnostic in most cases.

Therapeutic trial is a concept frequently overlooked in the assessment of conjunctivitis. In conjunctival inflammations severe enough to yield symptoms, but not severe enough to yield reliable diagnostic signs, a brief therapeutic trial often can be diagnostic. For example, the low-grade hyperemia and itching associated with mild allergy will resolve noticeably within a few seconds following topical application of an ocular decongestant (Figure 23.13). The same principle applies to minor tear-deficiency symptoms, except that several days may be necessary to complete the trial.

# CLINICAL SIGNIFICANCE

Tear deficiency probably is the most common cause of mild conjunctivitis, particularly in patients over age 50. Usually, the patient complains of chronic intermittent eye pains. Less commonly, the patient complains of intermittent tearing or "filmy" vision. In more severe cases, there may be filamentary keratitis; in less severe cases, there may be a normal cornea with decreased tear-film breakup time. In even milder cases, there may be nothing more than symptoms.

In the absence of obvious clinical signs, a positive diagnosis usually can be made by first ruling out the other possible etiologies (Table 23.2) and then obtaining subjective improvement with use of tear substitutes. Be sure to tell the patient to use the drops frequently throughout the day, perhaps as often as every hour. The patient can always reduce the dosage to equalize convenience with effectivity, but if not used often enough initially, they will be of no help. Similarly, if filamentary or diffuse keratitis improves in a few days with use of bland ointment, it was caused by tear deficiency and corneal exposure.

Allergic conjunctivitis may be classified as either mild or severe. In mild allergy, there is usually a complaint of subacute or chronic itching. There is only mild, diffuse conjunctival hyperemia, with chemosis being more clinically apparent. There is little or no tearing, no other discharge, and few if any inflammatory cells in the conjunctival smear. Often, the most positive clinical sign is a rapid improvement in signs and/or symptoms following instillation of a topical ocular decongestant.

More severe allergy is likely to present as an acute constant itching or irritation. Sometimes there is visible eyelid swelling and a white or clear stringy discharge. Biomicroscopy reveals both conjunctival hyperemia and chemosis along with papillae on the superior tarsus. The conjunctival smear contains either eosinophils or mononuclear cells, depending on the type of allergy. Eosinophils appear in immediate-type allergies. In this type of allergy, symptoms arise shortly after exposure to the allergen and resolve shortly after termination of exposure. Vernal con-

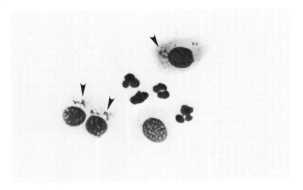

**FIGURE 23.12.**
Conjunctival smear showing epithelial cell cytoplasmic inclusion bodies (arrows) in chlamydial conjunctivitis (1000×).

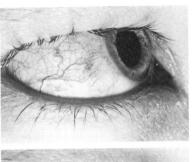

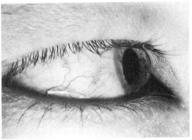

**FIGURE 23.13.**
Mild, allergic conjunctivitis before (top) and after (bottom) instillation of topical decongestant.

junctivitis and hay fever are examples of immediate allergy.

Mononuclear cells appear in delayed allergies. In delayed allergy, symptoms arise gradually several hours after initial exposure to the allergen and may persist for several days after termination of exposure. Poison ivy, drug allergies, and phlyctenular conjunctivitis are examples of this type. Topical decongestants are of little help in more severe allergies.

Phlyctenule and marginal keratitis are very similar in clinical presentation and natural course. Both conditions usually appear outwardly and symptomatically as a moderately severe external ocular inflammation. Biomicroscopy, however, reveals no discharge other than tearing and

Table 23.2
External Ocular Inflammation: Differential Diagnosis

| Condition | History | Gross Observation | Biomicroscopy | Other |
|---|---|---|---|---|
| Tear deficiency | Chronic, intermittent, sharp pains | Mild, diffuse hyperemia or negative | ↓ BUT; ↓ meibomian function; or negative | Positive trial with artificial tears |
| Allergic conjunctivitis (mild) | Chronic or subacute itching | Diffuse hyperemia | Chemosis > hyperemia | Improvement with decongestant |
| Allergic conjunctivitis (severe) | Acute itching or irritation | Lid swelling; white or clear, stringy discharge | Hyperemia; papillae | Eos/ Monos |

## Table 23.2
*(continued)*

| Condition | History | Gross Observation | Biomicroscopy | Other |
|---|---|---|---|---|
| Phlyctenule/ Marginal keratitis | Acute, constant pain or irritation | Localized hyperemia; tearing only | Marginal corneal infiltrate; ulcer | Few monos |
| Episcleritis, diffuse | Acute hyperemia with constant mild or intense pain | Localized or diffuse marked hyperemia; tearing only | Conjunctival chemosis | Negative smear |
| Bacterial conjunctivitis | Acute, constant pain | Yellowish, purulent discharge | Papillae; inferior corneal staining | Polys |
| Adenoviral conjunctivitis | Subacute, constant irritation | Lid edema and hyperemia; tearing; mucoid discharge | Follicles; diffuse corneal staining or infiltrate | Monos and epis > polys |
| Chlamydial conjunctivitis | Subacute, recurrent; may be urethritis | Hyperemia; tearing | Follicles (large); superior tarsal scarring | Polys and monos; cytoplasmic inclusion bodies |
| Herpes keratitis | Subacute irritation | Tearing; vesicles | Dendritic corneal ulcer | Corneal hypoesthesia |
| Recurrent corneal erosion | Acute, constant ache; usually improving by time of examination | Tearing; localized, mild hyperemia | Corneal erosion (small, resolving) | Recurrences |
| Iritis | Subacute, constant ache; photophobia | Tearing; miotic pupil; deep limbal hyperemia | Cells and/or flare in AC | ↓ IOP |
| Angle closure | Subacute, constant ache; nausea | Tearing; fixed, mid-dilated pupil | Venous engorgement; corneal clouding | ↑ IOP |

no palpebral conjunctival proliferation. The bulbar conjunctiva is obviously the most inflamed structure and the hyperemia may be either localized or diffuse. Corneal involvement, if present, appears as marginal infiltrate and/or ulceration. The conjunctival smear usually contains only a few mononuclear cells with even fewer, if any, epithelial cells and polymorphonuclear cells.

Both phlyctenule and marginal keratitis are considered to be microbial allergies of the delayed type. They are self-limiting with gradual resolution of several days to several weeks. Antibacterial treatment may help to prevent more severe inflammation if instituted early. Antiinflammatory treatment usually produces a dramatic improvement. A patient with an obvious phlyctenule may be referred for tuberculosis tests, but the result is usually negative.

Episcleritis has an outward appearance similar to that of phlyctenule and marginal keratitis. It differs in that it is idiopathic, more localized, and often recurrent. Episcleritis presents with acute hyperemia and either mild or intense pain. The hyperemia may be either localized at a muscle insertion (i.e., nodular episcleritis) or localized to one quadrant, or it may be present throughout the entire bulbar conjunctiva (i.e., diffuse simple episcleritis). There is usually considerable bulbar conjunctival chemosis with no discharge other than tearing. Severe cases may show corneal involvement in the form of marginal infiltrate and ulceration. The conjunctival smear is essentially negative.

Bacterial conjunctivitis usually starts with the introduction of a new and pathogenic bacterium to the conjunctival sac. The new pathogen rapidly proliferates and displaces the other nonpathogenic bacteria commonly found in the conjunctival sac. This rapid proliferation and production of toxins usually results in an acute inflammatory response. The patient complains of a constant burning or a foreign-body type of pain. Often there is a yellowish, purulent type of discharge. Biomicroscopy reveals palpebral and bulbar hyperemia with little or no chemosis or proliferation except for papillae on the superior tarsus. In most cases, biomicroscopy also reveals keratitis in the inferior quadrant of the cornea extending from the lower lid line down to the limbus. The conjunctival smear contains predominantly polymorphonuclear cells. The inflammatory response to bacterial infection usually leads to resolution after several days, but the process can be accelerated and potential complications minimized with antibacterial treatment.

Adenoviral conjunctivitis is characterized by a gradual onset, generally mild to moderate inflammatory presentation, and gradual resolution in spite of antibacterial treatment. Following introduction and incubation of the pathogen, the inflammatory response builds gradually over a period of several days. The patient usually complains of mild to moderate burning or irritation accompanied by tearing. Gross observation usually reveals eyelid swelling with mild hyperemia. Palpation of the preauricular and submandibular lymph nodes often shows there is lymphadenopathy. Biomicroscopy usually reveals follicle formation in the inferior palpebral conjunctiva. A gray white mucoid discharge can often be seen floating in the conjunctival sac. In less severe cases, there may be diffuse keratitis. In more severe cases, corneal involvement may appear as centrally located subepithelial infiltrates. In milder cases, the conjunctival smear contains predominantly mononuclear cells; in more severe cases, there may also be polymorphonuclear cells as well as numerous karyolytic epithelial cells.

Some adenoviral infections can be highly contagious. The classic appearance of epidemic keratoconjunctivitis includes central corneal infiltrates, but these do not usually appear until after the contagious phase has passed. Therefore, it is best to assume that every case of infectious conjunctivitis is highly contagious.

Chlamydial conjunctivitis is often associated with nongonococcal urethritis. The chlamydia organism is an intracellular parasite with viral and bacterial characteristics. It is spread venereally. The conjunctival inflammation is usually subacute, self-limiting, and recurrent. There is tearing and light mucoid discharge, with follicle formation and corneal infiltrate. There may be scarring of the superior tarsus after several recurrences. The conjunctival smear contains both mononuclear and polymorphonuclear cells.

Chlamydial conjunctivitis differs from adenoviral conjunctivitis in its history of recurrences. It differs from bacterial conjunctivitis in its failure to respond to topical antibacterial treatment. Its rapid response to treatment with systemic tetracycline is sometimes considered to be diagnostic. Herpes keratitis should be ruled out early in the assessment of external ocular inflammation. Corneal dendritic ulcer is said to be the classic sign of herpes infection, but bacterial corneal ulcers can also have a dendritic appearance. Herpetic ulcer is usually accompanied by relatively little subjective pain. There may be decreased corneal sensitivity, and often there are vesicles on the skin around the eye or mouth.

Two conditions that should be ruled out early in examination of the red eye are iritis and angle-closure glaucoma. The patient's description of symptoms can sometimes be misleading, but gross observations are quite reliable. Iritis usually presents with a miotic pupil, while angle-closure glaucoma presents with a fixed middilated pupil. In angle closure, the eye feels hard to the touch; in acute iritis, it usually feels soft. Biomicroscopy reveals cells and/or flare in iritis and corneal edema in angle closure. The differential diagnosis of these conditions is usually straightforward, but they should always be carefully ruled out before considering the other, more common causes of external ocular inflammation.

Conjunctivitis cannot always be differentially diagnosed in a single examination. Many inflammations are quite dynamic, and certain features may not appear until one or two days later. Therefore, it is often wise to think of initial diagnosis as tentative until the patient's second visit, when the response to treatment or the natural course without treatment can be evaluated. Conjunctival anomalies other than inflammation are generally benign and their clinical significance is usually obvious. Pigmentary anomalies should be seen in follow-up if there is any reason to suspect progression. Pterygia should also be seen in follow-up to determine if there is threat of encroachment into the pupillary zone. Symblepharon can be referred for possible treatment with steroids if there are signs of rapid progression. Anomalies such as pinguecula and amyloidosis have no pathologic significance.

If conjunctival aneurysms appear suspicious, look carefully for retinal aneurysms or dot hemorrhages near the fovea. These may be a sign of vascular disease. Spontaneous subconjunctival hemorrhages are common and have no pathologic significance; however, subconjunctival hemorrhage following trauma calls for a dilated fundus examination to rule out possible internal ocular complications. Also, high blood pressure should be ruled out. The appearance of telangiectatic conjunctival vessels near the rectus muscle insertions should prompt a search for other ocular signs of thyroid disease. An isolated area of dilated or congested conjunctival vessels could be associated with an internal ocular tumor; therefore, it would be prudent to dilate the eye for a peripheral fundus examination.

# References

Allen HF. Chlamydial eye disease. Int Ophthalmol Clin 1975;15(4):257–268.

Fedukowicz H. External infections of the eye: bacterial, viral, and mycotic. New York: Appleton-Century-Crofts, 1978; 2nd ed.

Laibson PB. Adenoviral keratoconjunctivitis. Int Ophthalmol Clin 1975; 15(4):187–201.

Laibson PB, Waring GO III. Conjunctival diseases and therapy. In: Dunlap EA, ed. Gordon's medical management of ocular disease. Hagerstown, Md.: Harper & Row, 1976;12:147–70;2nd ed.

Mamelok AE. Allergic conjunctivitis. Cutis 1976;17:244–248.

Miller SD. Hypersensitivity diseases of the cornea and conjunctiva with a detailed discussion of phlyctenular disease. Ophthalmic Semin 1977;2:119–165.

Naib ZM, Clepper AS, Elliott SR. Exfoliative cytology as an aid in the diagnosis of ophthalmic lesions. Acta Cytol 1967;11:295–303.

Reed K. Epidemic viral keratoconjunctivitis, diagnosis and management. J Am Optom Assoc 1983;54:141–144.

Schumann GB, Colin VF, Spinner PA. Eye cytology. Am Fam Physician 1980; 22:120–124.

Thelmo W, Csordas J, Davis P, Marshall KG. The cytology of acute bacterial and follicular conjunctivitis. Acta Cytol 1972;16:172–177.

Tullo AB, Higgens PG. An outbreak of adenovirus keratoconjunctivitis in Bristol. Br J Ophthalmol 1979;63:621–626.

# Larry M. DeDonato
# Barry J. Barresi
# CORNEA 24

*The cornea is an avascular and transparent tissue that, with the sclera, forms the outer tunic of the eye. Sixty-five percent of the eye's refractive power is provided by the corneal tissue. Because of the cornea's significant optical role in human vision, maintenance of its normal physiologic and anatomic characteristics is important.*

## BACKGROUND

The cornea is usually described as having five layers: epithelium, Bowman's layer, stroma, Descemet's membrane, and endothelium. Another structure has been identified, the basal membrane of the epithelium, which lies anterior to Bowman's layer.

The central corneal thickness in humans is about 0.52 mm. The epithelium is a layer of 5 to 10 cells in human corneas. The innermost of the epithelial cells are columnar and closely packed. As the cells migrate anteriorly, they flatten first into wing cells and finally into superficial squamous cells on the corneal surface.

The basement membrane lies over Bowman's layer. It serves as an area of attachment for the columnar corneal epithelial cells. The layer is an acellular region located posterior to the epithelial basement membrane. It is similar in structure to the stroma and cannot be separated from it. Bowman's layer is resistant to invasion of the cornea by microorganisms and is thought to offer resistance to trauma.

The *stroma* constitutes 90% of the corneal thickness and is the primary structural component. It consists mainly of collagen fibers, ground substance, and stromal cells. The collagen fibers run from limbus to limbus in bundles called *lamellae*. Mucopolysaccharide coats the fibers and fills the spaces between them. The hydrophilic (water-loving) nature of the mucopolysaccharides permits the relatively high water content (78%) of the corneal stroma.

The cells in the stroma are called *keratocytes*. They migrate into the area of a fresh stromal wound. These fibroblastlike cells participate in scar formation. Keratocytes accumulate products of inappropriate metabolism in many conditions, such as multiple myeloma, cystinosis, and in diseases of altered lipid and carbohydrate metabolism, such as sphingolipidosis and mucopolysaccharidosis.

Descemet's membrane separates the corneal stroma from the endothelium. It is composed of a meshwork of collagen fibers. Unlike Bowman's layer, Descemet's

317

membrane detaches easily from the stroma and regenerates after injury. It can proliferate into the hyaline warts seen in a number of pathologic conditions. Descemet's membrane usually thickens with age and sometimes is the site of metallic deposition. For example, copper is found in Descemet's membrane in patients with Wilson's disease and silver is found in those with argyrosis.

The endothelium is a single layer of hexagonal cells that borders Descemet's membrane. It shows great metabolic activity and is actively involved in corneal hydration maintenance. The endothelial cell density is about 3500 to 4000 cells/mm$^2$ at birth and decreases to approximately 2600 cells/mm$^2$ by age 80. The majority of endothelial cell loss occurs between birth and 30 years of age.

Following endothelial trauma, the surrounding endothelial cells slide over the injured area. There is no significant mitotic activity in the adult human endothelium.

The in vivo human corneal endothelium can be examined clinically by the use of specular reflection with the slit lamp biomicroscope (Figure 24.1).

The cells of the cornea require several nutrients, including oxygen, glucose, and amino acids. Because of the avascularity of the cornea and evidence that the limbal vasculature plays an insignificant role in corneal nutrient supply, the nutrients for the cornea must come from the tears and aqueous. The tears supply oxygen. The aqueous supplies oxygen also, as well as amino acids, glucose, and other nutrients.

## Corneal Wound Healing

Corneal wounds from foreign bodies, chemicals, contact lenses, and many other causes are commonly seen in optometric practice.

### EPITHELIAL WOUND HEALING

Epithelial cell repair begins soon after injury. Initially, there is a sliding of epithe-

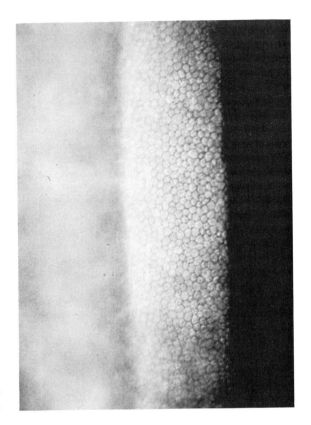

**FIGURE 24.1.**
Endothelial mosaic.

lial cells into the area of the wound. Once there is coverage of the wounded area, mitotic activity begins and continues until the epithelium regains its normal thickness. The main cells that slide are epithelial wing cells.

Reepitheliazation of abrasions and mild erosions usually proceeds rapidly with a smooth surface noted in less than 24 hours. Damage to the basement membrane, however, impairs healing and weakens epithelial-stromal adhesion. The consequence is persistent or recurrent epithelial defects, a condition called *recurrent corneal erosion*.

If the entire epithelium is removed, reepitheliazation is derived from cells of conjunctival origin. After the cells reach the corneal surface, they retain the appearance of conjunctival epithelium. There is a gradual change to cells that appear to be of corneal origin.

Epithelium derived from the conjunctiva may show some functional and morphologic differences. Particularly with extensive chemical or thermal burns, the patient may be plagued by persistent epithelial defects, neovascularization, or necrosis.

## BOWMAN'S LAYER AND STROMAL WOUNDS

Bowman's layer is unable to regenerate. The cells of the stroma, keratocytes, migrate to the wound area. Cellular proliferation and filament formation contribute to the growth of scar tissue. In severe wounds, scars can cause traction-induced corneal irregularity. If visual loss is due to this irregular topography of the cornea, and not to light scatter from the scar itself, a rigid contact lens often will provide adequate vision.

## DESCEMET'S MEMBRANE AND ENDOTHELIAL INJURY

Descemet's membrane is regenerated after injury. Injury to the endothelium will be followed by a spreading of preexisting cells over the injured area. If the endothelial cell density is reduced too much, the cornea will lose its ability to maintain hydration, and chronic edema will result.

# General Considerations

Two dominant considerations must be borne in mind with regard to pathology of the cornea. First, since the function of the cornea depends on maintenance of transparency and a smooth surface, minor changes, such as epithelial erosions or edema, that may be overlooked in other tissues, are of serious consequence in the cornea. In turn, structural changes, such as scarring, keratization, neovascularization and deposition, which further predispose the cornea to chronic and recurrent inflammation, also more seriously threaten corneal transparency and surface integrity.

# HISTORY

Presenting symptoms, past eye history, medications, and medical and family history should be fully investigated.

Presenting symptoms of corneal conditions include vision disturbances, discomfort or pain, photophobia, blepharospasm, and increased lacrimation. Conditions that cause roughened or irregular corneal surface or light scatter result in reduced acuity if the central cornea is affected. Some patients with corneal distortion will complain of shadowy vision, monocular diplopia, or polyopia. Reports of rainbows around lights or increased glare sensitivity suggest corneal edema. Spectacle blur after contact lens wear is due to central edema. In most cases, however, vision complaints are nonspecific.

Rather, it is the association of other signs, symptoms, and history that suggests a corneal condition.

Vision complaints, when concurrent with discomfort, point to infection or trauma. Mild epithelial irritation or edema may only yield symptoms of grittiness or a foreign-body sensation. Conditions like herpes simplex and neuropathic keratitis, as well as long-term contact lens wear, cause corneal hypoesthesia. These conditions may cause significant corneal disruption but produce only mild symptoms of discomfort. As a rule, however, the cornea is very sensitive. The epithelium is richly innervated, and significant pain, photophobia, and lacrimation will accompany corneal trauma and disease.

With vision disturbances and ocular discomfort, always investigate the chronology of events. Are the symptoms acute, chronic, or recurrent? Can a triggering mechanism be found? The patient's past eye history may be helpful. Past eye injuries, contact lens problems, or other conditions, like dry eye or chronic blepharitis, may point to a cause.

Corneal problems may be a manifestation of a systemic condition or an adverse drug reaction (Table 24.1). Knowledge of immunologic and collagen and mucous membrane conditions are most important.

Most corneal dystrophies are autosomally recessive. Family history should be investigated and consideration given to examining family members if the patient exhibits signs of a corneal dystrophy.

# EXAMINATION

Visual acuity measurements should be taken with the best subjective refraction in place. If good vision is not demonstrated, the test should be repeated with a pinhole. Corneal irregularity and edema will usually cause Snellen acuity changes, but pinhole acuity should be good. Testing of acuity with contrast sensitivity tests is a more valid indicator of visual change; however, these tests presently are expensive and cumbersome to administer in an office practice.

Visual loss from corneal irregularity, as with keratoconus, will usually be regained with application of a properly fitted rigid contact lens. When uncertain if alteration of the corneal topography is responsible for decreased vision, a rigid contact lens should be applied with the correct spherocylindrical overrefraction. The visual acuity is then compared to that with the spectacle refraction. A better visual acuity with the contact lens in place suggests a disrupted corneal topography. Mire distortion on keratometry also suggests an irregular corneal surface. Distortion of the retinoscopic reflex may also indicate disturbed corneal optics, although irregular optics in other regions of the ocular media may yield the same finding.

In gross observation, note any abnormalities of corneal size, lid position, or external inflammatory signs of the lids and conjunctiva. Corneal scars, pigmentation, and pterygia may also be prominent. Note any change in the corneal surface reflection. Normally, the reflections are round, regular, and located near the cornea center. With epithelial lesions, the reflection is often irregular and roughened. In pronounced dry eye, surface keratization may appear as a linear "corduroylike" pattern.

Assessment of corneal integrity and clarity is best accomplished with the slit lamp biomicroscope (Table 24.2). The high magnification and various illumination procedures enhance detection and qualification of corneal clinical signs. Both cell layer and topographic strategies are helpful in corneal assessment. Qualification of corneal lesions by site, depth, and topographic zone often is critical to diagnosis. Accurate assessment of the extent of lesions is also important to follow-up care.

It is best to systematically examine the cornea, layer by layer, starting from the precorneal tear film back to the endothelium (Table 24.3). The topographic distribution of corneal lesions often provides some diagnostic clues; if lesions are predominantly located in a particular region certain conditions are more likely at fault (see Table 24.4).

Sodium fluorescein and rose bengal offer an important adjunct to slit lamp exam of the corneal surface. Rose bengal will stain mucus strands and dead and damaged epithelium of the cornea and conjunctiva. Only a fraction of a drop is needed to highlight superficial lesions. Rose bengal is particularly helpful in quantifying

### Table 24.1
### Corneal Manifestations: Selected Systemic Diseases

| Disease | Clinical Signs |
|---------|----------------|
| Wilson's disease | Brownish green ring of copper in posterior peripheral portion of Descemet's membrane, clear zone located between ring (Kayser-Fleischer) and limbus |
| Hypercalcemia | Calcium band keratopathy of Bowman's lamina associated with hyperparathyroidism and idiopathic hypercalcemia |
| Multiple myeloma | Central crystalline opacities in anterior cornea seen in ages 50–70 |
| Fabry's disease | Vortexlike corneal opacities, deep epithelial and radiating from point slightly below the center of the cornea |
| Inflammatory disease | Interstitial keratitis with syphilis or tuberculosis |
| Diabetes mellitus | Spontaneous neurotropic corneal ulcers; predisposition to postvitrectomy corneal dysfunction |
| Nutritional disease | Xerophthalmia from vitamin A and protein deficiency |
| Presumed autoimmune diseases | Keratitis sicca associated with cicatrical pemphigoid, Stevens-Johnson syndrome, Lydell's disease, lupus erythematosus, rheumatoid arthritis |
| Dermatological diseases | Acne rosacea, ectodermal dysplasia, acrodermatitis, ichthyosis, eczema, psoriasis |
| Seventh nerve palsy | Corneal damage from exposure keratitis; early signs include rose bengal staining and punctate erosions. If persistent may lead to ulceration, vascularization, and ultimately to keratinization |
| Fifth nerve palsy | Corneal damage from neurotropic keratitis; early signs include vasodilation and edema of upper eyelid and conjunctiva; other signs include corneal edema, punctate epithelial defects, cell and flare in anterior chamber, and corneal ulceration |

superficial damage to the ocular surface caused by dry eye.

Sodium fluorescein dye permits eval- uation of the quality and quantity of precorneal tear film. This dye does not enter cells, but when attachments between ep-

Table 24.2
Recommended Slit Lamp Biomicroscopy
Observation Techniques

| | Direct | Sclerotic Scatter | Retro | Specular Reflection | Indirect |
|---|---|---|---|---|---|
| Angle between lamp & microscope | 45° to 50° | 45° or greater | 90° | 60° | Varies |
| Precorneal tear-film constituents | X | | X | X | |
| Foreign bodies, corneal nerves Hudson-Stahl line, etc. | X | | | | |
| Blood vessels, KPs, arcus senilis, and folds in Descemet's | X | X | XX | | |
| Endothelial dystrophy | X | | X | X | |
| Central corneal clouding | | XX | | | |
| Abrasions | X | X | XX | | |
| Edema | | XX | XX | | X |

Source:  Egan (1979)
Note:  X = commonly used.
       XX = preferred.

ithelial cells are disrupted, the dye passes between cells, and the yellow-green stain is noted.

The measurement of corneal thickness by pachometry can be used to evaluate the degree of corneal swelling or thinning for a variety of clinical conditions. Pachometry, however, is infrequently used in office practice.

# CLINICAL SIGNIFICANCE

In the previous discussion on examination emphasis was placed on the first three steps in the diagnostic process: (1) differentiate between normal variants and abnormal corneal appearance, (2) specify tissue level and other characteristics of any corneal abnormality, and (3) specify the visual consequences of any corneal abnormality.

The remaining steps to discuss are how to determine the etiology of the corneal signs or symptoms and to formulate a diagnosis justifiable by the evidence on hand. For the purposes of our discussion, the clinical significance of corneal conditions is reviewed under these headings: age-related changes, degenerations, congenital anomalies, dystrophes, pigmentation/deposits, and inflammation/structural change.

## Age-Related Changes
### CORNEAL ARCUS

Corneal arcus is a hazy, yellowish lipid deposit found in the corneal stroma. A clear interval separates the limbus from the bor-

Table 24.3
Corneal Assessment: Cell Layer Strategy

*Precorneal Tear Film*
| | |
|---|---|
| Evaluate | Uniformity and tear break-up time |
| Rule out | Rapid break-up, nonwetting patterns, mucus strands |

*Epithelium*
| | |
|---|---|
| Evaluate | Cell regularity, surface smoothness, and tissue clarity |
| Rule out | Punctate epithelial erosions (fine, coarse, or coalesced) |
| | Abrasion (geographic erosion with clear base) |
| | Ulcer (geographic erosion with cloudy, white base) |
| | Hazy "bedewing," focal or diffuse disruption (edema) |
| | Filaments (hypertrophied epithelium) |
| | Intraephithelial cysts (superficial) |
| | Superficial vascularization |

*Stroma*
| | |
|---|---|
| Evaluate | Cell regularity, uniform thickness, and tissue clarity |
| Rule out | Infiltrate (white anterior focal lesions) |
| | Scars (nebula, macula, leukoma) |
| | Haziness, thickening striae (edema) |
| | Uneven thickness |
| | Neovascularization |
| | Abnormal deposits |

*Endothelium*
| | |
|---|---|
| Evaluate | Cell regularity |
| Rule out | Guttate changes ("holes" in cell mosiac) |
| | Keratitic precipitates (punctate, mutton fat, or plaques) |
| | Cell density changes (endothelial photography) |
| | Abnormal deposits |
| | Bleb formation (contact lens wear) |

der of the arcus. The clear area is thought to be due to a tendency for the superficial lipid deposition to end at the termination of Bowman's layer.

In an elder patient, corneal arcus is usually benign; however, in Caucasian males younger then 50 years old and in black males younger than 40 who exhibit arcus, hypercholesterolemia should be ruled out.

## PINGUECULA

A pinguecula is a yellowish, usually triangular accumulation of degenerated conjunctiva adjacent to the limbus. It is more common to the nasal side. Pingueculae rarely are of concern. An exception would be the presence of poor wetting of the adjacent cornea, dellen formation, or dry eye symptoms.

## HASSALL-HENLE BODIES

Localized thickening of Descemet's membrane is common in the elderly. These nodules are called *Hassall-Henle bodies*. Histologically, they are the same as cornea guttata. They differ only in location and clinical significance. Hassall-Henle bodies are found in the peripheral cornea and are clinically unimportant. Cornea guttata are central and may be associated with an early Fuchs' dystrophy.

Hassall-Henle bodies and cornea guttata are seen as dark spots in the endothe-

## Table 24.4
### Corneal Assessment: Topographic Strategy

| Location | Possible Conditions |
| --- | --- |
| Central region | Contact lens edema<br>Epidemic keratoconjunctivitis<br>Groenouw's granular dystrophy (I)<br>Lattice and cystalline dystrophy<br>Cogan's microcystic epithelial dystrophy<br>Traumatic keratitis |
| Inferior region | Incomplete blink<br>Staphylococcal keratitis<br>Exposure<br>Entropion<br>Ectropion<br>Lagophthalmos<br>Keratitis sicca (interpalpebral) |
| Total surface—diffuse | Toxic (e.g., aerosol spray, chemical irritants)<br>Dust and airborne particles<br>Ultraviolet burns |
| Limbal (3 + 9 o'clock sign) | Limbal girdle of Vogt<br>Bridging dehydration (contact lens, pterygium) |
| Limbal (12 + 6 o'clock sign) | Early arcus |
| Limbal—Superior | Trachoma<br>Chlamydia<br>Atopic reaction (vernal catarrh)<br>Superior limbic keratoconjunctivitis<br>Molluscum<br>Neovascularization (contact lens induced) |
| Limbal—Circular (360°) | Mooren's ulcer<br>Terrien marginal dystrophy<br>Peripheral ischemic |

lial mosaic when viewed by specular reflection with the slit lamp biomicroscope.

### CORNEA FARINATA

Cornea farinata appear as small gray dots in the deep corneal stroma. It is usually a bilateral condition and does not interfere with vision. It is most easily seen in the central corneal area with indirect illumination. Cornea farinata is occasionally mistaken for cornea guttata. Examination of the endothelial mosaic by specular reflection reveals a normal endothelium, rather than the dark spots observed when guttata are present. Cornea farinata deposits are thought to consist of lipofuscin, a product of the degeneration of aged cells.

### MOSAIC (CROCODILE) SHAGREEN

Anterior mosaic shagreen is usually an age-related corneal change; however, juvenile and posttraumatic cases have been reported. Polygonal gray opacities appear in the region of Bowman's layer. There is little, if any, clinical importance, since the opacification rarely is great enough to affect vision.

Posterior mosaic shagreen is very similar to anterior mosaic shagreen except in its location. In the posterior variety, the polygonal opacities are observed in the deep stroma and Descemet's membrane.

# Corneal Degenerations

Corneal degenerations occur in conjunction with specific disease processes. They are not associated with a particular genetic pattern and may be unilateral or bilateral. Some of the more common corneal degenerations are discussed.

## BAND KERATOPATHY

Band keratopathy is the result of calcium deposition in Bowman's lamina and the anterior stroma. It occurs secondary to many systemic illnesses and ocular disease.

The calcific degeneration is seen most commonly in the interpalpebral area. A clear interval usually separates the calcium band from the limbus. Deposition of calcium in Bowman's lamina accounts for this because Bowman's lamina does not bridge the entire limbus. A swiss-cheese or frosted-glass appearance across the interpalpebral zone is typical.

## TERRIEN'S MARGINAL DEGENERATION

This is a relatively rare condition characterized by progressive thinning of the peripheral cornea. Large amounts of corneal toricity may be induced as the degeneration progresses. Typically, the thinning begins superiorly and is asymmetrically bilateral. Thinning occasionally becomes severe enough to warrant a corneal graft.

## SPHEROID DEGENERATION

Spheroid degeneration shows yellowish droplets in the subepithelial and anterior stromal regions of the cornea. It may be a primary ocular pathology or may be secondary to chronic corneal irritation or disease.

# Congenital Anomalies of the Cornea

Many corneal lesions are congenital. A discussion of some examples of aberrant development of the cornea follows.

### AXENFELD'S ANOMALY

Axenfeld's anomaly is an extension of iris strands across the angle. They insert into Schwalbe's ring. In approximately 50% of the patients with this growth, glaucoma develops (Axenfeld's syndrome). Axenfeld's anomaly has been associated with congenital glaucoma and a number of syndromes, such as Lowe's, Marfan's, Pierre Robin, and others.

### POSTERIOR EMBRYOTOXIN

Posterior embryotoxin is a centrally displaced and thickened Schwalbe's ring. It is often transmitted as an autosomal dominant trait and may be associated with corectopia and aniridia.

### MEGALOCORNEA

Megalocornea is a nonprogressive enlargement of the cornea, typically exhibiting a horizontal diameter of more than 14 mm. It is rarely secondary to congenital glaucoma and is most commonly transmitted as a sex-linked recessive trait. It has been reported to be associated with high astigmatism, myopia, and Krukenberg's spindles. There also have been associations with systemic afflictions, such as Marfan's and Alport's syndromes.

### POSTERIOR CIRCUMSCRIBED KERATOCONUS

Posterior circumscribed keratoconus is a localized noninflammatory thinning of the posterior surface of the cornea. It is not related to the usual form of keratoconus and does not often affect vision because the optical quality of the anterior corneal surface is usually unaltered. The difference in the indices of refraction of the cornea and aqueous are small, so disruption of the refractive properties of the cornea is minimal.

# Corneal Dystrophies

Corneal dystrophies usually appear during the first or second decade of life. Most are autosomally dominant, bilateral, and progress slowly. Fuchs' endothelial dystrophy and epithelial basement membrane dystrophy are most commonly seen by the optometrist. Granular, lattice, and fleck stromal dystrophies are less common, but are seen occasionally. (see Table 24.5). The remainder are rarely, if ever, seen in the general office practice. Waring, Rodrigues, and Laibson (1978) have written an extensive review on the subject. This section addresses the two corneal dystrophies seen most commonly in optometric practice: Fuchs' and epithelial basement membrane dystrophy. Keratoconus, although not typically defined as a dystrophy, is for convenience discussed here.

## EPITHELIAL BASEMENT MEMBRANE DYSTROPHY

Epithelial basement membrane dystrophy is also known as Cogan's microcystic dystrophy and map-dot-fingerprint dystrophy. Of the anterior corneal dystrophies, it is the most common (see Table 24.6).

This condition is probably inherited as an autosomally dominant trait and usually occurs after age 30. Patients typically complain of intermittent blurred vision and pain.

Recurrent epithelial erosion causes the pain. Approximately one-half of patients with recurrent epithelial erosion show signs of epithelial basement membrane dystrophy. It is asymptomatic in its early stages but eventually can cause irregular astigmatism and corneal epithelial erosion.

Its slit lamp appearance shows gray geographic patches seen best with diffuse illumination. Fingerprints are seen in retroillumination and represent fine refractile epithelial lines. These irregular geographic lesions are typically gray white in color and represent thickenings of basement membrane. Clear microcysts and puttylike intraepithelial opacities are also seen on retroillumination.

## FUCHS' ENDOTHELIAL DYSTROPHY

The most common endothelial dystrophy is Fuchs' endothelial dystrophy. Cornea guttata is an accumulation of collagen posterior to Descemet's membrane. They may represent a normal change associated with aging. When great in number, they form confluent patches, and there is corneal edema. At this stage, the condition is considered a Fuchs' dystrophy.

Fuchs' dystrophy occurs most commonly in postmenopausal women. It is generally bilateral but often asymmetric in its development. Ocular hypertension and chronic open-angle glaucoma may be more common in patients with Fuchs' dystrophy than in the general population.

In direct focal illumination with the slit lamp, guttata take on a golden brown appearance on the corneal surface. They are best seen with specular refraction; black dots are observed in the endothelial mosaic.

Most patients with cornea guttata remain asymptomatic. If corneal edema ensues, blurry vision and slight discomfort occurs, especially upon awakening. This probably is due to the hypotonic nature of the tears in the closed eye state, which shifts the cornea's osmotic equilibrium and results in an influx of water into the cornea. The increased hydration from the osmotic stress aggravates the already tenuous maintenance of the cornea's dehydration. Visual acuity decreases as the recurrent erosion of the corneal epithelium progresses.

**Table 24.5**
**Clinical Features of Selected Corneal Stromal Dystrophies**

| Dystrophy | Clinical Features |
|---|---|
| Granular dystrophy | Discrete, focal, white stromal dots<br>Anterior stroma<br>Concentrated in central cornea<br>Bilaterally symmetrical |
| Lattice dystrophy | Refractile lattice lines, white dots, central diffuse opacity<br>Anterior stroma<br>Central cornea, peripheral 2-3 mm clear<br>Bilateral |
| Macular dystrophy | Focal gray-white opacities, diffuse stromal haze, irregular Descemet's membrane<br>Entire stroma<br>Early central changes, by 2 or 3 decade extends to limbus<br>Bilaterally symmetrical, appears early in life |
| Central crystalline dystrophy | Combinations of minute crystals, diffuse gray haze, dense arcus, limbal girdle<br>Concentrated anterior stroma<br>Bilateral |
| Fleck dystrophy | Gray-white, dandruff-like specks<br>Throughout stroma<br>Varies from few to diffuse specking<br>Usually bilateral, may be asymmetrical or unilateral |

Source:   Adapted from Waring, Rodrigues, and Laibson 1978.

# KERATOCONUS

Keratoconus is a noninflammatory condition characterized by corneal thinning and protrusion. High amounts of irregular compound myopic astigmatism cause significant visual impairment.

The cause of keratoconus is not well known. Reports of familial incidence support the theory of a hereditary factor. Endocrine imbalance, thyroid disorder, allergy, vitamin deficiency, and eye rubbing have all been suggested as possible causes of the disease.

The visual symptoms of keratoconus are a result of the marked changes of the corneal topography. Patients report photophobia, polyopia, blurred vision, asthenopia, and headaches.

There are numerous clinical signs of keratoconus. In advanced cases, a bulge in the lower lid will be visible during down gaze (Munson's sign). Biomicroscopy shows vertical striate lines in the deep stroma. Increased visibility of the corneal nerves and corneal thinning are also seen. Fleischer's ring is a yellow brown to olive green ring that is found at the base of the cone. It probably is composed of hemosiderin at the level of Bowman's layer and is best seen with diffuse slit lamp illumination and cobalt blue light. Endothelial

Table 24.6
Clinical Features of Corneal Epithelial Cysts

| | Cogan's Dystrophy (Epithelial Basement Membrane) | Meesmann's Dystrophy | Bullous Keratopathy |
|---|---|---|---|
| Size and shape (mm) | Globular, elongated 0.02–0.9 mm | Globular, regular 0.01–0.05 mm | Globular, ovoid fused cysts 0.02–0.07 mm |
| Slit lamp | Diffuse debris Clustered blebs Gray lines, white microcysts | Opaque flecks Mix of clear and debris microcysts extending to limbus | Clear cysts in cloudy ground |
| Staining (Fluorescein) | Overlying punctate stain No staining of microcysts | Mild staining of microcysts | Moderate diffuse staining |
| | Associated tear-film thinning | Associated tear-film thinning | Associated tear-film thinning |

Source: Adapted from Bron and Tripathi 1973.

breakdown and rupture of Descemet's membrane are sometimes seen, but complete corneal rupture is virtually nonexistent.

The irregular toricity of the cornea will cause distortion of the retinoscopic reflex and keratometry mires. Scarring of the cone further disturbs the eye's optics.

# Pigment and Other Corneal Deposits

## HUDSON-STÄHLI LINE

The Hudson-Stähli line is a subepithelial deposition of an iron-containing pigment, which is probably hemosiderin. It is often simply a normal age-related change. It also occurs with chronic epithelial irritation, such as with exposure from sleep lagophthalmos. Other corneal trauma can also encourage the development of a Hudson-Stähli line.

## FLEISCHER'S RING

Fleischer's ring is found in patients with keratoconus. It is caused by hemosiderin in the basal epithelial cells. It appears as a brown ring near the base of the cone, and its appearance is enhanced by the use of the cobalt blue filter of the slit lamp biomicroscope.

## KAYSER-FLEISCHER RING

The Kayser-Fleischer ring is common in Wilson's disease. It is approximately 2 mm in width and typically extends to the limbus without a clear zone. Copper deposits in the posterior portion of Descemet's membrane and is usually yellow brown, although it occasionally appears more red, green, or blue. In the early stages, gonioscopy may be required to observe the pigment deposition.

## KERATIC PRECIPITATES

Keratic precipitates are inflammatory cells that adhere to the corneal endothelium. They become pigmented in some patients.

## GOLD

When systemic gold compounds are administered to patients with rheumatoid arthritis, deposition of gold granules may be found in the deep stroma. The granules will appear gold to purple violet. The gold deposition disappears when the medication is discontinued.

## MERCURY

Deposition of mercury in the deep stroma may occur in patients who are exposed to metallic mercury vapor or long-term use of mercury-based preservatives in topical ocular medications.

## COPPER

Chalcosis is the term commonly used to describe discoloration of ocular tissue by copper. Impregnation of corneal tissue with copper results in a blue green color in the area of Descemet's membrane. This type of deposition occurs with Wilson's disease, other hepatic diseases, and with exposure to metallic alloys that have high concentrations of copper.

## IRON

Siderosis is the impregnation of ocular tissues with iron. Iron shows an affinity for elastic tissue, so iron granules may be seen in Descemet's membrane and the deep stroma. A localized iron foreign body in the cornea forms a brownish red discoloration. "Rust rings" in the cornea may be removed surgically. Deferoxamine can be used to chelate corneal iron depositions.

## SILVER

Argyrosis is the discoloration of ocular tissue by silver. Silver can deposit in the cornea as the result of long-term use of silver-containing medications. These medications are no longer in use; however, silver deposition in the cornea can also occur with exposure to organic salts of silver. The cornea collects silver in Descemet's membrane and anteriorly in the epithelial basement membrane and anterior stromal collagen fibrils.

## CHLORPROMAZINE

Chlorpromazine is a phenothiazine drug used in the treatment of mental illness.

Fine yellow brown dots are found in the deep stroma and in Descemet's membrane. They are also sometimes seen in the epithelium. These deposits occur primarily in the palpebral fissure because of the greater exposure of this area to sunlight.

## EPINEPHRINE AND OTHER MEDICATIONS

Epinephrine ophthalmic drops can lead to dark deposits in the cornea.

Other medications such as chloroquine, indomethacin, and others can also cause corneal deposits that are visible on slit lamp examination.

# Inflammation and Associated Structural Change

Inflammation of the cornea usually results in leukocyte infiltration, corneal edema, and epithelial defects that stain with fluorescein. Ciliary and conjunctival injection, as well as corneal vascularization, may occur. Patient discomfort is also common.

Organisms that may infect the cornea include bacteria, viruses, fungi, and spirochetes. Inflammation also occurs with hypersensitivity reactions, nutritional deficiency, and with other conditions.

Given the serious consequences of bacteria, particularly *Pseudomonas*, and fungal corneal ulcers, careful corneal examination for inflammation is of utmost importance when there is a history of corneal trauma (see Table 24.7).

Inflammation of the cornea can be classified by morphological appearance. For example, a keratitis can be specified by the cell layer involved, topography of lesions, severity of signs, and presence of structural change. Corneal inflammation can also be classified by etiology. For example, infective, allergic, exposure/sicca, secondary syndromes, and idiopathic syn-

### Table 24.7
### Clinical Profile Selected Corneal Conditions

| Disease | Clinical Signs |
|---------|----------------|
| Herpes simplex keratitis | Either type I (ocular strain) or type II (genital strain) can cause ocular disease<br>Dendritic form: plaque or linear defect on epithelial surface with heaped up, ragged borders; may enlarge to geographic or maplike ulcer; patchy corneal anesthesia<br>Stromal and disciform stage: neovascularization under site of current or previous dendritic form, moderate uveitis typically present |
| Herpes zoster keratitis | Dendritic or superficial punctate keratitis similar to herpes simplex<br>Vesicles on tip of nose implicate nasociliary branch involvement and threat to cornea, iris, and ciliary body<br>Prolonged pain (postherpetic neuralgia) can occur secondary to original inflammation |
| Thygeson's superficial punctate keratitis | Coarse punctate, snowflakelike keratitis<br>Usually bilateral with remissions and exacerbations<br>Circular or oval gray lesions, slightly elevated, persistent stain with fluorescein<br>Absence of preauricular adenopathy and stomal disease<br>Only mild hyperemia with no follicles |
| Interstitial keratitis | Deep stromal inflammation (vascularization, infiltration) in the absence of epithelial involvement<br>Resolution with deep opacities and ghost vessels<br>90% of cases caused by congenital syphilis; other causes are tuberculosis and leprosy |
| Filimentary keratitis | Short stalks of hyperplastic epithelium with zones of focal epithelial erosions<br>Keratitis sicca and superior limbic keratoconjunctivitis most likely associations |

drome are all categories based on the type of inflammatory stimulus.

From an initial diagnostic point of view, the morphological manifestations are more convenient and practical than the etiologic classification. Inflammation of different etiologies often produces the same clinical picture. So, the diagnostic process suggested is to, first, make a morphological diagnosis based on clinical manifes-

tations. Second, consider etiologies most commonly associated with the particular spectrum of symptoms, patient history, and clinical signs presented by each case.

The schema of clinical manifestations of keratitis used here identifies four main types: (1) superficial keratitis, (2) stromal keratitis, (3) ulcerative keratitis, and (4) peripheral keratitis. For each main type, the conditions are further qualified by severity of inflammation, presence of structural change, associated signs, and suggested etiologies.

## SUPERFICIAL KERATITIS

Superficial keratitis is inflammation limited to the corneal epithelium, with the occasional exception that the process may cause subepithelial changes. Clinical signs include localized swelling, epithelial filaments, epithelial erosions, and subepithelial opacities.

Superficial keratitis combined with conjunctivitis is the most common presentation of corneal inflammation. The causes and clinical profile of keratoconjunctivitis, whether caused by infections, toxic agents, or dry eye, are best discussed in the broader context of lacrimal and conjunctival conditions (see Chapters 22 and 23).

While corneal inflammation typically occurs with at least some degree of concurrent conjunctivitis, some clinical conditions predominantly involve the corneal epithelium. For example, herpes simplex and herpes zoster present with focal, usually central, corneal inflammation. Chlymydia, vaccina, adenoviruses, and Thygeson's superficial punctate keratitis exhibit diffuse corneal epithelial inflammation (see Table 24.1).

1. *Epithelial changes.* In some cases of keratitis the earliest inflammatory sign is localized or diffuse epithelial disruption. These focal epithelial changes appear as whitish-gray clouding in areas of punctate corneal staining.

2. *Epithelial filament.* Another occasional sign with superficial keratitis is strands of coiled hypertrophied epithelial cells attached to the cornea. These filaments are often associated with mucous strands, especially in cases of keratitis sicca. Transitory filaments may also present with an infectious keratitis.

3. *Epithelial erosion.* The cardinal sign of superficial keratitis is epithelial erosion. These lesions may appear fine, course, or coalesced and present in a variety of topographic patterns. In addition to inflammation, fine epithelial erosions evidenced by punctate corneal staining with sodium fluorescein, may be induced by contact lens wear, lid abnormalities, dry eye, or a foreign body.

Fine punctate erosions, predominantly found in the lower quadrant, are commonly associated with staphylococcal blepharitis and acne rosacea (with or without blepharitis). A superior limbal confluence of fine epithelial erosions suggests trachoma, molluscum contagiosum, and inclusion conjunctivitis. These three conditions are associated with follicular conjunctivitis, but more severe structural changes such as pannus is more typical of trachoma. Molluscum contagiosum is implicated by the presence of the distinctive lid margin nodule.

When fine punctate staining is diffuse and across the cornea, suspect viral infection. Causal infections include the adenovirus (epidemic keratoconjunctivitis and pharyngoconjunctival fever), herpes simplex, herpes zoster, and systemic infections such as mumps, vacccina, rubella, and infectious mononucleosis. Thygeson's superior punctate keratitis (SPK) resembles the fine erosions of viral keratitis. The distinguishing feature of SPK is its periods of remission and exacerberation and that it presents without concurrent conjunctivitis.

Corneal epithelial erosions that are course and coalesced into a linear or branching pattern are typical of a latter stage of herpes simplex and herpes zoster keratitis.

4. *Subepithelial opacities.* Both herpes simplex and herpes zoster keratitis also may present with round, whitish-gray, subepithelial opacties. While subepithelial opacities may be seen with a number of types of infectious keratitis, their presence is a hallmark of epidemic keratoconjunctivitis (adenovirus 8).

Subepithelial opacities are thought to represent infiltrates of inflammatory cells.

They are found between the epithelial basement membrane and Bowman's layer, intraepithelial regions, and the anterior stroma. They are the result of an inflammatory response and appear as white or gray granules. Staining does not occur unless the epithelium above the lesion is damaged.

Leukocytes have been observed making amoeboid movement from the limbus into the cornea. Corneal infiltration depends on limbal vessel dilation and probably some substance that humorally mediates the movement of the cells into the cornea.

The presence of leukocyte infiltration with soft contact lens wear is significant. Klintworth (1977) observed that corneal vascularization was always associated with leukocyte infiltration. He suggested that leukocytes are a source of diffusable agents capable of causing directional vascular growth into the cornea. Peripheral corneal infiltration, therefore, should be considered a possible precursor to neovascularization.

Corneal infiltration is clinically significant because it indicates past or current inflammation, and it may be involved in the process of corneal vascularization.

## STROMAL KERATITIS

Inflammatory infiltration into the corneal stroma can be secondary to persistent epithelial inflammation. For example, in the course of stromal herpes simplex keratitis, repeated attacks of epithelial inflammation leads to inflammatory cell migration, stromal damage, neovascularization, and scarring.

In certain conditions, such as interstitial keratitis, the inflammatory process starts in the stroma. For example, in the absence of any significant epithelial signs, luetic interstitial keratitis typically exhibits bilateral widespread infiltration and vascularized patches in the deep stroma.

Other features of interstitial keratitis include a salmon-patch appearance of neovascular twigs or tufts and resolution over several months with the sequelae of deep opacities and ghost vessels. Possible etiologies of interstitial keratitis include congenital and acquired syphilis, tuberculosis, and, less commonly, herpes simplex, Cogan's syndrome, and relapsing fever.

## PERIPHERAL KERATITIS

Peripheral corneal conditions may occur with or without epithelial involvement. Peripheral stromal infiltrates are most commonly seen with concurrent microbial, usually staphylococcal, conjunctivitis. In this case, the inflammatory pathway most likely includes the overlying epithelium. The staphylococcal infiltrates, however, soon dominate the clinical picture. In addition, peripheral corneal ischemia with stromal thinning can occur secondary to long-standing microbial keratitis or other epithelial damage.

Primary conditions of peripheral corneal ischemia typically exhibit an intact epithelium in the presence of stromal edema, infiltrates, and significant stromal thinning. Marginal furrow or gutter dystrophy, Terrien's marginal dystrophy, and Mooren's ulcer are examples of primary peripheral corneal disease.

## ULCERATIVE KERATITIS

Corneal ulcers are serious. They require prompt recognition, definitive diagnosis, and swift and appropriate treatment.

Ulceration, the severe destruction of corneal tissue, occurs due to invasion of the cornea by a proliferating pathogenic organism. Corneal ulcers offer considerable potential for rapid corneal destruction and severe visual impairment.

In superficial keratitis the clinical features of the condition are the guideposts to diagnosis. With corneal ulcers, clinical features must also be qualified, but, given the high risk of rapid progression, prompt etiologic diagnosis is critically important. Thus, it is mandatory to complete a laboratory diagnostic workup in order to identify the causative organism and its antimicrobial sensitivity. Review of these necessary laboratory techniques and the clinical features of corneal ulcers are, however, beyond the scope of this book.

## STRUCTURAL CHANGE

Corneal scarring, keratinization, vascularization, and deposition are examples of structural changes that may occur secondary to corneal trauma and inflammation. All these changes threaten vision. The process of corneal vascularization is particularly important because its development is so often insidious and the process typically predisposes the cornea to recurrent and chronic problems (Figure 24.2).

Corneal avascularity is necessary to obtain good corneal optics. Vascularization of the cornea may occur with many external insults such as mechanical trauma, chemical burns, long-term contact lens wear, blepharitis, conjunctivitis, and keratitis. Corneal vascularization has been associated with peripheral corneal edema, leukocyte infiltration, limbal vessel engorgement, and damaged peripheral corneal epithelial cells.

Because of the potentially serious consequences of blood vessel growth into the

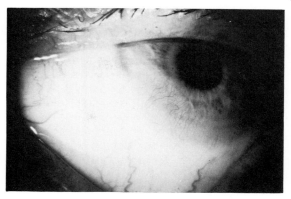

**FIGURE 24.2.**
**Corneal vascularization.**
Photo courtesy Rodney Gutner, O.D.

cornea, careful slit lamp observation for blood vessel growth, injection, infiltration, edema, and epithelial damage should assist the practitioner in identifying patients at risk for more extensive, and potentially sight-threatening, vascularization.

Removal of the causative agent often results in the regression of blood flow, although the so-called ghost vessels remain.

# References

Bier N, Lowther GE. Contact lens correction. Woburn, Mass.: Butterworths, 1976.

Curran RE, Kenyon KR, Green WR. Pre-Descemet's membrane corneal dystrophy. Am J Opthalmol 1974;77:711–716.

DeDonato LM. Corneal vascularization in hydrogel contact lens wearers. J Am Optom Assoc 1981;52:235–241.

Egan DJ. Biomicroscope information with contact lens application. Canadian J Optom 1979;41:(2)93–96.

Grayson M. Diseases of the cornea. St. Louis: C.V. Mosby, 1979.

Harris H. Role of chemotaxis in inflammation, Physiol Rev 1954;34:529–562.

Josephson JE, Caffery BE. Infiltrative keratitis in hydrogel lens wearers, Int Contact Lens Clin 1979;6:223–241.

Kenyon KR. Ocular ultrastructure of inherited metabolic disease. In: Goldberg MF, ed. Genetic and metabolic eye disease. Boston: Little, Brown, 1974; 139–185.

Klintworth GK. The contribution of morphology to our understanding of the pathogenesis of experimentally produced corneal vascularization. Invest Opthalmol Vis Sci 1977;16;281–285.

Kuwabara T, Perkins DG, Cogan DG. Sliding of the epithelium in experimental corneal wounds. Invest Ophthalmol 1976;15:4–14.

McDonald JE. Surface phenomena of tear films. Trans Am Ophthalmol Soc 1968;66:905–939.

Pinkerton RMH, Robertson DM. Corneal and conjunctival changes in dysproteinemia. Invest Ophthalmol 1969;8:357–364.

Rakes JA. Corneal neovascularization from extended wear lenses. J Am Optom Assoc 1983;54:259–261.

Robb RM, Kuwabara T. Corneal wound healing. I. The movement of polymorphonuclear leukocytes into corneal wounds, Arch Ophthalmol 1962;68:636–642.

Sanderson PO, Kuwabara T, Stark WJ, et al. Cystinosis: a clinical, histopathologic, and ultrastructural study. Arch Ophthalmol 1974;91:270–274.

Teng CC, Katzin HM. The basement membrane of corneal epithelium, Am J Ophthalmol 1953;36:895–900.

Waring GO III, Rodrigues MM, Laibson PR. Corneal dystrophies. I. Dystrophies of the epithelium, Bowman's layer and stroma. Surv Ophthalmol 1978;23:71–122.

# Barry J. Barresi
# SCLERA 25

*The sclera is a white connective tissue capsule that serves as the protective coat of the globe.*

## BACKGROUND

Constructed of collagen and elastic tissue, the netlike fibers of the sclera are resistant to wide changes in intraocular pressure and the pulling of extraocular muscles. The vascular supply to the sclera is minimal. With low metabolic activity, the tissue has a poor regenerative capacity, but is rarely diseased. Scleral disease most often develops as a passive response to disease or injury to adjacent ocular tissues, or it may be related to systemic disease, most notably the family of collagen-vascular conditions.

A thin, dense superficial layer, the episclera, is more vascularized than the scleral stroma. The innermost layer of the sclera, the lamina fusca, is dark and composed of numerous melanocytes. On occasion, the dark melanocytes pass through emissary foramina of penetrating ciliary arteries or nerves and form a dark spot observed on the scleral surface. These pigmented Axenfeld loops are normal but may be mistaken by the unwary as a foreign body or sign of intraocular melanoma.

Like body joints, the sclera is collagenous and subject to similar conditions. Of particular note is the association of scleritis with collagen-vascular disease, in particular rheumatoid arthritis (Host Response, Chapter 26).

In addition to inflammation, the sclera is subject to stretching, thinning, staphylomas, dehydration blue spots, pigment spots, and dilated episcleral vessels. Pigmentation of the overlying conjunctiva, such as with jaundice or ochronosis, may be mistaken for a scleral condition.

## HISTORY

Characterizing the type of discomfort experienced by a patient is the most important part of clinical investigation of scleral disease. Pain in the eye usually results either from exposure of nerve endings, such as with corneal abrasion, or by stretching of nerve endings, as with acute glaucoma. The pain of scleritis is severe because both pain mechanisms are operating. The severe pain of scleritis often refers to the temple and jaw. In contrast, episcleritis is not painful, but rather uncomfortable, hot, prickly, dry, or achy.

Scleral disease is typically bilateral with

335

recurrent attacks. Direct questioning should investigate suggestive attacks, alternation of visual acuity, and time course of onset. Occasionally, patients with scleral disease will complain of tearing and photophobia.

Investigate the past eye history for myopia, glaucoma, trauma, ocular tumors, and retinal detachment. Investigate the medical history for conditions associated with:

- Episcleritis and scleritis: psoriasis, rheumatoid arthritis, polyarteritis nodosa, vascularitis, gout. Review systems for evidence of collagen-vascular disease (e.g., general malaise, joint pain, morning stiffness, Sjögren's syndrome).

- Staphyloma and blue sclera: congenital and hereditary syndromes that affect skeletal and collagen development, such as Marfan's, osteo-genesis imperfecta, and Ehlers-Danlos.

- Dilated episcleral vessels: orbital vein occlusion, carotid cavernous fistula, hyperviscosity syndrome, cavernous sinus thrombosis, ophthalmic vein thrombosis.

# EXAMINATION

In gross observation of the sclera in daylight, look for abnormalities of color, shape, integrity, and surface vessels.

- Color: dark pigmentation is usually benign melanosis or migrated melanocytes at usually superiorly located scleral emissaria or Axenfeld loops. Pigmented intrascleral nerve loops may be painful to touch. Care should be taken to rule out pigmentation caused by a foreign body or extensions of malignant melanoma. Blue patches occur with local scleral thinning owing to myopia, recurrent scleritis, or more often, to congenital and hereditary syndromes. Rule out history of deafness, brittle bones, joint abnormalities.

- Shape and integrity: make sure the tissue is intact, free of thinning with uveal tissue in view, or swollen from inflammation. Slit lamp examination can help identify the depth of inflammation and specify level of involvement in the three vessel networks: conjunctival, superficial episcleral plexus, or deep arterial episcleral bed.

Adequate evaluation of scleral integrity may require blanching of superficial tissues with topical phenylephrine. Slit lamp examination with red-free light also is helpful in judging amount of congestion, vessel configuration, and presence of episcleral infiltration.

- Surface vessels: gentle pressure on the sclera can differentiate between movable vessels in the conjunctiva and superficial episclera from the stationary deep episcleral bed. A single dilated episcleral vessel over the lateral rectus muscle is characteristic of thyroid ophthalmopathy. With more diffuse, deep injection first rule out episcleritis, then consider orbital conditions (pseudotumor, abscess, carotid-cavernous sinus fistulas). Dilated, corkscrew epibulbar vessels that extend to the limbus suggest AV malformation.

In scleritis, careful slit lamp examination is important to rule out uveitis and secondary corneal disease (keratitis, limbic guttering, keratolysis). Other tests to assist in diagnosis of scleral disease and associated problems include:

- Visual acuity: keratitis or iritis secondary to scleritis may cause reduced visual acuity.

- Refraction: scleritis pain may induce ciliary spasm and a myopic shift. A posterior scleritis with macular swelling may cause a hyperopic shift.
- Tonometry: a secondary glaucoma may be precipitated by chronic scleritis and uveitis.
- Ophthalmoscopy: internal examination is necessary to rule out pars planitis, exudative retinal detachment, and fundus masses.

# CLINICAL SIGNIFICANCE

Primary diseases of the sclera are not frequently seen in office practice. Of the inflammatory conditions, episcleritis is more common than scleritis. Benign senile scleral changes can occur. Although tumors of other ocular tissues may affect the sclera, tumors of the sclera do not occur.

## Episcleritis

A benign and usually bilateral condition, episcleritis is characterized by the lack of severe pain. Rather uncomfortable, with a marked tendency to recur, episcleritis presents as a diffuse or modular mobile inflammatory swelling with marked conjunctival injection. Often the episcleritis attack is preceded by a viral infection or exposure to an allergen. The condition is self-limited, but attacks may be abated by use of topical steroids.

## Scleritis

Scleritis is a sight-threatening condition requiring early diagnosis and effective treatment. Most often a manifestation of systemic disease, scleritis more commonly presents bilaterally in women in the fourth to sixth decades of life.

Anterior scleritis is characterized by severe eye pain, which often radiates to the face, temple, and jaw. Inflammation of the eye builds gradually over days and becomes quite prominent. The area of bluish red hue may be localized or diffuse. Edema and necrosis of the sclera and injection of the deep episclerous vascular network are notable. The eye with scleritis is subject to a number of threatening secondary conditions: uveitis, glaucoma, and keratitis. These complications usually occur late in the disease. Early diagnosis and persistent systemic treatment with antiinflammatory agents offer the best chance for preserving the eye and minimizing any vision loss.

Posterior scleritis is even more uncommon in office practice than anterior scleritis. The diagnosis of posterior scleritis is difficult, however, and it may be mistaken for intraocular neoplasm, retrobulbal tumor, choroiditis, or central serous choroidopathy. In a series of patients from the Wills Eye Hospital (Benson et al. 1979), characteristic features of posterior scleritis were noted as follows: female, history of anterior scleritis or rheumatoid arthritis, fundus mass the same color as normal adjacent pigment epithelium, choroidal folds, vitreous cells, and ultrasonography finding of thickening of posterior coats of the eye. Corticosteroids for systemic and retrobulbar effect offer effective treatment.

## Degenerations

Senescent changes in the sclera are due to lipid and calcareous degenerations. These benign changes appear as a yellowish tinge with white flecks. Senile hyaline plaques, usually located between the insertion of the lateral or medial rectus muscle and the limbus, are translucent, slight depressions. The surrounding hyaline ring usually is hard and white.

# References

Benson WE, et al. Posterior scleritis, a cause of diagnostic confusion. Arch Ophthalmol 1979;97:1482–1486.

Cobo M. Inflammation of the sclera. Intern Ophthal Clinics 1983;23:159–171.

Watson PG. Diagnosis and management of scleritis. Ophthalmology 1980; 87:716–720.

Watson PG. Hazelman BL. The sclera and systemic disorders. Philadelphia: W.B. Saunders, 1976.

# Neal Nyman
# IRIS AND
# CILIARY BODY 26

*The uvea, the middle coat of the globe, can be divided into the iris and ciliary body anteriorly and the choroid posteriorly.*

## BACKGROUND

Lying between the outer protective corneoscleral shell and the inner neurosensory retina, the uveal tract is the densely pigmented, vascular layer of the eye. The primary function of the uveal tract is to provide nourishment for the entire globe. In addition, the muscles of the iris and ciliary body regulate the amount of light entering the eye and assist in refraction.

Disorders of the different regions of the uveal tract give rise to distinct clinical signs and symptoms. In this chapter the discussion focuses on disorders of the anterior portion of the uvea, the iris and ciliary body, but it is best to keep in mind that the etiology and pathophysiology of uveal disease is common to the entire uveal tract.

### Anatomy

The iris is a circular diaphragm lying in a frontal plane at the anterior end of the uveal tract. The anterior surface is divided into the peripheral ciliary zone extending from the iris root on the ciliary body to the collarette, and a central pupillary zone extending from the collarette to the pupillary margin. The ciliary zone is distinguished biomicroscopically by pitlike depressions known as *iris crypts* and by concentric ridges known as *contraction furrows*. Located at the pupillary margin is a dark fringe of pigment called the *pupillary ruff*. The sphincter muscle lies deep in the iris stroma, running circumferentially around the pupil near the margin and is innervated by parasympathetic fibers of the ciliary nerves. The dilator muscle, innervated by sympathetic fibers, extends radially from the sphincter muscle to the ciliary body, just anterior to the posterior epithelium.

The iris stroma is composed of an anterior limiting layer (anterior leaf), upon which the iris depends for its definitive color. It is a dense matting of connective tissue and chromatophores. In the blue iris it is thin with few cells; in the brown iris it is thick and densely pigmented. The bulk of the iris stroma consists of blood vessels, which for the most part run radially from the major vascular circle in the ciliary body to the minor circle in the collarette. In lighter colored irises, these vessels may be visible upon careful examination. The posterior epithelium is a densely pigmented cellular lining that curls around the pupillary margin, giving rise to the pupillary ruff.

The function of the iris is to regulate

the amount of light entering the eye. This is achieved by alterations in pupil size, which is controlled by the reflex activity of the sphincter and dilator muscles. In addition, the pigment epithelium serves as a barrier to incident light. The iris also provides nutrition to the anterior segment via diffusion of aqueous from the vascular stroma.

Posteriorly, the ciliary body appears as a ring approximately 6 mm wide. At the ora serrata the ciliary body is smooth and designated the pars plana. The inner surface, pars plicata, is ridged due to the presence of 70 to 80 ciliary processes. In sagittal section, the ciliary body forms a triangle, with its shortest side anteriorly. The anterior chamber angle, where aqueous drainage occurs, is formed here and the iris originates from this region.

The outer side of the triangle corresponds to the ciliary muscle and lies against the sclera. The ciliary muscles form the bulk of the ciliary body and consist of smooth muscle fibers arranged in meridional, radial, and circular fashion. With accommodation, contraction of the ciliary muscle slackens the suspensory ligaments. With decreasing tension on the lens capsule, the lens becomes more convex.

The inner layer of the ciliary body, the ciliary epithelium, is a double layer of cells. The innermost cells separate the ciliary body from the aqueous humor and vitreous body. This inner layer is nonpigmented, while the outer layer is heavily pigmented. The ciliary epithelium is responsible for the secretion of aqueous humor and may also be involved in the production of vitreous.

The uvea is made up of branches of the ciliary arteries, which pierce the sclera in the posterior pole. The posterior ciliary arteries arise as divisions of the ophthalmic artery, dividing into 10 to 20 short and 2 long branches. The two long posterior ciliary arteries travel forward in the suprachoroidal space to the ciliary body, where they anastomose with anterior ciliary arteries to form the major vascular circle of the iris, which supplies the ciliary body and iris, as well as the anterior portions of the choroid via the recurrent ciliary arteries. Tributaries from the major circle run radially to the collarette, where they form the minor vascular circle.

The venous return of the uveal tract is by way of two systems. The anterior ciliary veins accompany the anterior ciliary arteries as tributaries of the muscular veins. They carry blood from the ciliary muscle and the superficial plexuses, which accounts for only 1% of the venous return. The remainder of the uveal tract drainage is via the vortex veins.

In light of the rich vascularity of the uvea, it is not surprising that the most commonly encountered disorders are of an inflammatory nature and that the uvea is particularly likely to participate in systemic disease processes. The degenerative changes that occur in the uvea are primarily the result of vascular sclerosis, and the uvea is the most common intraocular site for metastatic tumors. Once a disease has become localized in the uvea, it often progresses rapidly—in large part because vascular tissue participates actively in pathologic processes. Because of the uvea's intimate contact with the rest of the eye and its function of providing nourishment to surrounding structures, uveal disease can disturb the metabolism of the eye severely enough to lead to complete destruction or atrophy of the globe.

Disorders of the uvea can disturb visual function via several routes: interference with the accommodative mechanism, transmission disturbances owing to the presence of exudates, blood, or other material in the media, or as a consequence of secondary open- or closed-angle glaucoma.

The uvea is involved in the following disorders: congenital and developmental anomalies, inflammation, degenerations and atrophies, cysts and tumors (neoplasms), and trauma.

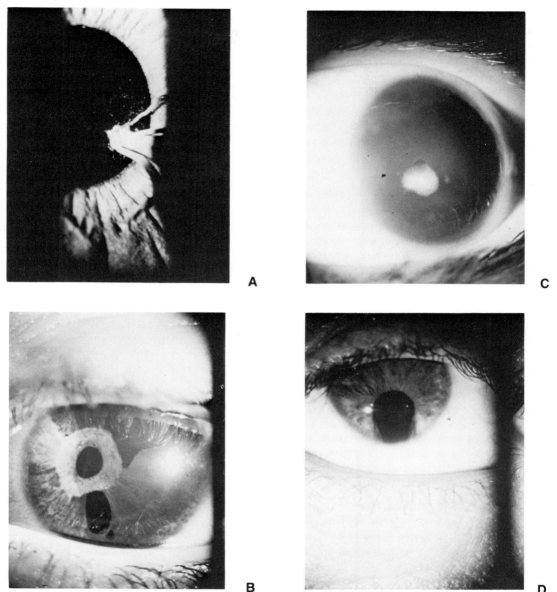

**FIGURE 26.1.**
Examples of congenital and developmental abnormalities of the anterior uveal tract. *A.* Persistent pupillary membrane. *B.* Polycoria. *C.* Aniridia. *D.* Iris coloboma.
Photos courtesy Jane Stein, Eye Institute, Pennsylvania College of Optometry.

# Congenital and Developmental Anomalies

These are conditions that affect the uveal tract at birth or later in life as the result of a hereditarily transmitted disorder (Figure 26.1) and Table 26.4). All of the various modes of inheritance are involved.

# Inflammation

Uveitis is the most prevalent of the disease processes affecting the uvea (12/100,000/year). If the inflammatory process is localized in the iris it is called an *iritis;* if it is localized in the ciliary body it is called a *cyclitis.* Most anterior uveitis presents as a combination of both and is referred to as *iridocyclitis.*

Historically, there have been several definitions of inflammation and several systems of classification of inflammatory disease. One definition of inflammation and a system of classification that derives from it have been proposed by Aronson and Elliott (1972). It has particular value for the study of ocular inflammation and is discussed in the following section. Understanding of these basic principles of inflammation is essential for proper clinical evaluation and management of anterior uveal disorders.

Inflammation is defined as "the interaction between a stimulus and a host, invariably resulting in some degree of structural change within the host" (Aronson and Elliott 1972). The inflammatory process is made up of the three interdependent variables of stimulus, host response, and structural integrity of the host tissue. Host exposure to an inflammatory stimulus results in a response in the host that has the function of restoring homeostasis and preserving structure. The interaction of stimulus and host results in varying degrees of inflammatory severity and thus varying amounts of structural alteration, depending on the quantity of the stimulus, its potency, and the duration of exposure to the host.

Any agent that can produce an inflammatory response in the host is considered an inflammatory stimulus. The following outline lists the major anterior uveal inflammatory stimuli:

I. Infectious agents
   A. Bacterial
   B. Viral
   C. Fungal
   D. Parasitic
II. Toxic agents (possess inherent properties that can damage host tissue)
   A. Chemical agents (e.g., acid or alkali burns)
   B. Physical agents
      1. Trauma
      2. Thermal injury
      3. Radiation
III. Environmental allergens (antigens)
IV. Endogenous allergens
   A. Autoantigens (lens-induced uveitis, sympethetic ophthalmia)
   B. Circulating antigen-antibody complexes

It should be noted that, clinically, uveitis may be the result of more than one inflammatory stimulus. For example, if an infectious agent gains access to the host, inflammation may result via the toxic effects of the invading pathogen and via the hypersensitivity response initiated by immune complexes present in the uvea itself or elsewhere in the humoral system of the host.

## HOST RESPONSE

Normal host response consists of the host's defense mechanisms, which function to eliminate the inflammatory stimulus and diminish its injurious effect on the host tissue. Abnormal host response refers to an increase or decrease in reactivity in the host response to inflammatory stimuli. The immune deficiency diseases and atopic diseases are examples of abnormalities of host response. The discussion of anterior uveitis will consider mechanisms of the normal host response only.

The normal host response can be thought of as a series of stages that comprise the defense system of the intact host. The first line of defense in the eye is the mechanical barrier of the lid, conjunctiva, and corneal epithelium. These structures serve as a physical barrier to the entrance of exogenous stimuli. Once a stimulus has penetrated the outer protective layer or entered the eye endogenously through vascular channels, a sequence of events mediated by the vascular and lymphatic systems takes place in an effort to eliminate the stimulus, inhibit its spread, and neutralize its toxic effects. These events lead to the activation of the final common pathways that produce the clinical picture of uveitis.

Because immunity plays an important role in the pathogenesis of uveal inflammation, the mechanisms of immunity will serve here as an example of host response. It is important to remember that nonimmune mechanisms can lead to a similar clinical presentation of uveitis via stimulation of final common inflammatory pathways.

The immune response consists of recognition and elimination of the inflammatory stimulus that is designated as an antigen. A broad collection of specific recognition cells are derived from lymphocytes and interact with their respective antigens, demonstrating a high degree of specificity, such that the interaction of only a few molecules is capable of triggering an impressive series of responses. Some of these molecules are found on the surface of lymphatic cells and account for cellular immunity, while others, called antibodies, circulate in the blood and interstitial fluid and mediate humoral immune reactions. After the initial antigen-antibody interaction, the immunologic signal is amplified via the release of a variety of pharmalogic factors, which enhance the local response, attracting additional lymphocytes and increasing vascular permeability in the area. Clinically, these changes man-

ifest themselves as vasodilation and edema. In humoral immunity (immediate hypersensitivity), the antigen-antibody complex combines with complement (a plasma protein complex), triggering the acute inflammatory pathway. This results in polymorphonuclear leukocytic chemotaxis and degranulation with subsequent lysosomal breakdown and release of hydrolytic enzymes, which facilitate phagocytosis of the antigen. If excessive amounts of these enzymes are released, autolytic breakdown of connective tissue occurs. The majority of structural changes that occur during the course of an inflammatory reaction can be explained by this phenomenon.

Once the host has been exposed to an antigen, immunologic memory develops. This is accomplished after initial antigen exposure by the production of specific antibodies on the cell surfaces and within the organized lymphatic tissues of the body. On subsequent exposures to the antigen, the "memory" of the original episode triggers an immunologic reaction that defends the host from antigen. It is particularly important to emphasize that immunologic memory cells can take up permanent residence at ectopic locations within the body where a previous immunologic encounter has taken place. It has been experimentally demonstrated that the uvea is such a site.

Lymphocytes with immunologic memory are present throughout the body. Thus, the host is alerted to foreign invasion even in its most distant parts. The immune response is somewhat indiscriminate: that is, it lacks the ability to assess the nature or extent of the threat posed by the antigen. This explains allergenic responses in a host with altered reactivity. It also helps to explain why it is so difficult to identify the etiologic agent in so many cases of anterior uveitis.

The final stage of host response is the regeneration and repair of injured connective tissue components. Regeneration is the process of replacement of injured tissue components with identical or functionally equivalent tissue, while repair refers to fibrous replacement of normal connective tissue following inflammation and results in scarring and neovascularization.

The last aspect of inflammation is structural alteration, which is defined as the change that occurs in normal tissue during the course of a primary inflammatory episode or subsequent to it. Structural change functions as an inflammatory modifier by permitting weak stimuli to become more significant as causes of inflammation. Depending on the severity of change that occurs, the eye is predisposed to recurrent or chronic inflammation. The repair stage of the host response is the histologic equivalent of structural alteration. Functionally, structural change of ocular tissue has been measured as increased vascular permeability. This increased permeability enhances predisposition toward subsequent inflammation by increasing the ability of the involved eye to concentrate inflammatory components. When structural change is mild to moderate, recurrent uveitis will result; when it is moderate to severe, chronic iridocyclitis is the outcome. The severity of structural change tends to increase after each exacerbation of active disease, so that recurrent iritis often progresses to chronic iridocyclitis.

The preceding discussion of inflammatory pathophysiology lays the groundwork for a consideration of the classification of uveal inflammation, a topic of much confusion historically. It is generally agreed that the most difficult etiologic diagnosis to arrive at when considering uveal inflammation is anterior uveitis. The reason for this is that the eye's direct exposure to the external world, in addition to the blood stream and other endogenous avenues, provides a myriad of points of contact for the entire spectrum of known inflammatory stimuli. This anatomic misfortune, coupled with the immunologic idiosyncrasies of the population, helps to explain why so many

cases of anterior uveitis remain labeled "etiology unknown." When a clinical etiologic diagnosis is made, it should be designated possible or probable unless there has been actual laboratory identification of the causative agent. Although anterior uveitis has traditionally been classified according to etiology, a system based on the operative pathogenetic mechanisms has been presented by Aronson and Elliott (1972). It is a clinically more useful tool, and it is presented in the following outline:

I. Primary uveitis
  A. Exogenous
    1. Acute iridocyclitis (no history of previous disease)
      a. Infectious agent
      b. Environmental agent (allergen)
      c. Medicamentosus (probable immunogenic)
  B. Endogenous-hematogenous origin
    1. Blood
      a. Congenital (in utero occurrence)
        (1) Infectious agent
          (a) Syphilis
          (b) Rubella
          (c) Cytomegalic inclusion disease
          (d) Toxoplasmosis
          (e) Herpes simplex
        (2) Nonreplicating stimuli (antigen-antibody complex disease)
      b. Acquired
        (1) Infectious
        (2) Nonreplicating
      c. Auto-allergic diseases
        (1) Lens-induced uveitis
        (2) Sympathetic ophthalmia
        (3) Chronic idiopathic
      d. Idiopathic uveitis
II. Structural change syndromes
  A. Recurrent iritis
  B. Iridocyclitis

1. Recurrent
2. Chronic
C. Chronic idiopathic syndromes
   1. Pars planitis (cyclitis)
   2. Heterochromic cyclitis (Fuchs' cyclitis)

# Degenerations and Atrophies of the Anterior Uveal Tract

Degenerative and atrophic changes of the iris and ciliary body affect both the stromal and pigmented epithelial layers Table 26.5). The primary pathophysiologic mechanism in these disorders is vascular sclerosis. The most common form of anterior uveal atrophy is the result of the natural aging process and will be referred to as senile atrophy or degeneration. Primary iris atrophies occur as senile changes or developmentally in early adulthood. Secondary anterior uveal atrophies occur after inflammation trauma, glaucoma, neurogenic disease, and ischemic processes.

# Cysts and Tumors of the Anterior Uveal Tract

Primary uveal cysts and tumors are classified according to their tissue of origin.

Secondary neoplasms occur as well (Table 26.8).

# Trauma

There are several incompletely understood mechanisms whereby trauma to the globe can produce anterior uveal tract disease. It is best to consider nonperforating or contusive injuries separately from perforating trauma (Table 26.6).

Contusive trauma may cause a sudden, transient increase of the intraocular pressure. If there is direct contusion of the cornea, a posterior displacement of the iris-lens diaphragm may occur, placing stress on the iris root and the suspensory ligaments of the ciliary body. The sclera and ciliary body may expand as a result of the concussion, placing stress on the uveal tissue. Another possible mechanism of injury is the creation in the aqueous of a pressure wave that concentrates its force at the iris root. As a result of damage to the ciliary epithelium, there is a breakdown of the blood-aqueous barrier and subsequent inflammatory reaction. Severe contusion can lead to scleral rupture.

Perforating trauma creates an entry point for exogenous stimuli, which may lead to a severe inflammatory response. If there is scleral rupture, severe complications may ensue.

# HISTORY

The purpose of this history is to identify and describe the patient's problem as specifically as possible and to orient the clinician toward a selective clinical examination to further clarify the nature of the problem. Careful qualification of the chief complaint will aid in the differential diagnosis of uveitis, conjunctivitis, and glaucoma. The major elements of the history in suspected anterior uveal disease are presented in Table 26.1.

## Inflammation

Inflammation is divided into primary and recurrent and/or chronic forms. The history usually is the best source of this information. If the disease falls into the primary category, the history is oriented toward identifying the nature of the inflammatory stimulus.

With regard to inflammation, the medical and environmental history often pro-

## Table 26.1
### History in Suspected Anterior Uveal Disorders

*Patient profile:* Age, sex, race, occupation, places of residence, avocations, pertinent interpersonal characteristics

*Chief complaint:* A brief statement in patient's own words describing the problem

*Qualification of chief complaint:* Onset; duration; course; quality; associated disturbances; precipitating, intensifying, relieving factors

*Ocular history:* Any trauma, previous inflammations (diagnosis and treatment), surgery, congenital or developmental anomalies

*Medical history:* Systems review, specific inquiry for rheumatoid disease, gastrointestinal, genitourinary, or granulomatous disease, allergies, recent URIs, lymph node swelling, or back pain

*Family history:* Ocular and medical—look for congenital, developmental, or other hereditary disorders

*Environmental history:* Any exposure to environmental toxic or immune agents, including medications and cosmetics

vide the clinician with clues as to the etiology or inciting agent. In primary exogenous uveitis, a history of recent trauma provides an explanation for the onset of inflammation. Uveitis associated with bacterial and viral infections, rheumatoid and immunologic disorders, parasitoses, or fungal infections present with either a history of past involvement (e.g., tuberculosis or syphilis), and/or active constitutional symptoms (e.g., joint pain, recent upper respiratory infection, or other flu-like symptoms) that alert the clinician to these etiologic possibilities. Allergenic inflammatory stimuli produce iritis accompanied by conjunctivitis in a patient with long standing history of seasonal allergy and/or a family history of atopy. Prolonged use of topical ophthalmic medications, such as epinephrine, may produce a uveitis of immune origin.

Primary endogenous uveitis is divided into congenital and acquired forms. The history is not of great help in identifying the inflammatory agent in these cases, although a history of maternal exposure to infectious agents may aid in the diagnosis of congenital endogenous infections. If the history reveals a systemic disease, such as sarcoidosis or syphilis, then the uveitis can be properly classified as an ocular manifestation of a systemic disease and appropriate management facilitated.

If the history suggests a recurrent or chronic uveitis, the role of the original inflammatory stimulus is not clinically significant, and the workup should be directed toward evaluating the degree of structural alteration present. Structural changes may render the eye responsive to a variety of inflammatory stimuli that, in a normal eye without structural alteration, could not initiate an inflammatory response.

The importance of an accurate problem-oriented history in the evaluation of uveal inflammation cannot be overemphasized. Even when the etiology is unknown, a thorough history will permit the clinician to make an informed decision as to whether further diagnostic studies are indicated. Coupled with a careful examination of the globe, the history is the clinician's most important guide to the formulation of an efficient management plan for anterior uveal inflammation.

# EXAMINATION

The following lists summarize the clinical examination of a patient suspected of having anterior uveal disease.

1. Visual acuity.
2. External examination.

   Pupil size, shape, reactivity.

   EOMs.

   Confrontation fields

   Gross inspection:color of irises; presence of injection, its distribution and severity (0–4); presence of discharge, its amount and type.

   Slit lamp evaluation (undilated and dilated pupil): using diffuse, focal and retroillumination, evaluate the lids, conjunctiva, cornea, iris, anterior chamber, lens, and vitreous, looking carefully for signs of anterior uveal disorders (see Tables 26.1–26.6).
3. Fundus examination (undilated and dilated pupil, direct and indirect ophthalmoscope): look especially for fresh or old chorioretinal lesions, retinal detachment, pars planitis, or mass lesions.
4. Gonioscopy: look for presence of inflammatory deposits, anterior synechiae, angle recession, vessel abnormalities, or mass lesions (generally only performed during the inflammatory episode if secondary glaucoma or mass lesion is suspected).
5. Intraocular pressure measurement.
6. Transillumination (direct and indirect): to rule out mass lesions and iris atrophy.

The clinician should strive to classify the disease as:

1. Primary versus recurrent or chronic (based on history and characteristic signs)
2. Exogenous versus endogenous
3. Iritis versus iridocyclitis versus cyclitis (based on distribution of inflammatory signs)
4. Mild, moderate, or severe (see Table 26.2)

**Table 26.2**
**Severity of Anterior Uveitis**

| Sign | Mild | Moderate | Severe |
|------|------|----------|--------|
| Cells | Grade 0–2 | Grade 2–3 | Grade 3–4 |
| Flare | " | " | " |
| KPs | Fine | Granular or mutton fat | Granular or mutton fat |
| Iris nodules | Rare | Occasional | Yes |
| Hypopyon | No | No | Yes |
| Vitreous involvement | No | Occasional | Frequent |
| Anterior synechiae | No | Occasional | Frequent |
| Posterior synechiae | Occasional | Occasional | Frequent |
| Sequelae | Few | Iris atrophy | Iris atrophy, glaucoma cataract, macular edema, retinal detachment, hypotony |

## Table 26.3
### Tests in Uveitis

| Test | Description | Indications | Comments |
|------|-------------|-------------|----------|
| Keratocentesis | Aspiration of fluid from anterior chamber by corneal puncture | 1. Specific microbial pathogens suspected as etiology<br>2. Specific antibody suspected in aqueous | The aqueous specimen can be cultured for bacteria, fluorescein antibodies to detect specific viruses. Cytologic and serologic examination of aqueous may be performed to detect cell types and antibodies |
| Blood tests | Used to test for antibodies that indicate patient's ability to respond to a given organism; most tests measure humoral immunity | History and clinical presentation suggest specific pathogen, e.g., syphilis | Tests for several antibodies are available; the most useful in anterior uveitis are those for syphilis, chlamydial infection (Reiter's syndrome), rheumatoid factor (antinuclear antibody) |
| General lab tests | ESR; CBC; WBC and differential; serum electrophoresis (SPEP); urinalysis (UA) | General health of patient may aid in diagnosis and management | Not routinely performed, but history and clinical presentation may indicate this type of workup |
| Skin tests PPD | Intracutaneous injections of soluble antigens prepared from microorganisms, tissue extracts, and other allergic materials. Tests measure delayed hypersensitivity | Tuberculosis suspected; occasionally other granulomatous disease is suspected | Positive result indicates exposure to the organism and delayed hypersensitivity to it; result does *not* conclusively prove the uveitis is related to it. Most important test is the PPD for tuberculosis |
| HLA typing | Cytotoxic analysis of the human leukocytic iso-antigen system | Acute or recurrent iridocyclitis in a patient suspected of having rheumatoid disease | HLA-B27 commonly associated with ankylosing spondylitis, Reiter's syndrome, colitis |

## Table 26.3
*(continued)*

| Test | Description | Indications | Comments |
|------|-------------|-------------|----------|
| X-ray studies | Chest | Granulomatous disease; | May reveal TB scars or hilar adenopathy associated with sarcoidosis |
| | Hands and feet | Granulomatous disease in association with joint pain; | May reveal sarcoidosis |
| | Spine | Uveitis associated with low back pain; | May reveal ankylosing spondylitis |
| | Temporomandibular joints | Joint pain | May reveal rheumatoid arthritis |

## Additional Tests in Uveitis

If the etiology remains unknown after ocular examination, then a decision must be made as to whether further diagnostic studies are indicated. While each case must be considered on its own merits, as a general rule, mild to moderate attacks of recurrent anterior uveitis in an otherwise healthy patient do not require further diagnostic workup. If, however, the history suggests associated systemic disease, or the clinical signs suggest a granulomatous process or a moderate to severe uveitis that poses a threat to vision, or if the prolonged use of nonspecific antiinflammatory agents (especially steroids) endangers the eye (via side effects such as cataracts or glaucoma), then a number of supplemental ocular and general medical tests are available. The general medical condition should be fully evaluated by the patient's primary care physician. Table 26.3 presents the most valuable supplemental studies available for the uveitis workup. These tests may be initiated by the primary eye care provider or as part of the general medical workup. Keep in mind that this list is not intended to be exhaustive, and depending on the specific aspects of a given case, there are several additional studies that may be helpful in arriving at a final diagnosis.

# CLINICAL SIGNIFICANCE

The diagnostic evaluation of congenital, developmental, degenerative, and traumatic disorders of the anterior uveal tract is straightforward, relying on accurate history and careful examination of the anterior uveal tissue (Tables 26.4, 26.5, 26.6).

## Inflammation

Traditionally, anterior uveitis has been divided into granulomatous and nongranulomatous types. According to this classification, nongranulomatous uveitis typically presents as a unilateral acute in-

Table 26.4
Congenital and Developmental Anomalies of the Anterior Uveal
Tract

| Name | Mode of Inheritance | Description | Comments |
|---|---|---|---|
| Aniridia | Autosomal dominant | Absence of iris (usually a small shelf of iris is visible gonioscopically) | Frequently associated with glaucoma |
| Pupillary anomalies: ectopic pupils | Autosomal dominant | | Must be distinguished from secondary pupillary anomalies |
| polycoria | | Decentered pupil | |
| miosis | | Multiple pupils | |
| | | Congenitally small pupil(s) | Most common cause of anisocoria |
| mydriasis | | Congenitally large pupil(s) | |
| persistent pupillary membrane | | Iris filaments arising from the collarette and branching in the anterior chamber and attaching to the lens capsule; may take form of epicapsular stars | |
| Coloboma | Irregular autosomal dominant | A missing wedge of iris tissue, usually inferiorly | Results from nonclosure of the fetal fissure; often accompanied by coloboma of choroid and optic nerve |
| Iridocorneal endothelial syndrome | Irregular autosomal dominant | Unilateral glaucoma, corneal endothelial proliferation, and iris stromal abnormalities. Clinical findings include posterior embryotoxin (centrally displaced; thickened Schwalbe's line); Peter's anomaly (central corneal opacity with associated posterior stromal defect; iris strands may attach to cornea) | Includes syndromes of essential iris atrophy; Chandler's syndrome; Axenfeld's syndrome; iris nevus syndrome; unifying concept is proliferation of corneal endothelium—unilateral, tendency to occur in women |

**Table 26.4**
*(continued)*

| Name | Mode of Inheritance | Description | Comments |
|---|---|---|---|
| Oculocutaneous albinism | Recessive or sex-linked (intermediate) | Deficiency of pigment of skin, hair, and eyes; iris hypopigmentation ranging from light blue with pink reflex to light hazel | Associated ocular abnormalities include nystagmus, subnormal acuity, strabismus refractive errors, and macular hypoplasia; the amount of iris hypopigmentation varies with the constitutive pigmentation of the patient, the age, and the amount of axial myopia |
| Heterochromia | Irregular autosomal dominant | Difference in iris color between two eyes or in different parts of the same eye | Must be distinguished from heterochromia associated with inflammation or atrophy |

flammation, characterized by pain, photophobia, cells, flare, ciliary injection, fine keratic precipitates, slightly reduced vision, and relative pupillary miosis (Figure 26.2). Etiology is thought to be noninfectious, usually unknown, perhaps immunogenic. Posterior synechiae may be present, as well as iris nodules. The course of the disease is acute and self-limiting, although recurrences are not uncommon. Granulomatous anterior uveitis is usually accompanied by posterior uveal involvement. The keratic precipitates are granular and "mutton fat" (greasy) in appearance. Onset is acute or insidious and etiology is thought to be infectious in most cases, although noninfectious diseases, such as sarcoidosis and sympathetic ophthalmia, may present as granulomatous uveitis as well.

Current opinion is that many types of uveitis fall strictly into neither category, some showing signs of both types, while others frequently change in character from week to week. The classification system still has value in certain syndromes and may aid the clinician in the search for etiology; therefore, it is presented here. Signs and symptoms of uveitis are summarized in Table 26.7.

# Neoplasms

In most cases, anterior uveal neoplasms are asymptomatic. Discovery of the lesion usually is made upon routine examination. Less frequently, a patient will become aware of an abnormal growth or discoloration of the iris and present specifically for evaluation of the problem (Figure 26.3). As has been mentioned, mass lesions of the iris and ciliary body may present as secondary inflammations or glaucoma, and the clinician should not overlook this aspect of the differential diagnosis in these conditions. The clinical characteristics of anterior uveal neoplasms are reviewed in Table 26.8.

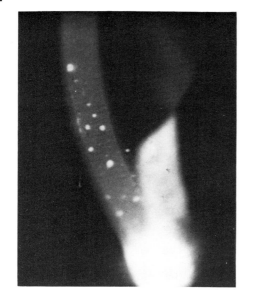

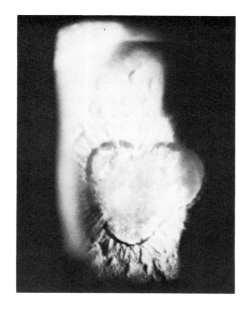

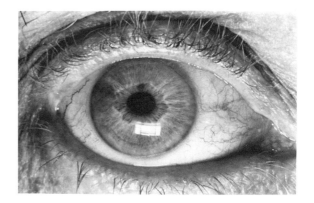

A

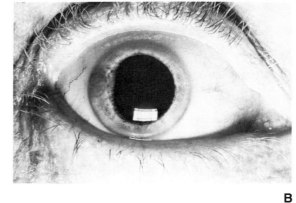

B

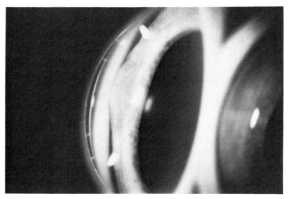

C

**FIGURE 26.2.**
Clinical signs of uveitis. *A.* Keratic precipitates.
*B.* Posterior synechiae (postdilation).
Photos courtesy Jane Stein, Eye Institute,
Pennsylvania College of Optometry.

**FIGURE 26.3.**
Iris melanoma. *A.* Increased pigmentation on
iris at 9 o'clock. *B.* Distortion of pupil after
dilation. *C.* Gonioscopic view.
Photos courtesy Rodney Gutner, O.D.

Table 26.5
Senile and Degenerative Changes of the Anterior Uveal Tract

| Structure | Type of Change | Clinical Appearance | Mechanism |
|---|---|---|---|
| Iris | Stromal atrophy | Overall thinning (especially pupillary zone), disappearance of iris crypts, thickened uveal meshwork; narrowing of anterior chamber angle | Sclerosis of stromal vessels |
| | Miosis | 3–4 mm pupil, sluggish light response | Sclerosis and hyalinization of stromal vessels and muscle |
| | Depigmentation | Pigment frill replaced by gray pellucid border, translucent stroma with retroillumination (often sector) Leads to granular pigment deposition on corneal endothelium, trabecular meshwork, and anterior lens surface | Secondary to sclerosis of stromal vessels |
| Ciliary body | Increase in bulk of ciliary processes Ciliary muscle atrophy Hyperplasia of nonpigmented epithelium Cystic degeneration of epithelium | Changes produce narrowing of posterior chamber with forward displacement of iris and shallow anterior chamber | Hyaline degeneration of vessels |

Many lesions of the iris and ciliary body, whether benign or malignant, appear clinically identical. Even malignant melanoma of the iris may appear as a remarkably slow-growing, benign lesion (spindle A type). Excisional biopsy of the iris is a readily available option, and newer surgical techniques permit excisional biopsies of the ciliary body in some lesions as well. In the past, many eyes have been enucleated because of suspicious lesions that have proven nonmalignant on path-ologic examination. With today's refined surgical procedures, conservative management is considered the wisest course.

The following guidelines are recommended as referral criteria for anterior uveal neoplasms:

1.  Size of lesion: excisional biopsy of iris lesions occupying less than two clock hours of the iris is usually adequate, since lesions in this category usually do not involve angle structures. There-

fore, lesions under two clock hours may be considered safe to follow for growth, assuming that careful slit lamp and gonioscopy has determined absence of corneal, angle, or ciliary-body involvement, and assuming the lesion does not originate close to the iris root, where earlier surgical intervention may be indicated.

Mass lesions of the ciliary body that are small and discovered during routine examination may safely be followed for growth; however, most ciliary-body lesions are not discovered until they produce symptoms (de-

creased vision, pain). By this time, the lesion probably is fairly large and should be referred for possible surgery.

2. Growth of lesion: slow-growing neoplasms of the iris under two clock hours in size should be followed for growth with photodocumentation or accurate drawings.

3. Signs of diffuse spread: any signs of diffuse spread, such as heterochromia, tumor seeds, or increased IOP, warrant immediate referral for surgical evaluation.

Table 26.6
Traumatic Sequelae-Anterior Uveal Tract

| Structure | Clinical Sign | Comments |
|---|---|---|
| Iris | Iritis | Mild reaction, flare and cells and occasional red blood cell in anterior chamber accompanied by transient decrease in intraocular pressure in involved eye |
| | Pigmentary dispersion | Pigment deposition on iris, corneal endothelium, trabeculum, and lens (may form Vossius ring on anterior lens capsule). Pigmentary glaucoma may subsequently develop |
| | Hemorrhage of iris stromal vessels | Infrequent, confined to small areas |
| | Pupillary miosis | Results from sphincter irritation, may be accompanied by accommodative spasm. Short lived in most cases |
| | Pupillary mydriasis | Transient sphincter paralysis. Short lived, though anisocoria may persist permanently |
| | Sphincter ruptures | May be partial or full thickness tear of iris stroma; mechanism uncertain. Clinical appearance varies from separation of small strand of iris stroma to notched defect of pupillary border |
| | Iridoschisis | Separation of anterior leaf layer of iris from iris stroma |
| | Iridodialysis | Separation of the iris root from the ciliary body and scleral spur. Range of severity related to force of traumatic contusion. May have associated hyphema |

**Table 26.6**
*(continued)*

| Structure | Clinical Sign | Comments |
|---|---|---|
| Ciliary body | Angle recession | Cleft in ciliary body between muscular fibers, clinical appearance varies from subtle separation of trabecular strands on gonioscopy and prominent ciliary-body band in one sector or 360° broadening of ciliary-body band with distinct scleral spur and associated peripheral anterior synechiae (examination must compare involved eye with noninvolved eye gonioscopically). Frequent cause of unilateral glaucoma from 2 mos–15 yrs posttrauma |
| | Cyclodialysis | Full thickness detachment of ciliary body from sclera; produces a cleft (small or wide) visible on gonioscopy; occurs rarely. Associated with hypotony (decreased intraocular pressure) |
| | Hyphema | Accumulation of free blood in the anterior chamber, usually encountered in children. Increased intraocular pressure in 1/3 of cases |

**Table 26.7**
**Signs and Symptoms of Uveitis**

| Sign/Symptom | Description | Pathogenetic Mechanisms | Associated with |
|---|---|---|---|
| Pain | Range from mild discomfort to severe pain; may be referred to ocular and periorbital region; aggravated by exposure to light and pressure | Irritation of ciliary nerves | Acute iritis and iridocyclitis |
| Photophobia | Range from mild light sensitivity to severe pain and blepharospasm | Trigeminal irritation due to ciliary spasm and/or corneal involvement | Acute or subacute iridocyclitis |
| Lacrimation | Not an important sign, associated with photophobia and varies in similar fashion | Trigeminal irritation of lacrimal gland | Acute or subacute iridocyclitis |

**Table 26.7**
*(continued)*

| Sign/Symptom | Description | Pathogenetic Mechanisms | Associated with |
|---|---|---|---|
| Blurred vision | Range from mild to moderate; related to severity of inflammation | Clouding of media due to exudates (KPs, cell, flare) in media. May also be associated with poor tear film, macular edema or other associated posterior lesions | All types |
| Small pupils | Relative miosis if compared to uninvolved eye; not always present | Vasodilation of iris vessels | Iritis and iridocyclitis |
| Conjunctival and ciliary injection | Pink to violet injection of circumlimbal episcleral vessels (ciliary flush), may extend to the conjunctival vessels in more severe cases; valuable sign in following progress of inflammation | Inflammatory vasodilation of radial episcleral vessels | Acute iritis and iridocyclitis |
| Keratitis and keratopathy | Peripheral superficial keratitis and/or corneal edema; band keratopathy associated with juvenile iridocyclitis, principally in association with juvenile rheumatoid arthritis | Extension of inflammation into peripheral cornea from limbal circulation (keratitis). Damaged corneal endothelium (edema). Progressive superficial deposition of calcium in cornea (band keratopathy). | Keratitis may be associated with all types; band keratopathy with JRA |
| Keratic precipitates (KPs) | Hemispheric deposits of inflammatory cells on the corneal endothelium, usually assuming a triangular area on lower half of cornea with base down. Range from fine white to giant waxy mutton fat. Pigment dusting is commonly | Inflammatory cells deposited on altered endothelium by centrifugal force of aqueous convection currents. Type of cell varies with type of inflammation | All types, mutton fat may be associated with granulomatous disease |

**Table 26.7**
*(continued)*

| Sign/Symptom | Description | Pathogenetic Mechanisms | Associated with |
|---|---|---|---|
| | associated with KPs, especially mutton fat KPs; classify according to type, size, distribution and number | | |
| Flare | Milkiness of aqueous humor, comparable to Tyndall effect. Range from faint to marked. Best observed with conical slit lamp beam in very dark room | Passage of light into protein rich aqueous, protein is transudate from inflamed uveal vessels | All types |
| Cells | Biomicroscopically visible inflammatory and pigmented cells in anterior chamber, retrolental space, and/or vitreous. Range from 0 to 4+ (50 or more cells per field) | Release of inflammatory cells from uveal vessels with altered vascular permeability | All types |
| Anterior chamber angle, iris and lens precipitates | White and mutton fat precipitates on trabecular meshwork, iris surface, and lens capsule | Same mechanism as keratic precipitates | Moderate to severe iridocyclitis |
| Fibrin (clot) | Coagulation of exudates in anterior chamber, range from slowing down of cellular movement in AC to clot formation in lower angle or pupillary zone. | Excessive accumulation of fibrin in AC | Severe acute iridocyclitis |
| Iris nodules, Koeppe, Busacca | Fluffy white nodular precipitates on inner surface of pupillary margin (Koeppe) or on surface of iris (Busacca) | Inflammatory cellular infiltration into iris stroma | Chronic iridocyclitis |
| Hemorrhage | Blood in anterior chamber (hyphema) | Hemorrhage of uveal vessels | Trauma, herpes, gonococcal uveitis |
| Hypopyon | Purulent exudate in the lower portion of anterior chamber | Purulent exudation from inflamed uveal vessels | Infectious uveitis |

Table 26.7
(continued)

| Sign/Symptom | Description | Pathogenetic Mechanisms | Associated with |
|---|---|---|---|
| Synechiae | Adhesions of iris to lens in pupillary zone (posterior synechiae), adhesions of iris to angle structures in ciliary zone (peripheral anterior synechiae) | Posterior synechiae are characterized by heavy exudation of protein leading to adhesions of iris to lens. Anterior synechiae result from shallowing if the AC as a result of pupillary block, organization of inflammatory exudates in angle, or edema and swelling of iris root | More common in chronic iridocyclitis |
| IOP variation | Low tension is characteristic of uveitis; glaucoma may develop as an early or late manifestation | Low tension probably due to decreased aqueous production. Interference with outflow via several mechanisms produces secondary glaucoma. | Low tension in acute iridocyclitis, glaucoma may be associated with all types |
| Iris atrophy | Diffuse, patchy, or focal atrophy of pigment epithelium | Prolonged inflammation of iris stroma and epithelium | Chronic iridocyclitis Nodular iritis |

### Table 26.8
### Cysts and Tumors of the Anterior Uveal Tract

| Lesion | Origin | Location | Pathophysiology | Nature | Clinical Characteristics |
|---|---|---|---|---|---|
| Epithelial cysts | Ectodermal | Iris and ciliary body | Congenital, post-inflammatory, post-traumatic, secondary to medicamentosa; most are formed | Benign | Common occurrence, may enlarge with age leading to secondary glaucoma |

**Table 26.8**
*(continued)*

| Lesion | Origin | Location | Pathphysiology | Nature | Clinical Characteristics |
|---|---|---|---|---|---|
| | | | by separation of pigmented and nonpigmented epithelial layers | | Posterior pigment layer frequently forms a heavily pigmented cyst |
| Epithelioma | Ectodermal | Iris | Simple growth of iris pigment epithelium | Benign | Common occurrence, frequently at pupillary margin, some lesions are cystic |
| Hyperplasia | Ectodermal | Iris and ciliary body | Secondary to degeneration, inflammation, or trauma; hyperplasia of pigmented and nonpigmented epithelium; hyperplasia of vessels and muscles may occur | Benign | May be difficult to differentiate from other neoplasms; should be monitored for growth |
| Medulloepithelioma (dictyoma) | Ectodermal | Ciliary body | Usually congenital, cell of origin is nonpigmented epithelium cell | Malignant (locally invasive) | Rare occurrence, appears as grayish-white mass arising in ciliary body and eventually presenting in pupillary area; may cause secondary glaucoma as presenting sign |
| Benign melanoma (iris freckle) | Neuroectodermal | Iris | Proliferation of normal uveal melanocytes | Benign | Very common, appear as discrete or clustered pigment spots on iris surface, more easily visible in light irides along the anterior border layer in the pupillary zone |

**Table 26.8**

*(continued)*

| Lesion | Origin | Location | Pathphysiology | Nature | Clinical Characteristics |
|---|---|---|---|---|---|
| Nevus | Neuroecto-dermal | Iris | Congenital melano-cytic cellular masses of spindle cell origin, con-genital but unpig-mented until puberty | Benign | Very common, may appear any-where on iris stroma, usually elevated; rarely undergo malig-nant conversion, may be associ-ated with ectro-pion uvea and irregularities of pupil |
| Neurilem-moma | Neuroecto-dermal | Iris and ciliary body | Originate from Schwann cell | Malignant | Very rare, clinically indistinguishable from malignant melanoma |
| Neurofi-broma | Neuroecto-dermal | Iris and ciliary body | Congenital, marked proliferation of Schwannian cells of ciliary nerves | Benign | May be seen in pa-tients with neu-rofibromatosis; frequently asso-ciated with glau-coma; very rare |
| Malignant melanoma | Neuroecto-dermal | Iris and ciliary body | Cell of origin is me-lanocyte, histolog-ically classified according to cell type:<br>1. spindle A<br>2. spindle B<br>3. epithelioid | Malignant | Rare, unilateral slow growing; most common primary intra-ocular tumor; more common over age 50; pig-mentation varies from amelanotic to heavily pig-mented. Spread by direct exten-sion, local or generalized me-tastasis. Second-ary glaucoma may occur. Tu-mors often nec-rotize giving rise to inflammation. Prognosis re-lated to cell type: spindle A: low mortality |

Table 26.8
(continued)

| Lesion | Origin | Location | Pathphysiology | Nature | Clinical Characteristics |
|---|---|---|---|---|---|
| | | | | | spindle B: mixed prognosis epithelioid: high mortality |
| Leiomyoma | Mesodermal | Iris | Unpigmented or slightly pigmented tumor of spindle cell origin | | Rare, difficult to differentiate from nevi and malignant melanomas, appears as grayish-white vascularized lesions on iris surface, usually inferior near pupillary border |
| Vascular tumors | Mesodermal | | Hemangioendotheliomas | Malignant | Very rare |
| Secondary malignant tumors | | Iris and ciliary body | May arise from intraocular structures via local invasion or metastatic from any organ in body, nature of lesion determined by primary tumor | Malignant | Most common site of origin is breast in women, lung in men; clinical presentation depends on site of primary lesion; usually presents in iris as pink or yellow mass located anywhere on iris |

# References

Aronson SB, Elliott JH. Ocular inflammation. St. Louis: C.V. Mosby, 1972.

Davson H. The physiology of the eye. New York: Academic Press, 1972.

Duane TD, ed. Clinical ophthalmology, v. 4. Philadelphia: Harper & Row, 1981.

Heath P. Tumors of the iris: classification and clinical follow-up. Trans Am Ophthalmol Soc 1964;62:51–85.

Hogan MJ, Kimura SJ, Thygeson P. Signs and symptoms of uveitis. Am J Ophthalmol 1959;47(5):155–170.

Hogan MJ, Zimmerman LE. Ophthalmic pathology: An atlas and textbook. Philadelphia: Saunders, 1962;2nd ed.

Last RJ. Wolff's anatomy of the eye and orbit. Philadelphia: Saunders, 1968; 6th ed.

Maumenee AE. Clinical entities in "uveitis": An approach to the study of intraocular inflammation. Trans Am Acad Ophthalmol Otolaryngol 1970; 74:473–504.

Moses R, ed. Adler's physiology of the eye. St. Louis: C. V. Mosby, 1970.

Pavan-Langston D. Manual of ocular diagnosis and therapy. Boston: Little, Brown, 1980.

Perkins ES. Diseases of the uveal tract. v. IX. In Duke-Elder S. System of ophthalmology. St. Louis: C. V. Mosby, 1977.

Silverstein AM. Immunogenic uveitis. Trans Ophthalmol Soc UK 1974; 94:496–517.

Van Metre TE. Role of the Allergist in diagnosis and management of patients with uveitis. JAMA 1966;195:167–172.

Yanoff M. Iridocorneal endothelial syndrome: unification of a disease spectrum. Surv Ophthalmol 1979;24:1–2.

# Morris Applebaum
# THE LENS 27

*The crystalline lens is a clear, avascular, biconvex structure located between the iris and vitreous. The lens contributes to the refractive power of the eye. The lens, zonules, and ciliary muscles function together in the process of accommodation.*

## BACKGROUND

The lens is derived from surface ectoderm. The basement membrane thickens to become the capsule. A single layer of cuboidal epithelium lying beneath the anterior capsule multiplies throughout life, and those cells at the equator elongate anteriorly and posteriorly to form lens fibers.

Lens fibers are produced throughout life, and new fibers are found anteriorly beneath the epithelium and posteriorly beneath the capsule. As new fibers are formed, the older fibers are forced inward, eventually losing their nuclei and becoming sclerosed.

The refractive index of the lens is higher than the surrounding aqueous and provides plus power to the eye. With contraction of the ciliary body, tension on the zonules and capsule are relaxed. The anterior capsule molds the elastic lens material to produce increased convexity, allowing the eye to accommodate for near objects. With age, the ability to accommodate declines, and presbyopia results.

New lens fibers are produced in layers called *lamellae.* Each fiber is less than one-half of the circumference of the lens, such that the ends meet along suture lines

rather than at the poles. During the fetal stage of development, these suture lines are Y-shaped, being erect anteriorly and inverted posteriorly. Those fibers that grow postnatally produce sutures that are increasingly complex and branching. The thickness and diameter of the lens increase with age, resulting in a displacement of the iris anteriorly and a shallower anterior chamber and a narrower angle.

The normal adult lens is described in terms of its clinical appearance with use of an optic section of the biomicroscope (Figure 27.1). The lens appears divided into segments with dark and light bands. Lamellae formed at different times have differing indices of refraction, and where these lamellae meet, the isoindicial surfaces produce increased light scattering and a bright band called a zone of discontinuity. The anterior light band is the anterior surface of the lens capsule. The second band separates the epithelium from the lens cortex. The third light band marks the anterior surface of the adult nucleus, the fourth the anterior surface of the fetal nucleus, and the fifth band the interface of the fetal and embryonic nucleus. The

**Anatomy of the Lens**

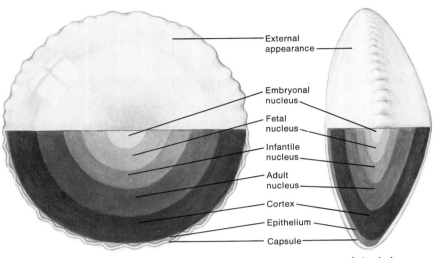

Anterior view                      Lateral view

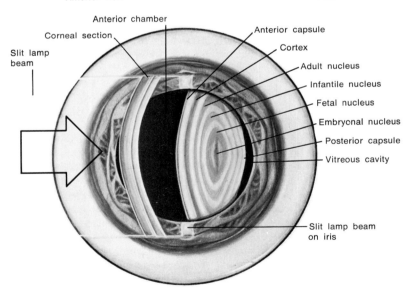

Clinical appearance on slit lamp examination

**FIGURE 27.1.**
**Anatomy of the lens and clinical appearance on slit lamp examination.**
With permission of CIBA Pharmaceutical Company, Division of CIBA-
GEIGY Corporation. From *Clinical Symposia,* illustrated by John A.
Craig, M.D. All rights reserved. Copyright 1974.

fifth band is bean-shaped and contains the Y-sutures. Posterior to the embryonic nucleus, the band pattern is seen in reverse order. The cortex and adult nucleus are very narrow in the infant.

The lens is subject to a wide range of abnormalities, including those of shape, size, location, and clarity. Any variance from optical clarity within the lens is called a cataract. Lens anomalies may be congenital, hereditary, developmental, or of senile origin. They may be associated with systemic or ocular disease, trauma or toxic substance, and produce ocular complications themselves.

Cataracts that form after age 30 to 40 are referred to as senile cataracts. Senile cataracts are pathologic, yet reflect an extension of the normal aging process of the lens. Senile cataracts can greatly affect vision and are a leading cause of blindness in the world. Their occurrence in the population increases with age, and some lenticular opacification is found in 96% of the population over 60 years of age.

Because of their location and differences in etiology, rate of progression, and effect on vision, senile cataracts generally are differentiated into three types: nuclear, cortical, and posterior subcapsular.

The nuclear cataract is an extension of the normal sclerosis of the nucleus. As the lens ages, the nucleus becomes increasingly yellowish in color, scatters more light, and has a higher index of refraction. As the sclerosis progresses, there is a shift toward myopia, with close vision becoming clear without reading glasses (the so-called second sight). As the sclerosis increases, the fetal nucleus may become more myopic than the adult nucleus, resulting in different refractive states in each zone and in polyopia.

With increasing pigmentation and opacification of the nucleus, hue discrimination, brightness, and form perception decrease, and visualization of fundus details becomes more difficult. In the advanced stages of nuclear sclerosis, the cataract may appear brown (brunescens)

or black (nigra). The thickness of the lens decreases with nuclear cataracts.

Cortical cataracts are referred to as soft cataracts in contrast to nuclear (hard) cataracts. The mechanism of cortical lens changes, in contrast to nuclear sclerosis, involves an increase in the water content of the lens and progressive cellular degeneration and opacification. In the earliest stages, direct illumination may reveal a few isolated vacuoles near the anterior adult nucleus. These contain liquid, are optically clear on transillumination, and do not affect vision. These may be stable or increase greatly in number.

In the cuneiform cataract, water enters the lens and may form clefts, separating the lens fibers radially, or lamellar separations. These are clear at first, or accompanied by lens edema, but they proceed to fill with cellular debris as the lens fibers degenerate. Opacification results in spokes or riders, which are generally located peripherally and have little or no effect on vision. This is the incipient or immature phase.

In the intumescent stage, water content increases and the lens swells, producing a shallower anterior chamber and increasing the risk of pupillary block and a narrow-angle glaucoma attack. The clefts increase and coalesce, and the lamellar separations increase to cause large wedge-shaped or bandlike opacities.

When the opacification increases to include the entire lens, the cataract is said to be mature. At this point, the lens appears uniformly opaque and yellow or white. The lens swelling has decreased and the anterior chamber is deepened.

If not removed, the lens will progress to the hypermature stage, in which the lens fibers dissolve and the fluid content is absorbed from the lens, leaving desiccated lens material in a shriveled lens capsule. Or, additional liquid enters the lens to produce a morgagnian cataract, in which the lens nucleus floats in the milky liquid within a very taut capsule. In the morgagnian cataract, the lens capsule can rupture or leak lens material into the anterior chamber to produce a phakalytic glaucoma, in which mononuclear phagocytes enter the anterior chamber and the debris blocks the trabecular meshwork, resulting in a rise in pressure.

Perinuclear punctate cataract is another form of cortical opacity in which dustlike opacities form on the surface of the adult nucleus. The effect on vision is related to the density of the opacification and proximity to the visual axis. These may remain stable for a time, but eventually lead to other cortical changes and total opacification.

The posterior subcapsular (cupuliform) cataract is a cortical cataract that commonly affects middle-aged adults. In the early stages, there is a granular appearance in the posterior pole adjacent to the capsule. It is only visible on retroillumination and appears as a distortion. This area enlarges to form a thin plaque of vacuoles and crystals.

The visual acuity is markedly affected by the posterior subcapsular cataract because of its axial location near the nodal point of the eye. Near acuity and acuity in bright light is most affected because of the associated pupillary constriction.

# Developmental Cataracts

Developmental cataracts are congenital or formed by age 3 months. There is a great variety of congenital cataracts that can have great or slight effect on vision; this text addresses those that have a significant effect. The etiology of the congenital cataract is often unknown but may be associated with certain prenatal conditions, including x-ray, drugs, diseases in the mother or embryo, or they may be hereditary.

The anterior polar cataract is a common congenital defect that is bilateral and symmetrical. It varies in size and may occlude the pupillary area. The opacity may extend from the capsule in pyramid shape into the anterior chamber (pyramidal cataract), or extend posteriorly through the cortex and adult nucleus. A variation of this is the reduplication cataract, in which the opacity is seen at the level of the anterior capsule and in lamellae posterior to the capsule, with clear material between. The opacity may be bipolar. Anterior polar cataracts affect vision depending on their size in relation to the pupil. Bipolar cataracts have a great effect because of the proximity to the nodal point.

Pyramidal cataracts are anterior polar cataracts ending in a pyramidal shape anteriorly and may be associated with a corneal opacity and a strand of material connected to the cornea, suggesting a keratitis or corneal ulceration in utero. They may be hereditary.

Posterior polar cataracts are nonprogressive and may be associated with hyaloid artery remnants. The shape varies widely and vision is greatly affected.

Remnants of the tunica vasculosa lentis are common and are seen anteriorly as pigmented spots on the lens capsule (epicapsular stars (Figure 27.2), or pupillary remnants that appear as pigmented strands extending from the iris collarette to the lens capsule, to the collarette at another point, or are free floating. Posteriorly, remnants of the hyaloid artery may remain attached to the posterior capsule (Mittendorf's dot) and is seen as a whitish dot 1.5 to 2 mm nasal to the posterior pole. It may have a threadlike attachment and does not interfere with vision.

# Juvenile and Presenile Cataracts

Cataracts that appear after 3 months of age through childhood are termed juvenile, while those in early adulthood are presenile. Juvenile and presenile cataracts resemble developmental cataracts, are stable or slowly progressive, and affect vision little.

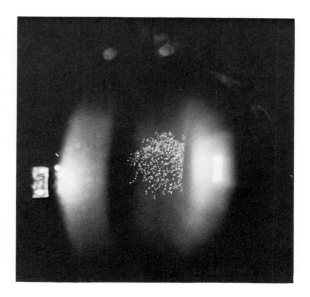

**FIGURE 27.2.**
Epicapsular stars. An embryonic remnant with
no associated disturbance of vision.
Photo courtesy John C. Townsend, O.D., and
Robert S. Vandervort, O.D., Southern
California College of Optometry.

The most common are the dilacerated cataract, which appears as a piece of teased out moss; the punctate (blue dot, cerulean) cataract, which appears as blue dots in the cortex and adult nucleus; and the coronary cataract, which appears as club-shaped opacities around the equator of the nucleus.

## Abnormalities of Shape and Size

Coloboma of the lens is associated with other developmental anomalies of the uveal tract and zonules. A flattening or indentation of the lens is seen peripherally and may be associated with opacities in the area. Colobomas are usually monocular.

Microspherokia is a rare bilateral anomaly in which the lens is small and spherical, has high refractive power, and is associated with subluxation and angle-closure glaucoma in the presence of a miotic pupil. It is associated with Marfan's and Weill-Marchesani syndromes.

Axial abnormalities of the lens surface occur anteriorly and posteriorly and may be conical (lenticonus) or hemispherical (lentiglobus). The refraction through the area is myopic, while the surrounding lens area is of normal refractive power.

## Anomalies of Lens Position

The lens is normally suspended from the zonules and centered along the visual axis. Ectopia lentis, a congenital defect of placement, is associated with Marfan's and other syndromes.

Displacement of the lens partially (subluxation) or completely (luxation) may be associated with trauma, intraocular inflammation, or hypermature cataract. Owing to loss of support by the lens, a tremulous iris is seen (iridodonesis).

With subluxation, the position of the lens may produce myopia and highly astigmatic errors, which are not easily corrected. If the lens is displaced sufficiently, the eye may be functionally aphakic and phakic simultaneously, with two different images. Corrections may be achieved with a high plus or high minus correction, with neither producing good image formation.

Dislocation of the lens may occur into the anterior chamber, pupillary aperture, or posterior chamber, with serious consequences.

Dislocation posteriorly produces an aphakic refractive status. Complications of a posterior displacement include choroidal scleroris, pigmentary degeneration, retinal detachment, iridocyclitis, secondary glaucoma, and if the capsule ruptures, phakotoxic uveitis, endophthalmitis, and sympathetic ophthalmia.

Dislocation into the anterior chamber usually is associated with serious sequelae, including pupillary block, synechiae formation, angle-closure glaucoma, iridocyclitis, and corneal endothelium damage.

## Syndromes Associated with Cataracts

Cataracts are associated with many hereditary and familial disorders, which include the syndermatoses (atopic dermatitis, Rothmund-Thomson and Werner's syndromes), diseases of bone (craniofacial dystoses, Paget's disease), and other syndromes, including Marfan's, Turner's, Laurence-Moon-Biedl, and Down's.

## Cataracts Associated with Metabolic Disorders

Systemic metabolic disorders, including galactosemia, diabetes mellitus, hypoparathyroidism, and cretinism, may produce cataracts.

Diabetes is associated with a rapidly maturing cataract, called a *snowflake cataract.* It occurs, most commonly in young, severe diabetics, beginning as a shift toward myopia, followed by the appearance of subcortical punctate (snowflake) opacities anteriorly and posteriorly, followed by vacuoles, water clefts, intumescence, and complete opacification. This may occur over a period of weeks or a few hours.

Senile cataracts are found more often in diabetics, occur at an earlier age, and progress at a more rapid rate. They are identical to other senile cataracts, may be associated with poor control of the diabetes, the duration of the condition, and occur more often in women.

Galactosemia, an inherited problem of galactose metabolism, produces a cataract of the cortex. The cataract commonly occurs within the first few days after birth and may be the first sign of this life-threatening disease, whose other symptoms include malnutrition, mental retardation,

diarrhea, and vomiting. Juvenile onset may occur in mild cases and can only be confirmed by a laboratory tolerance test.

## Traumatic Cataract

Blunt trauma or penetrating injury to the globe may result in cataract formation, dislocation of the lens, or rupture of the lens capsule. Cataract formation is usually posterior subcapsular, but may involve all or part of the lens and may be punctate or diffuse. A ring of iris pigment, Vossius' lenticular ring, may be seen on the anterior lens capsule.

If the lens capsule is ruptured, complete opacification may result. In the young, phakolytic enzymes may dissolve the lens substance, leaving the eye aphakic. In the older patient, the lens substance will not dissolve by action of the enzymes, and phakolytic glaucoma or phakoanaphylaxis may result. A traumatic uveitis may be seen and may produce posterior synechiae, iris bombé, and secondary angle-closure glaucoma.

Penetrating injuries may affect all or part of the lens. Iron that remains in the eye produces subcapsular brownish opacities, while copper produces a rapid complete cataract and loss of the eye.

## Complicated Cataract

Cataracts that form as the result of intraocular inflammation are known as *complicated* cataracts. Retinal detachments, retinitis pigmentosa, tumors, iridocyclitis, and glaucoma will produce cataracts.

Inflammations and degenerations of the posterior segment produce a posterior polar subcapsular and cortical cataract that initially appears as a polychromatic luster (Figure 27.3). This progresses to opacification into the cortex of a gray, dense cloud that may be round, stellate, or rosette shaped. It must be distinguished from the posterior subcapsular and traumatic cataracts.

In anterior uveitis, posterior syn-

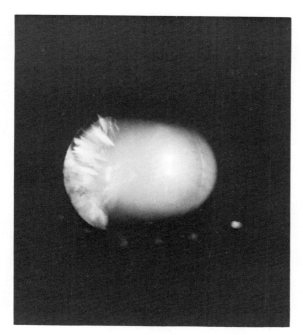

**FIGURE 27.3.**
Cortical cataract. Peripheral spoking viewed
after dilation.
Photo courtesy John C. Townsend, O.D., and
Robert S. Vandervort, O.D., Southern
California College of Optometry.

with microphthalmos, and miotic pupils. Defects of the ear and heart are associated. The cataract may be nuclear or total, and may be progressive after birth.

## Exfoliation and Pseudoexfoliation of the Lens Capsule

The lens capsule is composed of two layers. A separation of these layers produces a rare condition: exfoliation of the capsule. This usually is associated with exposure to heat, such as in glassblowers and furnace operators, although blunt trauma and iridocyclitis may produce this condition.

Pseudoexfoliation of the lens capsule is a degenerative, exudative condition in which a white, flaky substance is deposited on structures within the eye, including the iris, lens capsule, zonules, posterior cornea, and the angle.

It is most commonly seen on the anterior lens capsule and on the pupillary borders of the iris as dandrufflike flakes. With a dilated pupil, a ring is seen in which the material is missing because of the contact of the iris on the lens capsule. Pseudoexfoliation may be associated with glaucoma (glaucoma capsulare).

Another lens condition associated with glaucoma is called glaukomflecken. Following an attack of acute glaucoma, a necrosis of tissue occurs in the pupillary region, producing a white fleck arrangement of subcapsular opacities in the anterior cortex.

echiae, a thickened lens capsule, dense membrane formation across the pupil, and lens opacification may result. This process takes many years to occur and may be arrested with control of the inflammation.

## Embryopathic Cataracts

Transmission of diseases in utero can produce cataracts that are termed *embryopathic*. Syphilis, rubella, smallpox, and toxoplasmosis may be transmitted across the placental barrier.

Rubella that occurs in the mother during the first trimester of pregnancy can produce cataracts, pigmentary retinal degeneration, corneal opacities associated

## Drugs and Toxic Substances

Cataracts may be induced by certain drugs and chemicals and are called *toxic* cataracts. The chemicals include naphthalene, dinitrophenol, thallium, cobalt, and selenium. The drugs include morphine compounds, cholinesterase inhibitor miotics, corticosteroids, and phenothiazines.

Steroids produce posterior subcapsular and cortical opacities after prolonged use. Phenothiazines produce dustlike opacities in the anterior subcapsular region. There opacities resemble normal pigmentation that occurs commonly after age 60.

# HISTORY

The history of lens anomalies is based upon symptomatology, past eye history, family history, personal health, and drug history.

## Symptoms

Senile lens changes are the result of the location and extent of opacification and changes in refraction of the lens.

Nuclear cataracts (Figure 27.4) are associated early with symptoms of blurred vision at distance and clear vision at near as the nucleus develops a higher index of refraction. As the cataract progresses, symptoms include monocular diplopia, blur at all distances with best correction (owing to multiple foci), increased light scattering, and image distortion. The yellowing and opacification of the nucleus produces symptoms of hue discrimination and a need for more light, although in dull illumination the pupillary dilation may allow light to enter around the opacity.

Posterior subcapsular cataracts (PSC) produce visual distortion early in the course of opacification. The proximity of opacification to the nodal point and posterior surface irregularity produces great reductions in visual acuity. The patient will not be affected by glare from lights early in the cataract development. As the PSC changes progress, near vision will be greatly affected, as will vision in high illumination because of the associated pupillary constriction.

Cortical lens changes produce symptoms quite distinct from nuclear or posterior subcapsular cataracts. Since the cortical changes begin peripherally, there may be little or no visual effect. As changes progress, the patient will complain of glare and distortion with night and distance vision, while bright light and reading will constrict the pupil and reduce visual distortion. Vision will remain good as long as areas of clear lens remain, although glare may be a problem.

Patients may note dark spots in their vision owing to areas of opacification, which can be exaggerated by viewing through a pinhole or stenopeic slit held at

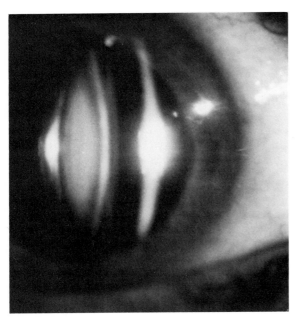

**FIGURE 27.4.**
**Moderate nuclear sclerotic cataract. (Grade 2 + ). Note increased contrast, dark ring around nucleus.**
Photo courtesy John C. Townsend, O.D., and Robert S. Vandervort, O.D., Southern California College of Optometry.

the anterior focal point (16 mm in front of the cornea).

## Eye History

A careful examination of the patient's eye history will alert the practitioner to the possibility of lens anomalies.

A history of trauma to the eye, either blunt or penetrating, may be associated with Vossius' lenticular ring, posterior subcapsular lens opacities, rupture of the lens capsule with local or generalized opacification, phakolytic glaucoma, phakotoxic uveitis, phakoanaphylaxis, and lens dislocations.

Episodes of acute closed-angle glaucoma can produce a fleck cataract in the anterior cortex (glaukomflecken).

A history of intraocular inflammation or retinal detachment may produce a complicated cataract.

A history of congenital anomaly will be associated with visual symptoms related to the location and density of the opacity or location of the lens. The stability of opacities may be judged by changes in visual acuity.

## Personal Medical History

Cataracts may be associated with general health problems, such as diabetes mellitus, galactosemia, hypoparathyroidism, and cretinism. Be alert to a history of any long-term drug use, particularly the phenothiazines and corticosteroids, or exposure to toxic agents and radiation.

## Family History

A family history of cataract will alert the practitioner to the possibility of cataract in the patient. History of any one of the many hereditary familial syndromes associated with lens anomalies is also significant.

# EXAMINATION

Examination for lens anomalies consists of a thorough evaluation of the lens, determination of the best visual correction, and assessment of ocular health in the presence of a lens anomaly.

Lens examination is best conducted under conditions of full pupillary dilation. The retinoscope is used to determine changes in refractive error, distortions in the media that produce scissors motions, and retroillumination to see small opacities where they appear as black spots in the field.

The direct ophthalmoscope is used to view the lens from a distance (20–40 cm), to view opacities and distortions by retroillumination, and to view the lens at close distances with a +20D lens by direct illumination. Opacities of the lens and displacement may be seen, but assessment of the axial location of an opacity is not possible with the ophthalmoscope. Indirect ophthalmoscopy allows good fundus visualization, even with significant lens opacification.

The ophthalmoscopic view of the fundus should be evaluated with respect to its correlation with best corrected visual acuities. The practitioner should routinely estimate the view of the fundus in terms of expected visual acuities. If the fundus view is better than the subject's visual acuity, the practitioner is alerted to investigate other causes of vision loss.

The use of the slit lamp is the best method for examining the eye for lens anomalies. With an optic section, the practitioner can identify the axial location of an opacity. Direct focal illumination with a wide beam allows assessment of the extent and density of opacification and pigmentation, while retroillumination allows assessment of distortion and density of opacification.

The slit lamp is also used to evaluate the depth of the anterior chamber, which becomes shallower with age and intumescent cortical changes. The anterior lens capsule is examined for pupillary remnants, Vossius' lenticular ring, exfoliation, pseudoexfoliation of the lens capsule, lenticonus, lentiglobus, and colobomas.

Visual acuities should be assessed prior to dilation through the best possible correction at distance and near with notation of the effects of changes of illumination and pinhole use.

In the presence of lens opacities that prohibit adequate examination of the ocular health by direct observation, a careful assessment of visual function is required.

Even in the presence of dense lens changes, the pupillary reflexes, direct and consensual, should be present. The absence of a Marcus Gunn pupil sign, and a pupil glow with transillumination is expected. A nuclear cataract nigra is an exception. If transillumination is not obtained, the possibility of an intraocular mass, retinal detachment, or hemorrhage exists, and ultrasonic examination is indicated.

Light perception should always be present, even with a dense cataract. Evaluation of retinal and macular function is important to predict outcomes of cataract extraction. Light projection in a dark room and the ability to distinguish two points of light are useful to evaluate the integrity of the visual field. The ability to count the number of holes in a retroilluminated disc held near the eye is an indication of normal macular function.

The entoptic phenomenon of the Purkinje "tree" of retinal blood vessels is useful in evaluating retinal function. A light is moved vertically back and forth over the closed lid. The patient will perceive a red field and the reversed pattern of the retinal vessels. Scotomas appear as black holes, and the vessels near the macula are seen most clearly. The perception of a bright light that appears to have a wet cobblestone look indicates an intact fovea.

The laser interferometer can be used to transmit interference fringe patterns through a cataract to evaluate visual acuities. The image is not affected by opacities of the media, and the ability to detect the separation in the fringe patterns is a measure of retinal integrity. ERGs are also useful in assessing retinal function.

# CLINICAL SIGNIFICANCE

The lens is normally an optically clear tissue. Any opacification of the lens is termed a cataract. The presence of a cataract requires the clinician to determine by history and examination its etiology and prognosis. The presence of a cataract may indicate the presence of ocular or systemic pathology that requires referral for further health assessment and treatment.

The majority of cataracts seen clinically are those associated with normal aging changes. Since cataracts are progressive, the clinician must appropriately classify the type and extent of the cataract (see Table 27.1). Progress of the cataract must be periodically assessed and appro-

priate changes in visual correction made to provide optimal function. If the cataract is affecting vision, ocular health must be assessed before visualization of the posterior structures becomes difficult. If vision is greatly affected and visualization of the posterior pole difficult, visual acuity and visual fields must be examined by special means to assess the integrity of the visual system in order to determine the prognosis of vision after cataract extraction.

In the presence of senile lens changes, patients must be counseled regarding etiology, visual loss, progression, and possible need for surgery. If surgery is indi-

**Table 27.1**
**Classifications of Cataracts**

| Grade | Cortical | Posterior Subcapsular | Nuclear |
|---|---|---|---|
| 1+ | Incipient stage<br>Occasional milky cleft peripherally<br>Visual acuity: minimal or no changes | Distortions best visualized with retroillumination<br>Subtle changes with direct illumination<br>VA: no change to 20/30; distortion and flare worse at near | Hint of cloudiness<br>Loss of definition in the nucleus<br>VA: trace of refractive error; shift toward myopia |
| 2+ | Intumescent stage<br>Coalescing spokes peripherally<br>VA: 20/25–20/80 with flare | Vacuoles and granules seen with direct illumination (early plaque) | Homogeneous nucleus<br>No Y sutures<br>Increased contrast with cortex/nucleus interface (dark ring around nucleus seen with slit lamp)<br>VA: 20/20–20/40; 1–3D change in refraction |
| 3+ | Intumescent stage (advanced)<br>Large wedge and band opacities extending to the central lens<br>VA: 20/100–FC | Increased area of plaques<br>Coalescence of vacuoles, granules, and crystals | Maximum contrast of nucleus<br>Increased opacification<br>VA: 20/30–20/80; polyopia<br>> 2D refractive error change |
| 4+ | Mature stage<br>Uniform milky white pupil<br>VA: FC to LP | Increased thickness of plaque extending into the cortex | Densely opaque nucleus<br>White to brown in appearance (usually brunescens)<br>VA: 20/100 or less |
| Advanced | Hypermature stage<br>Morgagnian Cataract | | Cataract nigra |

cated, a referral in a timely manner to allow the surgeon to examine the eye while the posterior pole can still be visualized is generally considered desirable. If surgery is contemplated, the patient should be counseled about the surgery and the postoperative care anticipated.

# References

Brandreth RH. Clinical slit lamp biomicroscopy. Berkeley: RH Brandreth, 1978.

CIBA Foundation Symposium 19. The human lens—in relation to cataract. New York: Associated Scientific Publishers, 1973.

Duke-Elder S. Diseases of the lens. In:

Duke-Elder S, ed. System of ophthalmology. St. Louis: C.V. Mosby, 1969;IX:3–378.

Greenberg DA, May LA. The senescent cataract patient: a management philosophy. J Am Optom Assoc 1982;53:125–129.

Luntz MH. Clinical types of cataract. In: Duane TD, ed. Clinical ophthalmology. Hagerstown, Md.: Harper & Row, 1982;I:73:1–20.

Olson L. Anatomy and embryology of the lens. In: Duane TD, ed. Clinical ophthalmology. Hagerstown, Md.: Harper & Row, 1982;I:71:1–8.

Phelps CD. Examination and functional evaluation of crystalline lens. In: Duane TD, ed. Clinical ophthalmology. Hagerstown, Md.: Harper & Row, 1982; I:72:1–23.

Morris Applebaum
Barry J. Barresi

# INTRAOCULAR PRESSURE 28

*The fluid pressure within the eye is called intraocular pressure.*
*Maintenance of intraocular pressure within a certain range is*
*necessary for normal ocular function.*

## BACKGROUND

### Aqueous Humor Dynamics

Aqueous humor is produced by active and passive filtration of fluid into the posterior chamber (Figure 28.1). The aqueous humor passes between the posterior border of the iris and anterior lens capsule through the trabecular meshwork, enters the canal of Schlemm, and drains through the collector channels into the episcleral venous system. The trabecular meshwork is located between the root of the iris at its attachment to the ciliary and corneal limbal junction. This is the recess of the anterior chamber angle.

The influence of aqueous humor dynamics on intraocular pressure is complex and not well understood. In simple terms, the control of intraocular pressure is a function of: (1) the rate of inflow of aqueous humor entering the eye, (2) the resistance to aqueous humor outflow, and (3) episcleral venous pressure. Intraocular pressure is constant when a steady state exists of inflow equaling outflow.

Normal intraocular pressure cannot be precisely expressed in numerical terms. Rather, normal intraocular pressure is a concept based on: (1) the distribution of intraocular pressure in a general population, (2) symptoms of eye pain or vision loss, (3) risk factors predisposing permanent damage to the eye, and (4) clinical signs of damage to the eye revealed by physical examination or tests of visual function.

Many factors can have a long-term influence or produce transient fluctuations in intraocular pressure (see Tables 28.1 and 28.2).

In three studies of intraocular pressure distribution in general populations, the mean intraocular pressure reported ranges from 15.91 to 17.18 (Table 28.3). Given the many factors that influence the definition of normal intraocular pressure, there is considerable overlapping of intraocular pressure distribution within nonglaucoma and glaucoma populations (Figure 28.2). The boundary between normal intraocular pressure and abnormal low intraocular pressure (hypotony) is also not precise. An intraocular pressure of less than 10 mm Hg is of concern. In those cases, however, other clinical signs of inadequate intraocular pressure dominate the clinical presentation.

## Production and Outflow of Aqueous Humor

**A. Anatomy of anterior and posterior chambers**

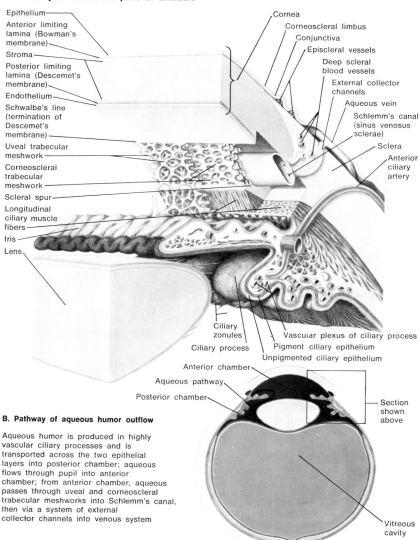

Epithelium

Anterior limiting lamina (Bowman's membrane)

Stroma

Posterior limiting lamina (Descemet's membrane)

Endothelium

Schwalbe's line (termination of Descemet's membrane)

Uveal trabecular meshwork

Corneoscleral trabecular meshwork

Scleral spur

Longitudinal ciliary muscle fibers

Iris

Lens

Cornea

Corneoscleral limbus

Conjunctiva

Episcleral vessels

Deep scleral blood vessels

External collector channels

Aqueous vein

Schlemm's canal (sinus venosus sclerae)

Sclera

Anterior ciliary artery

Ciliary zonules

Ciliary process

Vascular plexus of ciliary process

Pigment ciliary epithelium

Unpigmented ciliary epithelium

Anterior chamber

Aqueous pathway

Posterior chamber

Section shown above

Vitreous cavity

**B. Pathway of aqueous humor outflow**

Aqueous humor is produced in highly vascular ciliary processes and is transported across the two epithelial layers into posterior chamber; aqueous flows through pupil into anterior chamber; from anterior chamber, aqueous passes through uveal and corneoscleral trabecular meshworks into Schlemm's canal, then via a system of external collector channels into venous system

### FIGURE 28.1.
**Production and outflow of aqueous humor.**
With permission of CIBA Pharmaceutical Company, Division of CIBA-GEIGY Corporation. From *Clinical Symposia,* illustrated by John A. Craig, M.D. All rights reserved. Copyright © 1976.

Table 28.1
Transient Fluctuations in Intraocular Pressure

| Factor | Influence on Intraocular Pressure |
|---|---|
| Diurnal variation | Cyclic fluctuations throughout the day; peak may occur at any time of day; daily variation in the IOP by 5 mm Hg or more is abnormal (Drance 1972) |
| Postural variation | IOP increases when changing from sitting to the supine position |
| Exertional influences | Prolonged exercise lowers IOP and straining elevates IOP |

Source: Adapted from Shields 1982.

Table 28.2
Long-Term Influences on Intraocular Pressure

| Factor | Influence on Intraocular Pressure |
|---|---|
| Age | IOP distribution in general population shifts to higher pressures with advancing age |
| Sex | Increase in mean IOP with age is greater in females |
| Refractive error | Myopes tend to have higher pressures |

Table 28.3
Three Studies of Intraocular Pressure
Distributions in General Populations

| Study | IOP (mm Hg) (Mean) | Applanation Tonometer (S.D.) | Number of Individuals | Ages (yr) |
|---|---|---|---|---|
| Armaly (1965) | 15.91 | 3.14 | 2,316 | 20–79 |
| Loewen, Handrup, and Redeker (1976) | 17.18 | 3.78 | 4,661 | 9–89 |
| Ruprecht, Wulle, and Christl (1978) | 16.25 | 3.45 | 8,899 | 5–94 |

# Glaucomas

The glaucomas are a widely divergent group of disorders that represent the leading cause of irreversible blindness in the United States. Prevention of blindness from glaucoma requires early detection and proper treatment.

While the glaucomas are appreciated as a major public health problem, much controversy exists as to their definition, prevalence, etiology, and classification. For all forms of glaucoma, however, three common denominators are accepted as the basis of understanding these disorders: intraocular pressure, the optic nerve head, and visual fields.

Glaucomas differ as to the mechanism

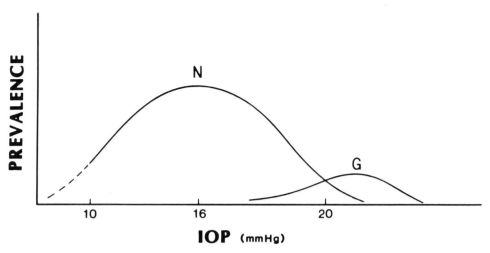

**FIGURE 28.2.**

Prevalence of intraocular pressure measurements in a normal (N) versus a glaucoma (G) population. Note how this theoretical distribution overlaps and illustrates the problem of defining a "normal" IOP.

of increased intraocular pressure. The elevation of intraocular pressure may be the result of hypersecretion of aqueous humor, mechanical blockage of the drainage system, or increased resistance to outflow in the absence of clinically observable ocular tissue changes. Many classification schemas for glaucomas have been developed. Underlying these schemas is an appreciation of the underlying cause of increased intraocular pressure, the concept of primary versus secondary glaucoma, and the clinical appearance of the anterior chamber angle. One such classification system by Shields (1982) is summarized in Tables 28.4, 28.5, and 28.6.

## Glaucomatous Optic Nerve Changes and Visual Fields

Glaucoma, regardless of the etiology of the increased intraocular pressure, is characterized by progressive cupping of the op-

**Table 28.4**
**Primary Glaucomas: Typically Bilateral with Genetic Basis**

*Primary open-angle glaucoma*
IOP consistently above 21 mm Hg in at least one eye
Open, normal appearing anterior chamber angle in the absence of other ocular or systemic abnormality causing increased IOP
Typical glaucomatous visual field or optic nerve head damage

*Primary angle-closure glaucoma; variety of forms, including*
Pupillary block glaucoma: acute, subacute, or chronic; a functional block due to resistance to flow of aqueous humor at point of contact between iris and anterior lens capsule. Resulting forward shift of peripheral iris can lead to complete or partial closure of the anterior chamber angle
Plateau iris: mechanical block of the anterior chamber angle by the last roll of iris if the pupil is dilated, but without pupillary block component

### Table 28.5
### Secondary Glaucomas

Unilateral or bilateral
Inherited or acquired
An associated ocular or systemic abnormality
Contribute to disease process

Glaucomas associated with:
1. Intraocular tumors
2. Disorders of the corneal endothelium
3. Pigmentary dispersion syndrome
4. Disorders of the lens
5. Retinal disorders
6. Ocular inflammation
7. Intraocular hemorrhage
8. Ocular trauma
9. Ocular surgery
10. Steroid-induced
11. Elevated episcleral venous pressure

Source: Adapted from Shields 1982.

### Table 28.6
### Developmental Glaucomas

*Primary congenital glaucoma*
Developmental abnormality obstructs aqueous outflow in the absence of other systemic or ocular defects

*Developmental glaucomas with associated anomalies*
1. Mesodermal dysgeneses of the anterior ocular segment
2. Glaucoma in aniridia
3. Glaucoma with congenital syndromes
4. Phakomatoses: Sturge-Weber Syndrome, von Recklinghausen's neurofibromatosis, von Hippel-Lindau disease, nevus of ota

Source: Adapted from Shields 1982.

tic nerve head, optic atrophy, and visual field loss. The mechanism of optic nerve damage has not been clearly delineated, but appears to be due to three basic mechanisms: (1) elevated intraocular pressure distorts and destroys supportive glial tissue; (2) elevated intraocular pressure shunts the circulation away from the vessels in the optic nerve head and superficial retinal vessels, producing anoxia; and (3) elevated intraocular pressure directly compresses the axons at the lamina cribrosa, interfering with the axoplasmic flow of material from the ganglion cell nuclei layer along the length of the optic nerve.

At some point in the natural history of glaucoma, damage to the optic nerve head is associated with characteristic visual field changes. The argument is often made that clinically observed glaucomatous damage to the optic nerve head or defects in the retinal nerve fiber layer always precede visual field loss. A perfect correction, however, does not exist, and a glaucomatous field defect may present clinically without the distinctive optic disc signs.

# HISTORY

The history can alert the clinician to the presence of glaucoma or to the possibility of its occurrence in the future. General features, presenting symptoms, and other historical information can be of considerable help in the differential diagnosis of glaucoma.

## Symptoms

Primary open-angle glaucoma is insidious, and symptoms usually are not associated with the disease until it is well established. As visual field loss becomes significant, the patient may report some difficulty with dark adaptation, blurring of vision, and difficulty with ambulation because of constricted peripheral vision.

In contrast to open-angle glaucoma, angle-closure glaucoma is characterized by profound symptoms. Acute angle-closure glaucoma may present with blurring of vision, colored halos around light, foggy vision, lacrimation, fullness around the eyes, severe pain about the eye, headache, nausea, vomiting, tooth pain, red eye, and stomach pain. The patient may appear prostrate, with facial pallor, cold extremities, and an irregular pulse. The cluster headache may produce symptoms that closely resemble an acute angle-closure attack, but intraocular pressure will not be elevated, and the absence of other clinical signs of narrow angle can rule out angle-closure glaucoma.

Subacute attacks of angle closure may produce episodic symptoms of blur, colored halos around lights, foggy vision, and mild pain intermittently, particularly at night and in dark surroundings. Severe pain is not expected. Intermittent partial angle closure may have no recognizable symptoms.

## Past Eye History

The many ocular conditions that can cause a secondary glaucoma (Table 28.4) should be kept in mind. Past history of a red eye, trauma, retinal detachment, cataract extraction, or retinal vein occlusion represents a red flag, alerting the clinician to rule out secondary glaucoma.

## Personal Health History

Hypertension can be indirectly related to the presentation of primary open-angle glaucoma. Hypertension may counteract elevated intraocular pressure by providing adequate perfusion of tissue. If the blood pressure is lowered by antihypertensive drugs, glaucoma may result from anoxia of the optic nerve. Severe hypotensive episodes owing to hemorrhage or surgery may produce anoxia to the optic nerve and resultant optic atrophy, which appears as a low-tension glaucoma. Diabetics are at greater risk both for primary open-angle glaucoma and for secondary neovascular angle-closure glaucoma.

As with past eye history, keep in mind the systemic conditions that are associated with the secondary glaucomas.

## Family History

Primary open-angle glaucoma is more prevalent among close relatives of glaucoma patients. Positive family history is a significant prognostic indication for primary angle-closure glaucoma. If a positive family history of glaucoma is elicited, it is helpful to qualify further. For example, in the relative's case, what was the age of onset of glaucoma, history of treatment (eye drops and/or surgery), acute attack or slow onset?

# EXAMINATION

The triad of intraocular pressure measurement, optic nerve head assessment, and visual field testing is the basis of assessment for glaucoma. Evaluation of the anterior segment and anterior chamber angle are also necessary to detect and classify glaucoma. Adjunctive procedures, such as tonography and provocative tests, are sometimes helpful, but are of limited clinical value.

## Tonometry

Glaucoma can occur at any age. It is best to perform applanation tonometry in all patients old enough to permit the procedure. While keeping in mind that normal intraocular pressure is a statistical concept and patients are at risk for low tension glaucoma, pressure readings over 21 mm Hg should be regarded as suspicious.

When a comprehensive assessment of risk factors, optic nerve head, and visual fields proves negative, the term *ocular hypertensive* may be applied to cases in which intraocular pressure is greater than 21 mm Hg.

# External Eye and Anterior Chamber

Circumcorneal injection (ciliary flush) may be present with angle-closure glaucoma or suggest the presence of iritis. In sudden elevations of pressure, a steaminess (edema) and irregularity of the cornea is a common feature associated with symptoms of blurred vision and colored halos around lights, while corneal anesthesia is a late finding in prolonged high pressure. The posterior corneal surface should be examined for pigmentary deposits (Krukenberg's spindle) associated with pigmentary dispersion syndrome and for keratitic precipitates indicative of an inflammatory process and possible posterior and peripheral anterior synechiae. With a history of trauma, evidence of blood staining should be evaluated.

Presence of a prominent Schwalbe's ring warrants gonioscopy to rule out mesodermal dysgenesis and the associated developmental glaucoma. Blisters and vesicles on the corneal endothelium should be noted, since both posterior polymorphus dystrophy and Fuchs' endothelial dystrophy can be associated with secondary glaucomas.

Careful observation is necessary to evaluate the anterior chamber for evidence of cells or flare. Increased protein and white blood cells released into the aqueous in iritis and uveitis may block the trabecular meshwork or be associated with posterior and anterior synechiae. Following trauma, red blood cells may be seen in the anterior chamber and produce elevated intraocular pressure. In addition, red blood cells may also be found in the anterior chamber associated with rubeosis iridis.

# Anterior Chamber Angle

Examine the anterior chamber angle to determine the presence of a narrow or closed angle. Estimation of the anterior chamber angle is done by means of a penlight, slit lamp, or gonioscope. By shining a penlight from the side of the cornea, a gross estimate of narrow angle is made. If the iris is bowed forward, a shadow is cast on the side of the iris opposite the light.

Using a slit lamp, an optic section of the cornea is viewed immediately adjacent to the limbus with the illumination 60° away from the microscope. The light is focused on the posterior cornea. The width of the aqueous-filled space between the corneal endothelium and the iris is compared to the width of the corneal section. With a ratio of one, the angle is said to be wide open; a ratio from ¼ to ½ is also open. These correspond to an angle of 20° to 45° and are incapable of closure. A ratio of ¼ is a moderately narrow angle (20°) and capable of closure, while a ratio of less than ¼ is a narrow angle of 10°, and angle closure is likely. If there is only a minimal space, the angle is almost closed and is called a slit angle. No aqueous space is seen in the closed angle. This should be estimated nasally, temporally, superiorly, and inferiorly.

The gonioscope allows viewing from the pupil along the anterior iris up to the corneal endothelium. In a wide-open (45°) angle, all of the structures of the angle recess are visualized. The structures seen in an open angle are

1. Angle recess and insertion of the root of the iris.
2. Ciliary body, if the iris attaches posterior to the scleral spur. It appears pale in light-colored eyes and brown in darkly pigmented eyes.
3. Iris process extending from the root of the iris to the scleral spur and occasionally Schwalbe's line. These are seen as thin fibers that follow the contour of the angle recess.

4. Scleral spur, which is seen as a whitish band.

5. Trabecular meshwork: a faint-bluish, glistening, translucent area in young people that fills with pigment that is most dense in the posterior portion. Schlemm's canal can be seen through the trabecular meshwork if it is filled with blood.

6. Schwalbe's line: a faint white line that represents the termination of Descemet's membrane. It is a shelflike projection into the anterior chamber on which pigment may collect.

The anterior chamber angle is evaluated by the degree to which these structures can be seen:

1. Open angle (35°–45°): All of the structures are visible; the iris plane is flat. Closure is not possible.

2. Open angle (20°–35°): The ciliary-body band and scleral spur are minimally visible or obstructed. The trabecular meshwork and Schlemm's canal are seen. Closure is not possible.

3. Narrow angle (20°): The scleral spur and the posterior trabecular meshwork is not visualized. Part of Schlemm's canal is seen. Closure is possible.

4. Narrow angle (10°): Only the anterior half of the trabecular meshwork is visible. Angle closure is likely.

5. Slit or closed angle: No angle structures are visualized; the angle is partially or completely closed.

With the gonioscope, examine the angle for excessive pigment in the trabeculum and on Schwalbe's line, for the whitish flakes of pseudoexfoliation, for peripheral anterior synechiae, and for congenital defects. Examine for anterior insertion of the root of the iris to detect a plateau iris. Tumors of the angle and neovascularization should be noted.

Traumatic recession of the angle, is seen as a cleft between the circular and longitudinal fibers of the ciliary body, and gives the appearance of a localized, deepened anterior chamber angle in the area of the tear. The iris attachment appears to be displaced posterior to the scleral spur. The iris processes in the area are discontinuous.

## Iris

The goal of assessment of the iris is to rule out posterior synechiae, secondary glaucoma of iridocorneal endothelial syndrome, pigmentary glaucoma, and rubeosis iridis.

Examine the iris with the slit lamp for evidence of angle closure, depigmentation, atrophic area, and paralysis. Areas of depigmentation, associated with increased trabecular pigment, and Krukenberg's spindle suggest pigmentary glaucoma. White flakes on the pupillary border are seen in pseudoexfoliation of the lens. Rubeosis iridis is associated with diabetes, central retinal artery, or vein occlusion, and can produce hemorrhages into the anterior chamber, resulting in a secondary glaucoma.

## Lens

Exfoliative syndrome, cataracts, and a dislocated lens can contribute to several forms of glaucoma. Characteristically, exfoliation materials on the anterior lens capsule may have three distinct zones: central translucent disc, clear surrounding zone, and a peripheral granular zone. This appearance should be distinguished from capsular delamination, which is characterized by thin, curled membranes that are separated from the anterior lens capsule.

Lens swelling in an advanced cataract can narrow the anterior chamber and contribute to angle-closure glaucoma. Subluxation or complete dislocation of the lens can lead to secondary glaucomas by a variety of mechanisms.

# Optic Nerve Head

The examination of the optic nerve head is a critical aspect in glaucoma examination. The optic nerve head can be examined by direct or indirect ophthalmoscopy, by slit lamp in conjunction with the Hruby lens or contact lens, and by fundus photography. The Hruby lens or fundus contact lens allows binocular viewing of the nerve head with greater magnification and stereopsis.

With regard to glaucomatous damage to the optic nerve head, an important parameter is the edge of the optic cup. This edge represents a change in the contour of the surface of the optic disc. While the area of the cup and the area of central disc pallor are frequently the same, this is not always the case. Hence the importance of using other monocular clues, such as surface vessel bending, to locate the edge of the optic cup.

Initial evaluation of the optic disc should include noting the cup/disc ratio (horizontal and vertical dimensions) and shape of the cup. Also note the contour of the cup. It may be cylindrical, dish-like, or steep nasally and sloping toward the temporal edge. The rim of neural tissue surrounding the cup should be pink and symmetrical to the outer edge of the optic disc.

Although the physiologic optic cup does vary considerably in size and shape, a distinguishing feature in normal eyes is that normal cups are typically symmetrical between fellow eyes and exhibit an evenness of the neural rim tissue. Additional features of disc changes suggestive of glaucoma are summarized in Table 28.7. Disc drawings and stereo fundus photos are of considerable value in monitoring any changes in the appearance of these parameters over time.

The peripapillary region should also be evaluated to rule out nerve fiber bundle defects. These dark stripes along the normal retinal axon striations represent areas of axonal bundle loss. These changes correlate highly with visual field changes, but

**Table 28.7**
**Signs of Glaucomatous Optic Atrophy**

*Glaucomatous cupping*
Alert to focal loss of neural rim at superior and inferior borders, the cup becomes more vertically oval than the disc
Alert to the progression of cupping beyond the area of pallor, use kinking of vessels or stereoscopic technique

*Vascular changes*
Alert to baring of the circumlinear vessel
Alert to splinter hemorrhages, in open-angle glaucoma is associated with higher incidence of field loss

are not specific to glaucoma and occur with other causes of optic atrophy (see Chapter 31). The best method for recording nerve fiber bundle defects is with a regular fundus camera, $2\times$ magnification attachment, Kodak Plus-X film, and a green filter.

# Visual Fields

Isopter contraction and baring of the blind spot are often cited as early glaucomatous visual field changes. Unfortunately, these early signs are not definitive and may be associated with other factors.

Arcuate or Bjerrum visual field defects are more characteristic of glaucoma. These defects in the nerve fiber bundle may occur anywhere along the path of fibers 5° to 20° around fixation. Hart and Becker (1982) suggest from their long-term follow-up study of 251 patients with chronic open-angle glaucoma and 826 patients with ocular hypertension that damage to the nerve fiber bundles occurs in three phases (Table 28.8).

While the subthreshold and threshold stages of primary open-angle glaucoma are prolonged, the late phase is characterized by extensive losses in visual fields. Hart and Becker (1982) propose a hypothetical model of the natural history of glaucoma damage based on the observation of a slow rate of irreversible, anatomic destruction of nerve fibers. They argue that the threshold stage, when defects first become manifest, actually occurs late in the disease process. Thus, since in phase 3 only a small number of fibers remain, little damage is needed to produce abrupt and extensive loss in visual fields.

## Tonography

The measurement of the facility of aqueous outflow using an electronically modified Schiøtz tonometer is diagnostic in open-angle glaucoma. After an initial measurement of intraocular pressure ($P_o$), the instrument is placed on the eye for 4 minutes and the drop in pressure measured. The facility of outflow ($C$) is determined by reference to charts. Normal facility of outflow is considered to be 0.28, while that of 0.18 or less is considered abnormal. A calculation of $P_o/C$ greater than 100 is abnormal, and above 125 is considered pathologic.

Table 28.8
Phases of Glaucomatous Damage to
Bjerrum Region

| Phase 1 | Subthreshold phase in which visual field appears normal, but IOP is markedly elevated |
| | Nonspecific visual field changes, such as isopter contraction, may be present |
| | Optic atrophy, afferent pupillary defect, deficient color vision, and reduced contrast sensitivity often present in the absence of field changes |
| Phase 2 | Threshold of detectable visual field defects |
| | Shallow, often transient defects |
| | Barely detectable with more sensitive perimetric test, static testing most sensitive, but less efficient than kinetic perimetry |
| Phase 3 | Manifest glaucomatous defects that progress despite treatment |
| | Extension of size and density of loss to cover entire Bjerrum area |

Source: Adapted from Hart and Becker 1982.

# CLINICAL SIGNIFICANCE

## Hypotony

Ocular hypotony may be associated with decreased resistance to outflow, such as would occur after a penetrating wound or as a complication of glaucoma surgery. Ocular hypotony can also occur in the presence of decreased aqueous production, which may accompany uveitis, ocular trauma, or retinal detachment. Systemic diseases, such as diabetic coma and uremic coma, may cause hypotony from metabolic disturbances. Drugs such as carbonic anhydrase inhibitors and cardiac glycosides inhibit aqueous formation. Drugs that raise the osmolarity of the blood, such as glycerol, urea, and mannitol, will lower intraocular pressure by osmosis.

Ocular hypotony is not a problem to normal ocular function unless the pressure is acutely low, in which case the lack of compensating pressure against the intraocular vasculature produces venous stasis and leakage of plasma into the ocular tissue. Subsequent degeneration and edema of the optic nerve head produces atrophy. The shape of the eye may be affected; other sequellae include corneal edema, vitreous clouding, and retinal folds.

## Primary Open-Angle Glaucoma

Primary open-angle glaucoma is the most common type of glaucoma. It is a bilateral disease that causes progressive optic nerve damage and visual field loss. The anterior chamber angle appears to be anatomically normal. The increased pressure, however, is due to resistance to aqueous outflow in the posterior trabeculum and Schlemm's canal. The existence of prolonged elevated intraocular pressure causes a degeneration and sclerosis of the trabeculum and the cells lining Schlemm's canal, which results in an increasing resistance to outflow.

Patients with primary open-angle glaucoma may exhibit normal pressure readings on one measurement. Within the trabeculum and ciliary body are neuropressure receptors that sense changes in intraocular pressure and produce a feedback loop to the ciliary body, which causes a fluctuating decrease in aqueous production. The diurnal variation in primary open-angle glaucoma is greater than normal (mean of $11 \pm 5.7$ mm Hg).

Myopic eyes are at greater risk of developing glaucoma in the presence of elevated intraocular pressure. The mechanism may be related to more vulnerability to pressure at the optic disc or the drainage system. Highly myopic eyes have shallower optic cups owing to the lamina cribrosa being closer to the retinal surface, tilted discs, and myopic degeneration around the disc. The myopic eye also has a lower scleral rigidity. The appearance of the optic nerve head may make it more difficult to assess changes in the cupping, while lower scleral rigidity produces a false low measurement of intraocular tension with some tonometers (Table 28.9).

The relationship of high blood pressure and elevated intraocular pressure has not been found to be significant; however, a patient with high intraocular pressure whose blood pressure is suddenly reduced by antihypertensive medications may be at risk. In these cases, the elevated intraocular pressure may prevent adequate perfusion of ocular tissues, and atrophy of the optic nerve may result.

Primary open-angle glaucoma may occur in the presence of normal intraocular pressure. This is termed low-tension glaucoma. In these cases a weakened vascular structure is more susceptible to compression by intraocular pressure.

In the presence of a central retinal vein occlusion, the fellow eye must be carefully evaluated for glaucoma and the affected eye must be watched for neovascular glaucoma.

Table 28.9
General Predisposing Factors: Primary Glaucomas

| Factor | Primary Open-Angle Glaucoma | Primary Closed-Angle Glaucoma |
|---|---|---|
| Age | Prevalence increased with age, but *not* limited to those over 40 years old | Increased prevalence with age corresponds to diminished depth and volume of anterior chamber |
| Race | More common among blacks | Less common among blacks |
| Sex | No definitive difference | More common among females than males |
| Refractive error | More common among myopes | More common in hyperopes |

# Primary Angle-Closure Glaucoma

In the normal eye, the iris and the cornea produce an anterior chamber angle of approximately 45°. In angle-closure glaucoma, abnormal position of the iris reduces the anterior chamber angle, occludes the angle, and blocks drainage of the aqueous humor through the trabecular meshwork.

Narrow angles, a bilateral, inherited trait, are often associated with the smaller hyperopic eye with its well-developed ciliary body, flatter cornea, anterior insertion of iris, and anteriorly displaced lens (see Table 28.9).

With age, the lens tends to swell, which displaces the iris forward and produces an increasingly narrow angle. Narrow-angle glaucoma is, therefore, more prevalent in the older population, with initial onset at age 55 to 60 years. Angle-closure glaucoma is more common in white women than white men, but equally distributed between sexes in the black population.

The mechanism by which the iris occludes the angle is usually associated with a pupillary block. The iris normally rests against the anterior lens surface. In the normal eye, with an open angle, the pressure of the iris against the lens is minimal. In the eye with a shallow anterior chamber, the forward position of the lens causes a greater pressure between the iris and the lens, resulting in a resistance to the flow of aqueous humor from the posterior chamber to the anterior chamber, which constitutes a functional blockage of the pupil. This increased fluid pressure causes the iris to bulge forward at its root, which is its weakest point anatomically. In the presence of a narrow angle, the iris is pushed up against the cornea and blocks the trabecular meshwork.

Pupillary block may occur in a variety of situations. With a mid-dilated pupil there is maximum contact between the iris and the lens, and the risk for pupillary block is greatest. Thus, the mid-dilated pupil offers the greatest risk of angle closure. There is sufficient iris-lens contact to constitute a pupillary block, and the iris is loose and able to bulge forward more easily. With a widely dilated pupil, there is minimum contact of the iris and lens, and pupillary block is unlikely. If the angle is very narrow, increased iris tissue at the angle may cause closure.

In plateau iris, an uncommon condition, the iris inserts quite anteriorly. In this case, the iris is seen to be in a flat plane, but the angle recess is quite narrow. Dilation of the pupil causes the iris to block the angle.

With angle closure, intraocular pressure may rise quickly up to that of the arterial pressure. This sudden rise causes significant ocular congestion and severe symptomatology. If the attack is not broken quickly, severe loss of vision can occur. The intraocular congestion caused by the sudden rise in pressure may produce exudation of protein, causing peripheral anterior synechiae and permanent obstruction of the angle in the area of the synechiae.

# Developmental Glaucomas

The most common type of congenital glaucoma, although rare, is primary congenital glaucoma. It is a genetically determined disease, usually bilateral, with increased pressure from dysplasia of the anterior chamber angle, with the iris inserting directly into the trabeculum. The angle is wide open, there is an absence of an angle recess, and the trabeculum is thickened. The presence of a membrane covering the trabeculum is debated. Glaucoma is associated with many other congenital anomalies and syndromes (Table 28.4). The effect of glaucoma on infants is significantly different than that in adults. The tissue of the infant eye is weak and capable of distention under pressure, producing enlargement of the cornea and sclera. The corneal enlargement can result in stretching and splitting of Descemet's membrane.

# Secondary Glaucoma

Glaucoma can occur secondary to systemic or ocular disease, effects of chemicals and drugs, and ocular trauma (Table 28.3). In an inflamed eye, the aqueous has a higher protein content, is more viscose, and contains cellular and inflammatory particulate matter. A viscose, cell-laden aqueous can block the pores of the trabecular meshwork and drainage canals. Initially, however, the intraocular pressure may drop because of suppression of aqueous production in the diseased ciliary body. If production of aqueous resumes in the presence of an increased resistance to outflow, then a severe rise in pressure occurs.

Intraocular inflammation may also cause anterior or posterior synechiae. Inflammatory exudation may cause attachments of the iris to the anterior lens surface (posterior synechia) or of the root of the iris to the cornea (peripheral anterior synchia). Synechiae may occlude the anterior chamber angle, causing a secondary angle-closure glaucoma.

Hyphema, whether spontaneous or traumatic, may block the outflow of aqueous and produce a severe rise in intraocular pressure. Hemorrhage into the anterior chamber or vitreous, which is not sufficient to block the outflow, may damage the drainage system by the products of the blood breakdown (hemosiderosis) and produce open-angle glaucoma. These patients need long-term follow-up care to rule out delayed presentation of glaucoma.

Angle recession from blunt trauma is often seen after the resolution of a traumatic hyphema. A secondary glaucoma may result from angle recession. It may occur shortly after the trauma and resolve, or may occur up to 10 years after the traumatic incident.

The lens may contribute to secondary glaucoma. A leaking hypermature cataract can cause phakolytic glaucoma. In this uncommon condition, phagocytes carrying lens material block the angle and cause a rise in intraocular pressure that may be impossible to control. The release of lens material into the eye, either spontaneously or owing to trauma or cataract extraction, may trigger a severe uveitis with a great inflammatory response, consequent tissue damage, and secondary glaucoma.

Postoperative secondary glaucoma may result after glaucoma surgery or cataract extraction. After glaucoma surgery there may be damage to the drainage system, formation of peripheral anterior synechiae, or a displacement of the iris-lens diaphragm, producing a complete angle closure known as *malignant glaucoma*. Following cataract extraction, secondary glaucoma may result from the formation of peripheral anterior synechiae associated with delays in reforming the anterior chamber and pupillary block caused by the vitrous occluding the pupil. A postoperative uveitis or hyphema may be produced. Injecting too much air into the anterior chamber may precipitate an iris bombé. The air bubble presses against the iris, preventing the aqueous flow through the pupil. Another possible complication is that the use of alpha chymotrypsin in cataract extraction can block the trabeculum, precipitating its inflammation and producing a temporary glaucoma. Epithelial downgrowth, as a complication of cataract extraction or a sequela of penetrating ocular traumas, can occlude the angle and cause glaucoma.

Pigmentary dispersion syndrome, with deposition of the iris pigment onto the lens, zonules, cornea, and the trabecular meshwork, is associated with a glaucoma. The iris pigment forms a characteristic pattern on the posterior cornea, a long, slender, vertical line centrally, which is known as *Krukenberg's spindle*. Whether the pigment actually causes the increased intraocular pressure is unknown, but the presence of pigment in the anterior chamber angle must be considered a risk factor for the presence of glaucoma.

Intraocular tumors may give rise to a unilateral glaucoma. The tumor may actually block the angle; however, malignant melanomas may cause increased intraocular pressure even when located in the posterior pole.

Another secondary glaucoma is caused by neovascularization of the iris, rubeosis iridis. It most often occurs as a sequela of proliferative diabetic retinopathy and/or central retinal vein occlusion. Less commonly rubeosis occurs with central retinal artery occlusion, malignant melanoma, and retinal detachments. The new vessels are fragile and hemorrhages into the anterior chamber occur frequently.

## Summary

Elevation of intraocular pressure produces glaucoma with its progressive optic nerve damage and visual field loss. Abnormally low intraocular pressure, ocular hypotony, results in loss of normal tissue shape, vascular leakage, and a loss of ocular function.

The glaucomas are a widely divergent group of disorders. Early detection and proper treatment are paramount to preventing blindness. A thorough case history investigating presenting symptoms, eye history, general health history, and family history will alert the clinician to the possibility of glaucoma and indicate those tests needed to fully assess its presence.

Acute angle-closure glaucoma is an ocular emergency; any delays in treatment risk permanent damage to the angle structures and dramatic vision loss. Ocular hypotony and subacute angle-closure glaucoma are ocular urgencies requiring prompt treatment to avoid further complications.

Routine periodic reevaluation of the patient at risk to glaucoma is needed to assess ocular structure and function. Photographs of the optic nerve provide the best method of documenting its appearance for comparison at a future date. Detailed visual field studies provide a quantitative measure of optic nerve function and glaucomatous damage. But, eyes with elevated IOP but normal fields cannot be assumed to have no damage. Patients at risk must be counseled as to the possibility of developing glaucoma and the need for periodic follow-up.

# References

Armaly MF. On the distribution of applanation pressure. I. Statistical features and the effect of age, sex, and family history of glaucoma. Arch Ophthal 1965;73:111.

Brandreth RH. Clinical slit lamp biomicroscopy. Berkeley: RH Brandreth, 1978.

Cockburn DM. Slit lamp estimate of anterior chamber depth. Am J Optom Physiol Opt 1982;59:904–908.

Cockburn DM. Prevalence and significance of narrow anterior chamber angles in optometric practice. Am J Optom Physiol Opt 1981;58:171–175.

Duke-Elder S, Jay B. Glaucoma and hypotony. In: Duke-Elder S, ed. System of ophthalmology. St. Louis: C.V. Mosby, 1969;XI:379–746.

Godio LB, Modesir RRK, Cullen AP. Ratio of the size of the optic cup to size of the disc. Am J Optom Physiol Opt 1981;58:367–371.

Hart WM, Becker B. The onset and evolution of glaucomatous visual field defects. Ophthalmology (Rochester) 1982;89:268–279.

Kass MA, et al. Risk factors favoring the development of glaucomatous visual field loss in ocular hypertension. Surv Ophthalmol 1980;25:(3):155–162.

Loewen U, Handrup B, Redeker A. Results

of a glaucoma mass screening program. Klin Monatsbl Augenheilkd 1976;169:754.

McDaniel DR, Tribbey CL, Tobias GS. Effects of moderate exercise on intraocular pressure. Am J Optom Physiol Opt 1983;60:154—157.

Nesterov A, Bunin A, Katsnelson L. Intraocular pressure. Moscow: MIR Publishers, 1978.

Ruprecht KW, Wulle KG, Christl HL. Applanation tonometry within medical diagnostic "check-up" programs. Klin Monatsbl Augenheilkd 1978;172:332.

Shields MB. A study guide for glaucoma. Baltimore; Williams & Wilkins, 1982.

# John W. Potter
# VITREOUS 29

*The vitreous is a highly transparent connective tissue structure composed of 99% water and 1% solids. It is a gel in its normal state, but in disease it becomes quite liquid.*

## BACKGROUND

The vitreous, an intriguing ocular tissue occupying two-thirds of the volume of the eye, is one of the most difficult ocular tissues to examine clinically. The major obstacle to the examination of the vitreous is that it is mostly water, and therefore only the fibers and membranes of the vitreous can be observed. When using the ophthalmoscope, only rather dense opacities in the vitreous can be observed against the red-orange choroidal glow. With the slit lamp microscope, however, fine fibers and membranes in the vitreous can be seen by the Tyndall effect. Even with the finest instrumentation and technique, the clinician is confronted with a tissue that is capable of changing morphology from semisolid to liquid in a brief period.

The vitreous body is roughly the shape of a hemisphere. The flatter portion of the hemisphere is adjacent to the lens, ciliary body, and the zonules. The curved, posterior section of the vitreous hemisphere attaches to the inner sensory retina. The vitreous base, an area of one disk diameter on either side of the ora serrata, separates the anterior and posterior vitreous. The anterior one-third of the posterior vitreous can be readily observed with the slit lamp

microscope through a dilated pupil; however, the examination of the remaining two-thirds of the vitreous requires special techniques. The ophthalmoscope may be used to view opacities in the vitreous, although magnification is limited with the ophthalmoscope and only retroillumination is possible.

The anterior vitreous is most easily observed in aphakic eyes. When the pupils are dilated, the entire vitreous will not tumble into the anterior chamber because the anterior vitreous is firmly attached to the vitreous base. The anterior face of the vitreous is actually a condensed membrane, glasslike, or hyaloid. The anterior hyaloid membrane attaches to the vitreous base, rests against anterior segment structures such as the ciliary body, and anteriorly attaches to the back of the lens. The anterior attachment to the lens is called *Wieger's ligament.*

The posterior hyaloid membrane surrounds the posterior vitreous. Cloquet's canal, a prominent structure in the posterior vitreous, runs from the back surface of the lens through the vitreous to the optic disc. The inner tubular part of the canal is optically empty, but the outer, sur-

391

rounding condensed membranes can easily be observed in the anterior portion of the vitreous in young eyes. These surrounding membranes are called *plicated membranes*. These membranes are quite mobile, especially upon eye movements. The remainder of the contents of the vitreous is composed of the fibers of the vitreous and accompanying optically empty areas.

The posterior hyaloid membrane attaches to the inner retina in three distinct locations. The strongest attachment of both the anterior and posterior vitreous is the vitreous base. The vitreous base extends one disc-diameter on either side of the ora serrata. Occasionally, there is some variability in the posterior extension of the vitreous base that is determined by the uniqueness of the vitreoretinal interface. The next strongest attachment of the vitreous occurs at the optic disc. This attachment is quite firm. In fact, if the posterior hyaloid membrane separates from the optic disc, the glial tissue connection of the vitreous to the optic disc may be torn off, staying adherent to the posterior hyaloid face. Next in strength of attachment is the macula. In this area, the attachment is about the size of the optic disc, but is oriented horizontally. It has been suggested that the vitreous may be attached to the crossings of retinal arterioles and venules, but this has not been proved. In addition to these normal attachments, the vitreous may be adherent to the retina at the site of vitreoretinal abnormalities associated with a variety of retinal and retinochoroidal diseases and disorders.

Because the vitreous is so intimately associated with the sensory retina, the majority of signs and symptoms of disease are related to the dynamics of these attachments. There are four symptoms that can be produced as a result of its relationship with the retina: floaters, light flashes, metamorphopsia, and blurred vision.

Since the majority of these symptoms can be produced as a consequence of aging changes within the vitreous, the natural responses of the vitreous to age will serve as a model for understanding how signs and symptoms in vitreoretinal abnormalities occur. With increasing age, or in the presence of any of a variety of intraocular inflammations, the vitreous responds by undergoing degenerative changes. When this occurs, two distinct processes take place: liquefaction and syneresis. Liquefaction represents the formation of optically empty spaces within the normal vitreous. Since these cavities are optically empty, they appear black with the slit lamp microscope because of a reduced or absent Tyndall effect. It is not possible to observe these pockets of liquid vitreous with the ophthalmoscope. These cavities within the vitreous are called *lacunae*. Syneresis represents a drawing together of particles within the vitreous, and when the fibers of the vitreous become more condensed, syneresis has begun. As the fibers condense further, they may appear to float freely within the liquefying vitreous. The clinical appearance of these broken fibers is called *fibrillary degeneration* of the vitreous. During the processes of syneresis and liquefaction, the patient may report the onset of floaters, which actually represent the condensing fibers of the vitreous casting their shadows onto the sensory retina. Within the liquefying vitreous, the floating, condensed fibers of the vitreous may cause annoying symptoms as they continue to become more mobile. Because the posterior hyaloid membrane attaches to the inner retina, the collapsing vitreous gel may cause the patient to see a phosphene, which is most often described as flashes of light. These flashes of light occur intermittently in the periphery of the field of view. For some unknown reason, the flashes of light reported by patients most often occur in the temporal field. The two symptoms of floaters and flashes of light are ubiquitous to diseases and disorders of the vitreous.

As liquefaction and syneresis are occurring, the vitreous may tug on the retina at its attachment at the macula. If this is severe enough to cause the outer layers of the retina to be disturbed, they may become distorted. If this occurs, the alignment of the visual receptors may become disoriented, resulting in symptoms of metamorphopsia. With metamorphopsia, it would seem that patients would also have an accompanying decrease in visual acuity. This is not the common manifestation, however. The patient may have a set of symptoms of visual disturbances with central vision; but the Snellen acuity may be only minimally altered.

Under certain circumstances, the vitreous may tug on the macula with such force that the macula may become so distorted that the patient can have a significant reduction in Snellen acuity. As long as hemorrhage is not present, the visual acuity may not be severely diminished. If a hemorrhage is present, the visual acuity may be remarkably reduced, and the patient may report a dense central scotoma.

Collapse of the vitreous generally begins with liquefaction in front of the macula. As a result of the collapse of the vitreous, the posterior hyaloid membrane becomes separated from the inner retina. When this occurs, posterior vitreous detachment has taken place. The clinician may now be able to observe the posterior

hyaloid face of the vitreous within the anterior one-third of the vitreous. In addition, the posterior face of the vitreous may have a round or oval glial ring attached. This ring represents the glial attachment of the vitreous to the optic disc (Figure 29.1).

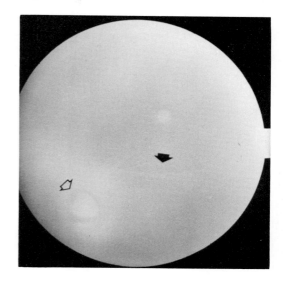

FIGURE 29.1.
Prepapillary annular opacity in posterior vitreous detachment; annular opacity *(hollow arrow)*, posterior hyloid membrane *(bold arrow)*.

# HISTORY

The interview and history of patients with diseases and disorders of the vitreous can present a significant challenge. Patients can report a variety of symptoms, and others will have significant abnormalities within the vitreous and few symptoms.

Many patients report floating opacities in their field of vision. These may represent abnormalities of the preocular tear film, and not the vitreous. To differentiate vitreous symptoms from preocular tear film symptoms, ask if the floaters move with blinking when the eye is stationary. Those

floaters in the preocular tear film will move about, while those in the vitreous will remain stable. Patients can have preocular tear-film floaters and vitreous floaters.

Patients with vitreous floaters may report them to be of various sizes, but usually they appear as small lines. The symptoms may represent either fibrillary degeneration in the vitreous or the prepapillary ring opacity from the optic disc. These symptoms are often vague in onset and tend to linger until the floater either settles out of the line of sight or local retinal adaptation occurs. Sometimes a patient may complain about a floater and, when the clinician examines the vitreous, the floater cannot be found. In other cases, the clinician may observe a large floater, and when the patient is questioned about this directly, the patient will not volunteer that any floaters can be seen.

Be very suspicious of a complaint of a sudden onset of a shower of small floaters if the event is associated with light flashes. This set of symptoms may represent the onset of a small hemorrhage in the vitreous. The shower actually represents red blood cells and pigment epithelium cells cast into the vitreous, associated with a break in the sensory retina. Isolated flashes of light with no associated symptoms can occur in healthy eyes and, rarely, can be due to compressive lesions and local ischemia within the visual pathway. Migraine photopsia, with or without headache, can mimic the light flashes caused by vitreoretinal traction (see Chapter 7).

Metamorphopsia and blurred vision are not temporary or fleeting, but they often follow episodes of either flashes of light or floaters. The best method to evaluate these symptoms is to examine carefully the macula and the posterior pole.

# EXAMINATION

After determining that the symptoms are vitreous or vitreoretinal in origin, use the ophthalmoscope and the slit lamp microscope to evaluate the vitreous. Begin the physical examination with an overall inspection of the vitreous, ideally with the binocular indirect ophthalmoscope through a dilated pupil. Initially view the posterior chamber without a condensing lens, alert to any gross floaters in retroillumination. Generally, it is easier to observe the prepapillary ring opacity in detail with the direct ophthalmoscope because of the advantages of magnification and precise focusing.

The next step is to evaluate the retina. Search for retinal abnormalities in all quadrants of the eye. It is often particularly rewarding to view the retina adjacent to the vitreous base, a likely location for retinal breaks. There are basically two kinds of retinal breaks: holes and tears. A hole is surrounded by an area of retinal detachment that causes the retina around the hole to appear gray in color. Since the hole is round, and is contrasted against the underlying burgundy-colored retinal pigment epithelium, retinal holes are sharply defined. Holes are generally less than one-quarter disc diameter in size.

Tears in the retina are larger than holes, and often appear to be about the size of one disc diameter. A tear will assume the shape of a horseshoe. As the retina in the tongue of the tear atrophies, the horseshoe shape expands, making discovery more easy. Tears or holes can occur in any quadrant of the retina, but the superotemporal retina is most often involved.

Search for vitreoretinal degenerations and abnormalites that can contribute to vitreous symptoms. The 20-diopter condensing lens is preferred for general inspection of the retina. The 30-diopter lens is helpful when a larger field of view is required. Occasionally, it is much easier to view the area of the vitreous base with the 30-diopter lens.

Depending upon the level of suspicion, scleral indentation can be implemented; it has two advantages. First, the technique can bring into view areas of the far retinal periphery. Second, scleral indentation technique permits the clinician to view fundus details dynamically. On occasion, indenting an area of suspicious retina can reveal subtle holes, tears, or areas of vitreoretinal traction.

The slit lamp microscope is a most valuable aid in diagnosis of diseases and disorders of the vitreous. The major advantages of the slit lamp over the ophthalmoscope are that the Tyndall effect enhances the quality of view, and magnification is variable. In addition, the clinician can employ a mirrored contact lens to examine the vitreous in greater detail and in difficult-to-observe locations. Initially, use a low magnification of 10 or 15 times. Direct the beam into the eye with a wide angle, maximizing the Tyndall effect, and view the fine fibers of the vitreous against a black background. The fibers of the vitreous will appear as gray white threads. In the presence of nuclear sclerosis cataract, the fibers may appear somewhat yellow in color. Membranes are more opaque than fibers and appear as gray white colored sheets. Especially in young eyes, it is possible to view the plicated membranes of Cloquet's canal. Because the vitreous is dependent upon gravity, the plicated membranes will appear to be on top of each other; however, if the patient looks up and then straight ahead, the clinician will have an opportunity to view the separated membranes to confirm that they are actually the plicated membranes of Cloquet's canal. This technique of examination is called the *ascension phenomenon*. With older patients, it becomes more difficult to view these plicated membranes. In older eyes, judge the appearance and quality of the vitreous fibers, which with increasing age will appear more opaque and fragmented. In the presence of inflammatory disease in the eye, or hemorrhage, examination of the vitreous may reveal white blood cells, pigment epithelium cells, or red blood cells.

Next, focus the slit lamp microscope back into the anterior one-third of the vitreous. Look here for the posterior hyaloid membrane from a posterior vitreous detachment. If separated from the inner retina, the collapsed posterior hyaloid membrane will appear gray white in color (like the membranes of Cloquet's canal) and somewhat irregular and wavy. In front of the posterior hyaloid membrane, the vit-

reous will consist of fibrillary degeneration, but posterior to the membrane the vitreous will be optically empty and black. When the patient is asked to look up, the posterior hyaloid membrane may move out of view for a few seconds, only to return again to its gravity-dependent position. The posterior hyaloid membrane can be viewed in several positions, while the plicated membranes of Cloquet's canal can only be observed in an area just behind the center of the posterior surface of the lens. By examining through a widely dilated pupil, taking full advantage of the ascension phenomenon and employing a variety of magnifications, the diagnosis of posterior vitreous detachment and other diagnoses can often be made without resorting to the mirrored contact lens.

The mirrored contact lens has the advantage of permitting the examiner to observe the vitreous in other views and to evaluate parts of the vitreous that otherwise would be unobservable because the pupil blocks them from direct view. The most common form of a mirrored contact lens for viewing the vitreous is the three-mirror contact lens; each mirror in the lens has a special function. The lens is inserted just like a goniolens: have the patient look up, apply the lens, and then have the patient look straight ahead. Use the center of the lens for viewing the anterior vitreous and the three mirrors for the periphery of the vitreous and retina. With each increase in steepness of the mirror angle, the view moves anteriorly, even to the point of examining the pars plana.

Two examination tips merit particular attention. Remember that the mirror will make objects viewed appear inverted in the anterior-posterior direction, but not laterally. Second, remember to have patience while learning the technique; take the time to relax so that the patient will relax as well. Use a comfortable elbow rest and wait to become dark adapted. A slow and gentle approach will make the examination of the vitreous cavity with the three-mirror lens much easier.

# CLINICAL SIGNIFICANCE

Four important clinical entities are discussed in this section: asteroid bodies in the vitreous, synchysis scintillans, cells and debris in the vitreous, and posterior vitreous detachment.

Asteroid bodies in the vitreous are commonly observed in clinical practice. They appear as small yellow or white spheres that frequently appear arranged in strings. They are generally unilateral, and although there may be so many asteroid bodies in the vitreous that the fundus may be obscured, the patient rarely, if ever, has symptoms of vision loss. The spheres are most mobile in eyes with posterior vitreous detachment. Following eye movements, the spheres return to their original configuration. Although asteroid bodies in the vitreous have been reported in association with diabetes mellitus, hypercholesterolema, and a variety of other disorders, these associations have remained unproved. It is most likely that asteroid bodies in the vitreous represent a local degeneration of vitreous fibrils, a theory supported by the presence of asteroid bodies almost exclusively in older eyes.

Much literature pertains to synchysis scintillans as a disorder of the vitreous to be differentially diagnosed from asteroid bodies. Synchysis scintillans is said to be a bilateral disorder that occurs in otherwise healthy eyes. The opacities appear as angular flakes that settle to the bottom of the eye when eye movements cease. There is considerable support for the conclusion that synchysis scintillans does not exist as a vitreous disorder to be differentially diagnosed from asteroid bodies in the vitreous. The documented cases of supposed synchysis scintillans are actually mislabeled cases of asteroid bodies or cholesterosis bulbi, a disorder of blind, severely damaged eyes.

The appearance of cells in the vitreous is of great clinical significance. White cells may appear in the vitreous of eyes with optic neuritis, pars planitis, and a variety of other uveal or optic nerve diseases. Clinically, they appear as if someone had shaken salt into the vitreous. When cells in the vitreous are noted, further examination should ensue; each case should be regarded with suspicion. It is often easy to determine the presence of cells in the vitreous because most of the diseases and disorders that precipitate such cellular response are unilateral, so that the fellow eye can serve as a control.

The appearance of pigmented cells in the vitreous should also be viewed with caution. They represent either red blood cells or pigment epithelium cells, caused by tears in the retina or other disorders that cause hemorrhage into the vitreous. When a patient complains of flashes of light or floaters, the clinician should be aware that pigmented cells in the vitreous strongly indicate that a retinal tear has occurred. Careful investigation of the retina should be pursued. One should note, however, that pigmented cells may appear in the vitreous in cases of resolved retinal inflammation or in normal aphakic eyes.

Posterior vitreous detachments occur as an age-related phenomenon, or as a result of insult to the vitreous from disease or trauma. In the decade of life between 50 and 60 years, approximately half of all patients will have posterior vitreous detachment. By the middle of the sixth decade of life, over 90% of patients will have had a posterior vitreous detachment. These separations of the posterior hyaloid membrane, with accompanying collapse of the vitreous, most likely occur within a few hours. In many patients there are no symptoms of light flashes or floaters. In others, however, symptoms are acute and can continue as long as there is traction of the vitreous on the inner retina. It is this traction that causes breaks in the retina. Acute posterior vitreous detachment is an important risk factor in the pathogenesis of retinal breaks and detachments.

It is important to note that half of all

patients who have a retinal detachment do not have a history of light flashes or floaters. It is most significant, however, that those patients with an acute posterior vitreous detachment with symptoms of light flashes and floaters are at greater risk to develop retinal breaks. In these patients it is important to examine zealously the vitreous and the retina. Once the presence of retinal breaks has been confirmed, consultation is advisable. Those patients without breaks noted at the time of examination should be monitored in 2 weeks, or sooner if symptoms increase. After the 2-week examination, the clinician should not dismiss the patient, but should continue maintenance care until clinical judgment determines that the risk of retinal breaks has abated.

# References

Foos RY, Roth AM. Surface structure of the optic nerve head. Vitreopapillary attachments and posterior vitreous detachment. Am J Ophthal 1973;76(5):662–671.

Hruby K. Slit lamp examination of vitreous and retina. Baltimore: Williams & Wilkens, 1967.

Linder B. Acute posterior vitreous detachment and its retinal complications. A clinical biomicroscopic study. Acta Ophthal 1966;87:7–108.

Potter JW. Does synchysis scintillans exist? South J Optom 1981;23(5):6–14.

Potter JW, Newcomb RD. Prevalence of asteroid bodies in a VA optometry clinic. J Am Optom Assoc 1980;51(1):19–25.

Potter JW, Semes LP, Thallemer JM. Prepapillary annular opacity in the diagnosis of posterior vitreous detachment. J Am Optom Assoc 1981;52(8):663–664.

Roth AM, Foos RY. Surface structure of the optic nerve head. 1. Epipapillary membranes. Am J Ophthal 1972;74(5):977–985.

Sigelman J. Vitreous base classification of retinal tears: clinical application. Surv Ophthal 1980;25(2):59–74.

Tolentino FI, Schepens CL, Freeman HM. Vitreoretinal disorders. Philadelphia: W.B. Saunders, 1976.

John W. Potter
Leo Semes

# OCULAR FUNDUS 30

*The ocular fundus is composed of the choroid, the vascular layer of the eye, and the retina, which is composed of the retinal pigment epithelium and the sensory retina. Enveloping the retina are two tissue layers that serve as important barriers. The internal limiting membrane separates the sensory retina from the vitreous while Bruch's membrane delimits the choroid from the retinal pigment epithelium. Certain diseases and disorders that affect the ocular fundus can lead to profound loss of visual function and, potentially, to total blindness. Such conditions require definitive diagnosis and management; others are benign and require only positive identification.*

## BACKGROUND

The ocular fundus consists of a limited number of tissues that respond to disease in a limited number of ways. Once the anatomy of the fundus (Figure 30.1) is understood, the task of relating its response to disease becomes easier.

The vascular choroid of the ocular fundus derives its arterial supply from the short and long posterior ciliary arteries. The short posterior ciliary arteries, which number between 15 and 20, enter the globe at the posterior pole. The long posterior ciliary arteries enter the globe more peripherally, and there are at least two per eye, generally at the 3 and 9 o'clock positions. The arterial supply divides into continually smaller calibre vessels until they end in a dense capillary network, the choriocapillaris, separated from the retinal pigment epithelium only by Bruch's membrane. These vessels are the sole nutritional source for the macula, the avascular portions of the sensory retina, and the vast majority of the peripheral retinal tissues.

About one-third of the choroid is made up of the choriocapillaris, which ends in small lobules about one-fourth disc diameter in size adjacent to the retinal pigment epithelium. A terminal choriocapillaris arteriole feeds each of these lobules.

If one were to remove the retinal pigment epithelium to view the otherwise intact choriocapillaris with the direct ophthalmoscope, the choriocapillaris would appear as a smooth, even, red surface. If one were to remove the retinal pigment epithelium and choriocapillaris, only the larger choroidal blood vessels would be observed, and they would appear as red

RETINA-CHOROID-SCLERA

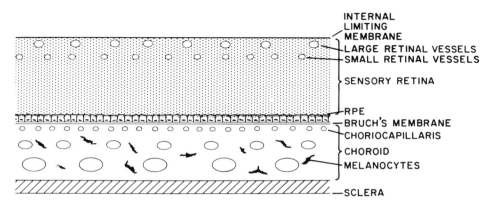

**FIGURE 30.1.**
Retina-choroid-sclera.

lines against a relatively white background, the sclera. The choroid is filled with melanin-containing pigment cells, melanocytes. Melanocytes, along with the choroidal blood vessels, prevent the ophthalmoscopic view from appearing white.

The venous return consists of somewhat larger calibre vessels that travel a course toward a vortex ampulla. These vortex vein systems number between four and six per eye and roughly define the equator of the globe. Clinically, the vortex system appears like a "red octopus," with the wide-angle view provided by the indirect ophthalmoscope. Frequently, there is a pigmented crescent at the scleral exit of the vortex ampulla. This crescent represents adventitial pigment.

Separating the choroid from the retina is Bruch's membrane, a clear cuticular layer that is not observable with the ophthalmoscope but is a very important tissue. Bruch's membrane extends from the ora serrata to the optic disc, and unless there is some break in this tissue, the choroidal and retinal circulations remain separate. At the limits of Bruch's membrane there can be normal communication between the choroidal and retinal

circulations, as in the typical cilioretinal artery. In older eyes, or in the presence of certain ocular diseases, the Bruch's membrane may develop cracks or breaks that can permit these two circulations to communicate.

Overlying the Bruch's membrane-choriocapillaris complex is the neuroectodermal portion of the retina, the retinal pigment epithelium (RPE). The retinal pigment epithelium is a single layer of cells, red brown in color, extending from the ora serrata to the optic disc. Each of the cells is tightly bound to its adjacent cells by zonula occludens. The retinal pigment epithelium is more tightly bound to Bruch's membrane than it is to the sensory retina, the second major portion of the retina. The potential spaces between the retinal pigment epithelium and Bruch's membrane and between the retinal pigment epithelium and sensory retina are frequently involved in ocular diseases that have an accumulation of serous or hemorrhagic components.

The retinal pigment epithelium, by virtue of being only one cell layer thick, betrays itself ophthalmoscopically in one of two ways. Absence of the pigment epithelium cells, such as following degeneration or atrophy, will allow a "window" view of the underlying choroid. If there is a proliferation of cells, such as postinflammatory reactive hyperplasia RPE, clumping will appear as dark, sharply demarcated black areas. This is in contradistinction to pigmented lesions in the choroid, which appear gray because of differences between the melanocytes in the choroid and the melanosomes in the cells of the retinal pigment epithelium. Since there are several layers of these melanocytes in the choroid, a pigmented lesion like a choroidal nevus viewed through the retinal pigment epithelium, which acts like a red brown filter, will have soft borders. This red brown cell layer also absorbs the red-free light of an ophthalmoscope, for example, attenuating visibility of pigmented lesions of the choroid or rendering them invisible.

Embedded in the retinal pigment epithelium is the outermost layer of the sensory retina, the rods and cones. Normally, the sensory retina is ophthalmoscopically transparent. The thickness of the sensory retina varies from about 0.5 mm adjacent to the optic disc to about 0.1 mm at the thinnest part, at the center of the fovea. The sensory retina consists of at least nine defined layers. The outermost layer of the sensory retina is the layer of rods and cones. The rods and cones are loosely attached to the retinal pigment epithelium. The term *retinal detachment* is technically a misnomer since it is the potential space between the layer of rods and cones and the retinal pigment epithelium that becomes manifest in retinal detachment.

The next layer inward from the layer of rods and cones is the external limiting membrane. This is not actually a true membrane since it is formed by the attachment of the sites of the layer of rods and cones and the Müller cells. The next inner layer is the outer nuclear layer, which contains the cell bodies of the rods and cones.

The next inner layer of the sensory retina is the outer plexiform layer. This layer is comprised of the axons of rods and cone

nuclei and dendrites of the bipolar and horizontal cells of the inner nuclear layer. In addition to its physiologic role, the outer plexiform layer of the sensory retina has numerous potential spaces within its structure of vertically arranged fibers. The vertical spaces are like cylinders, such that small amounts of blood can fill these potential spaces and appear clinically like dots or blots. If these small hemorrhages could be observed from the side, they would look like red cylinders instead of dots or blots. Deep hemorrhage in the retina and hard exudates are both located within this layer, as is extracellular retinal edema. Because of the nature of this layer, areas of capillary nonperfusion can produce rings of hard exudate.

The next layer inward is the inner nuclear layer, which contains the nuclei of the bipolar, Müller, horizontal, and amacrine cells. The next inner layer is the inner plexiform layer, which contains the nuclei of the bipolar cells with their synapses and the dendrites of the ganglion cells. The next layer inward is the ganglion cell layer, which varies in thickness from several cell layers about the macula to a single layer in the retinal periphery.

The next layer is the nerve fiber layer. It consists of the axons of the ganglion cells. As nerve fibers course toward the optic disc, their fine texture is almost always observable with the ophthalmoscope. This phenomenon is especially evident with the red-free filter. The nerve fibers arc above and below the macula, spreading in a fanlike fashion into the superior and inferior nasal retina. The larger retinal blood vessels are found in this layer and parallel the distribution of nerve fibers. Since these fibers are arranged in a striate fashion, hemorrhage or cotton-wool patches take on a flame-shape with feathered edges. In the periphery of the sensory retina, the nerve fiber layer is not as compact as in the posterior pole, and for this reason a hemorrhage would appear larger.

The innermost layer of the sensory retina is the internal limiting membrane. This acellular basement membrane extends all over the retina except at the optic disc. Reflections from the internal limiting membrane of the sensory retina are responsible for the appearance of the retinal reflexes so often observed with the direct ophthalmoscope. These water-silk reflexes diminish with age. Perhaps the most frequently observed retinal reflection is the foveal light reflex, which is produced by the sloping sides of the foveola. Depending on angle of this slope, the reflex may appear as a dot or a comma at the level of the retina, just in front of it, or seemingly cast toward the examiner. By the age of 50 years, many people will have lost the foveal light reflex. The presence or absence of a foveal light reflex may not be of diagnostic significance, except in two circumstances: the documented premature loss of a foveal light reflex, or a patient with a foveal light reflex in only one eye or a reflex that appears differently between the two eyes. These conditions only serve to raise a clinician's suspicion and are not specific determinants of ocular disease. Abnormalities in the internal limiting membrane can permit the proliferation of glial cells or the growth of new blood vessels beyond the retinal surface.

There are two blood supplies to the retina. First, the choriocapillaris provides nutrients to the macular portions of the retina, the outer two-thirds of the retina, while the central retinal artery and its branches provide nutrition to the inner third of the sensory retina. The central retinal artery originates from the ophthalmic branch of the internal carotid artery and divides into four branches as it enters the globe at the optic disc. One branch goes into each of the major four quadrants. The larger branches bifurcate into successively smaller branches until they form capillaries, which lie as deep in the retina as the inner aspect of the outer plexiform layer. The venous return is the mirror of the arterial distribution. Ophthalmoscopically, the veins are somewhat larger than the arteries and deeper red in color. At cross-ings between arteries and veins, the vessels share a common sheath.

Frequently, clinicians can take advantage of the ophthalmoscopic picture to relate to the anatomy, even though this is a clear tissue of small dimensions. An excellent way to demonstrate the ophthalmoscopic-anatomic correlation is via the relationship between hemorrhage and anatomy and exudate and anatomy. Hemorrhage in the vitreous is related to abnormalities in the internal limiting membrane; this type of hemorrhage frequently appears to be boat shaped. The boat shape comes from the influence of gravity on the extravasated blood and the nature of the intimate adhesion between the vitreous cortex and the internal limiting membrane. Flame-shaped hemorrhages occur in the nerve fiber layer. Dot and blot hemorrhages occur in the outer plexiform layer, and they would appear as cylinder shaped from the side.

The retinal pigment epithelium normally is a barrier to the passage of serous or formed elements from the choroidal circulation to the retina. Since there are potential spaces between the retinal pigment epithelium and both of its adjacent tissues, however, serous and hemorrhagic fluid can separate the sensory retina from the underlying pigment epithelium, or separate the retinal pigment epithelium from the underlying Bruch's membrane. These fluid separations between retinal pigment epithelium and Bruch's membrane appear like blisters, owing to the fairly tight bond between retinal pigment epithelium cells. Hemorrhage in the choroid appears dark and often spreads throughout the layers of the choroid in such a way that it actually appears deep in the fundus when viewed with the ophthalmoscope.

Exudates are commonly divided into the hard and soft types. Hard exudates are observed in the outer plexiform layer of the retina and are thought to be phagocytized lipid that has escaped from blood vessels. Because of the nature of the outer plexiform layer at the macula, hard exudates here appear ophthalmoscopically in a star-like fashion. Soft exudates, more frequently called cotton-wool patches, represent infarction of the nerve-fiber-layer axons.

Abnormalities within the retinal pigment epithelium are often elementary to note since the retinal pigment epithelium is only one cell-layer thick. An accumulation of retinal pigment epithelium cells appears black, informing the clinician that the tissue involved is retinal pigment epithelium. Absence of retinal pigment epithelium allows the clinician to observe the underlying choroid.

# HISTORY

An efficacious approach to the patient interview may yield information sufficient for a preliminary diagnosis of many fundus diseases and disorders. In order to take advantage of the interview and history of a patient, the clinician needs to use a strategy that will identify sufficient variables to make the task of examination a matter of confirming tentative diagnoses.

The vast majority of fundus diseases and disorders can be divided into two groups: those that cause a decrease in vision and those that do not. Each of these can be divided into two subgroups: of diseases that decrease vision, there are those that cause a decrease in central vision and those that cause diminishing peripheral vision; diseases that do not decrease vision may pose little risk of ever impairing sight or may have a significant potential for eventual loss of vision.

Poor or decreasing central vision is a common complaint among patients. Any changes in the integrity of the macula or any acquired abnormality can lead to immediate symptoms related to this sensitive area of the visual system. Perhaps the simplest way to plot the course of the interview is to ask the patient to talk about any vision loss. In dystrophic conditions, the onset of symptoms generally is gradual and fairly equal in both eyes. For almost all acquired diseases and disorders that cause poor central vision, one eye is affected earlier or more severely. When a young person has a complaint of equally poor central vision in both eyes, the clinician should immediately suspect a dystrophy. It is important to obtain other information from the young person and from the parents. At this point, it may be possible to establish diagnosis from an affected parent who has been examined previously. Many times, the early stages of retinal dystrophies are similar between relatives. Having a relative with the later stages, combined with history, is invaluable information. In addition, it may be possible to establish the mode of inheritance by questioning the parent. The clinician should also request information regarding sensitivity to light, quality of night vision, potential problems with color perception, and any other factors that the affected relative may have noted.

In the acquired macular diseases, it may be possible again to obtain enough information to classify the disease from the interview alone. Many of the symptoms that patients with acquired macular disease report are related to the accumulation of hemorrhage or serous fluid within potential anatomic spaces. When there is hemorrhage in the choroid, the sensory retina is secondarily affected as blood percolates through a compromised Bruch's membrane and the retinal pigment epithelium to damage the photoreceptors. If the hemorrhage is profound, then the retinal pigment epithelium may be elevated like a blister, since the retinal pigment epithelium cells are tightly bound together and firmly adhere to the Bruch's membrane. A fairly large elevation of the retinal pigment epithelium with hemorrhage can cause a patient many symptoms, and visual acuity can remain in the 20/40 to 20/200 range. Other symptoms prevail, however. Such an elevation of the retinal pigment epithelium will cause a moderate central scotoma and some alternation of color vision. Another important symptom to elicit is micropsia, which in the presence of hemorrhage is accompanied by metamorphopsia. Other helpful information can be obtained by asking the patient to compare the vision between his two eyes. Many patients will have already performed this step as a self-test.

In general, it is futile to try to establish exposure to parasitic or fungal fundus disorders until the objective examination of the eye has been completed. There are countless numbers of these exposures that can cause fundus disease, and one can spend much time and effort gathering information that will be discarded quickly once the objective examination of the eye is completed. In other cases, however, the previous health history is very valuable. Although rare, a previous history of a disease like pseudoxanthoma elasticum can alert the clinician to the possibility that the patient may exhibit angioid streaks. More frequently, a history of diabetes or hypertension will alert the clinician to the characteristic vascular changes.

Hemorrhage between the retina and the vitreous should be suspected when the vision is very poor and an Amsler grid defect is very sharp, and sometimes the patient will report red in his vision. When a patient with poor central vision reports seeing red color, the clinician should immediately suspect vitreous hemorrhage.

Retinal vascular disease can cause poor central vision. Diabetic retinopathy is by far the most common disease in this category. Either frank hemorrhage within the sensory retina or macular edema, secondary to vascular impatency, can be at the root of poor central vision. The main symptoms that these patients report are decreased vision and metamorphopsia.

Other retinal vascular disease, such as retinal vein obstruction, can cause similar symptoms. In the presence of a central retinal vein occlusion, central vision will be compromised.

If a patient complains about losing peripheral vision, the clinician is confronted with a different set of problems. Very few inherited diseases affect the peripheral fundus to cause symptoms. Perhaps the classic example of such a disease is retinitis pigmentosa. In this inherited fundus disease, night vision is affected initially; however, the symptom that the clinician is seeking in the history is poor mobility at night.

If a tumor (such as a choroidal melanoma) is present in the peripheral fundus, its growth will disturb the retina and eventually cause a defect in peripheral vision. It is very unlikely that a patient could have a melanoma in each eye at the same time, so the clinician should be aware of the possibility of intraocular tumor if part of the peripheral vision is defective in one eye. In the presence of retinal detachment, similar conditions prevail. A tumor usually grows slowly, however, whereas a retinal detachment generally progresses more rapidly. Pigmented tumors of the ocular fundus are extremely rare in black patients.

There are then two classifications of possibilities that remain: a patient may have a disease or fundus disorder that will not impair vision, and thus produce no symptoms, or a patient may have a disease with the potential to impair vision. Every clinician will encounter a variety of fundus abnormalities that are discovered on objective evaluation of the fundus and that do not threaten vision. The most significant hurdle for the clinician is to realize that even though the history may not reveal any symptoms of vision impairment, the patient may have significant vision-threatening disease. For example, angioid streaks can exist in a patient's eye and create no visual symptoms, but their discovery may provide the patient with the opportunity to receive additional health care that may identify systemic problems in need of treatment. Occasionally, a patient may be discovered with diabetic retinopathy and no diagnosis of diabetes; the clinician can then provide the patient with timely consultation for this systemic problem. Both of these fundus diseases can lead to permanent loss of sight in later stages.

The object of obtaining the patient history is to establish some guide to the objective examination of the eye. Many times the history can virtually make the diagnosis for the alert clinician. In the absence of symptoms, the clinician should take advantage of the anatomic layering within the ocular fundus to make the objective examination more meaningful. Finally, realization that certain diseases and disorders affect only one eye or one gender, are rare among specific races, and are age-group specific will help to establish the diagnosis.

# EXAMINATION

There are subjective and objective methods of evaluating the ocular fundus.

## Visual Field Assessment

One of the most frequently applied and most useful methods to evaluate subjectively the ocular fundus is visual field testing. Because of the consistent orientation of the nerve fibers of the sensory retina, it is possible to obtain certain patterns of visual field deficit that suggest specific fundus or visual system disorders.

A useful screening technique for evaluation of the visual fields is confrontation testing. It is performed unilaterally, as with all visual field testing, and begins with finger-counting fields. The patient covers one eye and has a fixation target, which can be the examiner's corresponding eye. The examiner extends fingers on each of his hands, in separate quadrants of the visual field, and asks the patient to report the number of fingers perceived. The examiner then confirms that the patient reports the correct number of fingers. The examiner can place the palms of his hands on either side of the line of sight in the presence of more significant defects in the visual field. Finally, the examiner can use the red caps on dilating eyedrop bottles as a more sophisticated level of visual field testing. The finger-counting, palm, and red-cap fields are useful screening techniques and are of great value in detecting the presence of gross lesions, such as clinical retinal detachments.

The tangent screen can be used for quantitation of visual field defects. It is an especially useful technique for lesions of the posterior pole, whereas the confrontation approach is more useful for the gross visual system lesions and certain peripheral retinal deficits. In general, the universal method for evaluation of the central visual field with the tangent screen is with the 2/1000 white target. With patience, the clinician can obtain very reliable results in a short time.

Patients with complaints of holes in the field of vision or positive findings on the screening tests deserve tangent-screen testing. Similarly, patients with history or objective signs of ocular trauma should be tested with the tangent screen. Following objective evaluation, patients suspected of having glaucoma or observable fundus lesions also merit a tangent-screen test.

A sophisticated method for evaluation of the peripheral visual field is Goldmann perimetry. This method can provide a great amount of information about the central and peripheral visual fields. A Goldmann-type perimeter allows evaluation of the visual field with different sizes and intensities of isopters. Indications for this type of evaluation are similar to those for tangent-screen testing. Keep in mind, however, the limitations of the tangent screen.

It is possible to evaluate the macular visual field with the Amsler grid. This checkerboard-patterned test-plate series can provide valuable information to the clinician. It is generally not necessary to present all of the plates to every patient to gather pertinent information. The most frequently used plate is the first one. The other plates can be used in certain situations to provide additional information. Although there are specific recommendations about how to use the Amsler grid regarding illumination levels, test distance, and specific questions, the most significant factor is consistency in testing.

Aside from initial evaluation, the Amsler grid can be used to note progress or alterations in the natural course of macular lesions. This can only be accomplished when testing procedures are consistent from visit to visit. Accompanying the Amsler grid is a notepad of charts on which to record results and which become a permanent part of the patient's file. Blank charts can also be used by patients for self-testing to detect the earliest alterations in macular function. This frequently is done for patients with diseases or disorders whose natural course includes exacerbations and remissions, such as presumed ocular histoplasmosis.

## Color Vision Assessment

Color vision testing subjectively evaluates retinal and optic nerve function. Although the color plates in booklet form are ideal for office testing of congenital color defects, they are not particularly useful for charting the color defects of acquired diseases. The plates are very sensitive to the known color confusions typical of congenital color defects, but they are not as sensitive as the panel D-15 for assessing acquired and subtle diseases, disorders, and dystrophies. The D-15 test can be used to detect and classify a great variety of color abnormalities, including congenital defects, and can be used to follow the natural course of a disease. The recording chart, like the Amsler grid, can become a permanent part of the patient's file. The Farnsworth-Munsell 100-hue test is a sensitive but tedious method to detect and follow acquired ocular and visual system disease.

## Photostress Recovery Time Test

One very simple test for macular lesions that is often overlooked is the photostress recovery time test. Surprisingly, this test is remarkably sensitive as an indicator of serous macular disease. Variations on the original procedure can be used for this test; again, however, consistency is the key to success. Let us assume that a patient has a serous macular disease in the left eye with 20/40 vision, metamorphopsia, and micropsia. When the clinician looks into the 20/20 right eye, the standard examination takes place, and in the left eye the clinician observes retinal abnormalities. Then the clinician has the patient cover the left eye and look down at the Snellen chart. Normal maculas will recover from photostress within a minute; abnormal, serous elevated maculas will take longer (Table 30.1).

It is not always necessary to measure the exact amount of time that it takes for the abnormal eye to return to its level of best visual acuity; the great difference between the two eyes is diagnostic in itself. In summary, it is important to remember that serous macular disease will have a grossly prolonged photostress recovery time and that it is the time difference between the two eyes that is important. A light is shone into the eye, and the time for recovery to best visual acuity is measured. In normal eyes this time is less than one minute; however, in abnormal eyes the time of photostress recovery is much longer. In photostress testing, the eye with

Table 30.1
Example of Abnormal Photostress Recovery Time

|  | Patient Symptoms | Photostress Recovery Time | Ophthalmoscopic Observations | Clinical Impression |
|---|---|---|---|---|
| OD | None | 3.0 sec | Unremarkable | Normal |
| OS | Decreased VA, "yellow spot in front of this eye," metamorphosia, micropsia | 2 min, 30 sec | Absence of foveal reflex, light-colored macular area, with slight elevation | Serous macular disease |

better vision serves as a built-in control. An increased photostress recovery time is indicative of a macular lesion rather than optic nerve disease.

## Self-Tests

Finally, a lot of information can be gained from patients by having them review their subjective symptoms, with the clinician applying some practical techniques. For example, when a patient with suspected serous maculopathy complains of micropsia, it is often easiest to have the patient make a size comparison of the E at the top of the eyechart. It is generally effective simply to ask the patient to make unilateral size comparisons by percentages. A common response in the presence of serous macular disease in one eye would be for the E to be about two-thirds the size of the E seen with the normal eye. The red green duochrome slide on the chart can be used as a gross color sensitivity test. All of these tests can be used by clinicians to gather valuable information for a diagnosis.

There are other methods in addition to these rather crude ways of evaluating visual function subjectively. Entoptic tests, such as that performed with Blue Field Entoptoscope,™ provides the clinician with the opportunity to assess macular function by having the patient observe his own leukocytes against a blue background.

Subjective assessment of retinal disease is difficult: symptoms are often overlooked if the visual decrease is unilateral,

pain is an infrequent accompaniment (except in some cases of tumor), and patients generally are poor observers. Therefore, diagnosis of diseases and disorders of the ocular fundus rests largely on the objective observations of individual clinicians.

## Objective Fundus Evaluation (Ophthalmoscopy and Contact Lens Biomicroscopy)

There are four ways in which clinicians view the ocular fundus: the binocular indirect ophthalmoscope, the monocular indirect ophthalmoscope, the monocular direct ophthalmoscope, and the slit lamp microscope in conjunction with a special fundus lens (Table 30.2). Each method makes a unique contribution to the diagnosis of any fundus disease or disorder.

The binocular indirect ophthalmoscope (Figure 30.2) has many advantages. Once the pupil has been dilated, the fundus can be viewed from ora serrata to ora serrata and beyond with the binocular indirect ophthalmoscope and scleral indentation when indicated. There are two main obstacles that novices with the binocular indirect ophthalmoscope will encounter. First, there is a tendency not to breathe when performing this type of ophthalmoscopy. Respiration at a regular rate will not cause the image to disappear or fall from

Table 30.2
Strategy for Ophthalmoscopic Evaluation

| Structure | Points of Evaluation |
|---|---|
| Optic disc | Margins<br>Cup/disc ratio<br>Optic cup margins and vessels |
| Retinal vessels | Continuity<br>Calibre<br>Crossings<br>Hemorrhage<br>New vessels |
| Macular area | Uniformity of RPE<br>Foveal reflex<br>Elevation<br>Hemorrhage<br>Exudate<br>Drusen |
| Other fundus | Pigmented lesions<br>Retinal breaks<br>Vitreoretinal abnormalities<br>"Window defects" |

view. The second obstacle is a tendency for clinicians to want to "crawl into the eye." Most clinicians want to treat this kind of examination technique like a direct ophthalmoscope and move closer to the patient as the fundus examination progresses. A working distance almost equal to the arm's length must be maintained for greatest efficiency with this kind of ophthalmoscopy. Another problem is the inverted image produced by this technique. This seemingly insurmountable problem can be eliminated by a slow and logical approach. For example, when one evaluates the posterior pole the inverted image can be dealt with by examining the patient reclined with the examiner situated positioned at the head of the patient facing toward the patient's feet. In this way, the inverted image appears as it would if the examiner were standing and facing the patient.

When situated in front of the patient, the clinician can project the inverted view of the ocular fundus to determine where any corresponding visual field defects will be plotted. If a lesion is located in the superior temporal portion of the condensing lens view of the posterior pole, then the field defect will likewise be plotted in the superior temporal quadrant. Perhaps the most significant key to mastering the inverted image is to realize that it is only this image produced by the condensing lens that is inverted. That is to say, the superior temporal fundus is still the superior temporal fundus, and only the view of the portion of the fundus under examination is inverted. Difficulties with the inverted image diminish as the examiner's technical skill increases.

Binocular indirect ophthalmoscopy is begun by viewing the red reflex from the choroid. This is done to search for gross lesions and to provide the patient with an opportunity to adapt to the intense light. After this initial period, a systematic examination of the fundus can begin. It is easiest to examine the superior nasal fundus of the right eye and superior temporal fundus of the left eye from the right side, with the patient reclined. Then the ex-

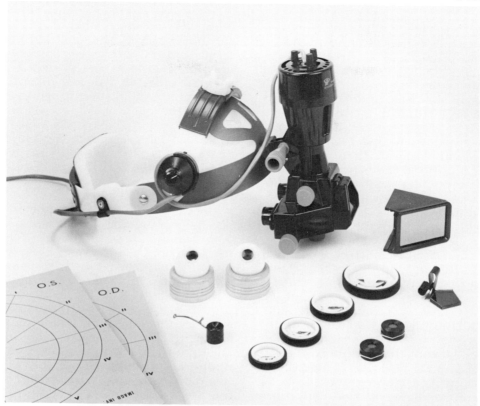

**FIGURE 30.2.**
**Binocular indirect ophthalmoscope and accessories for fundus examination.**
Photo courtesy Medical Instrument Research Associates, Inc., Waltham, Mass.

aminer can move clockwise around the patient to examine the inferior nasal fundus in the right eye. From this position, the left inferior temporal fundus is examined. The examiner can then move over to the left side of the patient and examine the inferior nasal fundus of the left eye, and the inferior temporal fundus in the right, all from the same position. The clinician can then move downward a bit to examine the superior nasal fundus of the left eye and the superior temporal fundus in the right. Finally, the clinician can move to the head of the patient, and examine both the posterior poles. This type of general strategy will help the clinician identify within the ocular fundus suspicious areas that can be scrutinized later in more detail. It is particularly important to develop a consistent routine of examination.

There are a variety of lenses, each with unique advantages, that can be used with the binocular indirect ophthalmoscope. The best general purpose lens is the 20-diopter lens, which provides a good-sized image with a comfortable working distance. The 30-diopter lens is very useful when the pupil does not dilate well or when a wider field of view is required, as in the presence of cortical cataracts. Because it produces the largest image, the 14-diopter lens is most useful for evaluating the posterior pole.

The system of binocular indirect ophthalmoscopy has advantages of steropsis, variable range of fields of view, increased resolution, and it allows examination of eyes with relatively opaque media. Armed with this basic information, the clinician can then apply other methods of fundus examination.

The monocular indirect ophthalmoscope offers several advantages when the pupils cannot be dilated. It will permit a larger field of view than the direct ophthalmoscope and does not cause the severe pupillary constriction of the binocular indirect ophthalmoscope. It is very useful when performing monocular indirect ophthalmoscopy to have the patient look into the field of view corresponding to the portion of the fundus that the examiner wants to view. This technique will enhance the view of the periphery. The aperture of the monocular indirect ophthalmoscope can be varied, and various filters can be used to gain additional information.

Probably the most widely used instrument for fundus examination is the monocular direct ophthalmoscope. Even its efficacy, however, is enhanced when the pupils are dilated. After the fundus has been viewed with one of the indirect ophthalmoscopes, the magnification of the direct ophthalmoscope allows examination for lesions at the posterior pole. As with the other techniques, direct ophthalmoscopy should be performed in a consistent manner.

Once lesions have been identified and their locations recorded, the slit lamp microscope can be used for stereoscopic study. The slit lamp is used with a lens that will neutralize the refractive power of the cornea, such as a preset Hruby lens, or the Goldmann three-mirror contact lens. It is helpful to remember that the slit lamp techniques can be as dynamic as those used in ophthalmoscopes. The patient's direction of gaze can be varied and the illumination changed such that the best image is obtained. The slit lamp techniques are useful in a number of ways, such as for observing detail stereoscopically, for detecting the Tyndall effect following ophthalmoscopy, and to elaborate upon vitreoretinal relationships.

In order to evaluate properly the ocular fundus, the clinician should be skilled at all of the forms of subjective and objective evaluation. With increasing numbers of patients and exposures to varieties of ocular abnormalities, the correlation and corroboration between subjective and objective examination will increase.

# CLINICAL SIGNIFICANCE

The clinical significance of diseases and disorders of the ocular fundus is their ability to cause a decrease in visual acuity, blindness, or even the loss of the globe. Perhaps the easiest way to think of such diseases and disorders is in terms of the type of vision loss encountered. Although many of these diseases and disorders can cause a loss of both central and peripheral vision, they primarily affect either central or peripheral vision. Vision loss can result from processes occurring within the choroid that affect the retinal pigment epithelium or the sensory retina.

## Central Vision Loss

Many of the diseases and disorders that cause loss of central vision do so by affecting the macula. A particular condition affecting the fovea and parafoveal area could potentially reduce visual acuity to the 20/200 level or poorer. In addition, a disease could affect an area near the fovea within the macular area and cause a loss of central vision. Finally, a disease or disorder could be general in its effect upon the posterior pole and cause a decrease of central vision, with or without an effect on foveal vision.

# Central Areolar Choroidal Dystrophy

There are a few choroidal dystrophies that can cause a loss of central vision. Central areolar choroidal dystrophy is an uncommon autosomal dominant disorder that initially affects the macular area in the teen years. It manifests as a fine pigment mottling, often without vision loss. The electro-oculogram is often abnormal; other electrodiagnostic studies are normal. Fluorescein angiography may enhance the clinical picture of mottling of the pigment epithelium. Later in life, these patients begin to develop an area of geographic atrophy of the retinal pigment epithelium, with eventual loss of the choriocapillaris. This area of geographic atrophy rarely exceeds four or five disc diameters in size, but correlates with a profound effect on central vision. As more of the choroid becomes atrophic, vision continues to decline. Eventually, the largest choroidal blood vessels are affected, appearing as yellow white lines.

Typical of dystrophies, central areolar choroidal dystrophy is bilateral. The differential diagnosis includes geographic atrophy of the retinal pigment epithelium as a manifestation of senile macular disease. This differential diagnosis should be straightforward. Although morphologically similar in their later stages, geographic atrophy of the retinal pigment epithelium in senile macular disease causes a loss of central vision later in life than central areolar choroidal dystrophy, and the former is almost always accompanied by drusen and peripapillary retinal pigment epithelial atrophy.

In addition, the diagnosis of serpiginous choroidopathy should be entertained as a differential. In an early familial study (Sorsby 1939) on central areolar choroidal dystrophy, the author included a peripapillary disorder that clearly was serpiginous choroidopathy. Serpiginous choroidopathy resembles central areolar choroidal dystrophy, but the former affects the peripapillary area first, while the latter affects the macula exclusively.

# Choroideremia

The later stages of choroideremia affect central vision (see Figure 30.3). Choroideremia is a rare, sex linked, and recessively inherited bilateral disorder that initially affects teen-aged males by impairing night vision. Later, the disorder demonstrates mottled pigment epithelium and choroidal atrophy in the midperiphery of the ocular fundus. At this stage, choroideremia often is confused with an atypical retinitis pigmentosa, but later in life the diagnosis becomes more obvious. Larger areas of the choroid appear atrophied until the macula is affected. At this time, the patients have poor midperipheral vision along with very poor central

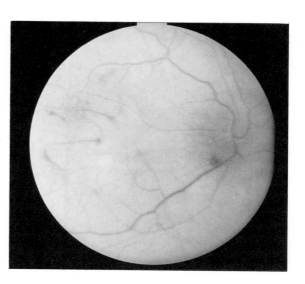

FIGURE 30.3.
Choroideremia.

vision. Female carriers do not have significant vision loss, but they often manifest pigment mottling at the macula and in the midperipheral retinal pigment epithelium. The most common differential diagnosis to consider is an atypical retinitis pigmentosa. It often may not be possible to confirm the diagnosis until some time passes, but other family members should be examined in an effort to clarify the morphologic spectrum and assist in the diagnosis. It is important to identify the affected males as well as the female carriers. The female carriers have the potential of having half of their daughters as carriers, with half of their sons affected with the disorder.

## Gyrate Atrophy

Another uncommon fundus disorder that primarily affects the choroid, at least initially, is inherited gyrate atrophy. The classic lesion of gyrate atrophy is the scalloped edge of atrophic choroidal lesion in the midperiphery of the fundus. These patients typically are myopic and have impaired night vision, and later in the natural course of the disease they will have poor central vision. Perhaps the most sophisticated manner in which the diagnosis can be established is via laboratory studies for plasma and cerebrospinal levels of ornithine, which are elevated in patients with the disorder.

Perhaps the best management for patients with inherited choroidal disorders is prevention through informed genetic counseling, and for those patients affected, vision rehabilitation through low vision care.

There are a great number of choroidal diseases and disorders of the posterior pole that can directly affect central vision. In addition, there are conditions of the choroid at the macula that can cause loss of vision by secondary effects upon the retinal pigment epithelium and sensory retina.

The vascular system in the choroid at the posterior pole is unique. The short posterior ciliary arteries that enter the globe about the optic disc and macula force blood into the choriocapillaris network. The resulting hemodynamic pressure probably is responsible for considerable stress in the submacular choroid. A large number of acquired choroidal diseases, disorders, and conditions affect the choroidal circulation at the posterior pole and may result in either a serous or hemorrhagic detachment of the overlying retinal pigment epithelium and sensory retina.

## Idiopathic Central Serous Choroidopathy

An acquired choroidal disease that epitomizes these relationships is idiopathic central serous choroidopathy. This disease is most commonly encountered in males between the ages of 20 and 50 years, and it is typically unilateral in presentation. These patients develop one or more small serous detachments of the retinal pigment epithelium; these detachments may occur in the area of the fovea. Subsequently, these patients may develop an overlying serous detachment of the sensory retina.

Ophthalmoscopy will fail to reveal a foveal reflex with the foveal involvement. With the binocular indirect ophthalmoscope, the detachment of the retinal pigment epithelium may be viewed as an elevated, lightly turbid discoloration. If the sensory retina is not detached over the pigment epithelium detachment, there may be an arclike salmon-colored reflex at the demarcation of the intact and separated pigment epithelium. The detachment of the retinal pigment epithelium typically is small, but occasionally there may be a detachment as large as two or more disc diameters. Since the attachment of the retinal pigment epithelium to Bruch's membrane is firm, a serous detachment of the retinal pigment epithelium resembles a blister.

Since the bond between the sensory

retina and the retinal pigment epithelium is tenuous, a separation of the sensory retina from the retinal pigment epithelium is more sloped in its margins and more difficult to detect with the ophthalmoscope. In such cases, the slit lamp microscope may be invaluable. With the slit lamp, the clinician may be able to observe the sensory retina elevated away from the underlying retinal pigment epithelium. The beam will be observed passing through the transparent sensory retina, and there will be a small gap between the sensory retina and the underlying retinal pigment epithelium. The underlying retinal pigment epithelium reflects the light back to the clinician. Occasionally, the clinician can cast the shadow of a blood vessel in the sensory retina onto the retinal pigment epithelium, which substantiates the diagnosis. This can be accomplished only rarely, but it is valuable evidence.

The fluorescein angiogram typically demonstrates some abnormalities in the retinal pigment epithelium. Fluorescein percolates through the abnormality in the retinal pigment epithelium to fill the sub-pigment epithelial space. If the sensory retina overlying the retinal pigment epithelium detachment is intact, the fluorescein will eventually fill in the space between the retinal pigment epithelium and sensory retina.

In almost all cases, the serous detachments resolve within 1 to 4 months. Because the retinal pigment epithelium is strained by the serous detachment, there often remains a subtle mottling or derangement of the retinal pigment epithelium. The foveal light reflex does not return.

Symptoms of vision impairment are so striking in idiopathic central serous choroidopathy that the diagnosis often can be strongly suspected on the basis of symptoms alone. A constant companion of idiopathic central serous choroidopathy, when it affects the fovea, is micropsia. Micropsia may even be the patient's major complaint. In addition, there is frequently some metamorphopsia. Often there will be some alteration of color perception and, rarely, a shift toward hyperopia. This refractive change is usually limited to less than three-fourths of a diopter.

In earlier literature, the symptom of acquired hyperopia in idiopathic central serous choroidopathy received more attention than it deserved. Upon closer analysis, the patients that have such serous detachments are often the same patients who are in the age group that becomes symptomatic with previously uncorrected hyperopia. In the majority of patients with acquired hyperopia in an eye with foveal involvement with idiopathic central serous choroidopathy, there is an equal increase in hyperopia in the fellow, normal eye, corresponding to the refractive error and not to the presence of disease.

The Amsler grid findings often are abnormal. The Amsler grid can be useful in detecting those serous detachments that are not affecting the foveal vision, which results in metamorphopsia, micropsia, color deficiencies, and acquired hyperopia. For those lesions that are at the fovea, the Amsler grid findings provide a reliable way to monitor the changes in vision function throughout the natural course of the disease.

For the lesions that involve the fovea, the photostress recovery time is one of the most sensitive methods to determine the presence of serous disease. Since idiopathic central serous choroidopathy is almost always unilateral, the difference between photostress recovery times in the two eyes often is remarkable. The eye without disease may have a photostress recovery of less than 30 seconds, and the eye with disease may have a photostress time of over 5 minutes. A history of micropsia, symptoms of occasional metamorphopsia, and prolonged photostress recovery often can lead to the diagnosis of serous disease affecting the fovea before ophthalmoscopy, slit lamp microscopy, or other objective means are employed. Symptoms of metamorphopsia, prolonged photostress recovery time, coupled with a general overview of the patient's feelings about vision recovery in bright light (subjective photostress recovery test) are accurate landmarks of the natural course of the disease. When the disease has resolved, mild metamorphopsia and color vision changes may remain, but the photostress time will return to under a minute. As many as one-third of patients affected with idiopathic central serous choroidopathy will experience a recurrence of the disease.

The etiology of idiopathic central serous choroidopathy is unclear, but it may be related to the hemodynamic pressure at the posterior pole. Because the etiology is unclear, and because the natural course of the disease is for the eye to retain good visual acuity and good visual function, treatment is reserved for the cases that are most troublesome. Medical therapy with systemic steroids is not generally an effective way to hasten the recovery of vision, and photocoagulation has a number of risks that prevent it from being considered the choice of treatment in all cases. For those patients that have a protracted course of disease, however, photocoagulation may hasten the visual recovery.

In patients over the age of 50 years, a serous detachment of the retinal pigment epithelium and sensory retina should be viewed with suspicion. Bruch's membrane often develops small imperfections with age. This loss of integrity may provide an opportunity for the choroid to grow new blood vessels beneath or even through the retinal pigment epithelium. These typically impatent new blood vessels may permit the serous components of the blood to percolate into the potential space between the membrane of Bruch and the retina. This subretinal neovascularization can be responsible for the serous disciform response in senile macular disease or for hemorrhage, resulting in a disciform hemorrhagic detachment of the retina.

# Senile Macular Disease

The clinical significance of subretinal neovascularization is an important consideration when discussing diseases and disorders that can cause a loss of central vision. Coupled with one or more other factors, subretinal neovascularization is a major component of a disease process that involves the choroid. Senile macular disease is a multifactorial disease that has become the leading cause of legal blindness in the industrialized world.

Senile macular disease may be thought of as a choroidal disease, but one must consider the other tissues that become involved. There are several manifestations of this disease: pigment derangement, pigment derangement and drusen, drusen, geographic atrophy of the retinal pigment epithelium, serous detachments of the sensory retina, hemorrhagic detachments of the sensory retina, and fibrovascular scarring. Changes in the choroid, Bruch's membrane, and retinal pigment epithelium are responsible for the disease complex. It is a disease that typically occurs bilaterally in older persons. One of the manifestations is pigment derangement: the retinal pigment epithelium at the macula appears mottled in affected patients. Visual acuity generally is only mildly affected, often better than 20/40. There also may be minor abnormalities in the Amsler grid findings.

Drusen (Figures 30.4 and 30.5) are one of the most interesting manifestations of senile macular disease, and virtually a constant companion of the disease. They appear as small yellow or yellow white nodules at the level of the retinal pigment epithelium about the macula; in addition, they may occur about the optic disc and in the equatorial retina. They represent localized discrete thickenings of Bruch's membrane, and they irritate the overlying retinal pigment epithelium to give the typical clinical appearance. Drusen may also

DRUSEN OVERLYING CHOROIDAL NEVUS

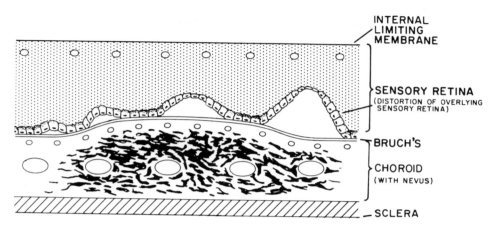

FIGURE 30.4.
Drusen overlying choroidal nevus.

increase in number with time. In addition, the drusen may coalesce to form larger drusen, or they may calcify, presenting a white color. In some cases, the drusen may disappear with time, leaving small areas of retinal pigment epithelium atrophy corresponding to their former location. When the drusen have resorbed, the clinician can view the underlying intact choriocapillaris, and retroillumination with the slit lamp or the direct ophthalmoscope will reveal these atrophic areas.

Histologically, drusen are products of degradation of the retinal pigment epithelium. It has been suggested that autolysis of retinal pigment epithelium cells is responsible for the appearance of drusen, and there is additional evidence that there is a contribution from other processes, including hyalinization between the retinal pigment epithelium and Bruch's membrane.

Fluorescein angiography often reveals many more drusen than does ophthalmoscopy. Drusen stain early in the angiogram and fade with the choroidal

fluorescence. In the presence of confluent drusen, the fluorescein may remain in the drusen after the background choroidal fluorescence has faded.

Drusen by themselves rarely cause much loss of visual acuity. Occasionally, a patient might have 20/40 visual acuity, but most patients have normal visual acu-

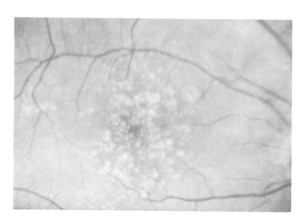

FIGURE 30.5.
Drusen.

ity. It is remarkable to watch drusen change with time: although they generally increase in number, they can undergo all of the previously mentioned changes, including appearing along with pigment derangement.

Assume for the moment that drusen produce an environment where there is a relative lack of oxygen being provided to the sensory retinal tissue. Recall that with age, Bruch's membrane may develop holes or cracks. If the choroid were to be exposed to this relatively hypoxic environment, it might be stimulated to grow new blood vessels to provide necessary nutrition to the sensory retina. If there are abnormalities in Bruch's membrane, there is the opportunity for the new blood vessels to gain access to the potential space between the retinal pigment epithelium and Bruch's membrane. The detection limits of the ophthalmoscope and fluorescein angiography do not allow early recognition of these neovascular buds.

The ophthalmoscopic appearance of a small arc of red beneath the sensory retina or a grayish discoloration beneath the retinal pigment epithelium, particularly in the presence of drusen, should raise the question of choroidal neovascularization. The presence of a small, shallow serous detachment of the retina, or an arc of red blood or pigment typically at the inferior aspect of the detachment, should similarly alert the clinician to the possibility of choroidal neovascularization. In addition, the presence of a yellowish exudate beneath a serous detachment should raise suspicion of subretinal neovascularization underlying the serous detachment.

Since the new blood vessels typically leak, subretinal neovascularization may cause a serous detachment of the retina. In addition, subretinal neovascularization may cause a passive extravasation of blood in an area that is typically about two disc diameters in size. With time, the extravasated blood is replaced with fibrous tissue, the so-called disciform scar. In other cases, a spontaneous hemorrhage may oc-

cur, which can elevate the retinal pigment epithelium and sensory retina. This blisterlike elevation of the retina with hemorrhage of subretinal neovascularization can be as large as six disc diameters. The large amount of blood, coupled with the pigmentation of the retinal pigment epithelium, causes the hemorrhage to appear dark olive or black and can be mistaken for malignant melanoma. At the edges of the detachment there may appear a red band of blood. This part of the hemorrhage appears red because it is in the thinnest portion of the detachment (Figure 30.6). With the direct ophthalmoscope it may be possible to highlight this red band with proximal illumination. Occasionally, the hemorrhage can percolate through the pigment epithelium and into the subsensory retinal space. This generally occurs at the top of the dome of retinal pigment epithelium detachment, and can even result in blood entering the retrovitreous space. A vitreous hemorrhage sometimes follows.

In all cases of hemorrhagic detachment, whether passive or spontaneous, when the fovea is involved the vision will be profoundly reduced. In time, and it may take several months, the hemorrhage will be replaced with fibrous tissue (Figure 30.7). The fibrovascular scar is always

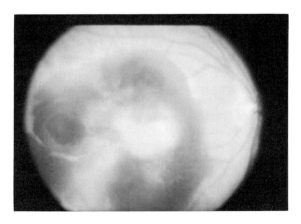

**FIGURE 30.6.**
Hemorrhagic maculopathy in senile macular disease.

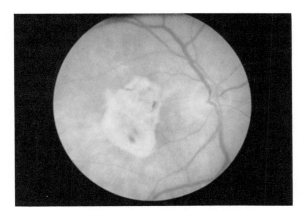

**FIGURE 30.7.**
**Fibrovascular scarring.**

smaller than the original hemorrhage. In some cases, cystoid macular edema occurs overlying the choroidal hemorrhage, and this carries a poor visual prognosis. In other cases, the fibrous scar can develop a vascular anastomosis between the retinal and choroidal circulations. Even if there is a fibrovascular scar in one eye, the clinician cannot be absolutely certain that secondary hemorrhage will not occur adjacent to the primary fibrous scar. In a very few cases, the exudative and reparative processes will continue until the majority of the posterior pole is involved. This fibrous tissue formation is similar to a disease in children of similar morphology, Coats' disease, except that this process is more appropriately termed *massive subretinal exudation.* Because of the reparative process, the prudent clinician should issue a guarded prognosis while assuring the patient that complete blindness is an extremely unlikely course of events.

Patients who have had a hemorrhagic detachment in one eye are at risk for a similar course in the fellow eye. If a patient has confluent drusen in one eye and a hemorrhagic detachment in the fellow eye, the risk of hemorrhagic detachment in the eye with confluent drusen is about 15% per year for 5 years.

There are some patients who develop areas of geographic atrophy of the retinal pigment epithelium following drusen resolution, resolution of serous detachment of the retina, or even occasionally after hemorrhagic detachment of the retina. There is atrophy of the retinal pigment epithelium in an area about two to four disc diameters in size, which permits a view of the underlying larger choroidal vessels. There often is atrophy of the choroid as well. The lesions are sharply demarcated, and central vision is poor when the fovea is involved. In almost all cases, there will be accompanying drusen and atrophy about the optic disc. Geographic atrophy of the retinal pigment epithelium is a fairly common manifestation of senile macular disease (Figure 30.8).

When reviewing the manifestations of senile macular disease, it becomes apparent that they can be divided into two distinct forms: nonexudative, predisciform or dry; and exudative, disciform, or wet. The nonexudative variety of senile macular disease can consist of pigment derangement, drusen, drusen and pigment derangement, and geographic atrophy of the retinal pigment epithelium. Unfortunately, there is little known preventive treatment for this form of the disease. Nearly one-third of the light that enters

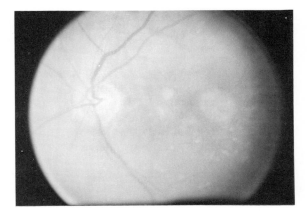

**FIGURE 30.8.**
**Geographic atrophy of retinal pigment epithelium.**

the eye can be absorbed by the melanin granules of the retinal pigment epithelium and the melanocytes of the choroid; much of this is converted to heat. One of the functions of the choroidal vasculature is to dissipate this heat. It may be that in the future there will be an ophthalmic lens for those patients with identified pigment derangement to reduce the amount of light absorbed at the level of the retinal pigment epithelium.

There is some evidence that drusen are inherited, and it is therefore unlikely that there will be any specific preventive treatment for drusen. Geographic atrophy of the retinal pigment epithelium may be the result of degeneration and atrophy of drusen, the result of resolution of serous or hemorrhagic detachment, or a focal atrophy of the choriocapillaris, and it is unlikely that there will be a preventive treatment for this manifestation of senile macular disease.

There has been some discussion of the possible role of nutrition and certain vascular therapies for the nonexudative manifestations of senile macular disease, but their roles remain unproved. At this time, the most appropriate management for the nonexudative senile macular disease is vision rehabilitation through low vision care.

The exudative manifestations of senile macular disease include serous and hemorrhagic detachments of the retina and fibrovascular scarring. It has been demonstrated that serous detachments of the retina without subretinal neovascularization carry no greater risk of vision loss in older patients than in younger patients. Serous and/or hemorrhagic detachments in the presence of subretinal neovascularization have a poor prognosis, however. There is some evidence from a recent clinical trial that patients over age 50 with metamorphopsia, drusen, and new subretinal neovascularization outside the fovea may be treated successfully with argon laser photocoagulation. To benefit, these patients must have visual acuity of 20/100 or better for argon photocoagula-

tion to be helpful in preventing further vision loss. Unfortunately, this acuity level excludes many patients. If argon laser photocoagulation is done on lesions within the immediate foveal avascular zone, it is unlikely that the lesion will improve as a result of possible foveal destruction by the heat from the argon laser.

It may be possible to identify with an Amsler grid patients at risk to develop serous or hemorrhagic detachments of the retinal pigment epithelium or sensory retina secondary to subretinal neovascularization. Those patients who are over 50 years of age and have drusen may be provided with an Amsler grid to be placed in a convenient place, such as on the bathroom mirror. Once a week the patient can look at the Amsler grid monocularly to attempt to note the onset of metamorphopsia. Such a preventive measure, with additional patient health education regarding some of the other manifestations of serous hemorrhagic disease, can serve as an important preventive measure. Once early subretinal neovascularization is identified, patients have an opportunity to receive treatment in a timely manner. Once significant serous detachment or hemorrhage has occurred, however, there is little likelihood that argon photocoagulation will have a positive effect on the natural course of the detachment.

Fibrovascular scarring is a later stage of the hemorrhagic process and is unlikely to be amenable to medical or surgical intervention. Many patients who have fibrovascular scarring respond well to low vision care.

The differential diagnosis of senile macular disease from other diseases and disorders should be straightforward. There are instances of drug toxicities and traumatic events that produce pigment derangement at the macula and which should be considered. A complete patient interview will be invaluable in these instances.

Drusen can be confused with hard exudates that occur in retinal vascular disease. This differential diagnosis has received far more attention than it deserves. Hard exudates form patterns within the retina and occur in retinal vascular diseases. Drusen almost always occur in both eyes in a similar pattern at the macula and lie at the level of the retinal pigment epithelium.

Geographic atrophy of the retinal pigment epithelium can be confused with central areolar choroidal dystrophy, but the former occurs in older patients with drusen and peripapillary atrophy. Central areolar choroidal dystrophy occurs in younger patients, and vision loss occurs at an earlier age. Larger serous or hemorrhagic detachment of the retina can be confused with melanomas of the choroid. Serous and hemorrhagic detachments change with time, and careful examination with retroillumination or indirect illumination with the slit lamp or the direct ophthalmoscope often will reveal serous or hemorrhagic components. In addition, there are other manifestations of senile macular disease in the affected eye and the fellow eye. Occasionally, a fibrovascular scar may be confused with an amelanotic melanoma of the choroid, but the same criteria hold true for the differential diagnosis of serous or hemorrhagic detachments of the sensory retina.

# Angioid Streaks

Although senile macular disease is an important cause of vision impairment, there are other choroidal and Bruch's membrane disorders that can cause loss of central vision. Angioid streaks represent linear breaks in Bruch's membrane. They occur in the collagenous and elastic portion of Bruch's membrane and tend to branch out into the fundus in a radiating pattern from the optic disc. Often, a streak will pass through the macula. The color of the streaks—red brown or olive—depends on how much of the overlying retinal pigment epithelium has thinned. Similar to some of the manifestations of senile macular

disease, the breaks in Bruch's membrane may provide the opportunity for choroidal neovascularization to penetrate to or through the retinal pigment epithelium. Like subretinal neovascularization in senile macular disease, the new vessels can passively or spontaneously hemorrhage. Trauma can be the catalytic event in spontaneous hemorrhagic detachment of the retina. If there is an angioid streak through the fovea, there is great risk of central vision loss from subretinal neovascularization and subsequent serous or hemorrhagic detachment with fibrovascular scarring.

Many patients with angioid streaks exhibit a mottling of the pigment epithelium in the midperiphery at the level of the retinal pigment epithelium: *peau d'orange.* Although angioid streaks might be assumed to be a straightforward diagnosis, one study (Shields et al. 1975) indicated that one-third of patients with angioid streaks had been wrongly diagnosed and often received inappropriate treatment. Patients with angioid streaks often have systemic disease, the most common being pseudoxanthoma elasticum, a connective tissue disorder. Some patients will be found to have Paget's disease, a chronic bone disease, and a few patients will be found to have sickle cell disease. When a clinician discovers a new patient with angioid streaks, a medical workup can determine the presence of systemic associations. Many cases occur in person without systemic diseases. Persons who are likely to suffer head trauma and have macular streaks should be told of the risk of developing a spontaneous hemorrhage. Persons with macular streaks need not completely alter their lifestyles because of their streaks, but such patients should have the opportunity to make an informed decision about the potential for vision loss. In fact, the very first patient reported (Doyne 1889) with angioid streaks suffered a loss of vision secondary to trauma. The differential diagnosis should be easy, but it is remarkable how often the diagnosis is missed since angioid streaks are uncommon. Argon laser photocoagulation has limited application in serous or hemmorrhagic disease processes secondary to angioid streaks.

## High Myopia

Patients with high myopia and its chorioretinal degenerative changes are at risk to lose their central vision (Figure 30.9). This can progress gradually, in association with thinning of the retinal pigment epithelium and choroid, and is often associated with lacquer cracks. Lacquer cracks occur because of irregular linear gaps in Bruch's membrane and the retinal pigment epithelium. An acute loss of central vision rarely occurs secondary to a serous or hemorrhagic detachment of the retina associated with subretinal neovascularization. When such a detachment resolves, a small pigmented clump abut one-half disc diameter in size remains and is surrounded by fibrous tissue or choroidal atrophy. Such a pigmented spot is called *Fuchs' spot* and is composed of fibrovascular tissue and accompanying retinal pigment epithelium proliferation.

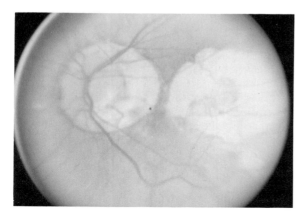

FIGURE 30.9.
High myopia.

## Presumed Ocular Histoplasmosis Syndrome

There are a variety of focal inflammatory conditions of the choroid that can cause a loss of central vision. Often, it is not possible to determine the precise etiologic condition that causes the choroidal inflammation, but the clinical portrait and laboratory tests often can provide information to support a presumptive diagnosis. Such a choroidal inflammatory disease can cause either a loss of central vision during the acute disease process with serous or hemorrhagic detachment of the retina overlying the focal inflammation, or later damage to the choroid, Bruch's membrane, and the retinal pigment epithelium. Such damage to these tissues can provide an environment favorable to subretinal neovascularization, which can result in serous or hemorrhagic detachment of the retina.

One of the most enigmatic of these choroidal diseases is the presumed ocular histoplasmosis syndrome. Systemic histoplasmosis is a chronic fungal infection almost always acquired through the respiratory tract, with primary focus in the lung and hematogenous dissemination to other tissues, including the eye. The spores are inhaled from the fungus found in soil. Systemic histoplasmosis is most often found in the eastern United States. Systemic histoplasmosis often occurs as a mild flulike disease, but occasionally a patient may have an acute pulmonary disease, which can last for 1 to 3 months. During hematogenic dissemination of the disease, small focal granulomas occur in the eye and are quickly destroyed, leaving atrophic scars in the choroid. At the sites of these choroidal granulomas, the choroidal vasculature is exposed to the retinal pigment epithelium and sensory retina.

There are four classic ophthalmoscopic signs that make up the spectrum of clinical findings leading to a diagnosis of ocular histoplasmosis. The first sign is a clear vitreous. Since ocular histoplasmosis is a choroidal disease, cells or flare in the vitreous would indicate a retinochoroidal inflammation. The second sign is the presence of punched-out spots in the midperiphery of the ocular fundus. These atrophic spots can number between 1 and 70, and like the other manifestations of the presumed ocular histoplasmosis syndrome, they are bilateral. The spots are always less than 1 mm in diameter. The third clinical sign of presumed ocular histoplasmosis is peripapillary choroidal atrophy. This peripapillary change differs from the typical atrophy secondary to other diseases in that there is often a crescent of pigment epithelium between the atrophy and the optic disc (Figure 30.10). Completing the clinical picture of ocular histoplasmosis is the presence of atrophic spots in the macula, which are morphologically similar to those spots in the midperiphery of the fundus. It is, of course, those spots in the macula that portend a loss of central vision. Since these areas of focal choroiditis provide an opportunity for choroidal neovascularization to occur, it is the maculopathy of presumed ocular histoplasmosis that prompts a patient to seek consultation. In general, those patients that do not have atrophic spots within two disc diameters of the fovea are at a low risk to develop symptomatic neovascular disease. The onset of serous or hemorrhagic detachment of the macula can cause metamorphopsia and blurred central vision.

Ophthalmoscopically, the clinician will observe a gray or olive green lesion about one disc diameter in size, which typically will have a pigmented signet-ring appearance about its circumference. The subretinal neovascular membrane that produces the ophthalmoscopically visible lesion rarely extends beyond one disc diameter from the gap in Bruch's membrane. It is, however, the geographic location of the neovascular membrane in relation to the fovea that is the most important determinant for central vision loss. For patients with neovascular lesions that involve the fovea, the prognosis is guarded. Patients with neovascularization and serous or hemorrhagic detachments may have remissions and exacerbations. The time period between episodes is typically about 4 years, but they can occur within a year or after a period of several years. In addition, the atrophic spots can grow in size, increase in number, and occasionally the peripapillary atrophic scarring can have a serous or hemorrhagic detachment as a complication of choroidal neovascularization of the site.

Since most patients with hemorrhagic detachments are in their twenties, thirties, and forties, the propensity for these patients to become legally blind in one or both eyes is fairly significant. If a patient has lost central vision in one eye, and has no atrophic spots at the macula in the fellow eye, there is about a 1 in 50 chance of having macular involvement in that fellow eye. If there are macular atrophic spots in the fellow eye, the chances are 1 in 4 for involvement in that macula.

Laser photocoagulation can be applied in some cases of serous and hemorrhagic detachments, but the overall prognosis for the preservation of central vision in those

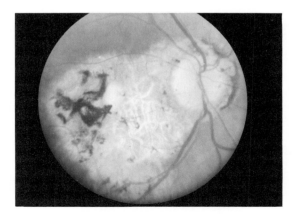

**FIGURE 30.10.**
Ocular histoplasmosis.

patients with foveal involvement with choroidal neovascularization is poor. The laser photocoagulation treatment of such lesions as peripapillary hemorrhages carries a much better prognosis. It is not uncommon to encounter legally blind patients in their early fifties or sixties who have bilateral fibrous scarring from ocular histoplasmosis. These patients deserve a complete low vision evaluation.

The differential diagnosis depends upon those other inflammatory diseases of the fundus that can mimic the clinical features of ocular histoplasmosis. The histoplasmin skin test is the most useful laboratory measure of the diagnosis of ocular histoplasmosis. The test is administered and interpreted much like the tuberculin skin test. A standard material is injected subcutaneously into the volar surface of the forearm. A positive reaction consists of a 5-mm or larger area of induration within 72 hours. Once a person has acquired skin sensitivity, it will remain throughout life, unless modified by severe illness, increasing age, or steroid therapy. There are two basic problems with the skin test: (1) in an area that is endemic for histoplasmosis, there will be a great number of false positives; and (2) the test is not always available in a timely manner, and it may not be cost-effective to pursue skin testing. Typically, the diagnosis can be established clinically by recalling the four classic fundus signs of ocular histoplasmosis: clear vitreous, punched-out spots in the midperiphery of the fundus, peripapillary atrophic scarring, and atrophic macular scars. Regardless of the sophistication of the diagnostic procedures, the clinician must always be aware that the ocular signs in question could be caused by another organism or condition.

## Serpiginous Choroidopathy

Another inflammatory condition of the choroid deserving attention is serpiginous choroidopathy. This condition is a focal inflammatory disease that involves the choriocapillaris and the retinal pigment epithelium. It is characterized by peripapillary and macular pseudopodal areas of choroidal atrophy in the inactive stages, and a yellow white discoloration of the retinal pigment epithelium in the active stages. The active lesions are adjacent to the inactive, atrophic areas and are typically observed in middle-aged persons. The lesions either produce scotomas or, if the macula is involved, poor central vision. Each active lesion can produce a posterior vitritis, and it may take a month or more for the active lesion to resolve. For many patients with bilateral involvement, the natural course of the disease ends with bilateral blindness.

## Acute Posterior Multifocal Placoid Pigment Epitheliopathy

A disorder that can be confused with serpiginous choroidopathy is acute posterior multifocal placoid pigment epitheliopathy. This disorder is ophthalmoscopically similar to serpiginous choroidopathy in its active stages. It is thought to involve primarily the retinal pigment epithelium and, secondarily, the choriocapillaris. Acute posterior multifocal placoid pigment epitheliopathy occurs in young people who may have had a previous viral infection or flu. The disease is characterized by the onset of creamy yellow colored patches throughout the posterior pole at the level of the retinal pigment epithelium. Central vision is at the 20/40 to 20/70 level. Since both eyes are simultaneously involved, these patients often can be differentiated from those with serpiginous choroidopathy, which involves one eye with active disease while the fellow eye harbors inactive lesions. The prognosis for resolution of the clinical signs and restoration of central vision function is excellent. The ophthalmoscopic picture generally begins to improve within 2 or 3 weeks of the diagnosis of acute posterior multifocal placoid pigment epitheliopathy, and shortly thereafter the central visual function returns. The end stages of this disease typically consist of mottled retinal pigment epithelium with a variety of clumps of pigmented cells and good visual acuity. This end-stage portrait can be contrasted with the end stage of serpiginous choroidopathy, which is characterized by extensive atrophy of the choroid with poor visual acuity.

## Choroidal Nevus

A choroidal nevus also may cause a loss of central vision. Most choroidal nevi occur within the posterior pole of the eye and rarely interfere with central vision function, although an occasional choroidal nevus may erode the overlying Bruch's membrane, irritate the retinal pigment epithelium, and eventually affect the sensory retina. Frequently, a choroidal nevus may precipitate the formation of drusen overlying the nevus. In addition, a loss of central vision can occur if the choroidal nevus produces an overlying serous detachment of the retina. A choroidal nevus can cause a loss of central vision also by the association with choroidal neovascularization, which can cause a hemorrhagic detachment of the retina. Such patients with a loss of central visual function need to be followed closely to determine if the natural course of the nevus might be indicative of a melanoma of the choroid.

## Choroidal Malignant Melanoma

A malignant melanoma of the choroid can cause a loss of central vision. This usually occurs by physical derangement of the photoreceptors or, more commonly, by serous detachment secondary to the choroidal neovascularization associated with the melanoma. Note the similarity between the mechanism for vision loss from benign nevus or melanoma disturbing overlying retinal structures and the vision-loss processes involved in senile macular disease. The discovery of a pigmented choroidal mass in the posterior pole of the eye is almost always in an asymptomatic patient. In either case, the clinician should be aware of the potential for the mass to be a malignant melanoma rather than a benign choroidal nevus. The following list delineates the characteristics of benign choroidal nevus versus those of malignant melanoma of the choroid.

1.  Benign choroidal nevi usually are less that five disc diameters in total area and, if elevated, less than 2 mm.

2.  Benign choroidal nevi often have drusen overlying them, whereas malignant melanomas often have overlying orange pigment (lipofuscin).

3.  Often a ring of hypopigmentation is observed about the borders of benign choroidal nevi.

4.  The borders of a malignant melanoma of the choroid are often lobulated, while the borders of benign choroidal nevi are even.

5.  A malignant melanoma of the choroid may have eroded Bruch's membrane to the point that the tumor can be viewed beneath the retinal pigment epithelium or sensory retina.

6.  A malignant melanoma of the choroid may have a greater thickness than benign choroidal nevi. This greater thickness can be manifested by a serous detachment in the presence of a lobulated choroidal mass. Most benign choroidal nevi appear flat.

7.  Angiographic evidence of choroidal neovascularization is much more indicative of benign choroidal nevi than a malignant melanoma of the choroid. The presence of large blood vessels within the tumor is indicative of a malignant melanoma of the choroid, however.

8. Visual field defects corresponding to the geographic location of benign choroidal nevi are rarely as large as the mass, but a visual field defect in the presence of a malignant melanoma of the choroid is generally as large or larger than the lesion.

9. The color of benign choroidal nevi generally is a uniform slate gray or light black, while it is typical for a malignant melanoma of the choroid to have uneven coloration.

10. Benign choroidal nevi rarely enlarge.

For those lesions that present diagnostic confusion the clinician should follow the patient using either fundus drawings or serial photographs. An enlarging mass with a color change, accompanied by a serous detachment of the retina and an enlargement of the visual field defect, should be viewed with suspicion (see Table 30.3).

Equivocal cases may benefit from investigation by fluorescein angiographic and/or ultrasonic techniques. In several studies, the misdiagnosis rate for lesions of the posterior pole that simulated a malignant melanoma of the choroid was almost 20%. The most frequent misdiagnosis was hemorrhagic senile macular disease. Clinicians should keep these points in mind, but should also be aware that a malignant melanoma of the choroid can be life threatening.

## Blunt Trauma

Blunt trauma to the globe can cause a patient to have a rupture of the choroid (Figure 30.11). These usually present with a positive history or signs of ocular contusion injury and the ophthalmoscopic appearance of hemorrhage in the subretinal space. The lesion will resolve with time, and the patient will be left with an arclike fibrous scar with overlying pigment clumping. Occasionally, a patient may develop choroidal neovascularization into the retina through a break in Bruch's membrane at the site of the rupture, and a subsequent serous or hemorrhagic detachment of the retina can occur over the rupture to the choroid.

Besides the diseases and disorders that

Table 30.3
Clinical Characteristics of Benign Choroidal Nevi versus
Malignant Melanoma of the Choroid

|  | Benign Nevus | Malignant Melanoma |
|---|---|---|
| Size | Usually <5 DD | Can be any size |
| Elevation | Usually <2 mm | May be slight (<0.5 mm) or can produce a solid retinal detachment |
| Overlying pigment configuration | Drusen (<4) | May have drusen (>4) and orange pigment |
| Borders | Smooth or feathery | More likely to be lobulated |
| Vasculature | Neovascularization (if any specific angiographic findings) | Has its own defined blood supply (large vessels seen on angiography) |
| Color | Slate gray to light black | Uneven |
| Progression | Very rarely enlarge | Likely to enlarge |

Note: Choroidal masses not falling strictly into one of these categories should be classified as suspicious nevi and observed with fundus drawings and serial photography.

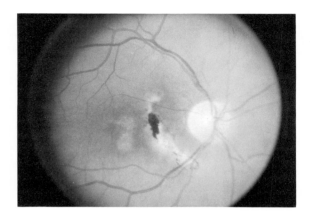

FIGURE 30.11.
Choroidal rupture.

are generally of choroidal origin, there are a variety of diseases and disorders that affect primarily the retinal pigment epithelium. Many of these are inherited, although acquired conditions can affect the retinal pigment epithelium.

## Vitelliform Macular Degeneration (Best's Disease)

One of the most morphologically striking fundus disorders to affect the retinal pigment epithelium is vitelliform macular degeneration, or Best's disease. This disorder of the retinal pigment epithelium is bilaterally inherited in an autosomally dominant mode. Ophthalmoscopic signs of vitelliform macular degeneration begin in the childhood years with a characteristic lesion of the macula, the so-called sunny-side-up egg. The lesion is at the level of the retinal pigment epithelium and is discrete with sharp borders. Later, vitelliform macular degeneration manifests itself as a "scrambled egg," as the yellow lesion begins to show signs of derangement. At this stage, the visual acuity decreases to 20/40 to 20/70. In adult life, there are occasional patients with vitelliform macular degeneration who develop serous and/or hem-

orrhagic detachments of the retinal pigment epithelium associated with choroidal neovascularization. In other cases of vitelliform macular degeneration the lesion may scramble into an area of geographic atrophy. In these later stages, the visual acuity is often poor.

In many patients, the diagnosis is quite apparent, but in others it may be elusive. In those cases that defy immediate diagnosis, the clinician should consider examining other family members for classic manifestations of the disease. Although most of the electrodiagnostic examinations are unremarkable, the electro-oculogram is often below 1.55.

## Foveomacular Vitelliform Dystrophy: Adult Type

Occasionally, a clinician may encounter a patient that is in middle life and has a lesion like that in vitelliform macular degeneration, but smaller than the typical one-disk diameter or larger lesion. These cases often present with good visual acuity, a lesion about one-third of a disc diameter in size with a small pigmented area in the center, and bilateral involvement. Many of these cases are not vitelliform macular degeneration, but foveomacular vitelliform dystrophy: adult type. Although foveomacular vitelliform dystrophy: adult type may be inherited in a similar mode to vitelliform macular degeneration, the clinical signs are different, as is the visual acuity. In addition, in cases of foveomacular vitelliform dystrophy: adult type, the electro-oculogram is essentially normal.

## Stargardt's Disease/Fundus Flavimaculatus

Another disorder of the retinal pigment epithelium that can diminish central vision actually has two names. For many years, Stargardt's disease and fundus fla-vimaculatus were thought to be different disorders. Both have yellow white flecks at the level of the retinal pigment epithelium symmetrically in both eyes as the hallmark of the disease. The former, however, oc-curs at the macula, while the latter typi-cally presents in the midperiphery. There is substantial evidence that these two dis-orders, Stargardt's disease and fundus flavimaculatus, are the same disease, an uncommon recessive disorder of the reti-nal pigment epithelium and sensory ret-ina. When the macula is involved, with what is referred to here as Stargardt's dis-ease, the ophthalmoscopic examination may reveal flecks at the level of the retinal pigment epithelium and sensory retina, which may not significantly reduce vision. In the early adult years, however, the le-sions typically begin to undergo disper-sion and derangement to manifest a beaten-metal appearance. At this time, vi-sual acuity is profoundly affected (20/100 to 20/400). If the macula is not involved, the prognosis for the retention of central vision is excellent. Most of the patients who suffer loss of central vision from Star-gardt's find help with low vision aids and vision rehabilitation. The morphologic portrait is the best way to make the di-agnosis; electrodiagnostic tests generally are of little assistance, except that the elec-tro-oculogram is abnormal in about half of the cases of Stargardt's disease.

## Retinitis Pigmentosa

Perhaps the most frequently encountered inherited disorder of the retinal pigment epithelium is retinitis pigmentosa. Symp-toms begin in early adulthood, and they are classic in that it is often possible to presume the diagnosis from the history alone. The major symptom in new cases of retinitis pigmentosa is impaired night mobility. Although most texts refer to this impaired night mobility as "night blind-ness," it is inappropriate for clinicians to put much faith in night blindness as a subjective complaint. Daily, clinicians en-counter patients who state that they have difficulty seeing at night, but it is the pa-tients who complain of impaired night mo-bility, or those from whom the clinician can elicit the complaint of impaired night mobility, that are likely to have retinitis pigmentosa. Later in life, the symptoms can include decreased visual field and im-paired central vision.

Objectively, the early fundus signs in-clude an olive discoloration of the retinal pigment epithelium and migration of ret-inal pigment epithelium cells into the ret-ina. The migration of retinal pigment epithelium cells generally occurs earliest in the midperiphery of the fundus. This is reflected in the classic ring scotoma plotted with visual field testing. Later, the retinal vessels become constricted and the optic disc shows wavy yellow atrophic pallor.

Electrodiagnostic tests are abnormal, specifically the electroretinogram. The electroretinogram is typically flat, and this can often be correlated to a patient's re-actions to a darkened room. Often, pa-tients manifest marked impairment of mobility under dim illumination. The cli-nician can use his own normal vision as the control.

The mode of inheritance in retinitis pigmentosa is often recessive, although there are some cases that are autosomally dominant or sex linked. The most severe form of retinitis pigmentosa is the X-linked disease manifested in males.

Management of patients with retinitis pigmentosa is oriented toward genetic counseling, vision rehabilitation with the use of low vision aids, and orientation and mobility training. In addition, it is not at all uncommon to encounter patients with retinitis pigmentosa that have a need for consultation for chronic bruises to their shins. The bruises arise from bumping into objects like coffee tables when the pa-tients have to make their way in a dark and unfamiliar room. Mobility is further hampered when visual field loss is present. Finally, one should always be on the alert for the onset of posterior subcapsular cataract in patients with retinitis pigmentosa, a well-known association.

# Rubella Retinopathy

There are a variety of acquired diseases and disorders of the retinal pigment epithelium, but perhaps the one most frequently encountered is rubella retinopathy. Mothers who acquire rubella in the first trimester of pregnancy are at risk to transmit to the fetus rubella-related abnormalities of vision. There are other systemic manifestations, but in the eye the most frequently encountered abnormalities are limited to mild, stationary mottling of the retinal pigment epithelium. Visual acuity is usually better than 20/40.

# Retinal Vascular Occlusion

There are a number of retinal vascular diseases that can affect central vision. They can generally be divided into two groups: those that involve the retinal arteries and arterioles and those that involve the venous vasculature.

## CENTRAL RETINAL ARTERY

A central retinal artery occlusion causes the most profound loss of vision of all retinal vascular diseases. The sudden reduction of the blood flow to the retina occurs most frequently from emboli from either the left side of the heart or from the arteries supplying the head. Most emboli contain either fibrin, cholesterol, or platelets. In central retinal artery occlusions, the cardinal symptom is a sudden painless loss of vision. About one-fifth of patients with acute central retinal artery occlusion will have no light perception. The majority of the remainder will have very poor vision. Patients with a patent cilioretinal artery, however, may have fairly good vision, albeit with a restricted visual field. Surpris-

ingly, many patients wait hours or days before seeking professional help.

The clinician will encounter a patient with a sluggish direct pupillary response. Ophthalmoscopically, the clinician may observe the emboli in the retinal arteries, usually at a bifurcation. Early in the course of central retinal artery occlusion, the clinician will observe a generally edematous or cloudy retina. The retinal arteries appear thin, and the retinal veins reveal sludging of the blood flow. In addition, many cases will reveal the classic cherry red spot within a few hours. This cherry red spot is observed at the fovea in patients with central retinal artery occlusion because the foveal retina is thin, permitting a view of the underlying red choroid. The remainder of the retina at the posterior pole is ischemic, preventing a view of the underlying choroid. Within a few weeks, the retina may look ophthalmoscopically normal, but because the retina cannot tolerate a loss of oxygen for very long, the visual acuity is poor. Unless immediate heroic measures prove successful, the presenting level of visual acuity is the best that can be expected.

## BRANCH RETINAL ARTERY OCCLUSION

There are cases where emboli affect the retina by causing a branch retinal artery occlusion. In these cases, the retina is affected only within the distribution of that occluded arterial branch. If the clinician encounters a patient with a central or branch retinal artery occlusion within an hour of the occlusion, there are a variety of procedures that can be attempted to reestablish vascular perfusion of the retina. The clinician can massage the eye to reduce the intraocular pressure or have the patient breathe an oxygen and carbon dioxide mixture. A variety of medications have been used in attempts to reperfuse the retina, including tolazoline, as well as surgical intervention with paracentesis. These emergency measures have met with limited success. A systemic workup is indicated.

## HYPERTENSIVE RETINOPATHY

Contrary to branch retinal artery occlusion and central retinal artery occlusion, hypertensive retinopathy rarely causes a loss of central vision. Although there are a number of well-known classifications of hypertensive retinopathy, including the Scheie classification, the Keith-Wagener-Barker classification, and Leishman's classification, the most successful method to evaluate the risk of hypertension in a patient without previous diagnosis is to use the sphygmomanometer. Once the diagnosis of systemic hypertension is established and the patient begins treatment, the clinician can follow the patient for hypertensive retinopathy on a yearly basis. Patients can lose central vision if the fovea is disturbed by a cotton-wool patch, intraretinal hemorrhage or exudates, or preretinal hemorrhage. In malignant hypertension, the clinician encounters severe hypertensive retinopathy signs that include the classic macular star and papilledema. These unfortunate patients have a predicted mortality within 36 months.

## DIABETIC RETINOPATHY

One of the most common causes of vision impairment and legal blindness in the industrialized world is diabetic retinopathy. The onset of diabetic retinopathy is related to the duration of the systemic disease. Approximately two-thirds of diabetics with duration of the disease of over 15 years will have diabetic retinopathy. Clinically, there are two types of diabetic retinopathy: background and proliferative diabetic retinopathy. The process that sets in motion diabetic retinopathy is related to the loss of intramural pericytes within the capillaries of the retina, and also closure of these capillaries. Capillary closure results in the release of suspected vasoproliferative factor(s) that stimulate a retinal neovascularization, leading to proliferative diabetic retinopathy. Diabetic retinopathy within

the retina is termed *background diabetic retinopathy.* The ophthalmoscopic signs of background diabetic retinopathy include microaneurysms, blot hemorrhages, cotton-wool spots, venous beading, hard exudates, and intraretinal microvascular abnormalities. Central vision is affected when background diabetic retinopathy involves the fovea with either hemorrhage or, more commonly, macular edema. Diabetic macular edema is the result of capillary permeability abnormalities. Clinicians will observe background diabetic retinopathy to wax and wane with time.

There is a phase in the natural course of diabetic retinopathy that is often called the *preproliferative diabetic retinopathy stage.* It is characterized by the appearance of cotton-wool patches, venous beading, and intraretinal microvascular abnormalities. Those patients that manifest these signs should be monitored very closely.

When the clinician suspects proliferative diabetic retinopathy, attention should be focused on the optic disc. Since no internal limiting membrane exists at the optic disc, it is here that new blood vessels from retinal neovascularization can easily grow onto the hyaloid face of the vitreous. These blood vessels can be recognized by their characteristic appearance as a frond of fine red lines. In proliferative diabetic retinopathy, the optic disc is involved almost 75% of the time; the remaining involvement consists of proliferative diabetic retinopathy elsewhere in the retina. It is convenient for clinicians to think of proliferative diabetic retinopathy as either neovascularization at the disc (NVD), or as neovascularization elsewhere (NVE).

When the vitreous contracts over these fronds of new blood vessels, frank vitreous hemorrhage can occur. As the vitreous hemorrhage resolves, the patient will manifest fibrous proliferation from these vessels. Although the hemorrhage into the vitreous temporarily blinds the patient, it is the fibrous proliferation that causes a permanent loss of sight. Fibrous tissue contracts along with the vitreous gel and causes a traction retinal detachment, which can lead to blindness. The onset of legal blindness from proliferative diabetic retinopathy is not only serious from a vision perspective: it is related to increased mortality.

There is little treatment for background diabetic retinopathy and, fortunately, it rarely reduces central vision. Argon laser photocoagulation sometimes can be used in prolonged cases of diabetic macular edema. It is not to be considered for most patients with background diabetic retinopathy and macular edema because the results are not consistently reliable.

For patients with proliferative diabetic retinopathy, however, the treatment of choice is argon laser photocoagulation in a panretinal pattern application. It has been demonstrated by the Diabetic Retinopathy Study Research Group (1979) that photocoagulation clearly is beneficial in certain cases of proliferative diabetic retinopathy. Eyes with three or more high-risk factors, as identified by the Diabetic Retinopathy Study Research Group, should be considered for such treatment. The four factors are presence of vitreous or preretinal hemorrhage, presence of new vessels, location of new vessels on or near the optic disc, and severity (density) of new vessels.

For some patients, vitrectomy may be beneficial. For the clinician with many diabetic patients, it is most beneficial to provide patients with health education regarding diabetic retinopathy and to follow these patients closely to detect the earliest signs of proliferative diabetic retinopathy, which are predictable by identification of preproliferative diabetic retinopathy.

## CENTRAL VEIN OCCLUSION

A profound loss of central vision can occur from a central retinal vein occlusion. There are two clinically recognizable types of central retinal vein occlusion: the venous-stasis occlusion and the ischemic occlusion. Both are characterized by dilated retinal veins and capillaries, vascular permeability, and capillary closure. Venous-stasis central retinal vein occlusion presents with a loss of vision to the 20/400 level or, frequently, better. This type of vein occlusion presents the bloody hemorrhagic appearance. Vision is compromised by the ensuing macular edema. The ischemic central retinal vein occlusion is characterized by much poorer vision and less hemorrhage, but often there will be cotton-wool patches. In ischemic central retinal vein occlusion, the clinical appearance is better but vision is worse.

There are three major complications of central retinal vein occlusions: retinal neovascularization, rubeosis iridis, and neovascular glaucoma. Neovascular glaucoma is perhaps the most serious consequence of central retinal vein occlusion. The period of greatest risk for developing this complication is within the first 3 months following the occlusion. There have been reports of this type of glaucoma, however, as early as 3 weeks and as late as 4 years after the discovery of the occlusion. The incidence of neovascular glaucoma, however, is less than 10% of all central retinal vein occlusions, but it is much higher in the group of patients with ischemic central retinal vein occlusion.

## BRANCH RETINAL VEIN OCCLUSION

Central retinal vein occlusions occur at sites proximal to the cribiform plate, whereas branch retinal vein occlusions occur at arteriovenous crossings distal to the cribiform plate. Because there are more arteriovenous crossings among the superior temporal vascular arcades, there are more branch retinal vein occlusions in that area of the fundus. Patients report with symptoms of central vision impairment depending on the degree of foveal involvement. The ophthalmoscopic picture is one of a fan-shaped area of hemorrhages and exudates emanating from a focus that is often an arteriovenous crossing.

Many of the patients presenting with branch retinal vein occlusion also suffer from systemic disease. The two most frequently associated systemic conditions are diabetes and hypertension. About 75% of patients with branch retinal vein occlusion are hypertensives. There is a variety of capillary abnormalities including variable permeability and capillary closure. When central vision is lost, it is due to macular edema. With resolution of the macular edema, vision often improves to better than 20/40 within 6 months. As the hemorrhage and exudate clear, the retina develops collateral venous drainage channels across the horizontal raphe. The presence of cotton-wool patches indicates a significant amount of capillary closure and should alert the clinician to the possibility that retinal neovascularization is imminent. In cases of branch retinal vein occlusion that have persistent macular edema or retinal neovascularization, argon laser photocoagulation can be considered as a treatment option. There is no known medical intervention that can alter the natural course of branch retinal vein occlusion. Branch retinal vein occlusion can occur in a patient with previously undiagnosed systemic disease. The clinical sign of branch retinal vein occlusion is justification for investigations for hypertension and diabetes.

## CYSTOID MACULAR EDEMA

The changes in capillary permeability that occur in many retinal vascular diseases lead to a distinct type of macular edema: cystoid macular edema. Because of the unique anatomic structure of the foveal area, serous exudation results in the formation of extracellular cysts about the fovea that appear like petals on a flower. The characteristic signs and symptoms of cystoid macular edema occur in about 5% to 10% of cataract extraction patients. The onset of cystoid macular edema after cataract extraction is between 1 and 3 months. Central visual acuity drops to the 20/40 to 20/70 level, and the condition usually resolves spontaneously in less than a year. Many patients with cystoid macular edema after cataract extraction resolve within a few weeks. The pathogenesis of cystoid macular edema is unknown, and the successful treatment for the condition is generally anecdotal.

It is often impossible for the clinician to observe cystoid macular edema with the indirect or direct ophthalmoscope, but with the slit lamp and a Hruby or contact lens the characteristic cystic pattern about the fovea is easily visualized. Regardless of whether the clinician can see the cysts with the slit lamp, a fluorescein angiogram will highlight the hyperfluorescent cysts.

# Ocular Toxoplasmosis

There are a variety of diseases that can affect central vision through inflammatory processes, but none is of greater significance than ocular toxoplasmosis. *Toxoplasma gondii* is a protozoa that is transmitted to the fetus congenitally or, less frequently, ingested in postnatal life. It has a predilection for the central nervous system. When the organism affects the retina, it produces a necrotizing retinitis. The lesion is characteristically less than five disc diameters in size, and appears whitish when active. The accompanying inflammation produces a vitreous reaction, which includes vitreous cells, condensations and, occasionally, membranes. The active inflammatory process usually resolves in about 3 months, leaving an atrophic scar with a hyperpigmented border (Figure 30.12). In some cases, a recurrent lesion can occur at a satellite site adjacent to the previous lesion. Small peripapillary lesions have the potential to produce large nerve fiber bundle defects.

The diagnosis is established by the clinical presentation, and only in active cases is laboratory work justified. Even in active cases, however, the clinician can never be certain that *gondii* is the etiologic

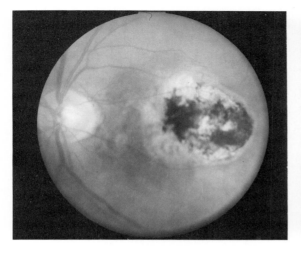

**FIGURE 30.12.**
Ocular toxoplasmosis.

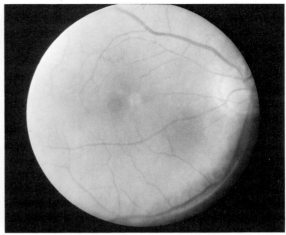

**FIGURE 30.13.**
Senile macular hole.

organism. The treatment of active ocular toxoplasmosis usually is reserved for macular lesions that diminish central vision. Pyrimethamine, sulfa, and steroids are often used in combination for macular lesions. There is no need to consider treatment for the inactive lesions of ocular toxoplasmosis. It is critical, however, for the clinician to diagnose differentially ocular toxoplasmosis, a retinochoroiditis, from ocular histoplasmosis, which is a primary choroidal disease. Each leaves its characteristic macular scar: ocular histoplasmosis leaves a fibrovascular choroidal scar, while the retinochoroidal scar from ocular toxoplasmosis is atrophic with hyperpigmented borders.

## Macular Hole

Idiopathic macular hole (Figure 30.13), without evidence or history of trauma, is a condition that affects the elderly population and results in loss of central vision. The onset of a senile macular hole does not appear to be related to any systemic condition. In general, the symptoms of the natural course of a senile macular hole consist of a slight diminution of vision and vague metamorphopsia. At onset, the patient may have ophthalmoscopically observable yellow deposits at the fovea. Later, a very small hole in the fovea develops. This hole enlarges until it is about one-third to one-half a disc diameter in size. This round macular break is often accompanied by a slight elevation of the surrounding retina. Visual acuity is usually 20/200 to 20/400 in the presence of a full-thickness senile macular hole. Since the retina is very thin at the fovea and the retinal pigment epithelium is dense, an atrophic senile macular hole may appear to be a deeper color than an atrophic hole in the periphery of the ocular fundus. This clinical picture will be most striking with a wide-angle view provided by the indirect ophthalmoscope. Circumstantial anatomic evidence and comparison to the mechanism of formation of operculated retinal holes suggest that senile macular holes result from abnormal vitreoretinal relationships.

Senile macular holes usually affect only one eye. Since no known medical or surgical management is feasible, patients with a macular hole and good vision in the fellow eye require education regarding the condition and assurance that the condition is rarely bilateral. Low vision therapy may be of some limited value to those unfortunate patients who develop bilateral macular holes or a macular hole in an only eye. There is no known preventive treatment for a senile macular hole.

In the presence of cystoid macular edema, visual acuity is better than 20/100. If a patient has developed a thinning of the fovea, a lamellar hole, visual acuity is 20/100 to 20/200. A lamellar macular hole is often difficult to diagnose with the ophthalmoscope or the slit lamp. Often, there are some abnormalities, but the presumed diagnosis and differential with a true hole in the fovea rests with the assessment of the visual acuity. In a true macular hole, visual acuity is 20/200 to 20/400. In many patients, the clinician can presume the type of abnormality by the visual acuity, and then often differentiate among cystoid macular edema, lamellar macular lesions, and full-thickness macular holes.

## Idiopathic Preretinal Macular Gliosis

There are a few surface abnormalities of the sensory retina, and predominant among them is idiopathic preretinal macular gliosis. These lesions most commonly occur temporal to the foveal and reduce central vision only when the fovea is involved. A preretinal macular gliosis usually will not alter the Amsler grid findings because the photoreceptors are below the wrinkled surface of the retina. Idiopathic preretinal macular gliosis appears as if the retina were puckered, and there is often a small glial wisp at the center of the pucker.

There is some histopathologic evidence that such lesions are caused by rents in the internal limiting membrane of the sensory retina that permit astrocytes to grow onto the surface of the retina. After this has occurred, the astrocytes contract, causing the characteristic pucker.

## Peripheral Fundus

The peripheral retina begins posteriorly at the equator, demarcated by drawing an imaginary circle connecting the ampullae of the vortex veins, and extends anteriorly terminating at the ora serrata. Because of the disorganized retinal layers in this region, this portion of the eye sees poorly or not at all. It is for this reason that diseases and disorders of the peripheral retina are often asymptomatic. Symptoms that include flashing lights, spots, or a cloud in the visual field, however, are significant.

Aside from the vortex vein ampullae demarcating the equator, several other anatomic structures provide useful landmarks for clinicians. The long ciliary nerves appear as long, lightly-colored streaks, often bordered by pencil-line pigmentation extending from the 3 and 9 o'clock positions posteriorly to the equator of each eye. They serve to divide the fundus into superior and inferior halves. Short ciliary nerves are similarly colored, but thinner, structures that are more likely to be branched. They are found at approximately the 11 and 1 o'clock and 5 and 7 o'clock positions of each fundus.

The most peripheral extent of the sensory retina, the ora serrata, appears more scalloped nasally than temporally, a feature useful for purposes of orientation. The entire ora is straddled by a translucent band, the vitreous base. This 2- to 3-mm wide portion of the vitreous is its firmest adherence to the retina. Clinically, the vitreous base is not strikingly evident in most patients. As with most vitreoretinal adhesions, however, the vitreous base can appear translucent or show the appearance of variable amounts of pigment dusting. An interesting management corollary is that retinal breaks occurring beneath the vitreous base are at extremely low risk of progressing to retinal elevation or detachment because the vitreous base's strong adherence to the retina denies access of fluid to the subsensory retinal space.

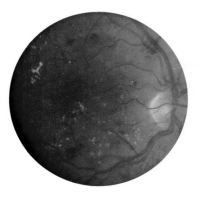

FIGURE 1. Background diabetic retinopathy

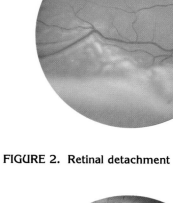

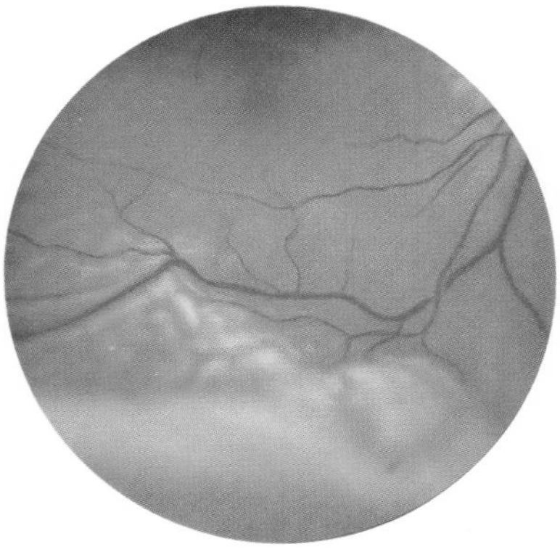

FIGURE 2. Retinal detachment

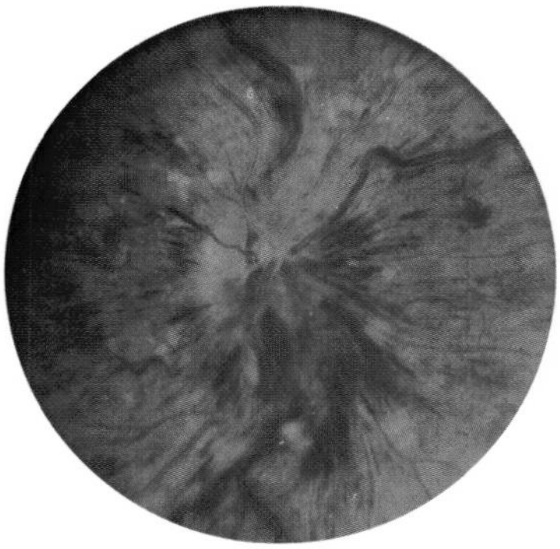

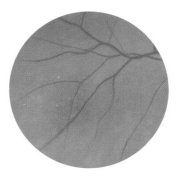

FIGURE 3. Central retinal vein occlusion

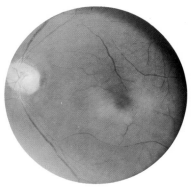

FIGURE 4. Central retinal artery occlusion

FIGURE 5. Choroidal nevus

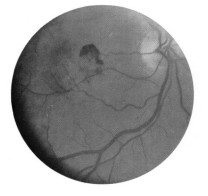

FIGURE 6. Subretinal evidence of choroidal neovascularization in senile macular degeneration

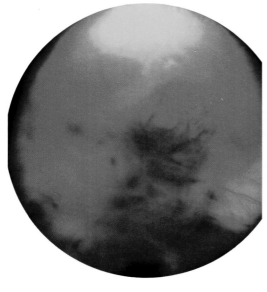

FIGURE 7. Equator-Plus photo of presumed ocular histoplasmosis

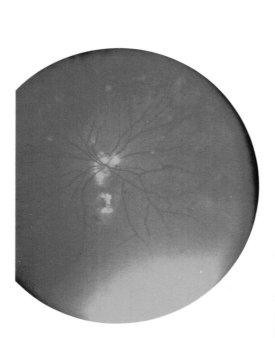

FIGURE 9. Myelinated nerve fibers (Equator-Plus)

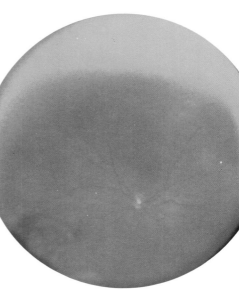

FIGURE 8. Equator-Plus photo of vitreous hemorrhage in proliferative diabetic retinopathy

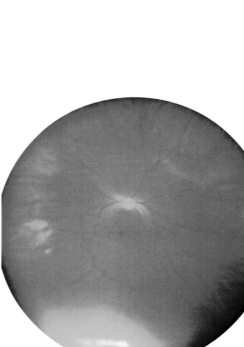

FIGURE 10. Malignant melanoma of the choroid (Equator-Plus)

Equator-plus photos courtesy of Arol Augsburger O.D. Publication of these photos was made possible by a grant from Medical Instrument Research Associates (MIRA), Waltham, Massachusetts.

# Retinal Detachment

Besides the diseases and disorders of the posterior pole that are known to be capable of diminishing central vision, there are a great number of conditions that can cause a loss of peripheral vision. The major mechanism of this loss is retinal detachment. In retinal detachment the sensory retina pulls away from the underlying retinal pigment epithelium, and consequently vision is reduced. There are three types of retinal detachments. The most common form of retinal detachment is the rhegmatogenous retinal detachment. Rhegmatogenous retinal detachment results from a break in the sensory retina that permits fluid vitreous to pass beneath the retina, peeling it away from the underlying retinal pigment epithelium. The second type of retinal detachment is the nonrhegmatogenous retinal detachment, or a detachment without a break in the retina. These occur secondary to the presence of fluid from the underlying choroid, which is permitted to gain access to the subretinal space or a solid mass elevating the retina. The third type of retinal detachment is the traction detachment. In this type of detachment, the sensory retina is separated from the underlying retinal pigment epithelium by the contraction of fibrous tissue that has grown into the vitreous. The most frequent cause of traction retinal detachment is secondary to proliferative diabetic retinopathy.

Virtually every clinician has encountered retinal detachment. A common experience is for a patient to report to the office with very poor vision in one eye and no other symptoms. The clinician examines the affected eye, observing the somewhat opaque retina obscuring visualization of the underlying choroid. The retinal vessels are disturbed and are wavy, and frequently the retina is mobile with eye movements. Most of these patients are in midlife, and about one-half of them will recall seeing either flashes of light or floaters in the previous weeks or months before losing sight. Generally, the onset is more rapid in an aphakic eye, and the detachments are more severe. In many of these patients, the intraocular pressure may be lower in the affected eye, and there may be pigment cells in the anterior vitreous.

All rhegmatogenous retinal detachments are preceded by retinal breaks. There are two types of rhegmatogenous retinal detachments: clinical and subclinical. The subclinical retinal detachment is a localized detached retina about a retinal abnormality, and a clinical retinal detachment is one where the retina has separated to produce a larger detachment that diminishes the visual field. Not all retinal tears produce retinal detachments. The prevalence of retinal tears in the general population is about 4%, and the prevalence of retinal detachments is about 10 per 100,000 person years. That is to say, a retinal tear has about a 1 in 70 risk of causing a clinical retinal detachment.

There are many influences that make the natural course of any retinal break unpredictable. Some of the factors that tend to alter the potential of a retinal tear to produce a retinal detachment are the size and number of the breaks in the sensory retina, the type and location of the retinal break, the nature of any existing vitreoretinal traction, the nature of the vitreoretinal interface, intervening trauma, and the presence of symptoms.

# Retinal Breaks

There are two frequently encountered kinds of retinal breaks (full thickness rents in the sensory retina): round (holes) and linear (tears). An atrophic retinal hole is a round break in the sensory retina that can result from a spontaneous breakdown of retinal tissue. An atrophic retinal hole is generally less than one-quarter disc diameter in size, and has no evidence of vitreous traction. On the other hand, a retinal tear (linear retinal break) is produced by traction of the vitreous on the retina. A retinal tear is often horseshoe shaped, and is typically less than one disc diameter in size. Concentrated vitreous traction can produce a round retinal break known as an *operculated retinal hole.* The operculum represents a plug of cystic retina residing on the hyaloid face of the detached vitreous. This very localized portion of retina has been completely torn free from the surrounding retina, resulting in this special case of round break. The mechanism is identical to that which results in a horseshoe tear. In either instance, if vitreous traction causes a retinal break (hole or tear), a vitreous detachment must have occurred. The nature of this detachment is either local (partial) or complete.

There are two rarer types of retinal breaks: dialyses of the retina and giant retinal tears. Dialyses are produced by breaks in the sensory retina at the ora serrata. They commonly occur in young people and present at the inferior ora serrata in most cases. There is often a history or manifestation of ocular trauma. Giant retinal tears are uncommon and involve at least 90 degrees of the fundus.

There are many diseases and disorders of the peripheral fundus that predispose a patient to lose peripheral vision. Not all of them will result in a complete loss of peripheral vision, but each may contribute to a loss of peripheral vision if they separate the sensory retina from the underlying retinal pigment epithelium or result in a splitting of sensory retinal layers. In addition, retinal vascular diseases that affect the peripheral fundus can cause a loss of vision, whether via the retinal detachment route or via hemorrhage into the vitreous, occluding the visual axis.

## Cystoid Degeneration

Perhaps the most commonly encountered and most innocuous degeneration of the peripheral retina is typical peripheral cystoid degeneration or microcystoid degeneration. The characteristic appearance of cystoid is a salt-and-pepper band proceeding posteriorly and circumferentially from the ora serrata with advancing age. Rarely, it can extend posteriorly to the equator. Studies on large patient populations have shown the presence of cystoid in all eyes of patients over the age of 8 years; it has been reported in eyes as young as 6 months. As is typical of many degenerations, bilaterality and symmetry are the rule.

The clinical course of cystoid degeneration appears to be one of benign progression. Retinal tears rarely develop; round atrophic holes only occasionally appear. Retinal breaks (tears or holes) developing within areas of cystoid are generally beneath the vitreous base and, therefore, are at low risk of progressing to retinal elevation or detachment. Retinal breaks discovered on routine ophthalmoscopy within areas of cystoid degeneration can be monitored at 3-month intervals. This should be extended to 6 months if no progression can be documented at several successive intervals. The patient should be made aware of the signs and symptoms of retinal detachment (flashing lights, floating spots, cloud over vision).

The rounded domes of typical peripheral cystoid degeneration seen with microscopic examination represent spaces between the inner plexiform and outer nuclear layers of the retina. Pillars of retinal tissue separate these "blisters."

In a histopathologic study of over 2000 eyes, two types of peripheral cystoid degeneration were encountered. The first was the typical peripheral cystoid degeneration that has just been described. The second type was reticular peripheral cystoid degeneration, and it occurred in about 20% of cases. Reticular peripheral cystoid degeneration occurs typically in the inferior fundus and differs from typical peripheral cystoid degeneration in that it often extends posterior to the equator of the globe, and it appears as a reticular or arborized pattern to the thickened retina. It involves the inner layers of the retina, including the inner plexiform layer, the nerve fiber layer, and the internal limiting membrane of the retina.

Histologic evidence further suggests that acquired retinoschisis (laminar splitting of intact retinal layers) may develop from cystoid degeneration. Acquired retinoschisis is another peripheral retinal disorder that is intraretinal.

## Acquired Retinoschisis

Acquired retinoschisis is most frequently observed in the inferotemporal quadrant and is continuous posteriorly from sites of cystoid degeneration. The salient clinical feature of this peripheral retinal disorder is the observation of glistening white dots on the inner elevated surface. These are best studied with the biomicroscope in conjunction with a three-mirror contact lens. Retinal elevation results from a laminar separation between the inner nuclear and outer plexiform layers of the retina of intact retinal layers. This results in two distinct retinal layers. Acquired retinoschisis occurs typically in patients over the age of 40 years and is bilateral and symmetrical in about 80% of cases.

The typical lesion of acquired retinoschisis rarely produces visual symptoms, although affected patients can manifest absolute field defects with careful sensitive peripheral-field testing. It is interesting that although these patients have an absolute visual field defect, it is very unlikely that a clinician will encounter a patient with acquired retinoschisis and visual symptoms. Over time, the lesions may change somewhat, either expanding, shrinking, or shifting, while the visual field defect remains almost the same.

Although acquired retinoschisis has a straightforward clinical appearance, eyes have been enucleated for acquired retinoschisis that was thought to be a malignant melanoma of the choroid. In one study, about 7% of eyes mistakenly enu-cleated for malignant melanoma of the choroid harbored acquired retinoschisis instead. This is unfortunate and should not occur at the hands of prudent clinicians. Binocular indirect ophthalmoscopy should provide the clinician with the appropriate tool for differential diagnosis.

A malignant melanoma of the choroid, regardless of whether it is melanotic or amelanotic, is a mass lesion. It is not possible to view the underlying choroid, and there is often an overlying gravity-dependent nonrhegmatogenous retinal detachment. In acquired retinoschisis, the retinal bullous is transparent, smooth, and tense. With the binocular indirect ophthalmoscope, it is possible to view the underlying choroid through the lesion. In addition, acquired retinoschisis is almost always contiguous posteriorly with peripheral cystoid degeneration, whereas a malignant melanoma of the choroid commonly stands alone.

There may be some difficulty, however, for clinicians to differentially diagnose acquired bullous retinoschisis from retinal detachment. In acquired retinoschisis, the lesion is transparent, immobile, and has a smooth and taut inner layer. In addition, acquired retinoschisis produces an absolute visual field defect. In retinal detachment, the detached retina is often gravity dependent, wavy in appearance, and the retina is frequently opaque. The visual field defect produced by retinal detachment is relative. Using the nature of the visual field defect as a pivotal diagnostic point, however, has its pitfalls. The other clinical characteristics should weigh more heavily in the clinician's judgment. Transillumination may also be of some diagnostic value.

In acquired retinoschisis, both the inner layer of the schisis and the outer layer can develop retinal holes. These holes are difficult to observe with either the binocular indirect ophthalmoscope or the slit lamp microscope. Because a statistically greater number of outer-layer breaks progress to retinal detachment, they bear closer monitoring than inner-layer breaks. In rare cases, these holes may contribute to a retinal detachment. In this rare event, laser photocoagulation and a scleral buckling procedure can be considered. In other cases where consultation with a retinal specialist can be considered, there should be evidence of progression beyond the equator of the globe, which would reduce the visual field to within 20 degrees of the fovea or an associated rhegmatogenous retinal detachment. It is not at all common for a lesion in acquired retinoschisis to require this type of treatment.

## Paving-stone Degeneration (Primary Chorioretinal Atrophy)

Paving-stone degeneration is a misleading descriptive term for small (0.1–1.5 mm), discrete, nonelevated, pale yellow lesions occurring in the peripheral retina of about 20% of patients over the age of 40 years (Figure 30.14). The individual lesions are generally separated from the ora serrata by a narrow band of intact retinal pigment epithelium. Since the localized loss of choriocapillaris and inner retinal layers results in a flat or subtly depressed lesion, a more appropriate proposal is primary chorioretinal atrophy. The typical lesions are round, demonstrating varying degrees of choriocapillaris atrophy with subsequent atrophy of the retinal pigment epithelium resulting in a hyperpigmented border. Most common inferiorly, these bilateral discrete lesions may coalesce into a chain separated by incomplete pigment septa. Although the size and number of the lesions increase with age and eyeball length, no sequelae have been reported.

It is thought that the lesions of paving-stone degeneration may be caused by partial occlusion of terminal arteries of the choriocapillaris. The size of the lesions is approximately the size of a lobule of a choriocapillaris bed, and similar lesions have been produced in rabbit eyes by occluding some recurrent ciliary arteries. Although the choroid and retinal pigment epithelium are involved, the sensory retina is rarely affected. Because there is little or no involvement of the sensory retina, paving-stone degeneration rarely causes or contributes to a loss of peripheral vision.

"PAVINGSTONE" DEGENERATION
(PRIMARY CHORIORETINAL ATROPHY)

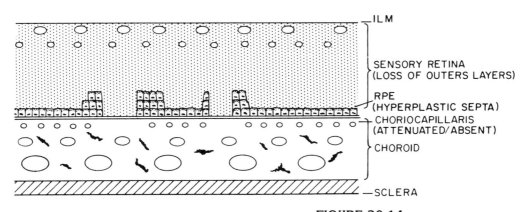

**FIGURE 30.14.**
"Pavingstone" degeneration (primary chorioretinal atrophy).

# Focal Pigment Proliferation

There are a great number of patients who have varying degrees of focal pigment proliferation throughout the peripheral fundus. This focal pigment proliferation can occur in many patients in the equatorial region of the ocular fundus. Occasionally, a patient may develop a retinal tear in association with one of the manifestations of focal pigment proliferation.

In some cases, the pigment disturbance will be observed in association with vitreous traction about peripheral retinal blood vessels. This situation can result in vitreous hemorrhage or retinal tear when an acute posterior vitreous detachment occurs (see Chapter 29).

The key to management is positive diagnosis. Differentials include postinflammatory scars (variable size, shape, and location, presence of postinflammatory material in overlying vitreous), lattice degeneration (elongated shape, inner retinal layers involved), and round atrophic retinal breaks (red in color, often bordered by a cuff of subretinal fluid).

# Reticular Pigment Degeneration of the Midperiphery

An entity whose clinical picture can be easily confused with retinitis pigmentosa is peripheral tapetochoroidal degeneration (or reticular pigment degeneration of the midperiphery). The granular or spiculated appearance of the midperipheral fundi of patients over the age of 40 years and with negative history should arouse no concern for the clinician. Often the entire circumference of the midperiphery is involved. Loss of melanin granules from an intact retinal pigment epithelium is responsible for the striking bilateral clinical picture. Aside from history, the clinician will observe normal-calibre retinal vessels and full visual fields when the need arises to identify reticular degeneration of the midperiphery.

# Drusen

Drusen in the peripheral fundus frequently are seen in the same patients who exhibit them in the posterior pole. This condition is not known to be related to systemic disease, nor correlated with serious retinal or visual sequelae.

# Retinal White-with- and White-without-Pressure

There are two clinical disorders that are vitreoretinal in nature that can predispose to retinal detachment and a subsequent loss of vision. They can be discussed together: white-with-pressure and white-without-pressure. The characteristics of white-with-pressure and white-without-pressure are observed with the binocular indirect ophthalmoscope. When the clinician indents the globe, the chorioretinal indentation appears orange in color. In the presence of white-with-pressure, the indented area appears to have a gray white film over it. In eyes where this phenomenon is observed without scleral indentation, the gray white film is termed *white-without-pressure*. This white-without-pressure is simply a more advanced form of white-with-pressure. Both of these lesions are located almost exclusively in the peripheral fundus between the equator of the globe and the ora serrata. In patients with a more pigmented fundus, it is often easier to visualize either white-with-pressure or white-without-pressure.

These ophthalmoscopic portraits of white-with-pressure and white-without-pressure are most likely to be produced by one of two mechanisms related to vitreoretinal adhesion: a detached posterior vitreous can tug on the sensory retina (especially in the vicinity of the vitreous base) to produce an edematous atrophic sensory retina, the characteristic lesion;

or the vitreous gel could contract to a sufficient degree without detachment to produce a similar condition to that just mentioned where vitreoretinal adhesion causes retinal edema and atrophy.

Retinal white-with-pressure or white-without-pressure generally are innocuous findings. Clinicians should observe the posterior border of the lesion for retinal breaks, however. It is this location where a retinal break would occur, although such breaks are quite uncommon. The posterior border of this lesion characteristically has a red outline. This convenient landmark can be carefully scrutinized for breaks or scalloped edges (which seem to predispose to breaks).

## Lattice Degeneration

Perhaps the vitreoretinal condition that deserves the greatest attention is lattice degeneration (Figures 30.15 and 30.16). Because of the intimate relationship between the vitreous and the sensory retina, a lesion that involves the vitreoretinal interface, such as lattice degeneration, could logically contribute to or cause a retinal detachment. In lattice degeneration, there are a great number of variations in clinical presentation. There are, however, many characteristics that are shared by all of the various morphologic varieties. Lattice degeneration occurs in patches that are more round in configuration nearer the posterior pole, and narrower near the ora serrata. The more peripheral lesions of the lattice degeneration are parallel to the ora serrata and frequently are oriented along a retinal vessel in the peripheral fundus. The classic configuration of lattice degeneration would be bilateral symmetrical lesions that are about two disc diameters long and one disc diameter wide; however, there can be great variation in this classic clinical picture.

Most lattice degeneration occurs in the vertical meridian, and over 80% of lesions have abnormal retinal pigment disturbance as a clinical sign. In addition, an equal percentage of patients with lattice degeneration have retinal white flecks on the inner surface of the thinned retina. Thinning of the sensory retina is a constant companion of lattice degeneration, and frequently there can be observable

LATTICE DEGENERATION

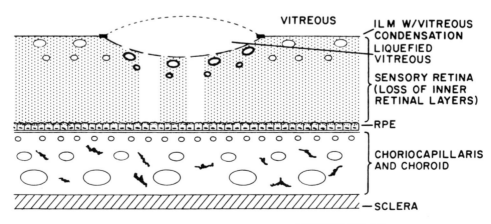

FIGURE 30.15.
Lattice degeneration.

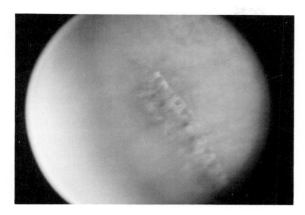

**FIGURE 30.16.**
Lattice degeneration.

erosions of the retina and retinal holes. Finally, many lesions have arborizing white lines within the boundaries of the lesion. It is from this pattern that lattice degeneration gets its name. The white lines represent sheathed or partially occluded retinal venules and, occasionally, retinal arterioles.

The relationship of the vitreous to the retina in lattice degeneration is quite intimate. Overlying the lesion, the vitreous is liquified, and at the edges of the lesion it is tightly bound with a condensed membrane. This condensed membrane borders the lesion. In some cases, the clinician can observe retinal white-with-pressure or white-without-pressure along the posterior border of lattice degeneration. This represents the condensation of vitreous surrounding the lesion.

Because of the intimate relationship between the vitreous and the retina in lattice degeneration, it is clear that lattice degeneration can be involved in the onset of retinal holes, tears, and detachments. Lattice degeneration may be a direct cause of about one-fourth of all retinal detachments, and it is present in up to 40% of detachments. In young myopes, the onset of retinal detachment associated with lattice degeneration generally comes from atrophic retinal holes within the lesions.

In older patients, the onset of retinal detachment associated with lattice degeneration is related to tears along the edges of the lattice degeneration. These tears are caused by vitreoretinal traction and become manifest following an acute posterior vitreous detachment.

Since lattice degeneration is related to retinal detachment, the clinician should consider that prophylactic treatment of an associated retinal hole or tear could prevent the onset of retinal detachment. For lesions that do not manifest a retinal break, clinicians should be prudent in judging the need for prophylactic treatment. A partial list of circumstances where prophylactic treatment is to be considered includes:

1. Ophthalmoscopic and slit lamp biomicroscope evidence of progression of the lesion, *in association with flashes of light and floaters.*

2. Progressive cataract, which could impair visualization of the lattice degeneration in the presence of observable progression of the lesions.

3. An aphakic eye.

4. Extensive lattice degeneration above the horizontal meridian when the fellow eye has suffered a retinal detachment.

5. The eye with lattice degeneration is the only eye.

6. The lattice degeneration occurs in an eye with systemic disease that is associated with retinal detachments.

All eyes with lattice degeneration and associated *symptomatic* retinal tears should be considered for prophylactic treatment. In many cases, the first eye will have had a retinal detachment, and the clinician must consider the efficacy or prophylactic treatment of lattice degeneration in the fellow eye. In these cases, the presence of a retinal tear certainly would benefit from prophylactic treatment.

# References

Benson WE. Prophylactic treatment of retinal breaks. Surv Ophthalmol 1977; 22:41–47.

Byer NE. Lattice degeneration of the retina. Surv Ophthalmol 1979;23:213–248.

Cox MS, Schepens CL, Freeman HL. Retinal detachment due to ocular contusion. Arch Ophthalmol 1966;76:678–685.

Davis MD. Natural history of retinal breaks. Arch Ophthalmol 1974; 92:183–194.

Diabetic Retinopathy Study Research Group. Four risk factors for severe visual loss in diabetic retinopathy. Arch Ophthalmol 1979;97(4):654–655.

Doyne RW. Choroidal and retinal changes: the result of blows on the eyes. Trans Ophthalmol Soc UK 1889;9:128.

Foos RY. Senile retinoschisis. Trans Am Acad Ophthalmol Otolaryngol 1970; 74:33–51.

Gass JDM. Problems in the differential diagnosis of choroidal nevi and malignant melanomas. The XXXIII Edward Jackson Memorial Lecture. Am J Ophthalmol 1977;83(3):299–323.

Glaser JS, et al. The photostress recovery test in the clinical assessment of visual function. Am J Ophthalmol 1977; 83(2):255–260.

Gutman FA, Zegarra H. The natural course of temporal retinal branch vein occlusion. Trans Am Acad Ophthalmol Otolaryngol 1974;78:178–192.

Horton RO, Bartlett JD. Presumed ocular giardiasis and vitelliform macular lesions. J Am Optom Assoc 1983;54:23–27.

Kanski JJ. Complications of acute posterior vitreous detachment. Am J Ophthalmol 1975a;80:44–46.

Kanski JJ. Giant retinal tears. Am J Ophthalmol 1975b;79:846–852.

Karlin DB, Curtin BJ. Peripheral chorioretinal lesions and axial length of the myopic eye. Am J Ophthalmol 1976; 81:625–635.

Lindner B. Acute posterior vitreous detachment and its retinal complications. Acta Ophthalmol 1966;87 (suppl.):1–108.

Maumenee AE, Emery JM. An anatomic classification of diseases of the macula. Am J Ophthalmol 1972;74(4):594–599.

McMahon TT, Rosenthal BP. X-linked juvenile retinoschisis. J Am Optom Assoc 1983;54:55–61.

Mims JL, Shields JA. Follow-up studies of suspicious choroidal nevi. Trans Am Acad Ophthalmol Otolaryngol 1978; 85(9):929–943.

Morse PH, Scheie HG, Aminlari A. Light flashes as a clue to retinal disease. Arch Ophthalmol 1974;91:179–180.

Newcomb RD, Potter JW. Clinical investigation of the foveal light reflex. Am Acad Optom Physiol Opt 1981;58 (12):1110–1119.

O'Malley PO, et al. Paving-stone degeneration of the retina. Arch Ophthalmol 1965;43:169–182.

Potter JW. Hemorrhagic detachment of the retinal pigment epithelium in senile macular disease. South J Optom 1982;24(7):16–20.

Potter JW, Dobson S. Differential diagnosis of choroideremia. Rev Optom 1981;118(11):85–95.

Potter JW, Norden LC, Spruance RD, Ziegler D. Angioid streaks: ocular findings and associated systemic conditions. South J Optom 1983;1:1–17.

Potter JW, Thallemer JM. Geographic atrophy of the retinal pigment epithelium: diagnosis and vision rehabilitation. J Am Optom Assoc 1981;52 (6):503–508.

Rosenthal ML, Fradin S. The technique of binocular indirect ophthalmoscopy. Highlights of Ophthalmology 1967; 9:179–257.

Rutnin U, Schepens CL. Fundus appearance in normal eyes. Am J Ophthalmol 1967;63:764.

Schepens CL, Marden D. Data on the natural history of retinal detachment. Am J Ophthalmol 1966;61:213–226.

Shields JA. Current approaches to the diagnosis and management of choroidal melanomas. Surv Ophthalmol 1977; 21(6):443–463.

Shields JA, Federman JL, Tomer TL, et al. Angioid streaks. I: Ophthalmoscopic variations and diagnostic problems. Br J Ophthalmol 1975;59:257–266.

Sorsby A. Choroidal angiosclerosis with special reference to its hereditary character. Brit J Ophthalmol 1939;23:433–444.

Spencer LM, Foos RY. Paravascular vitreoretinal attachments. Role in retinal tears. Arch Ophthalmol 1970;84:557–564.

Tasman WS. Posterior vitreous detachment and peripheral retinal breaks. Trans Am Acad Ophthalmol Otolaryngol 1968;72:217–224.

Tillery WV, Lucier AC. Round atrophic holes in lattice degeneration—an important cause of phakic retinal detachment. Trans Am Acad Ophthalmol Otolaryngol 1976;81:509–518.

Watzke RC. The opthalmoscopic sign of "white with pressure." Arch Ophthalmol 1962;66:812–823.

Weidenthal DT, Schepens CL. Peripheral fundus changes associated with ocular contusion. Am J Ophthalmol 1966; 62:465–477.

# J. David Higgins
# OPTIC NERVE 31

## BACKGROUND

Patients with optic nerve dysfunction often show visible optic atrophy and any number of associated neurologic impairments that suggest the nature and site of the pathologic process. In these cases the diagnosis usually is strongly suggested on the basis of the clinical exam. Many cases of incipient optic nerve failure are not so revealing, however, and the problem becomes one of localizing the lesion in the eye or visual system.

Before an intense workup for optic nerve dysfunction is contemplated it is wise to consider the entities listed in Table 31.1. These nonneurologic entities are included here to remind the examiner of the most likely ocular disorders when a case of "unexplained" reduced vision presents.

## HISTORY

Suspicious complaints of optic nerve dysfunction include loss of contrast, despite good Snellen acuity, and a feeling that colors are not as vivid as they used to be. Here, the patient complains that the vision seems "faded or dim." Difficulty seeing at night may especially cause the patient to seek care.

Occasionally, a sense of field loss or impaired depth perception may be the complaint. Stereopsis in these cases is usually measured to be normal, but unequal optic nerve conduction speeds (Pulfrich phenomenon) have affected the perception of moving objects. Alternatively, a bitemporal chiasmal defect may cause difficulty with judging the distances of objects away from fixation because of loss of binocular input to cortical cells.

Patients with nerve sheath tumors occasionally note their vision to fade on eccentric eye movements. Transient obscurations of vision occur with nonperfusion of the optic nerve, and occasionally occur when patients with multiple sclerosis view bright scenes. Frequent visual fading with changes of posture is characteristic of decompensating papilledema.

# EXAMINATION

With or without suspicious symptoms, the tests listed in Table 31.2 are useful when unexplained loss of vision compels consideration of an optic nerve disorder.

Snellen acuity measures only one small area of the visual spectrum: that of high contrast/high spatial frequency. Patients with optic nerve dysfunction may have difficulty seeing the edge of the road in twilight and still maintain near perfect Snellen acuity; thus, it can be important to test resolution under conditions of reduced contrast. A qualitative assessment of this complaint can be obtained by washing out contrast on the projected acuity chart. This can be easily accomplished if the projector is equipped with an iris diaphragm in a dimly lit exam room. If not, one can use a rheostat or a homemade diaphragm cut out of cardboard to accomplish the same

purpose. Using this simple technique, it is possible to make it difficult for a normal observer to see the 20/30 line. A patient with an optic nerve disorder seeing 20/20 on the regular chart may now have difficulty seeing the 20/200 line under the altered conditions.

A similar function can be assessed by introducing a neutral density 2.00 filter (1% transmission) before the suspect eye. While a functionally amblyopic eye will suffer a decrement of no more than two lines of visual acuity, a much more severe drop is characteristic of optic nerve disorders.

It is also possible to use neutral density filters to demonstrate subjectively and quantify a difference in optic nerve conduction speed between the two nerves. If one observes a pendulum swinging in the frontoparallel plane, the introduction of a neutral density filter before a normal eye will slow down afferent conduction speed in the eye so that increasing "central disparity" is produced as the pendulum accelerates down its arc. The stereoscopic effect so produced appears to make the pendulum move out of its plane, becoming slightly closer to the observer when it crosses in the left to right direction, for example, and slightly further away on its

**Table 31.1**
**Ocular Causes of Occult Visual Loss**

Common
    Congenital bilateral amblyopia
    Microtropia/monofixation syndrome
    Hysteria/malingering in children and
        adolescents
    Incipient keratoconus

Less common
    Central serous retinopathy
    Cystoid macular edema
    Incomplete (tyrosine positive) albinism

Rarer
    Early Stargardt's (juvenile) macular
        degeneration
    Macular cysts in congenital retinal schisis
    Ocular albinism
    Cone dystrophies

Very rare
    Rod monochromaticism/cone
        monochromaticism
    Congenital stationary nyctalopias (vision
        normal when dominant)
    Leber's congenital retinal dystrophy

**Table 31.2**
**Tests Useful in Diagnosing Occult Optic**
**Nerve Dysfunction**

Normal macular function suggested via photo-stress test and careful fundus exam
Decreased contrast sensitivity
Neutral density 2.00 filter
Pulfrich phenomenon
Pupillary escape/Marcus Gunn pupil
Subjective brightness comparison
Pupil cycle test
Acquired color vision defect, usually deutanlike
Red desaturation
Visual field testing
VER latencies

right to left return. This perceived elliptical wobble is called the *Pulfrich effect.* A patient with slowed optic nerve conduction might therefore observe and complain of the phenomenon without the benefit of neutral density filters. By introducing a variable density filter before the good eye it is possible to quantify the defect by recording the percent transmission that causes the pendulum to appear to again swing from side to side in a single plane. One may similarly quantify a Marcus Gunn pupil by placing neutral density filters over the good eye until pupillary escape is no longer seen.

Pupillary measures of conduction failure are surprisingly sensitive as objective measures of optic nerve lesions (observations of pupillary escape (Marcus Gunn pupil) can be made with the swinging flashlight [see Chapter 18]). A subjective variant can be performed by allowing the patient alternatively to fix a white index card. In such cases, patients with optic nerve disorders may appreciate a dimming of white when the cover is switched to allow the suspect eye to fix. The card may now take on a less lustrous dull gray brown or "parchment" appearance.

The pupil cycle test is performed by positioning the patient comfortably in front of the slit lamp. In a nearly dark room a horizontal beam of about 1 mm in diameter is raised to just partially enter the pupil. The patient gazes over the examiner's shoulder at a penlight. An assistant points the light slightly downward to illuminate a stopwatch rather than directly at the patient. Blinking is allowed. When the slit lamp beam is raised to just enter the pupil a constriction will occur that will cause enough miosis to completely obstruct further passage of light through the pupil. At this point, redilation occurs and the beam again enters the pupil such that an indefinite series of constriction/dilation cycles then occur. Assuming a normal iris and third nerve, it can be seen that the major determinant of the length of a cycle is determined by optic nerve conduction speed. The usual procedure is to start the pupil cycling and upon a full miosis announce "start" so that the assistant activates the stopwatch. Thirty successive cycles are then counted, at which point the examiner announces "stop" to complete the measurement period. The upper limit of normal for 30 cycles is 29 seconds, and/or no more than a 2-second difference between the eyes. If an eye fails to cycle rhythmically, this itself is evidence of optic nerve failure. When borderline values are obtained it is wise to repeat the test several times, averaging the results. The test is analogous to the visual evoked potential as an objective measure of nerve conduction speed. Its obvious advantage is that it can be done as a routine test in the office. Furthermore, it is an entirely objective indicator.

Compared to the early stages of retinal disease, the color vision in early nerve conduction defects is usually disproportionately reduced vis-à-vis the acuity. Because of the frequency of congenital color defects, it is good practice to obtain baseline monocular color visions on all initial exams. With the pseudoisochromatic plates, optic nerve disorders usually simulate deutan defects, although any pattern of findings is possible. Glaucoma and dominantly inherited optic atrophy are more likely to be accompanied by blue yellow failure, however. Patients with definite subjective symptoms of faded color vision may occasionally pass pseudoisochromatic charts; for this reason it is a great advantage to also have available in the office the Farnsworth D-15 or, better, the 100-hue test.

Because of its small isopter size, red stimuli often allow patients to make important qualitative judgments of papillomacular bundle impairment, by far the most important and frequently disturbed area of visual field function in neurologic lesions. A common technique is to show the patient two red objects, one brightly saturated and the other less saturated (i.e., faded, chalky, more pastel, or pink), so as to demonstrate desaturation. Then the brightly saturated object is alternatively fixed by the good and suspect eye. Subjective reduction in color vividness in the suspect eye strongly argues for an optic nerve lesion. In such cases the redness of the test object may actually *increase* as the target is moved away from fixation, which clearly demonstrates a relative central scotoma—the hallmark of optic nerve disease.

Since chiasmal lesions are often associated with reduced central acuity, it is important to also look for temporal hemicentral defects by passing the red target temporally across the midline just above and below fixation. A sudden diminution of color intensity should always be given credence, even when formal visual field testing of larger isopters is normal. Always

remember to test the good eye when optic nerve disease is suspected, as uncovering upper temporal field loss or red desaturation in this eye represents an anterior junction syndrome and possible parasellar mass.

Contrast sensitivity is difficult to test formally in office practice. A new edition of the Arden plates, which are very useful for this purpose, may be available.*

Finally, the evaluation of the visual field in both eyes is a mandatory procedure when there is a possibility of optic nerve disease. While arcuate and altitudinal defects are sometimes associated with optic nerve disorders, the hallmark of compression lesions are the central scotoma and the temporal field cut. Visual fields are discussed in Chapter 32.

# CLINICAL SIGNIFICANCE

The causes of optic nerve dysfunction are legion. Apart from common local processes and demyelinating disease, a large variety of hereditary, toxic, metabolic, degenerative, and other disorders may be present. Table 31.3 lists some of the salient features of these disorders.

Local processes include inflammation, ischemia, developmental abnormalities, and masses (granulomas, abscesses, tumors, and aneurysms). Masses are the most important lesions and often have the most occult presentation. Compressive lesions as far back as the anterior tracts can be associated with a loss of central acuity. Perichiasmal masses account for one-fourth of all brain tumors and commonly cause visual acuity decrements.

The most frequently occurring and important masses affecting optic nerve function are the gliomas, meningiomas, and aneurysms. *Gliomas* are the most common of the brain tumors. Those affecting the optic nerves and diencephalon chiasm occur most frequently in young children,

approximately 20% of whom will have signs or family history of neurofibromatoses (Figures 31.1 and 9.3). Those affecting the optic nerves often show a period of rapid expansion associated with proptosis. Those affecting the chiasm are often associated with monocular or seesaw nystagmus and failure-to-thrive syndrome (emaciation, pallor, and hyperactivity). When the optic nerve is affected, the optic foramen usually is seen to be asymmetrically enlarged on CAT scan or optic nerve polytomes. In young children, strabismus probably is the most common presentation when more striking signs are lacking.

*Meningiomas* are the second most common brain tumor. They are slightly more frequent in neurofibromatoses and may occur at any age; however, they occur much more frequently in women, especially in middle age. They are usually slow growing and keep little company except headache and progressive visual loss. Often optic nerve meningiomas are overlooked simply because the patient states

* American Optical Co., Southbridge, Massachusetts.

Table 31.3
Causes of Optic Nerve Failure

| Cause | Description |
|---|---|
| Hereditary optic atrophies | Dominant (most common). Positive family history; slow onset of mild to moderate (20/40–20/80) visual loss in childhood; often with temporal pallor and excavation; may show tritan color defect.<br>Leber's congenital recessive dystrophy. Disc pallor may predominate or precede retinal pigmentation; suspect in any infant with nystagmus; watch for intense eye rubbing (oculodigital sign). Diagnosis is via markedly abnormal ERG in an otherwise healthy infant.<br>Leber's pseudo X-linked optic neuropathy. Young adult, usually male, always via maternal inheritance, sudden onset of dense central scotomas affecting both eyes within several months; active disc signs are mild degree of erythema, peripapillary retinal edema and telangiectases.<br>Juvenile recessive optic atrophy. Severe onset of bilateral optic atrophy in childhood. Diabetes mellitus follows around age 10. |
| Toxic substances | Hydrocarbons (e.g., methanol, carbon tetrachloride)<br>Heavy metals (e.g., lead, arsenic)<br>Antibiotics (ethambutol, isoniazide, sulfonamides, choramphenicol, etc.)<br>Nonsteroidal antiinflammatory agents (Clinoril, Motrin, Naprosyn)<br>Miscellaneous (digitalis derivatives, Placidyl, Antabuse, ergots) |
| With retinal pigmentation and deafness | Congenital syphilis<br>Refsum's disease (recessive)<br>Usher's syndrome (recessive)<br>Alstrom's syndrome (recessive)<br>Hallgren's syndrome (recessive)<br>Cockayne's syndrome (recessive) |
| Secondary to compression | Infantile hydrocephalus<br>Thyrotropic disease<br>Paget's disease in the elderly<br>Hypercalcemias |

**Table 31.3**
*(continued)*

| Cause | Description |
|---|---|
| | Crouzon's disease and other craniofacial dystoses |
| | Masses (tumors, aneurysms, granulomas) |
| Nutritional | $B_{12}$ and/or folic acid deficiency in pernicious anemia or after gastrectemy. Optic neuropathy may precede anemia, decreased vibratory sensitivity, and stomatitis. |
| | Thiamine and generalized vitamin deficiency as seen in alcoholics and depressed elderly patients living alone; onset may be relatively acute and accompanied by ataxia, ptosis, nystagmus, sixth nerve, and gaze paresis. |
| With hereditary ataxia | Menke's (kinky hair) disease. A sex-linked disorder of copper metabolism. |
| | Friedreich's ataxia. Cerebellar ataxia usually recessively inherited; relatively common with onset in first or second decade along with sensory loss and nystagmus; optic atrophy not common. |
| | Marie's ataxia. Rarer, dominantly inherited ataxia where optic atrophy is a prominent component; onset in third to sixth decades; often with downbeat nystagmus. |
| Lipid storage diseases | Autosomally recessive metabolic disorders more common in Jews and presenting in infancy or childhood with psychomotor retardation, hepatosplenomegaly, and variable cherry red spots. Optic atrophy prominent in Tay Sachs, Sandoff's, and, to a lesser extent, Niemann-Pick variations. ERG is normal. |
| Leukodystrophies (white matter degenerations) | Chiefly autosomal recessive inherited dysmyelinating metabolic disorders producing ataxia, weakness, nystagmus, mental deficiency, seizures, and death. Most common |

**Table 31.3**
*(continued)*

| Cause | Description |
|---|---|
| | disorder by far is metachromic leukodystrophy, where onset may be delayed to adolescence. Optic atrophy is also common in the sudanophilic dystrophies, Krabbe's disease and Canavan's sclerosis, in which infantile onset predominates. In children, adrenoleukodystrophy in boys (sex linked) may mimic Shilder's disease. |
| Ceroid lipofuscinoses (gray matter degenerations) | Chronic juvenile form (Batten-Mayou disease). Autosomally recessive and most common neurodegenerative disease of children. Relatively acute visual loss at ages 6–7, along with mental deterioration and, later, seizures. Trophic macula and occasional peripheral pigment clumping more evident than optic atrophy. ERG is reduced.<br>Acute infantile form (Bielchowsky's disease). Atrophy of nerve head more evident vis-à-vis macular changes, but ERG is still markedly diminished. Usually no nystagmus as seen in Leber's disease. |
| Demyelinating disease | Multiple sclerosis in young to middle-aged adults.<br>"Diffuse" scleroses (Shilder's disease). Probably severe multiple sclerosis variant in children with cortical predilection including blindness or hemianopia; course is usually relentless and fatal over several years, with optic atrophy, retardation, pyramidal signs, and deafness prominent.<br>Postviral demyelination. Usually follows acute exanthems or immunization in children by 7–10 days; often with visible bilateral optic nerve involvement (papillitis). Visual outcome is often excellent. May also follow other viral infections in adults as well, such as upper respiratory |

**Table 31.3**
*(continued)*

| Cause | Description |
|---|---|
| | illness, mononucleosis, and zoster. |
| | Progressive multifocal leukoencephalopathy. An unfortunate viral syndrome of massive progressive demyelination in cancer patients and/or others on immunosuppressive therapy. |
| | Subacute sclerosing panencephalitis. A fatal (over months) syndrome of children owing to infection with measles virus some 6–7 years earlier. Early signs are mental and personality deterioration and often increased startle response, including enhanced blepharospasm. Optic atrophy is usually a late sign, but early macular changes sometimes occur. |

the vision in one eye has been "a little off" for 10 or 15 years; such a story hardly is a substitute for an acceptable diagnosis. Those affecting the anterior visual system usually arise from the nerve sheath, planum of the sphenoid, tuberculum sella, sphenoid ridge, and occasionally from the olfactory groove. Optic nerve sheath tumors, as with the gliomas, may present with a compressive disc edema rather than optic atrophy (Figure 31.2). They therefore may be mistaken for optic neuritis, especially if steroids produce (short-lived) improvement in vision.

Patients with optic nerve meningiomas occasionally will note their vision to fade on eccentric gaze. Opticociliary shunts on the disc may occur as with any chronic local compressive disorder (see section on optic nerve atrophy later in this chapter), but are most characteristic of larger meningiomas. The most important neuroradiologic sign is localized growth of new bone (hyperostosis). When this sign is absent, meningiomas in the parasellar area are often difficult to demonstrate even with CAT scan; angiography, air studies, and even exploratory surgery may be required if there is strong clinical suspicion (slowly progressive loss of vision).

Olfactory groove meningiomas are the textbook cause of the Foster Kennedy syndrome: progressive loss of vision and optic atrophy in one eye followed by disc edema in the other as the tumor enlarges (atrophied discs do not become edematous). Anosmia is a classic accompanying sign and is tested on each side by occluding one nostril and then the other to aromas such as cloves or coffee. Since any frontal lobe tumor may be relatively silent neurologically, it is good office practice to test for anosmia in any case of occult visual loss when even minimal frontal lobe signs are evident.

Supraclinoid variety *aneurysms* are important causes of visual loss. While occasionally affecting the ophthalmic artery, the more common locations are the anterior communicating-anterior cerebral artery junction above, and the internal carotid lateral to the nerve (Figure 31.3). Congenital berry aneurysms rarely produce symptoms in youth. The supracli-

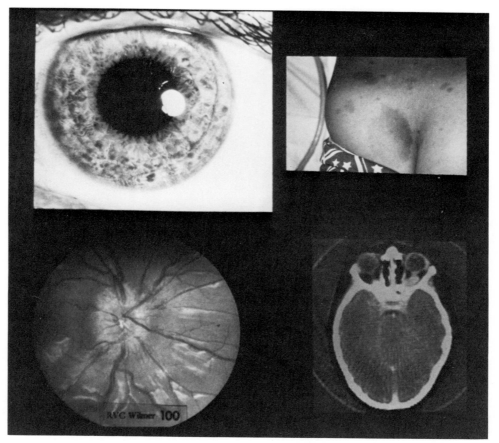

**FIGURE 31.1.**
Optic nerve glioma in neurofibromatosis. Clockwise from upper left:
*1.* Multiple iris nevi. *2.* Café au lait spots. *3.* Enlargement of optic nerve
on CAT scan. *4.* Compressive disc edema.
Reprinted by permission of the publisher, from Miller NR and Fine SL.
The ocular fundus in neuro-ophthalmologic diagnosis. In: Sights and
sounds in ophthalmology, vol. III. St. Louis: C.V. Mosby, 1975.

noid varieties are most common in middle-aged women and, unfortunately, are usually asymptomatic prior to rupture. Suspicious company would include reduced acuity, periorbital pain or numbness, altitudinal field defects (which may vary from day to day), and the presence of an orbital bruit audible to the Bell stethoscope. Anterior communicating artery aneurysms have a particular tendency to rebleed, so a baseline field is always in order.

The reader is directed to the neuroophthalmologic literature for discussion of the less common masses that may arise in the area of the optic nerves.

*Demyelinating disease* is a cause of occult visual loss. In children, excepting those with fulminant meningitis, optic neuritis most commonly follows the onset of an acute viral illness, mumps, or chicken pox by about 10 days. It is often accompanied by visible papillitis, which may be

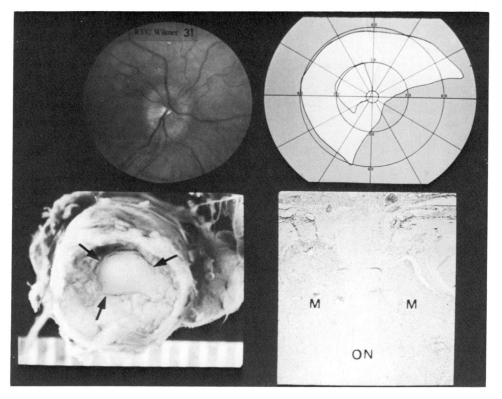

**FIGURE 31.2.**
Meningioma of the optic nerve sheath. Clockwise from upper left:
*1.* Blurred disc margins. *2.* Temporal field cut. *3.* Gross specimen of
nerve sheath tumor. Patient was a 43-year-old woman with 20/30 vision,
a color defect, and a Marcus Gunn pupil.
With permission from the original color. Miller NR and Fine SL. The
ocular fundus in neuro-ophthalmologic diagnosis. In: Sights and
sounds in ophthalmology, vol. III. St. Louis: C.V. Mosby, 1975.

bilateral and usually resolves with little visual sequela. Postviral demyelination may follow an upper respiratory infection (URI) in adults as well, with viral vestibularitis, Bell's palsy, and optic neuritis being the most common presentations. In young adults, however, the possibility of multiple sclerosis must always be considered. Less common demyelinating syndromes reflect inherited enzyme defects, adrenal leukodystrophy, subacute sclerosing panencephalitis in children, and progressive multifocal leukoencephalopathy in the immunosuppressed.

In a classic case of optic neuritis owing to multiple sclerosis, vision reduces (over hours) accompanied or preceded by an ache in the eye on extreme lateral or up gaze. There is usually little or no sign of papillitis. Vision typically worsens for a few days with many of the tests of optic nerve function being markedly positive before returning to near normal levels in several weeks, with or without steroid treatment.

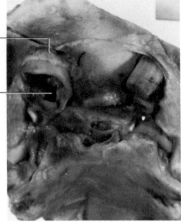

Severe flattening of nerve

Diffuse aneurysm of carotid

**FIGURE 31.3.**
Compression of left optic nerve into dural fold over intracranial opening of optic foramen. Masses in this area may produce altitudinal field defects. Patient complained only of headaches during the week prior to fatal rupture of this suprasellar carotid aneurysm.
Reprinted by permission of the publisher, from Lindenberg R, Walsh FB, and Sacks JG. Neuropathology of vision: an atlas. Philadelphia: Lea & Febiger, 1973.

The diagnosis is suggested by age, prior history of other typical demyelinating attacks (Table 31.4), and by the presence of increased white cells and gamma globulin fraction in the cerebrospinal fluid. The myelin-basic protein and oligoclonal banding are usually not helpful tests in patients with isolated retrobulbar neuritis.

Nerve conduction testing for subtle defects is becoming more important in early diagnosis. Visual, auditory, and somatosensory evoked potentials may show prolonged latencies even in asymptomatic patients. With improved diagnostic methods it is likely that as many as 50% of patients suffering an isolated attack of retrobulbar neuritis will be classified as having multiple sclerosis. A second episode of retrobulbar neuritis has the same prognostic significance.

While a significant demyelinating focus in the optic nerve usually results in compression of the papillomacular bundle with acute onset of central visual loss, this need not always be the case. Visual evoked response (VER) latencies are often abnormal in asymptomatic fellow eyes of patients suffering from optic neuritis, and some or all of the tests in Table 31.2 may be abnormal in patients who have had acute visual complaints. In some of these patients, careful fundoscopy will disclose ganglion cell defects, and visual fields may disclose asymptomatic arcuate defects or a "swiss cheese" field, where multiple areas of target dimming or disappearance are evident. Therefore, careful assessment of optic nerve function is strongly recommended in patients who have experienced suggestive nonocular episodes or who present with an achy eye on EOMs, for example. About 10% of patients with multiple sclerosis will show some evidence of venous sheathing periphlebitis. Papillophlebitis and pars planitis are also slightly more common in patients with multiple sclerosis. Visual fading with exercise and overheating (Uhthoff's sign) and in conditions of intense illumination are typical of patients with established multiple sclerosis, but are usually not very helpful in making the initial diagnosis.

A discussion of all the entities of Table 31.3 is beyond the scope of this book. As is suggested by the table, considerable attention must be paid to the associated signs and symptoms in a case of apparent optic nerve failure. Careful fundoscopy, assessment of family history, toxic history, cerebellar function, and so forth all become important in the case of subnormal acuity of any duration when accompanied by suggestive findings on an optic nerve test battery. Do not assume a benign cause in even a 20/20 eye when, for example, a color defect is uncovered and an ND 2.00 filter reduces the vision to 20/100. This dictum remains true even in the presence of lens opacities, senile macular degeneration (SMD), anisometropia, or any other nonneurologic accompanying disorder that ordinarily would explain reduced vision.

Table 31.4
Historical Inventory of More Common Signs and Symptoms in
Suspected Multiple Sclerosis

| Sign | Characteristics |
| --- | --- |
| Cranial nerve neuritis | Bell's palsy<br>Viral vestibularitis<br>Optic neuritis—acute or subacute |
| Cranial nerve weakness | Transient dysarthria<br>Swallowing difficulty<br>Diplopia, especially sixth nerve |
| Brain stem/long tract | Leg weakness, especially bilateral<br>Gaze palsy, INO, gaze nystagmus<br>Incontinence |
| Cerebellar signs | Gait ataxia<br>Dysmetria/clumsiness<br>Change in handwriting<br>Eye movement disorders |
| Peripheral neuropathy | Stocking/glove paresthesia<br>Pins and needles<br>Balance difficulty/positive Romberg<br>Bandlike constrictions of trunk/extremities |
| Neuralgia | Sciaticlike shooting pains<br>Periorbital neuralgia |
| Miscellaneous | Uhthoff's sign: symptoms worsening with exercise/warm baths<br>Photopsia on eye movement or startling noises<br>Visual fading in bright light<br>Lhermitte's sign of electrical sensations on neck flexion<br>Acute onset of mental symptoms<br>Perioral myokymia on closure of eyes |

# Disc Edema

*Clinically visible swelling of the optic disc accompanied by extravasation of fluid. Papilledema specifically refers to disc edema caused by raised intracranial pressure.*

## BACKGROUND

The superficial ganglion cell layer of the disc is nourished by branches of the central retinal artery. In the prelaminar region, only two or three twigs off the short ciliary arteries anastamose with choroidal recurrents to form the circle of Zinn, which is of great pathophysiologic importance in perfusing this critical area (Figure 31.4): ciliary artery ischemia is a major cause of disc edema.

Especially in smaller, often hyperopic discs, the normal orthograde axoplasmic flow from ganglion cell bodies may suffer from a physiologic block in passing through strictures of the lamina cribrosa. This can result in benign swelling of the nerve fibers producing a picture of pseudopapilledema. In such discs, optic nerve drusen often become manifest in adult life, possibly as a byproduct of chronic extravasation from partial axoplasmic blockage. They are discussed in the next section of this chapter.

The subarachnoid space is patent in most individuals to the level of the lamina cribrosa (Figure 31.4). With increased intracranial pressure, cerebrospinal fluid is forced into the nerve sheath and impairs both axoplasmic transport and the delicate prelaminar circulation. While ischemia in this area is certainly sufficient to cause visible disc edema, it may be that in papilledema the first local pathologic change is axoplasmic block. The swollen axons themselves may contribute further to the ischemic process, producing a vicious circle of further blockage, swelling, ischemia, and finally leaking of fluid extracellularly visible to fluorescein angiography (Figure 31.5). The full picture of venous stasis, exudation, and disc hemorrhages probably is due to impaired perfusion. Impairment of venous egress through the cranial sinuses may play a role when large masses or sudden major obstruction of ventricular flow occurs; however, even after subarchnoid hemorrhage, dilated veins follow the picture of axonal swelling only after several days.

While a number of ocular and systemic diseases can produce disc edema, the most important causes are those that produce papilledema. In some individuals, however, the subarachnoid space terminates retrolaminarly, and no disc swelling will be evident even with major cerebrospinal fluid obstruction. Also, myopic discs, the discs in senility and, especially, atrophied discs will show reduced or perhaps no swelling even when intracranial pressure is quite high. Furthermore, while papilledema is almost always bilateral in its fulminant stage, it may often appear unilaterally or asymmetrically in its incipient stage. The absence of disc edema or its asymmetry then cannot always be re-

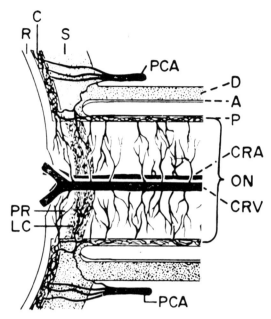

**FIGURE 31.4.**
Blood supply to optic disc. Prelaminar regions
(*PR*) are supplied by recurrent collaterals from
choroid and by direct branches of posterior
ciliary arteries (*PCA*). Other abbreviations:
*A*, arachnoid; *C*, choroid; *CRA*, central retinal
artery; *CRV*, central retinal vein; *D*, dura;
*LC*, lamina cribrosa; *OD*, optic disc; *ON*, optic
nerve; *P*, pia; *R*, retinal; *S*, sclera.
Reprinted by permission of the publisher,
from Hayreh SS. The optic disc. In: Davidson
SJ. Aspects of neuro-ophthalmology. London:
Butterworth, 1974.

the skull, as in Paget's disease, can be a
cause. Most often, however, cerebral edema
is the culprit, such as following rapid
elevation of the blood pressure (hypertensive encephalopathy) or in benign intracranial hypertension (pseudotumor
cerebri). These conditions may present
with papilledema in a patient with severe
morning headache and no focal neurologic
signs or symptoms.

Benign intracranial hypertension often
occurs idiopathically in young obese
women, but may also occur in vitamin A
intoxication, in those on steroids or birth
control pills, or those weaned too quickly
from long-term steroid treatment. In children, the cause may be an idiosyncratic
response to tetracycline, but if the history
is negative in a lethargic or irritable child,

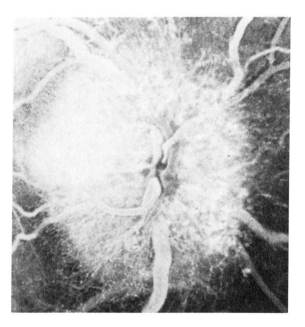

**FIGURE 31.5.**
Markedly abnormal capillary leakage on
fluorescein angiography in true disc edema.
Reprinted by permission of the publisher,
from Cartlidge NEG, Ng RCY, and Tilley PJB.
Dilemma of the swollen optic disc: a
fluorescein retinal angiographic study. *Br J
Ophthalmol* 1977; 61:385–389.

lied on to rule out raised intracranial pressure. Indeed, in chronically raised
intracranial pressure disc edema is probably more often absent than present.

Symptomatic papilledema need not always reflect the direct effects of an obstructive mass on ventricular flow. In a
nonelastic cranium, any mass attaining
significant size can by itself produce the
picture of papilledema; if it is in a relatively
silent area of the brain (e.g., nondominant
frontal lobe), the patient may have little or
no symptoms except headache. Alternatively, compression from the thickening of

the possibility of lead poisoning must be borne in mind. Such a child may present to the eye practitioner because of school problems, enlarged pupils, or accommodative paresis.

It is possible to have dilated ventricles with normal cerebrospinal fluid pressure (low tension hydrocephalus). This is a disease of the elderly to be suspected whenever a relatively acute onset of a gait disturbance and dementia presents, especially if accompanied by incontinence.

In most cases, the signs and symptoms of papilledema will be accompanied by other focal symptoms that suggest a localized mass. Posterior fossa masses are particularly likely to cause obstructive hydrocephalus early in their course because of the narrowness of the aqueduct of Sil-

vius. If focal signs are entirely absent, an intraventricular mass is still a possibility. Consider colloid cyst of the third ventricle, astrocytic hamartoma in Bourneville's disease, and most important in eye practice, occult craniopharyngioma filling the third ventricle.

No matter what the cause, the old maxim of "one stick in the back is worth a thousand peeks at the disc" no longer applies with today's advanced methods of detecting ventricular obstruction. If raised intracranial pressure is seriously entertained, it must be remembered that the sudden lowering of spinal fluid pressure with a tap can result in a downward pressure gradient, causing herniation of the brain through the foramen magnum and the sudden death of the patient.

# HISTORY

The history when disc edema is suspected is guided by a thorough knowledge of its many possible causes as discussed in the section on clinical significance. First investigate the possibility of raised intracranial pressure caused by a mass lesion. In such cases, severe headache is usually present, especially on awakening or after lying down. It is almost invariably worsened transiently by activities that suddenly increase thoracic venous pressure (stooping, lifting, straining, coughing, bowel movement). Early morning vascular headache, in contrast, is momentarily abated during a valsalva maneuver. General central nervous system signs might include lethargy or irritability, decreased mentation, and vomiting, which is especially significant when without nausea. Nonlocalizing focal CNS signs would include sixth or seventh nerve weakness and, more rarely, a bitemporal field defect or internal third nerve palsy.

While those general signs might also accompany malignant hypertension or pseudotumor cerebri, much more ominous signs would be those of a focal neurologic nature, especially those of the posterior fossa (pyramidal signs, difficulty with balance or gait, intention tremor, oculomotor disturbances, dysarthria, etc.). Bradycardia is particularly ominous.

While mild visual complaints or photophobia may occasionally accompany papilledema, transient failure of vision upon changes in posture signifies major disc decompensation; even in benign intracranial hypertension, heroic measures such as optic nerve decompression may be in order to save the sight. As a general rule, patients in whom papilledema is strongly suspected should be admitted to the hospital as soon as possible.

When headache or focal neurologic complaints are not a major part of the disc edema presentation, then the cause quite likely is not a neurologic disorder. Here the focus of the history will relate to the patient's general condition or to the eye itself. As such, the general entities discussed under clinical significance will guide the history.

# EXAMINATION

With several exceptions, the various causes of disc edema produce a similar picture. The diagnosis of early disc edema is via the ophthalmoscope; enlargement of the blind spot and fluorescein leakage are not early signs. While blurring of the disc margin is an early sign, it is not especially helpful unless a change has been noted from a previous observation. This is because many normal discs show somewhat blurred margins, especially nasally, and blurred disc margins are characteristic of congenitally anomalous discs. Much more significant is peripapillary retinal edema. The normal ganglion cell layer just off the disc margin is almost perfectly transparent; it loses considerable transparency only when axons are swollen. Thus a "gray out" of fine retinal detail and loss of clarity of the vessels and their reflexes is very suggestive. Similarly, the fine ganglion cell striations normally well seen in the arcuate zones in all but very blond fundi may fill in and disappear as the fibers approach the nervehead (Figure 31.6). This also strongly suggests peripapillary edema. These observations of increased opacification of the ganglion cell layer are enhanced using the red-free filter of a bright ophthalmoscope.

Severe edema of the disc may produce concentric ripples in the retina between the disc and macula, Wise's lines. A resulting bitemporal depression in the fields may falsely lead the unexperienced clinician to suspect a chiasmal syndrome. Large craniopharyngiomas are the only perichiasmal mass that commonly produce papilledema.

While disc erythema is said to be an early sign, it often is not; in any case, it is difficult to judge and is commonly present in congenitally blurred discs. Much more helpful is the telangiectatic appearance of the small disc vessels—these normally appearing threadlike structures become significantly and often unevenly

engorged, providing further confirmation of true disc edema.

If one looks closely at the light reflexes on the veins as they emerge from the disc, one may expect to see a venous pulse in about 80% of the population. Loss of a preexisting spontaneous venous pulse certainly is a significant sign. In the usual case, however, one does not have the luxury of knowing whether the patient in question had spontaneous venous pulses in the past. Absence of this pulse, especially on light digital pressure to the globe, certainly is suggestive, but not definitive. More significant is the presence of venous pulsation in arguing against disc edema. In one review, none of 43 patients with documented increased intracranial pressure had spontaneous venous pulses, even though 33 of these discs had no other signs

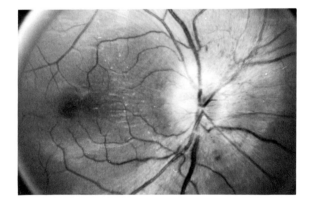

**FIGURE 31.6.**
Peripapillary retinal and disc edema in papillophlebitis. Note obscuration of vessels, their reflexes, and the ganglion cell striations near the disc.
Reprinted by permission of the publisher, from Newman N. The prechiasmal afferent visual pathways. In: Burde RM and Karp JS. Clinical neuro-ophthalmology: the afferent visual system. International Ophthalmology Clinics 17. Boston: Little, Brown, 1977.

of disc edema. Thus the presence of a spontaneous pulse is good evidence against papilledema (assuming the IOP is not elevated); its absence is far from diagnostic, but is merely confirmatory evidence.

A disc swelling becomes more marked as the unmistakable picture of fulminating papilledema develops, with several diopters of swelling, disc hemorrhages, venous stasis, peripapillary retinal hemorrhages, and exudation. Even here, normal or near normal acuities are expected. To estimate the degree of swelling the examiner focuses the ophthalmoscope on the raised margins by going from plus to minus. Retinal detail several millimeters away should now be blurred, and the examiner further reduces plus until clarity is first obtained. The dioptric difference can be used to measure and follow changes in the degree of swelling. Chronic disc edema eventually produces a picture of secondary optic atrophy with overlying gliosis; visual loss usually starts as field contraction, often most severe nasally, and may proceed to no light perception. When this picture is due to pseudotumor cerebri, optic nerve decompression or lumbar-peritoneal shunt becomes an emergency vision-saving procedure.

# CLINICAL SIGNIFICANCE

There are many other causes of disc edema besides increased intracranial pressure. Probably the most frequent cause (at least to the internist) is congestive heart failure. When characteristic headaches and/or focal neurologic signs are not prominent, it is well to consider other causes. An unnecessary referral to the neurologist may lead to expensive and invasive tests that delay accurate diagnosis. Be familiar with the nonneurologic causes of disc edema to manage most efficiently these presentations. The following breakdown is useful in approaching disc edema.

causes of unilateral disc edema associated with reduced vision—chiefly that caused by local compression or Leber's optic neuropathy. Generally speaking, papillitis is strongly suggested by the *acute onset* of visual loss, central scotoma, Marcus Gunn pupil, and variable eyeache on eccentric gaze. Vitreous cells are confirmatory and often are best seen without a Hruby lens, after a minute or two of dark adaptation, by moving the slit lamp as far forward as possible and having the patient move the eye.

## Inflammatory Disc Edema (papillitis)

Bilateral papillitis ophthalmoscopically simulating papilledema occasionally occurs in the young, where it may follow on the heels of a viral illness and be accompanied by other symptoms of postviral encephalitis such as headache, confusion, fever, stiff neck, etc. Acute methanol and lead poisoning may produce a similar picture. The major area of confusion is distinguishing unilateral papillitis from other

## Local Compression

Compressive disc edema cannot be forgotten as a common presenting sign of local masses and is the most important papillitis look-alike (see Figures 31.1 and 31.2). Although suggested by insidious progressive loss of vision, the onset of visual loss with masses can be relatively acute, as when infarct and swelling occur within the tumor, or when compressive ischemia reaches a critical threshold level. As in most optic nerve disorders, the presentation usually will be of the central scotoma variety, with reduced color vision, positive Marcus Gunn pupil, and so forth. The vision and disc edema may improve initially on steroids, further strengthening an erroneous diagnosis of papillitis. Papillitis should be accepted when the history is suggestive (e.g., very acute onset, symptoms of multiple sclerosis, photophobia, eyeache on lateral gaze); when the swelling is segmental or dominated more by exudation and "filling in" of the cup than major edema and stasis; and when inflammatory cells are seen in front of the disc. Company suggesting compression should always be looked for in questionable presentations. Suspicious findings would include a temporal field defect in the affected eye or its partner (perhaps suggesting parasellar mass); EOM signs, conjunctival congestion or proptosis (orbital apex or superior orbital fissure mass); opticociliary shunt (meningioma); orbital bruit (possible aneurysm); the presence of predisposing conditions such as sarcoid (question granuloma); neurofibromatosis (question glioma); frontal bossing, bone pain, and hearing loss (Paget's disease). Infiltrative tumors, such as with leukemic or lymphomatous disease, should also be considered, as should infiltrative thyroid (Graves') disease.

## Leber's Optic Neuropathy

The sudden onset of a dense, central-cecal scotoma, with an afferent pupillary defect in an otherwise healthy young adult male without historical evidence of demyelinating disease, suggests Leber's optic neuropathy. Here, disc signs are minimal with mild peripapillary edema, slight erythema, and perhaps a few telangiectatic small vessels being evident off the disc margin. In the United States, the disease has a marked male preponderance (pseudo X-linked), being transmitted only by the usually asymptomatic female. Thus, where a positive family history is evident, the disease usually will involve siblings or uncles

on the maternal side. Although bilateral, the onset in the two eyes often is not simultaneous. The pathogenesis of the disease is not understood, and there is no accepted treatment—despite earlier reports of success with high dose hydroxycobalamine. Leber's disease is the only common nontoxic cause of bilateral optic neuropathy with central-cecal scotomas.

## Hypoxic/Ischemic Causes

Poor disc perfusion and/or anoxia is the most important common denominator in a large variety of systemic disorders that may present with disc edema. While severe anemia itself rarely may be accompanied by disc edema, a variety of hematologic conditions that may be accompanied by secondary anemia are especially pertinent. Often these are accompanied by hyperviscosity states, further embarrassing optic nerve nutrition (e.g., the leukemias, polycythemias, macroglobulinemias, plasma cell dyscrasias, cryoglobinemas, hemoglobinopathies, etc.). When hyperviscosity complicates a primary hematologic condition, there often will be evident venous abnormalities (dilation, tortuosity, calibre irregularities, increased nicking, and perhaps retinal hemorrhages).

The picture of venous stasis and disc edema also accompanies arterial nonperfusion. In small vessel disease, one thinks primarily of diabetes and hypertension, but inflammatory disease in giant cell arteritis or the collagen diseases must be considered as well in the elderly (Figure 31.7). Disc edema in arterial insufficiency syndromes, however, more commonly presents with acute disc infarct and "pale edema," to be discussed later in this chapter.

Cardiopulmonary causes of hypoxia (congestive heart failure, severe emphysema, cystic fibrosis) often are accompanied by a secondary polycythemia and represent a relatively common class of disc edema. All of these systemic disorders become more suspect when general and focal

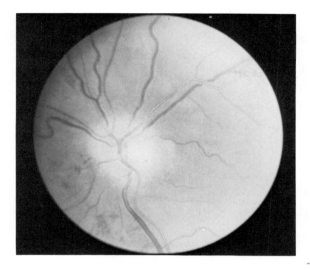

**FIGURE 31.7.**
Pale edema of disc obscuring peripapillary vessel detail following optic nerve infarct. Note extent of retinal arteriole sclerosis in this patient with coexisting diabetic retinopathy. Diagnosis: anterior ischemic optic neuropathy.
Reprinted by permission of the publisher, from Larson HW. The ocular fundus: an atlas. Philadelphia: W.B. Saunders, 1976.

neurologic signs are absent or are an incidental finding amid a variety of suggestive systemic signs and symptoms. For example, disc edema in a ruddy-faced chain smoker with cynotic extremities, venous stasis retinopathy, clubbed fingernails, and severe dyspnea certainly suggests emphysema, despite complaints of headache and dizzy spells.

There are very few occult eye disorders that present with disc edema. Rapid changes of IOP cause axoplasmic block, so disc edema may therefore accompany angle-closure glaucoma or acute hypotony, such as may follow blunt trauma, penetrating eye injuries, surgery, or an idiosyncratic response to drugs (sulfonamides, diuretics). The patient whose optic nerve is adversely affected by drugs usually presents simply with reduced vision and/or optic atrophy, but disc edema is part of

the picture of acute heavy metal or hydrocarbon toxicity—lead or methanol poisoning, for example.

The most easily missed ocular cause of disc edema would be chronic cyclitis/pars planitis, where a relatively asymptomatic eye with good vision may have little external or anterior chamber signs. Usually a few cells and vitreous opacities arouse interest, and the diagnosis is made using the indirect ophthalmoscope, with which a substantial vitreous reaction usually is seen inferiorly near the ora serrata. This disorder is a good example of the general need for a complete eye exam whenever an apparently isolated defect exists. It would be more then embarrassing for the eye practitioner to refer a patient with pars planitis to the neurologist to determine the cause of disc edema (Figure 31.8).

## Hypertensive Encephalopathy

Disc edema in hypertension usually reflects acute vascular decompensation owing to a sudden marked rise in blood pressure, such as may occur with kidney disease or pheochromocytoma. Often, the disc is not erythematous in comparison to the amount of edema observed (Figure 31.9). In contrast to patients with essential hypertension, patients with hypertensive encephalopathy are likely to suffer from headache, especially the early morning variety, as well as the general and focal signs and symptoms of cerebral edema. The diagnosis is suggested by markedly elevated blood pressure in the company of retinal signs indicating acute vascular decompensation: a fundus with a minimally erythematous and raised disc, but covered with arteriole irregularities, superficial hemorrhages, and cotton-wool spots. If the disc signs dominate the retinal signs in the presence of only moderate hypertension, one must remember that posterior fossa masses are themselves causes of hypertension. Here the presence of any suspicious neurologic company would

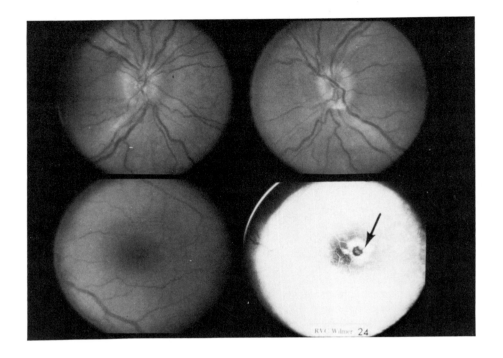

**FIGURE 31.8.**

Bilateral disc edema in a 13-year-old patient shunted for suspected pseudotumor cerebri (*top photos*). Although macula looks reasonably normal (*bottom left*), fluorescein angiography demonstrates cystoid macular edema (*bottom right*). Both the disc and macular edema proved to be secondary to unsuspected pars planitis.
Reprinted by permission of the publisher, from Miller NR and Fine SL. The ocular fundus in neuro-ophthalmologic diagnosis. In: Sights and sounds in ophthalmology, vol. III. St. Louis: C.V. Mosby, 1975.

strongly argue for immediate neurologic consult rather than a hypertension workup by the internist. When hypertension is the cause of disc edema, one expects to see some abatement of the disc signs by the second week following normalization of the blood pressure.

## Papillophlebitis (Big Blind Spot Syndrome)

The onset of unilateral disc edema with little or no visual symptomatology in a healthy, usually young adult is poorly understood. These patients have no neurologic symptoms, normal cerebrospinal fluid pressure, and little evidence of a primary optic nerve compressive or inflammatory disorder. The key to the diagnosis is its unilaterality, the absence of symptoms in a healthy patient, and especially the dilated venous tree extending far into the periphery, perhaps accompanied by some hemorrhaging (Figure 31.10). In some patients, signs of vasculopathy are present, such as sheathing of the disc veins or perivascular cuffing in the periphery,

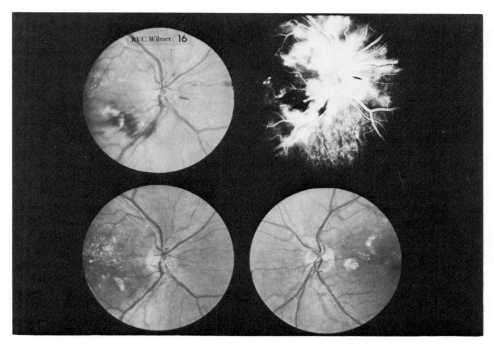

**FIGURE 31.9.**
Disc edema without marked erythema in presence of hypertensive retinopathy (*top left*). Fluorescein demonstrates incompetence of the vasculature (*top right*). *Bottom photos* show resolution save hard exudates in maculas with treatment.
Reprinted by permission of the publisher, from Miller NR and Fine SL. The ocular fundus in neuro-ophthalmologic diagnosis. In: Sights and sounds in ophthalmology, vol. III. St. Louis: C.V. Mosby, 1975.

which should lead to consideration of multiple sclerosis or inflammatory vascular disease owing to sarcoid, lupus, or even syphilis. If the patient is taking estrogens, prudence would advise their discontinuation. Papillophlebitis tends to resolve over a period of months, with or without steroids, with little or no visual sequelae. In older patients, the picture of benign papillophlebitis should prudently be considered that of impending retinal central vein occlusion and a referral made for treatment if indicated (e.g., lowering in the IOP if elevated, better control of hypertension, etc.).

# Acute Anterior Ischemic Optic Neuropathy (Disc Infarct)

The picture of pale disc edema accompanying sudden loss of vision or a field defect in a patient past 50 years represents ciliary-vessel infarct of the optic nerve. Depending on the extent of involvement, visual loss may be mild (e.g., arcuate defect) but is much more commonly severe (altitudinal or total). Similarly, the disc edema may be segmental, altitudinal (superior disc/inferior field much more often

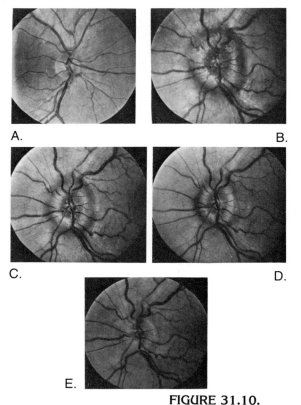

A.

B.

C.

D.

E.

**FIGURE 31.10.**
Normal right eye (*A*) compared to marked disc edema of fellow eye (*B*) in papillophlebitis. Note dilation of venous tree even as recovery begins over ensuing months (*C, D, E*).
Reprinted by permission of the publisher, from Miller N. The big blind spot syndrome. In: Smith JL. Neuro-ophthalmology update. New York: Masson Publishing USA, Inc., 1977.

involved), or total. Attacks often occur in patients with preexisting small vessel disease (diabetes and especially hypertension), commonly upon awakening. Limited histopathologic study suggests this disease may be due to a drop in critical perfusion pressure rather than to thrombosis; in several cases that have come to autopsy, however, platelet emboli have been found as well, and it has occurred in migraine. For this reason, the cardiac status and the patency of the great vessels should be as-

sessed in affected patients. The most important disease occasionally underlying ischemic optic neuropathy is temporal arteritis, which must always be ruled out in the elderly.

In some patients, the distinction between chronic progressive primary glaucoma and acute ciliary infarct can become blurred. Cardiovascular diseases and involutional changes are risk factors for both diseases, and the observation of a disc margin hemorrhage might be considered a sign of decompensating glaucoma by some, and as segmental ischemic optic neuropathy by others. If an arcuate defect with a disc hemorrhage is followed in several weeks by a notch in the disc rim, it would be reasonable to consider this pic-

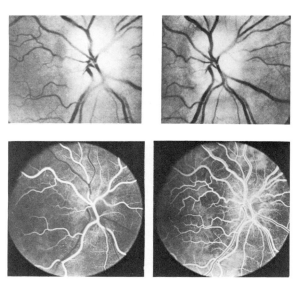

**FIGURE 31.11.**
Stereophotographs of pale disc edema in a case of optic nerve infarct (*above*). Arterial and early arteriovenous phases of fluorescein angiography (*below left* and *right*) show lack of early disc leakage concomitant with circumpapillary ciliary nonperfusion in choroid.
Reprinted by permission of the publisher, from Hayreh, SS. Anterior ischemic optic neuropathy. New York: Springer-Verlag, 1975.

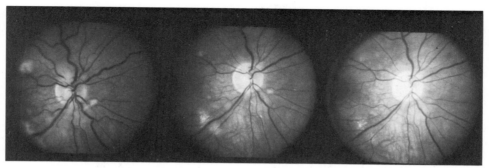

**FIGURE 31.12.**

Segmental pale disc edema, venous stasis, and cotton-wool spots in a case of lupus vascularitis (*left*). Patient was a young woman with little complaint save joint pain. Note development of optic atrophy concurrent with resolution of signs of acute retinal ischemia (*middle and right photos*).

Reprinted by permission of the publisher, from Miller NR and Fine SL. The ocular fundus in neuro-ophthalmologic diagnosis. In: Sights and sounds in ophthalmology, vol. III. St. Louis: C.V. Mosby, 1975.

ture one of segmental infarct. In either case, the optic disc decompensation would strongly suggest lowering of even moderately elevated IOP to assist disc perfusion. Peripapillary retinal atrophy (glaucomatous halo) is also paralleled by acute peripapillary and disc nonperfusion via fluorescein after optic nerve infarct (Figure 31.11). Indeed, even the peripheral retina (watershed zones of the short ciliary arteries) shows areas of nonperfusion and subsequent degeneration after an attack of ischemic optic neuropathy. One wonders whether the correlation of retinal detachment and its predisposing vitreoretinal degenerations, with history of cardiovascular disease and aging, also reflects in part an impaired ciliary perfusion mechanism.

The picture of ischemic optic neuropathy generally is one of pale edema, perhaps accompanied by a few telangiectatic vessels and a splinter hemorrhage or two. When secondary to temporal arteritis, visual loss tends to be severe, not as likely to be accompanied by hemorrhages, and the edema is likely to be markedly pale. One might also observe acute ischemic signs in the retinal vascular tree as well, such as venous stasis accompanied by cotton-wool spots. In general, the patient's age and the constitutional symptoms suggest the need for an ESR and/or biopsy to rule out this disease. In younger patients, especially women, always consider a collagen vascular arteritis in this disease (Figure 31.12).

The final picture of optic atrophy when it results from ischemic insult is sometimes of a cavernous nature and may mimic glaucoma—that is, with glial retraction, pallor, and cupping. Regardless of etiology, all patients suffering from an episode in one eye are at long-term risk for contralateral infarct; this possibility is especially real with temporal arteritis and may occur within hours or days. When the patient history is unrevealing, those presenting with acute loss of vision and disc swelling in the second eye can be distinguished from those with Foster Kennedy syndrome by the presence of cupping; compressive optic atrophy rarely shows cupping. It is rare to have a second episode in an incompletely affected optic nerve, which may be of some slight consolation to the patient. Patients suffering a delayed infarct not long after cataract surgery face a 50% risk of a second attack if the fellow eye is operated on.

It can be appreciated that the primary eye practitioner confronting disc edema treads a very thin line. Signs of raised intracranial pressure and/or focal CNS signs constitute a near emergency referral to neurology. On the other hand, failure to recognize disc edema secondary to other disorders can place the patient in jeopardy and perhaps delay the correct diagnosis of an important systemic condition. Finally, the picture may represent pseudoedema, and referral will have unnecessarily and adversely affected the patient economically, psychologically, and perhaps physically.

# Pseudo Disc Edema

*Pseudo disc edema presents as blurred and elevated margins
that simulate disc edema but do not leak fluorescein. Relevant
entities include congenital hyaloid/glia remnants, myelination
of ganglion cells, and anomalous elevated disc with or
without drusen.*

## BACKGROUND

The smaller the disc radius, the greater is axonal layer thickness at the rim. Since the axons are not perfectly transparent, the margins of smaller, usually hyperopic discs, may appear raised and blurred. A smaller scleral canal in these eyes may result in increased laminal constriction of axons, mild physiologic axoplasmic block, and thus further blurring of the disc margin.

A second association of the small disc is its tendency to manifest drusen later in life. Many of these discs probably have buried drusen in the disc substance as well, although these may be hidden from ophthalmoscopic view. While superficial drusen are usually easily diagnosed, it is the small disc without drusen or the disc with buried drusen that cause the most trouble in differentiation from true disc edema. Since drusen are a distillate of axoplasm, one theory holds that drusen, rather than being a cause of pseudo disc edema, are actually the effect: the result of chronic extracellular axoplasmic leakage from swollen axons in the small disc. Drusen, however, are common at autopsy (1/100 cases) and are frequently observable clinically (1/300 cases), in large as well as small discs. They are less frequent in dark-skinned patients and relatively rare in blacks.

## EXAMINATION

The approach to the suspiciously blurred disc is twofold: first, look for telltale signs of congenital disc anomaly or drusen; second, rule out the signs, symptoms, and causes of true disc edema. Thus, while the disc may be somewhat erythematous, it should not contain telangiectatic vessels on its surface. The peripapillary retina should retain its normal nerve fiber striations up to the margin and remain transparent with no obscuration of the small vessels surrounding the disc. A spontaneous venous pulse is very helpful in confirming pseudo edema.

Small discs, discs with centrally emerging vessels through a small central cup, and discs showing multiple early branching are consistent with the diagnosis of a benign anomalously blurred disc. The observation of a similar appearance to the disc in other family members is helpful, as blurred discs often run in families.

Often a hint of drusen may be suggested in the disc substance. Such buried drusen are made more visible with red-free light and especially with focal illumination at the disc margin. For this examination, the streak aperture of the ophthalmoscope may be used, but it is much better accomplished using the slit lamp and a contact fundus lens. Here the ganglion cells at the margin act as miniature light cables, conducting back toward the nonilluminated disc and often causing a focal glow to be evident at the site of buried drusen (Figure 31.13). This phenomenon is similar to the sclerotic scatter principle used to enhance epithelial edema in contact lens wearers.

When drusen are near the margin, the disc contour may be somewhat irregular. Also, discs blurred from drusen often have a somewhat yellow cast, as opposed to the more erythematous picture of true disc edema. When the drusen are superficial, they usually have the typical refractile appearance shown in Figure 31.14 and present no problem in diagnosis.

Although enlargement of the blind spot and arcuate defects accompany disc drusen, the presence of reduced vision, an afferent pupil, or temporal field cut suggests a more serious compressive cause of the apparent edema. For example, infiltrating meningiomas occasionally present at the disc, simulating drusen.

The diagnosis of pseudo disc edema obviously is only capable of being accepted when systemic or ocular conditions causing disc swelling are absent and when there are no general or focal neurologic symptoms or signs suggesting raised intracranial pressure. In addition, consider that drusen are common enough to coexist occasionally with entities producing disc edema, such as a brain tumor.

Rarely, fluorescein angiography or other special tests may be necessary to make the diagnosis when the clinical ap-

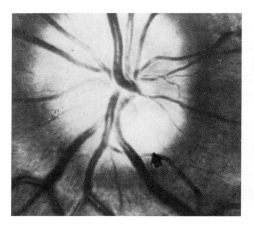 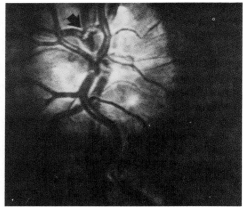

**FIGURE 31.13.**
"Hint" of drusen (*arrow*) in congenitally anomalous disc with centrally emerging vessels (*left*). *Right photo* shows use of focal illumination to enhance buried drusen. Note lack of cup, central emergence of vessels, and anomalous branching evidenced by superior venous trifurcation (*arrow*).
Reprinted by permission of the publisher, from Savino PJ and Glaser JS. Pseudopapilledema versus papilledema. In: Burde RM and Karp JS. Clinical neuro-ophthalmology: the afferent visual system. International Ophthalmology Clinics, 17. Boston: Little, Brown, 1977.

pearance itself is not definitive. The absence of early leakage and the presence of late focal staining of the drusen make the diagnosis (Figure 31.15). Using a bright ophthalmoscope and cobalt filter, it is often possible to observe the drusen "autofluoresce" in the office without the need to instill fluorescein.

In most cases, therefore, a good clinical exam will obviate the need for fluorescein when the patient shows no evidence of raised intracranial pressure.

If for some reason the patient is not able to tolerate fluorescein, computerized tomography or ocular ultrasound usually will make a definitive diagnosis, if necessary.

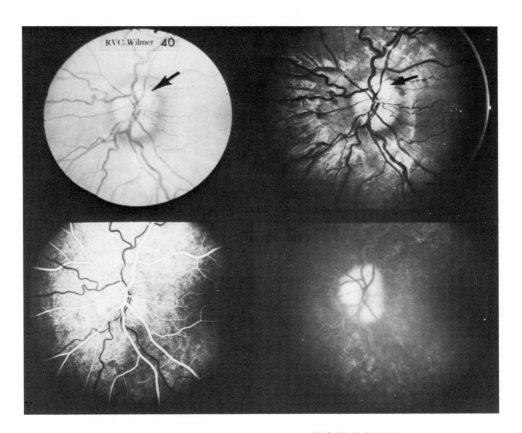

**FIGURE 31.14.**
**Bilateral refractile superficial disc drusen in a patient with failing vision (*top photos*). Disc pallor and marked arteriolar attenuation is compatible with a diagnosis of drusen associated with pigmentary retinal degeneration, which was evident in the peripheral fundus (*bottom photos*).**
Reprinted by permission of the publisher, from Miller NR and Fine SL. The ocular fundus in neuro-ophthalmologic diagnosis. In: Sights and sounds in ophthalmology, vol. III. St. Louis: C.V. Mosby, 1975.

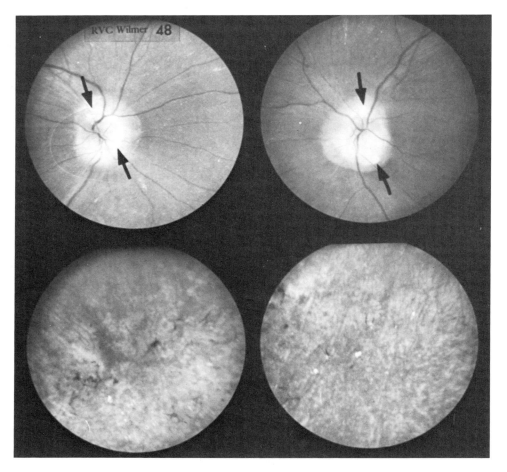

**FIGURE 31.15.**
Blurred disc with centrally emerging vessels (*top left*). Red-free photograph enhances buried drusen (*arrow*) and shows retention of normal clarity of small vessels off the disc margin (*top right*). Fluorescein angiography demonstrates competent disc vasculature in early phases (*lower left*) and focal staining of the buried drusen in late phase (*lower right*). Diagnosis: congenitally anomalous disc with buried drusen.
Reprinted by permission of the publisher, from Miller NR and Fine SL. The ocular fundus in neuro-ophthalmologic diagnosis. In: Sights and sounds in ophthalmology, vol. III. St. Louis: C.V. Mosby, 1975.

# CLINICAL SIGNIFICANCE

Recognizing the anomalously elevated disc can spare the patient an unnecessary, expensive, and potentially risky neurologic workup. Always inform the patient of the finding to prevent future diagnostic dilemmas.

The role of drusen in causing a fortuitously discovered field defect must also be appreciated. Such defects may be slowly progressive and occasionally result in significant disability. Disc drusen are also occasionally associated with disc margin hemorrhages and, rarely, subretinal or even subhyaloid hemorrhages occur. Transient ischemic attacks seem to be more common in elderly patients with drusen of the discs.

Finally, drusen are reported to be associated with a number of conditions, and may thus be of some significance in their diagnosis. Drusen are common in retinitis pigmentosa and sickle cell anemia (Figure 31.14). When seen with angioid streaks,

Paget's disease and especially pseudoxanthoma elasticum are suggested; an alkaline phosphatase should be ordered and skin folds examined to help rule out these diseases. Drusenlike inclusions also seem to be more common in tuberous sclerosis and von Recklinghausen's disease, but these may represent small astrocytic disc hamartomas rather than true drusen.

In summary, a variety of clinical features usually make it possible to differentiate congenitally blurred discs from those with true edema (Table 31.5). In the majority of cases, the experienced examiner may confidently make this important differential diagnosis in the office.

Table 31.5
**Helpful Features in Diagnosing Congenitally Blurred Discs**

| | |
|---|---|
| Rule out: | Signs and symptoms of raised intracranial pressure, such as morning headache, focal CNS signs, projectile vomiting, etc. |
| | Signs of true disc edema, such as significant erythema, disc telangiectases, opacification of papillary retina, etc. |
| | Signs of local compression, such as color defects, afferent pupil, temporal field cut, etc. |
| Look for: | Clarity of the nerve fiber layer striations and small vessels off the disc margins |
| | Spontaneous venous pulsation |
| | Signs of congenital anomalous disc, such as small size, lack of cup, multiple anomalous early vessel branching |
| | Presence in other family members |
| | Irregular contour to margin in waxy disc |
| | Suggestion of buried drusen: enhanced by red-free light, focal illumination, autofluorescence to cobalt light |
| | Suggestive associated conditions (RP, sickle cell, etc.) |
| | Special testing (rarely necessary) by fluorescein, ultrasound, CAT scan |

# Developmentally Anomalous Optic Discs

*Recognition of the developmentally anomalous disc is important in explaining reduced vision, ruling out important occult associated anomalies, and in differentiating active disc processes.*

## BACKGROUND

Developmental abnormalities of the optic nerve tend to fall into two categories: dysplastic and colobomatous. Dysplastic optic nerves contain fewer than the normal number of ganglion cells and may range from a mild hypoplasia to total absence of disc tissue. These defects may be uniocular or binocular, isolated or related to a microphthalmic or highly hyperopic eye, and sometimes reflect a more widespread disorder of central nervous system development. Colobomas (Figure 31.16) generally reflect a more limited abnormality related to defective closure of the fetal cleft. They may be uniocular or binocular, and in the case of the latter often show a dominant pattern of inheritance or represent part of a major syndrome involving multiple CNS malformation. When not involving the entire nerve, they usually occupy an infranasal position where they may often be associated with a similar defect in the choroid, sometimes the iris, and occasionally the lens. Optic nerve pits are very small colobomalike defects.

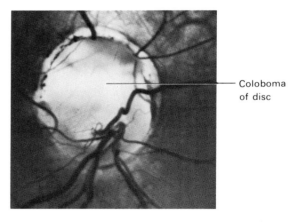

Coloboma of disc

**FIGURE 31.16.**
**Atypical coloboma involving superior aspect of disc.**
Reprinted by permission of the publisher, from Lindenberg R, Walsh FB, Sacks JG. Neuropathology of vision: an atlas. Philadelphia: Lea & Febiger, 1973.

# EXAMINATION

Major dysplasia is obvious and is a leading cause of severely reduced vision in infants. Mild optic nerve hypoplasia is more subtle and can be associated with near normal visual acuity. Here the scleral canal is often of normal size, producing the so-called double ring sign (Figure 31.17). This disorder is often recognized more by the vessels appearing to be relatively large rather than the disc small. The vessels often emerge eccentrically from the disc and may appear excessively tortuous, especially in the fetal alcohol syndrome. When uniocular and associated with hyperopia, the small size may be thought to be optical and defective vision ascribed to refractive amblyopia, a diagnosis not compatible with the depressed field limits that often are observed.

A more common disc variant, which is often bilateral, is the excessively oval and tilted optic disc that often is associated with myopic astigmatism (Figure 31.18). These torsional or inverted discs often show a left-right inversion of the normal angle of entrance of the retinal vasculature and also are often accompanied by an inferior conus and ectatic (Blonder) appearance of the infranasal fundus. When torsion is marked, vision may be slightly subnormal and an upper bitemporal field defect is often found paralleling the inferior nasal retinal ectasia. Such field defects slope across the midline without the characteristic stepping seen in chiasmal syndromes.

While sporadically occurring colobomas are usually without significance beyond the vision and field defects, optic pits have an unfortunate propensity to become associated later with subretinal serous leakage and prolonged flat detachment

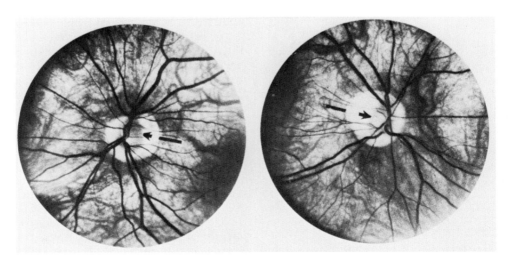

**FIGURE 31.17.**
Myopic fundi with small optic disk associated with reduced vision. *Arrows* show actual border of the neural tissue surrounded by normal-sized scleral canals, double ring sign of optic nerve hypoplasia. Courtesy Dr. J. Bjork. Published with permission from the American Journal of Ophthalmology 1978; 86:524–529. Copyright by the Ophthalmic Publishing Co.

of the macula, leading to loss of vision. The source of the fluid is thought to be vitreous. Typically, pits appear as small, round, or oval gray zones on the inferior temporal aspect of the nerve and sometimes are observed to have a vessel emerging from their depths (Figure 31.19).

# CLINICAL SIGNIFICANCE

The significance of colobomas when bilateral is the possibility of familial transmission by either the autosomally dominant or recessive mode. The significance of the pit is to realize the eye is at future risk and to look for its presence in cases of serous maculopathy to distinguish it from the more benign central serous choroidopathy.

Dysplastic and hypoplastic optic nerves are more likely to be associated with other significant related defects. When associated with nonfamilial aniridia of any extent, the possibility of a serious kidney neoplasm must always be ruled out (Wilms'

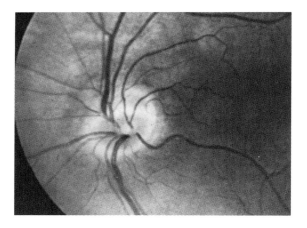

**FIGURE 31.18.**
Congenitally tilted disc. Commonly observed in myopic astigmats, these discs may be associated with superior bitemporal field depressions, erroneously suggesting a chiasmal syndrome.
Reprinted by permission of the publisher, from Lindenberg R, Walsh FB, Sacks JG. Neuropathology of vision: an atlas. Philadelphia: Lea & Febiger, 1973.

nephroblastoma). Thus, these children must always be referred.

While dysplastic and hypoplastic nerves may be isolated findings, the examiner must always be attuned to the possible presence of other CNS abnormalities when the child's physical, behavioral, and intellectual development seems abnormal. Evidence of other midline intracranial defects should be sought. One such accompaniment is aplasia of the septum pellucidum (opticoseptal dysplasia or the de Morsier syndrome), which normally separates the lateral ventricles (Figure 31.20). Porencephalic cysts occur in as many as 40% of the cases and agenesis of the corpus callosum is sometimes seen as well. Pituitary malfunction with multiple endocrinopathies represents another possible aspect of the spectrum of midline defects. Growth hormone assays and a complete endocrinologic workup are especially called for if the child's stature is small for his age.

Another very significant midline defect that may be associated with the hypoplasia syndrome is that of basal encephalocele, in which CNS tissue protrudes down into the nasopharynx. Obviously, this could result in the direst outcome if it is tampered with through confusion with a polyp or other entity.

CNS defects are more likely to accompany optic nerve hypoplasia when the syndrome is bilateral, and external midline defects are also present (flat face on profile, saddle bridge, cleft lip or palate). Cytomegalic inclusion virus, youthful pregnancy, and maternal use of insulin, Dilantin, LSD, and barbiturates have all been implicated as possibly having significant associations with optic nerve hypoplasia. The most frequent cause is

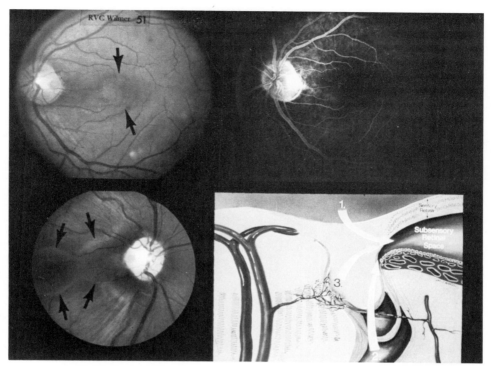

**FIGURE 31.19.**

Optic disc pit at 3 o'clock with serous elevation of sensory retina but no pinpoint leak through Bruch's membrane to fluorescein (*top left* and *right*). *Bottom left photo* clearly shows extension of serous detachment from disc into macula in a second case associated with optic disc pit. *Bottom right* indicates possible sources of the subretinal fluid: vitreous (*1*), CSF (*2*) and serum (*3*). Experimental evidence favors vitreous. Reprinted by permission of the publisher, from Miller NR and Fine SL. The ocular fundus in neuro-ophthalmologic diagnosis. In: Sights and sounds in ophthalmology, vol. III. St. Louis: C.V. Mosby, 1975.

undoubtedly maternal alcoholism. Other ocular features of the fetal alcohol syndrome include blepharophimosis (100%), retinal vessel tortuosity (94%), hypoteliorism (82%), and epicanthus (47%). Keratometer readings typically exceed 47 diopters. The small palpebral fissures combined with a saddle bridge, short upturned nose, flat midface, and thin upper lip produce an almost pathognomonic face (see Figure 31.21). Major aspects of the syndrome include small stature, mental retardation, other CNS defects, and a host of developmental anomalies in other organs. There is no treatment for this unfortunate syndrome except efforts to prevent its recurrence in the same family and a search for significant systemic malformations.

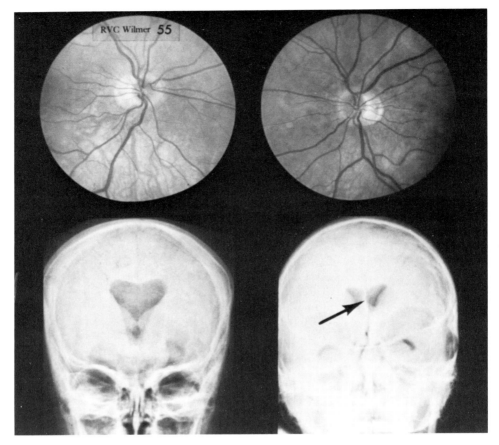

**FIGURE 31.20.**
Bilateral optic nerve hypoplasia in a 16-year-old patient with agenesis of septum pellucidum, which normally separates lateral ventricles (*lower left*). Compare septal defect to intact septum in normal CAT scan (*arrow, lower right*).

Reprinted by permission of the publisher, from Miller NR and Fine SL. The ocular fundus in neuro-ophthalmologic diagnosis. In: Sights and sounds in ophthalmology, vol. III. St. Louis: C.V. Mosby, 1975.

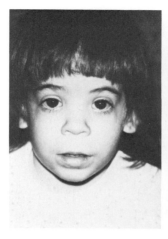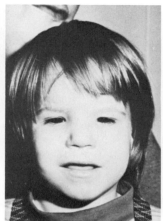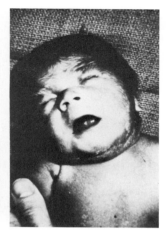

**FIGURE 31.21.**
Regardless of age, the face in fetal alcohol syndrome is remarkably consistent. Note short palpebral fissure, epicanthus, broad bridge, short upturned nose, and thin upper lip.
Left photo reprinted by permission of the publisher, from Clarren SK and Smith DW. Fetal alcohol syndrome. *N Engl J Med* 1978; 298:1063–1067. Middle and right photos reprinted by permission of the publisher, from Jones KL and Smith DW. The fetal alcohol syndrome. Teratology 1975; 12:1–10. Copyright A.R. Liss, Inc.

# Optic Atrophy

*Optic atrophy refers simply to death of ganglion cells manifested in the clinical or pathologic examination of the optic nerve.*

## BACKGROUND

Since the ganglion cells gather at the disc to form a brain tract rather than a peripheral nerve, lesions anywhere in their course will lead to anteriorgrade or retrograde degeneration visible on inspecting the disc. Thus, cell body death in the retina, or axonal lesions in the nerve head, nerve proper, chiasm, and even optic tracts will result in optic atrophy.

Primary optic atrophy is defined as optic atrophy not associated with disease of the disc proper, but rather owing to lesions of the retrobulbar aspect of the nerve prior to the geniculate, or occasionally caused by massive retinal degeneration, as in retinitis pigmentosa or Leber's congenital retinal dystrophy. Primary atrophy is characterized by simple pallor of the disc.

Secondary optic atrophy refers to atrophy associated with a disc process such as papillitis or prolonged disc edema. Such prior disc disease often is manifested by gliosis of the nerve head, which gives the disc a veiled or dirty appearance.

Cavernous optic atrophy refers to a loss of retrolaminal axons and glial support, with fibrotic retraction of the lamina as in glaucomatouslike cupping. Cavernous optic atrophy usually, but not always, reflects anterior optic nerve head ischemia. Outside of obvious causes, such as glaucoma and acute anterior ischemic optic neuropathy, the remainder of the cases are often lumped into the category of low tension glaucoma when visual field loss exists.

## EXAMINATION

The hallmark of optic atrophy is pallor of the optic disc. Because of the preponderance of macula fibers in the nerve, optic atrophy often is most manifest as temporal pallor. This may be sometimes difficult to judge in equivocal cases, and the discs must be closely compared when an optic nerve lesion is suspected. Refer to the beginning of this chapter for tests and findings suggesting an optic nerve lesion, as visible atrophy may be absent even if the patient is symptomatic. On the other hand, and especially after demyelinating lesions, temporal pallor may be unequivocally present even though vision is 20/20. Typically, pallor develops in 2 to 4 weeks, depending on the distance from the disc where the ganglion cell lesion has occurred. Therefore, it is sound medicolegal practice to get disc photos in trauma patients to document the onset of optic atrophy.

As a rule of thumb, the normal nerve usually shows 10 to 12 threadlike vessels on its surface in youth, and 8 to 10 in the aged. Thus, the loss of the expected number of such vessels is also confirmatory of optic atrophy (Kestenbaum's sign).

It is also possible to study the ganglion cells themselves as they approach the optic nerve. In all but the blondest eyes, these cells form visible semirelucent fasciculations, which appear ophthalmoscopically as glistening fine striations best seen in the arcuate areas just off the disc margin at 10 to 12 o'clock and 6 to 8 o'clock for the right eye. Since the ganglion cell layer is less transparent to red-free light, it is best observed using the blue green filter of a bright ophthalmoscope.

Besides the normal striations, the presence of a normal ganglion cell layer also slightly obscures visible detail in deeper structures such as vessel reflexes, the smaller arterioles, and retinal pigment epithelium granulation. When this layer is atrophied, the examiner will have the feeling that such structures stand out in bold relief. This may be hard to judge on an absolute basis, but can be easily appreciated when a sector defect is present in the midst of normal cells or by comparison with the good eye. Ganglion cell defects (Figure 31.22) usually mirror field defects. Clinically, they have been most useful in documenting actual disc decompensation in early glaucoma, where they may actually precede a plottable-field defect and thus signify the need for treatment. Additionally, slit defects have been documented in multiple sclerosis and may represent asymptomatic defects corresponding to subacute demyelinating placques where the patient has not been aware of a central visual disturbance.

# CLINICAL SIGNIFICANCE

Secondary optic atrophy usually points to prior inflammation or swelling of the disc with its many attendant causes. In cases of chronically elevated intracranial pressure, field contraction, visual loss, and secondary atrophy often mean a poor prognosis even if decompression is attempted.

Cavernous optic atrophy also suggests a limited number of possibilities. If cupping or segmental disc pallor or notching follows on the heels of an acute loss of vision or disc margin hemorrhage, the cause has been acute infarct of the optic nerve (as previously discussed) (Figure 31.23). If the patient is relatively asymptomatic, and cupping is manifest in the absence of elevated pressure, glaucoma is still the main suspect. In such cases the tension may be intermittently elevated, suggesting the need for diurnal monitoring, tonography, or even a water or darkroom provocative test. Strongly suspect glaucoma in the presence of suspicious company of narrow chambers, thyroid opthalmopathy, pseudoexfoliation, pupillary iris atrophy, anterior chamber pigment dispersion, or developmental anomalies of the anterior segment. Finally, if the Schiøtz tonometer has been used, the scale reading may be inaccurate because of low ocular rigidity, as in high myopia or Graves' disease.

Often the attempt to prove elevated pressure as the cause of suspicious cupping is unrewarding. In such cases, the finding may be due to congenitally cupped discs, but the examiner should attempt to rule out an ischemic cause either historically (prior acute blood loss, precipitous loss of blood pressure, cardiac arrest, etc.) or ongoing (carotid stenosis, collagen vasculitis, or syphilitic microvascular disease). Even if this search is unrewarding, the presence of field loss should call for the diagnosis of low-tension glaucoma. Such patients rarely develop major field loss, however. In patients with significant peripapillary atrophy and strong history of multifocal vascular disease, perhaps a

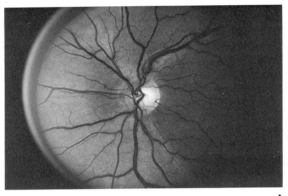

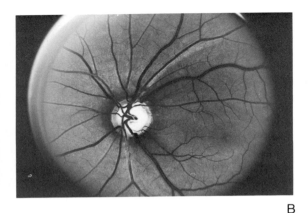

A

B

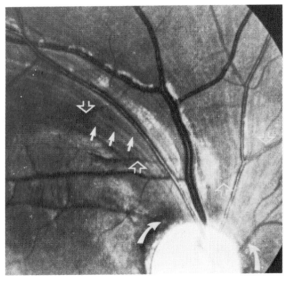

C

### FIGURE 31.22.

*A.* Slight temporal pallor with dramatic loss of papillomacular bundle evident in ganglion cell layer of fundus in 1:30 to 4:30 sector. Note loss of retinal relucency and increased visibility of small vessels in this area. Patient suffered from a toxic amblyopia. *B.* Arcuate nerve fiber layer defect between 1 and 2 o'clock in glaucomatous cupping. Note notch in neural rim corresponding to area of ganglion cell loss and field defect. *C.* Optic atrophy after trauma, with thinning of ganglion cell layer between curved arrows. Rake or slitlike defects are most prominent in arcuate areas (*solid arrows*). Small vessels (*open arrows*) are obscured upon entering normal nerve fiber layer.

Photos A and B reprinted by permission of the publisher, from Newman N. The prechiasmal afferent visual pathways. In: Burde RM and Karp JS. Clinical neuro-ophthalmology: the afferent visual system. International Ophthalmology Clinics 17, Boston: Little, Brown, 1977. Photo C. Reprinted by permission of the publisher, from Bell F and Behrens M. Observation of retinal nerve fiber layer degeneration after optic nerve injury. In: Glaser JS. Neuro-ophthalmology. St. Louis: C.V. Mosby, 1977; vol. IX.

more accurate label would be chronic arteriosclerotic (ciliary) cavernous optic neuropathy (Figures 31.23 and 31.24).

When reduced central vision accompanies abnormal disc cupping and pallor, the possibility of a mass lesion must be explored even though cavernous optic neuropathy is atypical for tumors. A much more likely cause when bilateral would be dominant optic atrophy, usually associated with temporal excavation, some form of a central scotoma, and often tritanopia

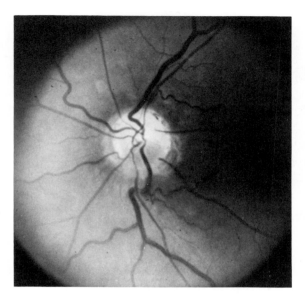

**FIGURE 31.23.**
Segmental disc pallor superiorly after attack of anterior ischemic optic neuropathy associated with inferior altitudinal field loss. Note saucerization of superior disc evident by bends of vessels on rim; also note venous enlargement, suggesting poor retinal perfusion. Reprinted by permission of the publisher, from Burde RM. Ischemic optic neuropathy. In: Glaser JS. Neuro-ophthalmology. St. Louis: C.V. Mosby, 1973; vol. VII.

(Figure 31.25). As children, these patients may have near normal vision, and even older relatives manifesting the disease often retain usable vision (20/60–20/100).

The causes of primary optic atrophy are legion and of great importance to the practitioner. Table 32.3 outlined some of the more prominent causes; more complete tabulation is available in major neuroophthalmologic sources. Fortunately, it is rare for an optic nerve disorder to cause visible optic atrophy without also producing a loss of central vision and a demonstrable central scotoma, or at least a suspicious temporal field defect. Chiasmal or tract defects may exist in the presence of 20/20 vision, however. Some form of temporal field defect will usually be manifest (if looked for) in the case of the chiasm, and a contralateral homonymous field defect will be present in the case of the tracts. Since crossing fibers predominate in the chiasm, and these occupy a bandlike distribution in the middle third of the nerve head, the presence of band atrophy is highly characteristic of lesions at the chiasm or in the tracts (Figure 31.26). In the case of a tract lesion, band atrophy will be manifest in the contralateral eye, which usually will show pupillary escape even when the visions are equal in each eye. This type of pallor always demands a field exam.

For patients in whom optic atrophy is suspected, it is important to be aware of characteristic symptoms and test findings. Of equal importance is an awareness of accompanying symptoms that indicate disease in the area of the anterior pathways. Standard texts on neurology extend this discussion. Recognition of suspicious company drastically changes the interpretation of slightly substandard vision or an unexplained color defect that might otherwise by passed off in a busy practice. Unfortunately, many diseases in the region of the anterior visual pathways have little company. The practitioner's suspicions alone often form the basis of special studies, the most important of which are optic canal and sella polytomes, in addition to VER latencies, standard x-rays and, of course, the CAT scan. Even if these are unrewarding, definitive subjective and/or objective signs of optic nerve failure alone call for special studies, such as arteriography for an occult aneurysm, air studies looking for dents in the third ventricle from meningioma, or even exploratory surgery. A pathognomonic finding strongly suggestive of a slow growing compressive optic nerve lesion (e.g., meningioma) is that of opticociliary shunts. These shunts become dilated when chronic impairment of central retinal vein flow exists, apparently serving as an egress for blood from the disc via the choroidal route (Figure 31.27).

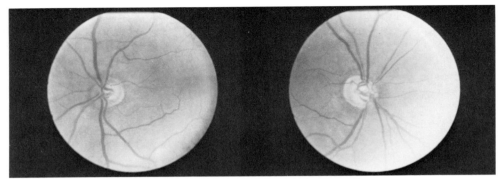

**FIGURE 31.24.**
Major asymmetry of cup-disc ratios in patient with chronic hypertension but equal intraocular pressures. Note more prominent peripapillary atrophy around suspect disc, suggesting poor ciliary perfusion. Always suspect vascular insufficiency in this type of presentation and ausculate carotid bifurcation.
Reprinted by permission of the publisher, from Donin JF and Keane JR. Diagnostic problems in neuro-ophthalmology. New York: Famous Teachings in Modern Medicine, Medcom, Inc., 1973.

# References

## Overview

Arden GB. The importance of measuring contrast sensitivity in cases of visual disturbance. Br J Ophalmol 1978; 62:198–209.

Butler WM, Taylor HG, Diehl LF. Lhermitte's sign in cobalamin (vitamin B-12) deficiency. JAMA 1981;245:1059.

Cohen MM, Lessel S, Wolf PA. A prospective study of the risk of developing multiple sclerosis in uncomplicated optic neuritis. Neurology 1979;29:208–213.

Davis FA, et al. Movement phosphenes in optic neuritis: a new clinical sign. Neurology 1976;26:1100–1104.

Finn JE, Mount LA. Meningiomas of the tuberculum sellae and planum sphenoidal: a review of 83 cases. Arch Ophthalmol 1974;92:23–27.

Gass JDM. Diseases of the optic nerve that may simulate macular disease. Trans Am Acad Ophthalmol Otolaryngol 1973;83:763–770.

Glaser JS. Office and laboratory testing of visual function. Trans Am Acad Ophthalmol Otolaryngol 1977;83:797–804.

Glaser JS, Laflamme P. The visual evoked response: methodology and application in optic nerve disease. In: Thompson HS. Topics in neuro-ophthalmology. Baltimore: Williams & Wilkins, 1979;189–218.

Glaser JS, et al. The photostress recovery test in the clinical assessment of visual function. Am J Ophthalmol Otolaryngol 1977;83:255–260.

Hoyte CS. Autosomal dominant optic atrophy. Ophthalmology (Rochester) 1980;87:245–251.

Miller SD, Thompson HS. Pupil cycle time in optic neuritis. Am J Ophthalmol 1978; 85:635–642.

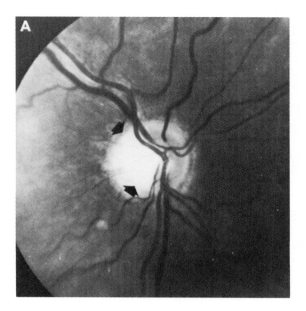

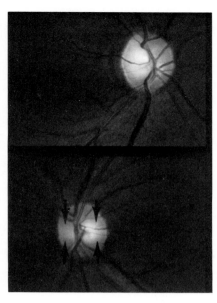

**FIGURE 31.25.**
Temporal excavation and pallor in a case of dominant optic atrophy. Disease is suggested by family history, mild progression of acuity loss, tritanopia, and typical disc appearance. Reprinted by permission of the publisher, from Glaser, JS. Neuro-ophthalmology. Hagerstown, Md.: Harper & Row, 1978.

**FIGURE 31.26.**
Right optic tract lesion with hint of pallor in right optic nerve (*top*). Left optic nerve shows a wedge of pallor extending through central third of disc (*between arrows, bottom*). Such band atrophy indicates degeneration of the decussating fibers at the chiasm that enter the contralateral optic tract. Reprinted by permission of the publisher, from Miller NR and Fine SL. The ocular fundus in neuro-ophthalmologic diagnosis. In: Sights and sounds in ophthalmology. St. Louis: C.V. Mosby, 1975; vol. III.

Sokol S. The Pulfrich stereo-illusion as an index of optic nerve dysfunction. Surv Ophthalmol 1976;21:18—44.

Thompson HS. Afferent pupillary defects: pupillary findings associated with defects of the afferent arm of the pupillary light reflex arc. Am J Ophthalmol 1966;62:860—873.

# Disc Edema

Chester EM, et al. Hypertensive encephalopathy: a clinicopathological study of 20 cases. Neurology 1978;28:928—939.

Ellenberger C Jr. Ischemic optic neuropathy as a possible early complication of vascular hypertension. Am J Ophthalmol 1979;88:1045—1051.

Hayreh, SS. Anterior ischemic optic neuropathy. New York: Springer-Verlag, 1975.

Hayreh SS. Anterior ischemic optic neuropathy. V: Optic disc edema as an early sign. Arch Ophthalmol 1981;99:1030—1040.

Hinzpeter EN, Gottfried N. Ischemic papilledema in giant-cell arteritis. Arch Ophthalmol 1976;94;624—628.

Kelter JL, et al. Pseudotumor cerebri. Surv Ophthalmol 1979;23:315—322.

Levin BE. The clinical significance of

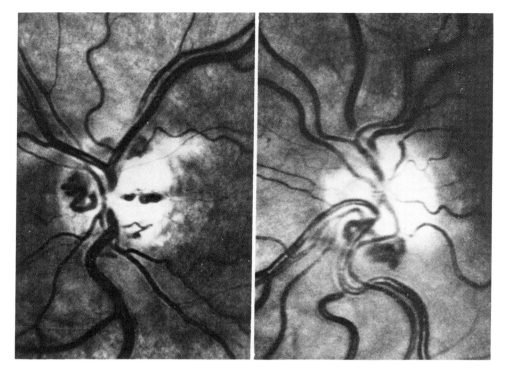

**FIGURE 31.27.**
Optic atrophy associated with enlarged opticociliary shunts draining venous blood from the disc to choroid. Opticociliary shunts always suggest a chronic compressive optic neuropathy, usually owing to meningioma, as in the two cases shown.
Reprinted by permission of the publisher, from Frisen L, Hoyt WF, and Tengroth BM. Optico-ciliary veins, disc pallor and visual loss. *Acta Ophthalmol* 1973; 51:241–249.

spontaneous pulsations of the retinal vein. Arch Neurol 1978;35:37–40.

Miller NR. The big blind spot syndrome: unilateral optic disc edema without visual loss or increased intracranial pressure. In: Smith JL, ed. Neuro-ophthalmology update. New York: Masson, 1977;163–170.

Smith JL, Hoyt WF, Susac JO. Ocular fundus in acute Leber optic neuropathy. Arch Ophthalmol 1973;90:349–354.

Trobe JD, Glaser JS. Quantitative perimetry in compressive optic neuropathy and optic neuritis. Arch Ophthalmol 1978;96:1210–1216.

Tso MOM, Hayreh SS. Optic disc edema in raised intracranial pressure. IV: Axoplasmic transport in experimental papilledema. Arch Ophthalmol 1977; 95:1458–1462.

Weinstein JM, Feman SS. Ischemic optic neuropathy in migraine. Arch Ophthalmol 1982;100:1097–1100.

## Pseudo Disc Edema

Rosenberg MA, Savino PJ, Glaser JS. A clinical analysis of pseudo-papilledema. I. Population, laterality, acuity, refractive error, ophthalmoscopic characteristics and coincident disease. Arch Ophthalmol 1979;97:65–70.

Sachs JF, Choromokos E. Drusen of the optic disc. In: Smith JL, ed. Neuro-ophthalmology update. New York: Masson, 1977;145–154.

Savino PG, Glaser JS, Rosenberg MA. A clinical analysis of pseudo-papilledema. II: Visual field defects. Arch Ophthalmol 1979;97:71–75.

Spencer WH. Drusen of the optic disc and aberrant axoplasmic transport. Am J Ophthalmol 1978;85:1–12.

# Developmentally Anomalous Optic Discs

Anonymous. Small optic discs. Br J Ophthalmol 1978;62:1–2. (Editorial)

Clarren SK. Recognition of fetal alcohol syndrome. JAMA 1981;245:2436–2439.

Goldhammer Y, Smith JL. Optic nerve anomalies in basal encephalocele. Arch Ophthalmol 1975;93:115–118.

Gonzalez ER. New ophthalmic findings in fetal alcohol syndrome. JAMA 1981;245:108.

Graham MG. Wakefield GJ. Bitemporal visual field defects associated with anomalies of the optic discs. Br J Ophthalmol 1973;57:307–314.

Lieblich JM, et al. The syndrome of basal encephalocele and hypothalmic-pituitary dysfunction. Ann Intern Med 1978;98:910–916.

# Optic Atrophy

Chumbley LC. Brobaber RF. Low tension glaucoma. Am J Ophthalmol 1976; 81:761–767.

Frisen L, Hoyt WF. Insidious atrophy of retinal nerve fibers in multiple sclerosis. Arch Ophthalmol 1974;92:91–97.

Frisen L, Hoyt WF, Tengroth BM. Optociliary veins, disc pallar and visual loss: a triad of signs indicating spheno-orbital meningioma. Arch Ophthalmol 1973;51:241–249.

Gittinger JW, et al. Clinical challenges: glaucomatous cupping-sine glaucoma. Surv Ophthalmol 1981;25:383–390.

Hogan MJ, Zimmerman LE, eds. Ophthalmic pathology: an atlas and textbook. Philadelphia: W.B. Saunders, 1962; 2nd ed.

Quigley H, Anderson DR. Cupping of the optic disc in ischemic optic neuropathy. Trans Am Acad Ophthalmol Otolaryngol 1977;83:755–762.

Radios RL, Anderson DR. The mechanism of disc pallor in experimental optic atrophy: a fluorescein angiographic study. Arch Ophthalmol 1979;97:532–535.

Trobe JD, et al. Nonglaucomatous excavation of the optic disc. Arch Ophthalmol 1980;68:1046–1050.

Wirtschafter JD. Diagnosis of optic atrophy. Perspect Ophthalmol 1980;4:223–251.

J. David Higgins

# POSTOPTIC NERVE VISUAL PATHWAY 32

*The visual field defect is the cardinal sign of sensory neurovisual pathology.*

## BACKGROUND

Nerve fibers from the nasal hemiretinas, representing temporal visual space, cross in the optic chiasm to join fibers originating in the temporal retina of the ipsilateral eye. These ganglion cells then course backward and upward around the cerebral peduncles via the optic tracts to the lateral geniculate body in the posterior-lateral thalmus (see Figure 32.1). Lesions in the chiasmal area have a predilection for affecting the crossing fibers, producing characteristic temporal field defects in one or both eyes that may be associated with a loss of visual acuity, optic atrophy, and sensory pupillary abnormalities. Lesions confined to the tracts involve the right or left hemifields of both eyes, are not associated with loss of central visual acuity, but may be accompanied by visible optic atrophy and/or pupillary abnormalities.

Second-order afferents leaving the lateral geniculate constitute the visual radiations and course backward around the inferior horn of the lateral ventricles, first through the temporal lobe (anterior-ventral radiations) and then through the deep parietal lobe to finally reach the striate cortex in the occipital lobe. Lesions past the geniculate tend to produce very similar (congruous) areas of visual loss in the con-

tralateral hemifields of both eyes; in adults they are never associated with visual acuity decrement, optic atrophy, or clinical pupillary abnormalities. Inferior retinal fibers tend to course inferiorly throughout the entire pathway posteriorly, so that lesions affecting their ventral aspect tend to be associated with defects in the superior visual field, and vice versa. The normal field extends 50° superiorly, 60° nasally, 70° inferiorly, and 90° temporally, excluding brow and nose artifacts. The anatomy of the visual system at each stage on the way to its final cortical termination is discussed in succeeding sections.

Because of the great anterior-posterior expanse of the visual system in the brain, approximately 50% of brain tumors are associated with visual field defects. About 25% of these visual defects are totally unrecognized by the patient, more so with postgeniculate lesions. An additional 25% of patients with visual defects have only indirect and incomplete knowledge of their field defect, surmised by losing their place reading, bumping into objects, and so forth. Thus, half the patients feel they actually see in areas of the field where memory alone is in fact completing visual space. So strong is this tendency that patients

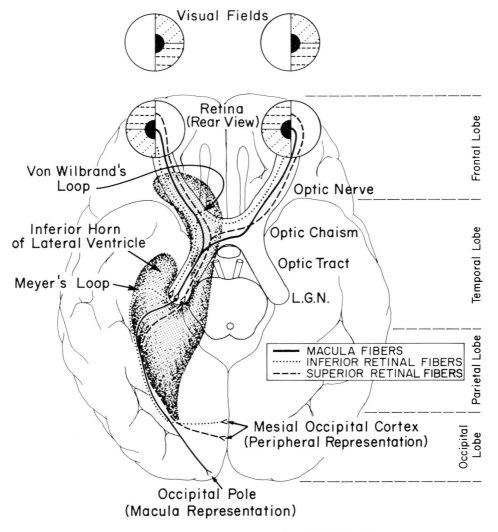

Visual Fields

Retina
(Rear View)

Von Wilbrand's
Loop

Inferior Horn
of Lateral Ventricle

Meyer's Loop

Optic Nerve

Optic Chaism

Optic Tract

L.G.N.

MACULA FIBERS
INFERIOR RETINAL FIBERS
SUPERIOR RETINAL FIBERS

Frontal Lobe

Temporal Lobe

Parietal Lobe

Occipital Lobe

Mesial Occipital Cortex
(Peripheral Representation)

Occipital Pole
(Macula Representation)

FIGURE 32.1.
Ventral view of the brain and retinotopic projection. Retinal and field
orientations shown as if seen by examiner looking through transparent
tangent screens into fundi. For example, fibers shown in right optic tract
subserve right temporal hemiretina and left nasal hemiretina,
but correspond to patient's left visual fields.

will insist they see their complete face in the mirror, even though it is objectively possible to demonstrate total absence of vision on one side of fixation. It is this *negative* characteristic of field defects that puts the responsibility on the optometrist for either doing routine field screening or being very sensitive to the accompanying clinical signs and symptoms that suggest the need for a field exam. Unfortunately, the sensory pathways starting at the chiasm course through relatively "silent" areas of the CNS, where lesions do not tend to produce obvious defects compared to posterior fossa lesions. Moreover, even when accompanying symptoms are present, it is characteristic for cortical defects not to be properly appreciated by the patient (agnos-agnosia). This can become so exaggerated as to incorrectly suggest a generalized dementia, such as in a patient with parietal lobe disease properly cleaning, shaving, and dressing only one-half of his body, or even denying visual disability in the presence of complete cortical blindness (Anton's syndrome).

Although the characteristics of a plotted field defect sometimes suggest the location of a lesion, often they do not. It is, therefore, helpful to know the signs and symptoms associated with disease sur-rounding the visual fibers at each level in the nervous system. For example, the detection of an isolated asymptomatic homonymous field defect in an alert elderly patient probably deserves little more than a call to the family physician; the same presentation in a patient who tends to get lost in familiar surroundings suggests a parietal rather than occipital lobe lesion and much greater likelihood of a cranial mass. Furthermore, with asymptomatic visual fields defects, it is often difficult to assess the onset or progression by the ocular history alone. Related symptoms may be more easily addressed. The following sections present some nonvisual signs and symptoms often associated with regional brain disease affecting the visual fields.

# EXAMINATION

The examination of the visual fields can take many forms, ranging from crude qualitative methods to the most sophisticated psychophysical testing. Fortunately, since the great majority of the visual system is devoted to macular function, the central isopters are by far the most revealing in neurologic testing. Thus, the tangent screen still represents the most useful and widely used instrument in neuroopthalmologic office testing. The multiple-isopter sophisticated static "salad bowl" instruments are more valuable in assessing the early changes in a variety of ocular diseases producing peripheral defects, such as glaucoma and the hereditary retinal degenerations.

There are numerous indications for visual field testing, and their application depends largely on the suspicions of the examiner regarding associated complaints. Besides unexplained loss of acuity or actual field symptoms volunteered by the patient, *any potential neurologic sign or symptom calls for assessment of the visual fields.* In this light, the indications are far ranging and encompass the areas of suspicious headache; unexplained photopsias; at-risk patients; and any perceived change in intellectual, affective, motor, sensory, perceptual, language, or neuroendocrinologic function. The practitioner must be sensitive to the use of the specialized neuroopthalmologic tools: for example, a mood change may reflect frontal lobe disease; difficulty finding words suggests temporal lobe disease; hypothyroidism may be secondary to a pituitary adenoma; and migraine symptoms may represent an arteriovenous malformation. As "a diagnosis not suspected is never made," so, too, is it a clinical truism that sophisticated technology does not replace clinical suspicion: the perimetrist usually finds only what he already suspects to be there.

Because of the ephemeral nature of plotting visual fields, attention to technique deserves discussion. Patients have widely varying response criteria as to how "sure" they must be before making a decision that a target is truly "seen." For most patients, the best initial target is one that (at 25°–30° eccentricity) is just visible near the limits of the tangent screen, usually a 3/1000 W. Depending on room illumination, patient reliability, age, refractive error, and visual acuity, this selection may have to be modified. It is a good practice initially to use static on-off presentations near the edge of the screen to give the patient the idea of what is meant by first becoming "just aware" of the target's presence versus gross movement of the wand. This may be accomplished by using a projected light on a gray screen or by rotating the standard black wand so as to hide the traditional white target. Plotting the blind spot from inside out (invisible to visible) also helps in giving the patient the proper set early in the exam.

The general set is to ensure that the patient looks steadily at the fixation spot while expanding his attention to the test objects in his side vision. It goes without saying that the examiner must monitor the quality of the patient's fixation, as most patients will unconsciously look into the area where the yet unseen target is anticipated. Plotting the fields is so demanding, especially in the elderly, that they should be scheduled early in the exam or on a revisit when the patient is fresh. It is critical for the examiner to generate some enthusiasm and demand active responding on the part of the patient (e.g., "see, see, see, gone"). Besides noting the actual disappearance of the test object, the patient should also be instructed to report any sudden brightness diminution or blinking of the test object.

Despite such attempts to produce consistent response sets, one frequently obtains circularly constricted fields of 5° to 15° in both eyes, and the fields may shrink with further testing (fatigue or "spiral" fields). Assuming the eyes have been thoroughly examined (i.e., no glaucoma, retinal pigmentary degenerations, etc.), such fields almost never represent neurologic disease but are highly characteristic of neurotic depression; occasionally they represent a generalized depression in visual function, such as that produced by aspirin, quinine, or mercury toxicity and, most commonly, congenital amblyopia. If such fields are tubular (i.e., they retain their same linear size when target size and test distance are doubled), then the patient is not being straightforward. Usually this is due to a semiconscious attempt to exaggerate visual complaints and/or to attempt a false consistency in reporting. Occasionally, tubular fields may represent the intentional deception of the malingerer or be a true report of a deranged perception in hysteria. In any case, the principle focus would be outside the neuroophthalmologic realm in the case of bilateral tubular fields.

As opposed to the circularly constricted field, the presence of vertical stepping is the hallmark of postoptic nerve visual field defects. For example, in chiasmal disease an abrupt discontinuity in the isopters just on the temporal side of the midline is almost pathognomonic. Such abrupt midline steps are much more valuable in confirming significant neurologic lesions than vaguer depressions in the peripheral limits of the fields, which can have many causes (including the brow and nose). Because such steps are much more likely to show up closer to fixation than vice versa, it is important to inspect the central isopters by using small or colored targets.

Another method for checking for abrupt midline discontinuities in sensitivity is to pass the target laterally back and forth across the midline above and below fixation while questioning as to sudden decreases of target brightness on one side or the other (see Figure 32.2). Because the isopters for red appreciation are small, a favorite technique is to have the patient compare the redness of a test object on either side of the midline at several distances above and below fixation. A convenient way to explain what is meant is to show the patient the bottle caps of a new versus old bottle of Mydryacil or Cyclogel, as an old bottle cap fades and becomes chalky and gives the patient the idea of

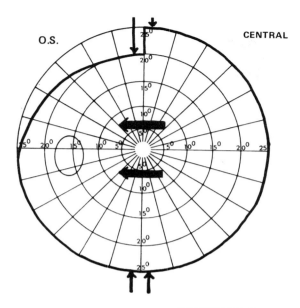

O.S.                    CENTRAL

**FIGURE 32.2.**
The hallmark of neurologic field loss is the midline step. This may be tested for by introducing stimuli on either side of the vertical meridian looking for a discontinuity in the field limits; or alternatively by passing the test target laterally through the paramacular areas searching for a sudden diminution of brightness/color saturation just as one passes into the suspect hemifield.

what is meant by desaturation. Experience has shown that the abrupt desaturation of red in the central temporal hemifields is not to be disregarded as a sign of chiasmal disease, even though the peripheral isopters to larger targets are normal.

While the above techniques are more qualitative than quantitative, it is important to make some attempt at varying target size when a field defect is actually uncovered (Figure 32.3). For localization purposes, it is often necessary only to change to very large targets, such as a 5 × 8 index card. For example, what appears to be a complete bitemporal field defect to a 3/1000 W actually may retain some superior vision with the index card; this

suggests a lesion at the chiasm from above—more likely a craniopharyngioma than an adenoma, for example. What appears to be a complete homonymous R field defect actually may be incomplete and show definite signs of dissimilarity (incongruity) between the eyes; this strongly implicates pathology at the level of the optic tracts. Without using the larger target, no localizing information whatsoever is available from the plot, except that it is retrochiasmal on the left side of the brain (Figure 32.4). In general, field defects that increase significantly in size as target size is decreased are said to have "sloping margins" and suggest mass lesions rather than ischemia.

In elderly or demented patients, who are most likely to harbor field defects, it is often beneficial to use a quick simultaneous comparison technique in place of the tangent screen. Such a routine may be essential at the bedside as well as being useful for screening purposes. Unequal visual acuities suggesting optic nerve disease usually are associated with some form of dimunition of the central isopters. By having the patient fixate a mydryacil bottle cap with one eye and then the other, red desaturation may be uncovered in the suspect eye. A definitely positive response suggests a form of central scotoma, which is the hallmark of optic nerve disease. Have the patient try to confirm that the red gets brighter as the bottle cap moves slightly away from fixation. Such an inversion of isopters is indicative of anterior (optic nerve or chiasm) lesions and may be present even when the standard office color plates are passed.

For briefly assessing the chiasm, each eye is tested separately while the patient fixates the examiner's eye and simultaneously compares the appearance of the examiner's fingers held at comparable locations in both hemifields. In the periphery, the examiner may simply ascertain whether both hands are equally distinct or whether the patient notes slight movements on one side or the other. As the

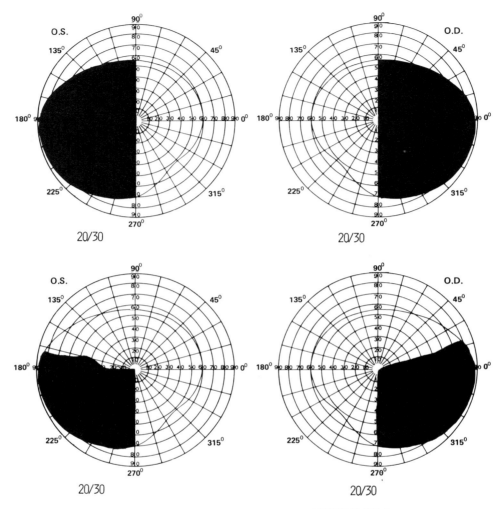

**FIGURE 32.3.**
Complete bitemporal hemianopia plotted with small targets (*above*)
reveals some sparing in superior quadrants when replotted with larger
stimuli (*below*). The additional information now suggests compression
from above, as with pharyngioma.

midperiphery areas are tested, the awareness of the number of fingers (one, two,
or three) present on each side of the midline can be assessed. In the paramacular
areas, the examiner can assess whether
the patient can tell whether the nails are
facing him or away from him on each side,
and the clarity and pinkness of the nail

beds can simultaneously be compared.
Such testing, while only qualitative, better
ensures fixation, is rapid and nonfatigu-
ing, and sometimes even produces a definite and repeatable difference in
simultaneous perception, whereas the
same patient may be totally unsure of when
a target on the tangent screen is first seen

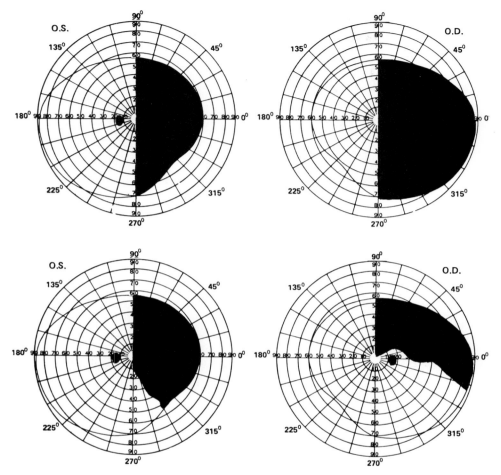

**FIGURE 32.4.**
Complete homonymous hemianopia plotted with small targets has little
localizing value (*above*). When replotted with larger targets (*below*), the
defect is now seen to be denser superiorly and markedly incongruous,
being worse in the eye on the side of the lesion. A left optic tract lesion
is now suspected.

and produces a worthless, fatigue-laden field.

For assessing retrochiasmal defects, the same procedure using the examiner's hands may be employed as just described for chiasmal lesions. In some cases, as when an obvious parietal lobe stroke has occurred, the examiner may only check for a homonymous defect, allowing the pa-

tient to keep both eyes open. Lesions in the radiations are especially likely to produce an inattentive patient with poor fixation. In the patient with parietal lobe disease, the presence of an inattentive visual hemifield (extinction phenomenon) may be suspected by the tendency of the patient reliably and accurately to shift gaze to fixate one hand but ignore the other in simultaneous comparison testing. Such patients may give full fields when the inattentive hemifield alone is probed using standard tangent screen methods, and the important defect can go undetected.

In young children and infants, the problem of fixation is considerable and the fields may have to be gross, as in simply observing refixations when a shiny object is unobtrusively moved in from the side. Alternatively, the examiner can stand behind the child and move his face around into the child's view in all four quadrants. Finally, in testing the aspects of one hemifield, the examiner can turn the child's face so that the eyes are fully contraverted and cannot be further rotated in the attempt to cheat by looking where the test object is anticipated.

# CLINICAL SIGNIFICANCE

The significance of a field defect depends on its configuration, selected aspects of the neurologic status, and the assessment of the patient as a whole. These are discussed in following sections.

# The Optic Chiasm

*Optic nerve ganglion cells serving the nasal hemiretinas
decussate shortly after entering the cranium to become
associated with uncrossed temporal retinal fibers of the
contralateral eye. The structure in which the output of each
optic nerve is so mixed as to form right and left optic tracts,
serving the left and right hemifields, respectively, is called the
optic chiasm.*

## BACKGROUND

Because the position of the chiasm can vary considerably in its anterior-posterior position, sellar area masses may affect the optic nerves, chiasm, or even optic tracts (Figures 32.5 and 32.6). Situated above the chiasm is the third ventricle, in its floor the hypothalamus, and extending into the pituitary stalk the embryonic rest cells (Rathke's pouch), from which craniopharyngiomas arise.

The anterior cerebral arteries and their communicating branch occupy a promi-

nent position anterior-superior to the chiasm, along with the tuberculum sella and planum. The carotid arteries follow the inferior lateral aspect of the optic nerves back and up toward the chiasm before becoming the middle cerebral arteries laterally. Anterior and inferior to the chaism lies the sphenoid sinus.

Disease in these anterior structures is often associated with progressive visual loss in one eye and a temporal field defect in the contralateral eye, usually denser superiorly. The explanation of this "anterior junction syndrome" is that lower fibers from the uninvolved optic nerve cross in the anterior aspect of the chiasm and loop into the opposite optic nerve before coursing backward toward the tracts. This Von Willebrand's loop is shown in Figure 32.1.

The most important inferior relation to the chiasm is the pituitary gland, although its exact anterior-posterior position with respect to the chiasm varies from person to person. Below and laterally lie the cavernous sinuses and their contents, cranial nerves III to VI, and the carotid artery. On occasion, an adenoma will break through into the sinus, causing ocular motor palsies, but most often, headaches,

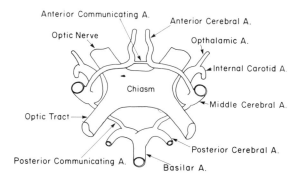

**FIGURE 32.5.**
**Top view of chiasm showing relationship with
circle of Willis.**

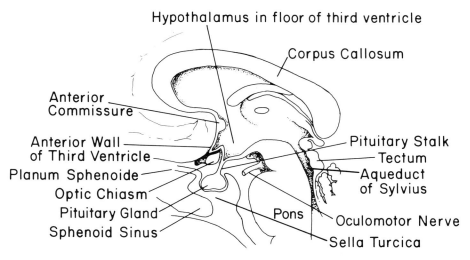

FIGURE 32.6.
Lateral view of brain emphasizing parasellar structures.

endocrinopathies, and isolated visual involvement are the presenting complaints. Inferior and rostral to the chiasm lie the infundibulum, posterior communicating arteries, and third nerves. Pressure from behind, as from a Rathke's pouch tumor, is likely to impinge on the crossing macula fibers, yielding bitemporal hemicentral scotomas early in course. Since the pituitary fossa lies a full centimeter or so below the chiasm, it is unusual for small adenomas to affect vision early in their course. Roentgenographic changes (ballooning of the sella and thinning of dorsum) usually are evident by the time vision is affected. Visualizing focal thinning and slanting of the floor with small tumors often requires tomograms.

# HISTORY AND EXAMINATION

The chiasm is located in a relatively silent area of the brain, as far as prominent focal neurologic signs and symptoms are concerned. For this reason, the visual fields are a bulwark in diagnosing disease in this area. Even in the case of adenomas, which must attain some size before affecting vision, patients are surprisingly asymptomatic; alternatively, their headaches and affective/endocrinologic complaints may not have been properly interpreted early in the clinical course. This is unfortunate, since noninvasive studies such as x-ray or prolactin assay may have revealed the tumor prior to the patient visiting the eye doctor. At this stage, radical surgery or irradiation may be needed, whereas transphenoid microsurgery years earlier may have saved the patient lifelong replacement hormone therapy. Worse, the patient may present with a hemorrhage or infarct in the tumor or pituitary apoplexy; severe headache, muscle palsies, and visual loss may herald a life-threatening event.

For the optometrist then, a readiness to plot the fields in patients complaining of headache or neuroendocrinlogic symptoms is of paramount importance (Figure 32.7).

The hallmark of parasellar disease is the temporal field defect manifest to a variable extent in one or both eyes. The special

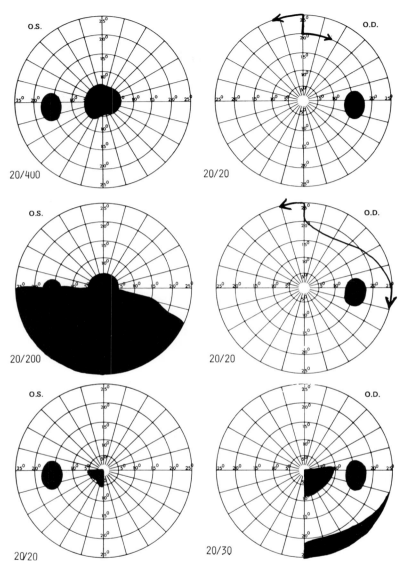

**FIGURE 32.7.**
Some chiasmal syndromes: *Top.* A central scotoma takes on new
significance when one uncovers an upper temporal defect in the good
eye (anterior junction syndrome). *Middle.* altitudinal defect suggests an
ischemic process until a junction defect is plotted in good eye,
suggesting a mass lesion in the area of the intracranial opening of the
optic foramen (see Figure 32.3). *Bottom.* Bitemporal hemicentral
scotomas are often the earliest sign of chiasmal compression and are
easily missed on the perimeter.

sensitivity of crossing nasal optic nerve fibers has been explained variously as being due to the stretching of the crossing fibers, vulnerability of their microvasculature, and so forth.

Testing focuses on searching for abrupt vertical stepping at the midline near fixation, using small or red-colored targets. The papillomacular bundle is very sensitive to compression in the chiasm as well as optic nerve. Thus, even with normal peripheral field limits, the abrupt desaturation of a red object as it crosses the midline into the paramacular temporal field is a chiasmal syndrome until proved otherwise. Such sharp discontinuities, which "respect the midline," are not typical of most pseudochiasmal entities causing sloping bitemporal depressions (Table 32.1 and Figure 32.8). The usual causes that may simulate a mass lesion are

1. Bilateral central-cecal scotomas in toxic optic neuropathies and Leber's optic neuritis
2. Peripapillary retinal edema in disc swelling of any cause
3. Third ventricle dilation in increased intracranial pressure
4. Demyelinating disease
5. Torsion of optic nerves with inferior nasal retinal ectasia
6. Sector retinitis pigmentosa
7. Ethambutol toxicity; rarely chloroquine
8. Bilateral optic nerve hypoplasia
9. Bilateral drusen of the optic nerves

Chiasmal defects are often associated with decreased visual acuity in one or both

Table 32.1
Localizing Symptoms Suggesting the Anatomic Site
of Homonymous Hemianopia

| | Optic Tracts | Temporal Lobe | Parietal Lobe | Occipital Lobe |
|---|---|---|---|---|
| Frequency | 2% | 25% | 33% | 40% |
| Mass/ischemia ratio | Mass common if chiasmal signs; stroke common if no chiasmal signs | 90% | 50% | 25% |
| Pupillary signs | Marcus Gunn pupil common | None | None | None |
| Acuity | May be decreased with parasellar mass | Normal | Normal | Normal |
| Optic atrophy | Band atrophy opposite lesion | None | None | None |
| Bell's reflex | Normal | May be conjugate away from lesion | May be conjugate away from lesion | May be conjugate away from lesion |
| Opticokinetic nystagmus | Always symmetrical | Always symmetrical | Almost always asymmetrical | May be asymmetrical with parietal lobe extension of mass |
| Photopsias | Rare | Common | Less common | Somewhat common |

**Table 32.1**
*(continued)*

| | Optic Tracts | Temporal Lobe | Parietal Lobe | Occipital Lobe |
|---|---|---|---|---|
| Suggestive field defects | Incongruent with greater field loss on side of lesion | Superior wedge defects | Lower quadrantanopia. Extinction phenomena | (1) Bilateral homonymous field defects<br>(2) Homonymous paracentral scotomas<br>(3) Temporal crescent defects<br>(4) Complete quadrantanopias with sharp borders |
| Congruity | Marked incongruity the rule | May be incongruous | Completely congruent | Completely congruent |
| Macula sparing of 5° or more | Rare | Not common | Fairly common | Very common |
| Suggestive company | Sellar signs (amenorhea, acromegaly, seesaw nystagmus, etc.). Lower extremity pyramidal signs | Complex seizures<br>Fluent aphasia<br>Dementia<br>Prosopagnosia<br>Hallucinations | General:<br>Dysgraphesthesia<br>Astereognosis<br>Finger agnosia<br>Lower facial weakness<br>Nondominant:<br>Visual-spatial agnosia<br>Ideomotor apraxia<br>Dominant:<br>Alexia and agraphia without aphasia<br>Bilateral disease:<br>Visual agnosia<br>Balint's syndrome | Riddoch phenomenon<br>Anton's syndrome<br>Normal mental status<br>Alexia without agraphia<br>Prosopagnosia<br>Acquired cortical color deficiencies<br>Kaleidoscopic photopsias |

Source: Smith 1962.

eyes and may be associated with a Marcus Gunn pupil in the more severely affected eye. (Remember always to do the field in the good eye.) Optic atrophy may also be manifest as temporal pallor in one or both eyes. When the crossing fibers are significantly affected, however, pathognomonic band atrophy may be seen (Figure 32.9). Here, the pallor extends as a wedge through the central one-third of the nerve head, leaving the superior and inferior poles pink. Optic atrophy obviously implies a poor prognosis for visual recovery.

Because a significant bitemporal de-

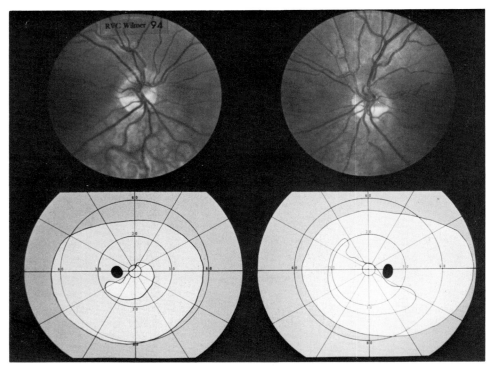

**FIGURE 32.8.**
Marked torsion of the optic nerves with inferior conus, visible inferior
retinal ectasia, and upper corresponding bitemporal field defects
simulating chiasmal syndrome. Note the smooth transition of the
isopters across the midline without the typical abrupt step typical of
sellar area masses. Diagnosis: benign congenitally tilted discs.
Reprinted by permission of the publisher, from Miller NR and Fine SL.
The ocular fundus in neuro-ophthalmologic diagnosis. In: Sights and
sounds in ophthalmology. St. Louis: C.V. Mosby, 1975; vol. VIII.

fect leaves only uncrossed fibers from each eye to course back to their respective ipsilateral hemispheres, loss of binocular cell input may present as poor fusional ability and complaints of poor depth perception, despite normal findings on office tests, which look only at macular function. Occasionally, bizarre disassociations of the eyes may take place, depending on the direction of a preexisting phoria; thus, the two intact hemiwords may slide into an overlapped position, be separated by a zone of nothingness, or show a vertical step at the midline. With complete bitemporal de-

fects, objects past the fixation point fall on the nasal hemiretinas, so that an expanding wedge of blindness exists behind the object of regard.

Finally, the observation of seesaw (one eye going up while its partner goes down) or monocular vertical nystagmus always makes one suspect a perichiasmal lesion and should bring the patient to the tangent screen. Always suspect an anterior third ventricle glioma when these eye movement anomalies are present in an emaciated child.

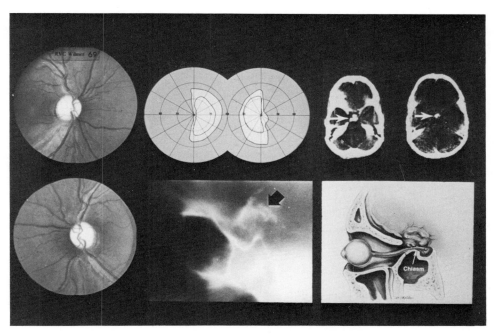

**FIGURE 32.9.**
Bilateral optic atrophy more bandlike in OD (*above*). Patient was a 9-year-old with headaches, 20/30 visions, and bitemporal field loss. Serial CAT scan (*upper right*) shows suprasellar density appearing as calcification on lateral skull film (*below, middle*). Schematic shows anatomic locus of the tumor (*below, right*). Diagnosis: craniopharyngioma.
Reprinted by permission of the publisher, from Miller NR and Fine SL. The ocular fundus in neuro-ophthalmologic diagnosis. In: Sights and sounds in ophthalmology. St. Louis: C.V. Mosby, 1975; vol. VIII.

# CLINICAL SIGNIFICANCE

With a chiasmal syndrome, the presence of a mass is much more likely than in any other type of visual field loss. Vascular disease is a truly rare cause of bitemporal field defects; however, senile atherosclerotic aneurysmal desiccation of the carotid arteries has been reported as an occasional cause of temporal and even binasal defects. Since those arteries lie laterally they will impinge on the uncrossed fibers (nasal defects), but more often they will disrupt the integrity of the more sensitive crossing fibers (temporal defects).

Trauma is an occasional cause of tearing of the chiasm, and multiple sclerosis cannot be overlooked, although chiasmal syndromes in demyelinating disease are not common. Outside of a fulminant basal meningitis in an obviously sick patient, other inflammatory causes are quite rare.

Focus more on the chronic subacute granulomatous diseases such as tuberculosis, syphilis, and sarcoid.

Of suspected masses, suprasellar aneurysm is the most important to discover and is suggested by periorbital pain and/or numbness, bruits, varying field defects, and signs of actual leakage, such as severe headache and stiff neck, especially in older patients. Of particular interest is the anterior cerebral-anterior communicating artery aneurysm, where a temporal field defect and/or acuity loss tend to be more severe ipsilaterally and may be complicated by an altitudinal field component inferiorly, simulating an attack of ischemic optic neuropathy (Figure 32.7). These aneurysms are more frequent in women and tend to rebleed; they always call for a thorough baseline field plot.

Parasellar tumors are the most frequent causes of a chiasmal syndrome and account for 25% of all CNS neoplasms. Meningiomas in this region tend to arise from the planum, tuberculum sella, or occasionally encroach on the chiasm from the sphenoid wing. These masses are most common in middle-aged women, rarely produce endocrinopathy, and if hyperostosis is not evident on x-ray, the mass may be missed unless air studies are done. Slowly progressive visual loss often is initially unilateral, and headache may be the only accompanying symptom.

Craniopharyngiomas arising from above the chiasm tend to produce early inferior temporal field defects, which are often quite asymmetrical compared to adenomas. Occasionally, craniopharyngiomas will first affect a single optic nerve or even the optic tracts producing a homonymous hemianopic defect. Asymmetrical visual acuity reduction and optic atrophy are also common. In children and adolescents, these growths tend to calcify, producing the pathognomonic picture of suprasellar calcification on x-ray film (Figure 32.10). Besides headache, affected children may manifest diencephalic/pituitary dysfunction, such as being of small

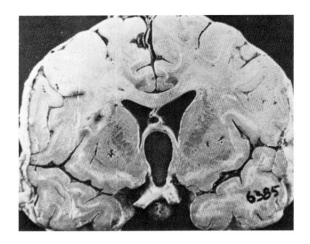

**FIGURE 32.10.**
Craniopharyngioma appearing as dark mass filling third ventricle and producing hydrocephalus, evident from dilated lateral ventricles. Note location of chiasm below third ventricle. Besides headache, a personality change was the only obvious symptom in this 45-year-old woman.
Reprinted by permission of the publisher, from Cogan D. Neurology of the visual system. Springfield, Ill.: Charles C Thomas, 1966.

stature and thirsty. These tumors account for nearly 10% of childhood CNS tumors and often are accompanied by delayed sexual development as well.

Although their peak incidence is in youth, craniopharyngiomas also occur again in old age (25% in patients past the age of 40), where the tendency to calcify is not nearly so common. These growths tend to have a cystic component that may produce a variation in successive field plots, suggesting aneurysm. Since craniopharyngiomas may occlude the third ventricle (Figure 32.10), they represent the only perichiasmal mass commonly associated with increased intracranial pressure; signs of increased intracranial pressure are the most common presentation in children, whereas visual symptoms predominate in older adults.

Since the chiasm directly underlies the third ventricle, obstructive hydrocephalus may occasionally produce inferior bitemporal defects as a false localizing sign, such as when a posterior fossa mass abruptly closes off the aqueduct of Silvius (Figure 32.11). With pseudotumor cerebri, the chiasm may actually herniate into the sella.

Gliomas affecting the chiasm are not common and tend to occur in young children. They should be suspected in any chiasmal syndrome accompanied by stigmata of von Recklinghausen's disease. Diencephalic gliomas are recognized as a cause of failure-to-thrive in infants (emaciation, pallor, and hyperactivity). The presentation of a history of "not recognizing parents" in an emaciated child should be taken seriously.

Pituitary adenomas (15% of all intracranial tumors) are the classic cause of chiasmal syndromes. As they usually im-

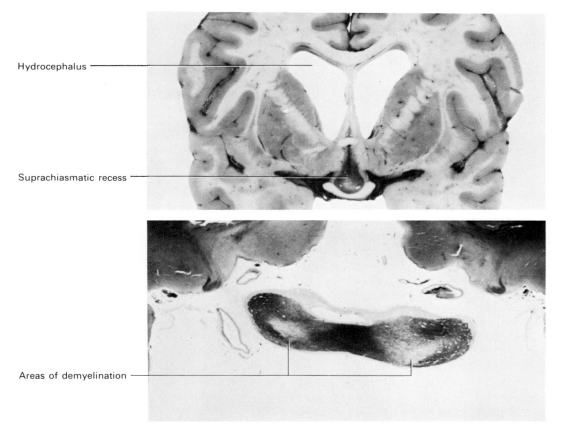

Hydrocephalus

Suprachiasmatic recess

Areas of demyelination

**FIGURE 32.11.**
Chiasmal destruction from dilated ventricular system in hydrocephalus. Patient was a 27-year-old woman with a cerebellar astrocytoma, found dead in bed due to brain herniation. Bitemporal field loss may rarely be a false localizing sign in raised intracranial pressure.
Reprinted by permission of the publisher, from Lindenberg R, Walsh FB, and Sachs JG. Neuropathology of vision: an atlas. Philadelphia: Lea & Febiger, 1973.

pinge on the chiasm from below (Figure 32.12), upper bitemporal defects are the rule early in their course, and both eyes tend to show rather symmetrical field loss. The earliest field defects tend to occur in the macular region, so the exam is not complete without checking for diminution of brightness/red saturation as one crosses the midline temporally just above and below fixation. This screening test should be part of the workup of every patient with even minor loss of acuity in one or both eyes.

Although adenomas are commonly thought to be tumors of middle age, they may occur at any time. In the classic cytologic scheme, about 75% of all adenomas are considered nonsecretory (chromophobe), producing symptoms chiefly by compressing functioning tissue. Symptoms of panhypopituitarism may include fatigue, thirst, loss of body hair, loss of libido or actual impotence in men, and most important, amenorrhea in women. Symptoms of secondary hypothyroidism are common, such as coarseness and dryness of the skin, fatigue, weight gain, constipation, neuropathies, cold intolerance, coarseness of the hair, puffiness of the fin-

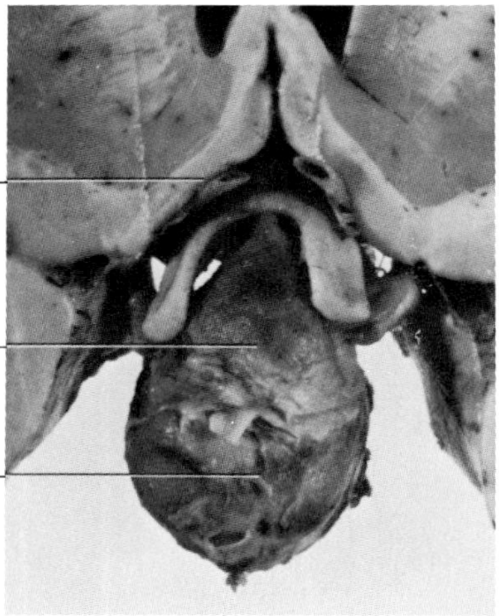

Anterior cerebral artery

Suprasellar pituitary adenoma

Intrasellar pituitary adenoma

**FIGURE 32.12.**
Large pituitary adenoma illustrating extent of growth necessary to cause chiasmal compression and visual symptoms. Finding was incidental at autopsy in a farmer found gored by a bull in a field. One may rightly wonder who saw better—the farmer or the bull?
Reprinted by permission of the publisher, from Lindenberg R, Walsh FB, and Sachs JG. Neuropathology of vision: an atlas. Philadelphia: Lea & Febiger, 1973.

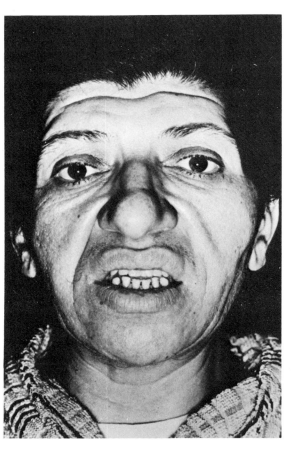

**FIGURE 32.13.**
Coarsening of the features typical of acromegaly (see Figure 9.2).
Reprinted by permission of the publisher, from Cogan D. Neurology of the visual system. Springfield, Ill.: Charles C Thomas, 1966.

gers and lids, mental apathy, anemia, and dysarthria. In children, decreased growth, smooth, pale wrinkly skin with fine, brittle hair, and decreased development of the genitals and secondary sex characteristics may predominate.

Eosinophilic tumors account for 22% of adenomas in the classic scheme, with associated hypersecretion of growth hormone producing giganticism in youth and acromegaly in adults (Figure 32.13). Increased prominence of the hands and feet (gloves and shoes do not fit), frontal bossing, and prognathism are characteristic. Diabetes insipidus is relatively common, as is glycosuria; these symptoms may be misinterpreted until visual loss brings attention to the pituitary gland. Lethargy, weakness, and coarseness of the skin are also common complaints, and prolactin levels are elevated in about one-third of patients.

Finally, basophilic tumors are the rarest (2% of the cases) and produce a Cushing's syndrome. Although headache may bring the patient to the eye doctor, these tumors are small and do not produce visual loss, and rarely produce roentgenographic changes. It is now known that basophilic tumors occasionally secrete TSH, LH, and FSH as well.

The classic scheme notwithstanding, mixed secretory tumors also exist. The most important nonclassic tumor, however, is the prolactinoma, which may produce gynecomastia, galactorrhea, and amenorrhea in women. Galactorrhea is, however, the most common complaint. Prolactinomas account for 35% of the cases of amenorrhea/galactorrhea and have a modal onset in the thirties. These tumors have an unfortunate tendency to grow and affect vision in pregnancy.

Visual symptoms are not the most common presenting complaint in women (only 15%); it must be emphasized, however, that these tumors can attain large size in men and, therefore, commonly present to the eye doctor. Impotence and decreased libido are usually present, and gynecomastia occurs in about 25% of patients.

While other causes of chiasmal syndromes exist (sphenoid mucocele, multiple sclerosis, empty sella syndromes and others), they are not very common, and the reader is directed to the general neuro-ophthalmologic literature for a more complete discussion.

# The Optic Tracts

*Retinal ganglion cells serving the contralateral visual field exit the chiasm and course in the optic tracts up and around the cerebral peduncles to synapse in the lateral geniculate body of the thalamus.*

## BACKGROUND

Since the tracts are short, run outside the brain substance proper, and are supplied by early branches of the middle cerebral arteries, they are the least common site responsible for homonymous field defects.

Important relations anteriorly are the chiasm, then the third nerves and posterior communicating arteries. Running alongside the cerebral peduncles, the optic tracts first cross the descending pyramidal motor fibers and then the ascending sensory lemniscus prior to terminating in the lateral geniculate amid other sensory nuclei (Figure 32.14).

Deep to the tracts lie basal ganglia nuclei, where lesions tend to produce resting motor defects such as tremor, chorea, and athetosis. Because of more aggressive treatment of hypertension, hemorrhage of the lenticular striate branch of the middle cerebral artery is not as prominent a cause of tract/basal ganglia syndromes as in the past. Hemorrhage or thrombosis of the middle cerebral arteries may produce the common stroke picture of hemiplegia, hemianopia, and aphasia (if on the dominant side); hemisensory defects occur if the posterior tracts and medial lemniscus are involved. More distal middle cerebral artery thrombosis affecting the parietal radiations also produces hemianopia and hemiplegia. Here the weakness usually is much more severe in the hands, arms, and lower face, as opposed to tract/peduncle lesions, while the trunk and lower extremities usually are equally affected.

## EXAMINATION

Both optic atrophy and pupillary escape may be seen with tract lesions. The pupillary afferents leave the tracts about two-thirds of the way through their course, which may be helpful also in localization of a hemianopic field defect. As with any postchiasmal lesions, one expects 20/20 vision, even with total hemianopia when a lesion is limited to one tract.

The principal field defect is complete hemianopia in the contralateral visual fields, splitting fixation. This has little localizing significance. When incomplete, optic tract defects are commonly associated with incongruous field defects, usually more extensive in the eye ipsilateral to the lesion and denser superiorly. Thus, any "apparent" total hemianopia should always be rechecked with very large targets to see whether some residual field exists

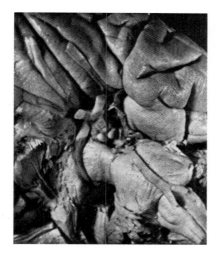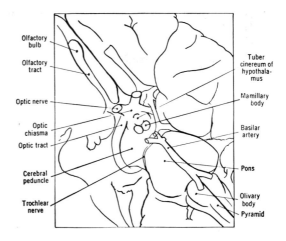

**FIGURE 32.14.**
Right temporal lobe removed to show the compactness of the optic tract in its short course around the cerebral peduncle toward its destination in the lateral geniculate body.
Reprinted by permission of the publisher, from Gardner E. Fundamentals of neurology. Philadelphia: W.B. Saunders, 1963; 4th ed.

in either eye and to look for incongruity, an important localizing sign.

Anterior tract defects may involve macular fibers crossing at the rear of the chiasm to the opposite tract. Thus, both hemimacular fields of the eye ipsilateral to the tract lesion may be involved; reduced visual acuity contralateral to the hemianopia thus strongly implicates early optic tracts as the site of the lesion. With very incongruous defects, or when reduced visual acuity exists, a Marcus Gunn pupil may occur, with pupillary escape seen in the more severely affected eye, again usually ipsilateral to an anterior tract lesion.

Since optic tract lesions involve ganglion cells, some degree of optic atrophy will result in several weeks. This usually is most evident as either temporal pallor or band atrophy (Figures 32.15 and 32.26) in the eye contralateral to the tract defect and represents another helpful localizing sign.

As the papillomacular bundle at this level is again sensitive to early compressive lesions, contralateral homonymous hemicentral scotomas occasionally occur—the only site where this occurs outside of a lesion at the very tip of an occipital pole (Figure 32.16).

When faced with complete hemifield defects in both eyes and with good acuity, reliance must be made on associated clinical findings to localize the lesion to the tracts. Besides disc pallor, a positive Marcus Gunn pupil in the eye ipsilateral to the hemianopia suggests optic tract involvement.

In summary, tract defects tend to produce specific neurologic company. In contrast, neurologic company is absent in occipital lobe hemianopia, and complex integrative defects are present in radiation lesions involving the parietal lobe.

When sensorimotor anomalies accompany a hemianopia, an important ocular test helping to rule out hemispheric (parietal lobe) lesions is the retention of sym-

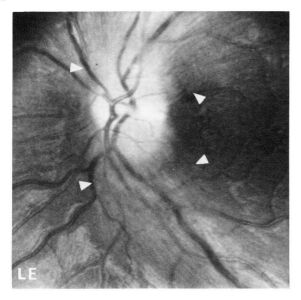

**FIGURE 32.15.**
Disc and peripapillary edema at poles (*between arrows*), divided by a central wedge of optic atrophy. Patient suffered from a mass lesion producing raised intracranial pressure; however, compression of contralateral optic tract resulted in retrograde degeneration of the ganglion cells to the disc. Photograph thus demonstrates band atrophy and that atrophic discs do not swell, despite raised intracranial pressure.
Reprinted by permission of the publisher, from Paul TO and Hoyt WF. Funduscopic appearance of papilledema with optic tract atrophy. Arch Ophthalmol 1976; 94:467–468. Copyright 1976, American Medical Association.

metrical opticokinetic nystagmus. If positive, the eyes will show jerky nystagmus of about the same quality and degree, no matter in which direction the stimulus is passed before the eyes. Also, small tract lesions usually do not show spasticity of conjugate gaze, an eye sign typical of cortical involvement. This test is performed by having the patient attempt to close the eyes against the resistance of the examiner's fingers and watching the Bell's reflex. In only 2% of normal eyes will this reflex have a conjugate component to one side or the other. A conjugate Bell's reflex is considered confirmatory for a lesion in hemisphere contralateral to the conjugate excursion.

Considering all the eye, pupillary, field, and other possible neurologic company, one can often decide whether a homonymous field defect represents an optic tract lesion. If so, it is important to try to decide if the anterior (parasellar) tracts are involved, as a mass then becomes much more likely. Thus, ipsilateral visual acuity loss, youth, hemicentral scotomas, insidious onset and progression, hypothalamic or pituitary signs (e.g., amenorrhea), gross inconjugacy with the denser field defect in the ipsilateral eye, and absence of hemisensory signs more likely implicate the early tracts; whereas age, history of vascular disease, sudden onset of the defect with major company (headache, aphasia, hemiparesis equal or greater in the lower extremities, hemisensory defects, absence of pupillary defects) argue for senile stroke.

# CLINICAL SIGNIFICANCE

Aside from paroxysmal stroke with major deficits beside the fields, the major clinical significance in the detection of an optic tract hemianopia is in the minimal symptomatic patient with a possible mass lesion. Here, craniopharyngiomas (35%), adenomas (15%), and aneurysms (15%) occur most often. Demyelinating disorders and other causes are rare. Craniopharyngiomas and the adenomas are discussed in the preceding section. Aneurysm of the posterior communicating artery or at the origin of the middle cerebral artery occasionally will produce some degree of homonymous defect. Suggestive company, if any, might include some de-

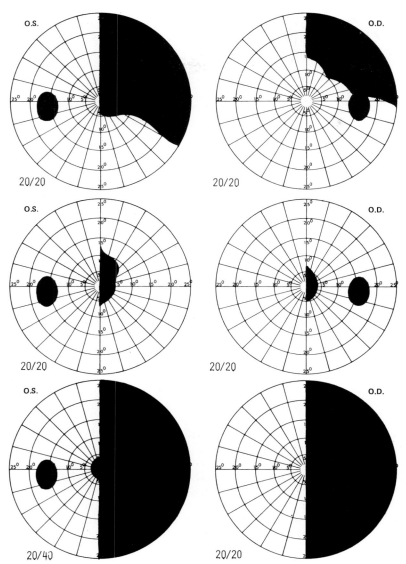

**FIGURE 32.16.**
Some optic tract field plots. *Above.* Markedly incongruous defects denser in the eye ipsilateral to the lesion usually reflect tract pathology. *Middle.* Homonymous hemicentral scotomas are usually occipital in origin. Without a history of trauma, however, always suspect a tract locus, especially if incongruous or when endocrine signs are evident. *Below.* Complete homonymous hemianopia is nonlocalizing. If associated with acuity loss, optic atrophy or pupillary escape, a tract lesion is to be strongly suspected, however.

gree of third nerve involvement (lack of full constriction to bright light in the ipsilateral eye, or even accommodative weakness), orbital bruit, evidence of contralateral pyramidal tract involvement such as flexion and lack of swing of the arm, stiffness, swinging or hyperactive tendon reflexes in the leg, a positive Babinski, and perhaps headache.

# Anterior Temporal Lobe Radiations

*Following ganglion cell synapse in the lateral geniculate body, second order fibers course back toward the occipital cortex. The most anterior and inferior of these optic radiations pass through the temporal lobe.*

## BACKGROUND

Upon leaving the lateral geniculate, the inferior horn of the lateral ventricle necessitates a looping of the inferior radiations into the anterior temporal lobe (Figure 32.1). The more dorsal of the anterior radiations, and their entire posterior continuation, course through ventral parietal lobe, which lies deep to the middle temporal gyrus; thus, posterior temporal lobe masses may occasionally compress the posterior radiations as well. The relatively isolated anterior loop, Meyer's loop, gives rise to the homonymous superior quadrantic field defect pathognomonic of anterior temporal lobe pathology.

Lesions in the anterior radiations produce contralateral homonymous field defects not accompanied by visual acuity loss, pupillary abnormalities, or optic atrophy. Such defects are often poorly appreciated by the patient and tend to be accompanied by relatively sophisticated neurologic defects.

Since a common presenting symptom of brain tumors is seizure, the practitioner must be aware that even relatively unformed, migrainelike photopic episodes may represent an irritable cortical focus from a mass. A field exam is always in order in the presence of suspicious photopsias. The complaint of seeing a nonexistent person or inanimate object occasionally occurs when radiation lesions deafferent the occipital lobes—a phenomenon similar to phantom limb pain. Intense sensory persistence of a just previously fixated object in a blindfield is also a recognized phenomenon (palinopsia). Such hallucinatory experiences, especially when confined to one hemifield, should not be passed off as psychogenic, but rather suggest a field defect or drug side effect, the most important being to digitalis and its derivatives.

## EXAMINATION

Temporal lobe field defects are less common than parietal lobe involvement and much rarer than occipital lobe hemianopias. They usually are quite congruous unless the optic tracts are also involved. Suspicion of a temporal lobe defect is important, as a tumor is much more likely than with occipital lobe defects. Approximately 80% of the masses here produce field defects; if the nondominant temporal lobe is involved, visual symptoms are likely to present.

The characteristic field defect in temporal lobe disease is the homonymous superior quadrantanopia. If incomplete, this defect is likely to be manifest as a wedge "pie-in-the-sky" defect extending close to fixation (Figure 32.17). Such defects underscore the importance of looking for steps with suspected CNS pathology just to either side of the vertical meridians, as they may otherwise be missed. Temporal lobe field defects usually extend to fixation.

Besides variable degrees of dementia, tumors in the anterior radiations on the dominant side are likely to be associated

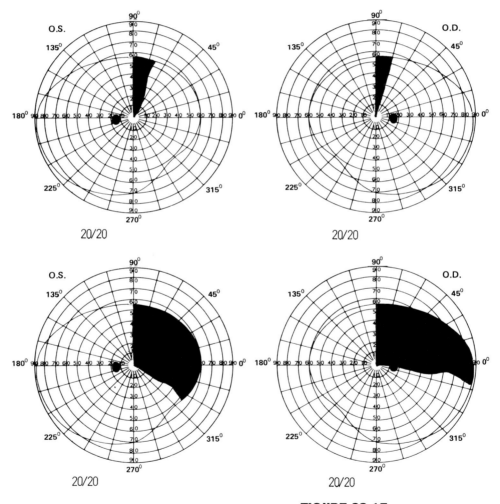

**FIGURE 32.17.**
"Pie in the sky" defect (*above*) is nearly pathognomonic for a temporal lobe lesion. Slightly incongruous defects that are denser above and encroach on fixation also suggest temporal lobe pathology (*below*).

with "fluent" aphasia; the patient may retain ease of speech production but may not make good sense, and speech comprehension is impaired. Such focal defects can slip by a harried examiner or be misinterpreted as senile dementia. Some degree of alexia and agraphia usually accompany such aphasia, and the patient may then complain of difficulty reading with little comprehension that it is not his vision per se that is at fault.

Tumors in this area are often associated with complex seizures that may involve time-sequenced auditory or visual hallucinations, disagreeable odors (uncinate fits), episodes of absence, automatic movements (lipsmacking, eyewinking), and occasionally even more bizarre episodes, such as directed aggression or déjà vu experiences. A specific type of agnosia may occur with lesions of the nondominant temporal lobe where even the most familiar faces cannot be recognized, despite 20/20 vision (prosopagnosia). This most interesting defect is also seen in nondominant occipital lobe lesions when fibers from the remaining "seeing" hemisphere crossing over to the nondominant temporal lobe are also damaged—a disconnection syndrome. With an occipital lesion, the patient is likely to have difficulty discriminating colors.

Occasionally, a temporal lobe tumor will compress the brain stem to produce a partial or internal third nerve palsy; Hutchinson's pupil is much more likely to occur with rapidly expanding supratentorial masses, such as subdural hemorrhage. Memory loss or auditory agnosia usually reflects bilateral temporal lobe involvement, such as may occur with occlusive vascular disease.

Finally, temporal lobe lesions are often associated with a conjugate Bell's reflex toward the uninvolved hemisphere on forced lid closure; they do not, however, cause asymmetric opticokinetic nystagmus characteristic of parietal lobe disease.

# CLINICAL SIGNIFICANCE

The significance of suspecting a temporal lobe disorder is the increased possibility of a brain tumor rather than a stroke. Demyelinating disease is quite rare as a cause of lesions in the radiations. Abscesses, however, may present with a progressing picture suggesting a tumor; infections from otitis and SBE have a temporal lobe predilection. In these more acute presentations, recognition of early involvement of the central nervous system by noting typical field defects and associated company may be lifesaving.

# Parietal Lobe Radiations

*The major extent of the optic radiations traverses the ventral parietal lobe in a vertically oriented fan that rotates to become more horizontally oriented as it approaches the occipital-parietal lobe junction.*

## BACKGROUND

The entire temporal-parietal radiations are supplied by the middle cerebral artery, the artery most commonly involved in thromboembolic stroke. Often such strokes affect the more dorsal terminal vessels (watershed zone) and spare the visual field. At the parietal-occipital lobe junction, the inferior radiations receive variable anastamoses from the posterior cerebral artery, making the more superior fibers more at risk.

In general then, inferior quadrantanopias suggest parietal disease (Figure 32.18), although not necessarily at the parietal-occipital junction, as the most anterior superior radiations pass solely through the parietal lobe. Nevertheless, complete homonymous hemianopias are at least as common as inferior quadrantanopias and even superior, non-wedge-like, quadrantanopias occasionally occur.

As in the temporal lobe, field defects tend to be negative, unassociated with visual acuity loss, optic atrophy, or pupillary phenomena. They may, however, be accompanied by photopsias, hallucinations, hemifield metamorphopsia, and palinopsia.

The parietal lobes are primary cortical reception areas for somasthetic information; lesions here produce cortical defects of the tactile sense rather than numbness.

In middle cerebral artery stroke this is best appreciated in the face and hand, which are represented in the superior-lateral surface (watershed zone) of the parietal lobe. Lateralized attention defects often occur, so that a wisp of cotton appreciated in unilateral testing is not felt when both sides of the face or both hands are simultaneously stimulated (extinction phenomenon). *Astereoagnosia*, or the inability to tactually recognize objects in the hand opposite the lesion, is highly characteristic of parietal dysfunction. Position sense may be affected, and the patient may be unable to tell whether a contralateral digit is being passively flexed or extended by the examiner (be careful to grasp the digit firmly on the lateral aspects so as not to give pressure cues). If looked for diligently, the examiner may also note a deficit in fine touch or two-point localization. Middle cerebral strokes often simultaneously infarct the lateral surface of the frontal lobes, producing pyramidal motor signs that typically are most severe in the lower face and arms.

Nondominant parietal lobe disease, in addition to producing somasthetic and kinesthetic defects, tends to produce two additional major disabilities that should be recognized. The first is *visuospatial dysagosia*, or a loss of the normal appre-

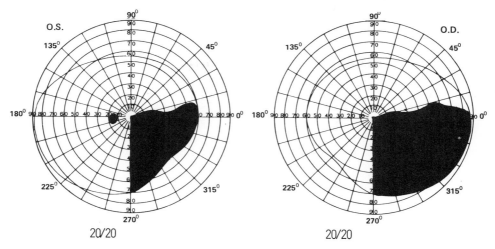

**FIGURE 32.18.**
Although complete hemianopia also is common, congruous defects denser below and approaching fixation suggest parietal lobe disease. Look for diminished opticokinetic nystagmus on moving the tape to the side of the lesion (*left*) to confirm a parietal lobe locus.

ciation of three-dimensional spatial orientation. Affected patients tend to become easily lost even in familiar surrounds and have difficulty in drawing objects in proper relationship. Often this is accompanied by some degree of ideomotor apraxia. Here, skilled sequential behaviors seem difficult to retrieve, and common tasks, such as getting dressed, become inappropriately carried out despite the absence of paresis.

Perhaps the best illustration of a nondominant parietal lobe syndrome is by way of quoting a case report of Dr. David Cogan (1979):

> This 64-year-old, right-handed man's initial symptom was loss of way in familiar territory. This was first evident on driving his car home from the office and in sailing his boat in well-known waters. The disability increased so that he mixed up rooms in his house. Nevertheless, he was alert in other fields and continued to perform surgery. He volunteered in jest: 'I can still do an appendectomy if I can find my way to the hospital.'

> Other difficulties consisted of a mild dressing apraxia as evident in putting his shoes on the wrong foot and in being unable to find the proper pant leg.

> Examination disclosed a left homonymous hemianopia with sparing of the central area . . . He was able to read well but could not draw a simple map, diagram the position of the organs in the abdomen, or the floor plan of his house, and made left-sided errors in inserting the numbers in a clock face or in drawing the petals on a daisy . . .

> Pneumoencephalography disclosed a cerebral tumor in the lower parietal region and the right. Biopsy indicated glioblastoma multiforme.

Dominant parietal lobe lesions tend to produce defects in symbolic behavior in addition to the somasthetic defects discussed. In temporal lobe lesions, alexia and agraphia are common but are accompanied by obvious aphasia. In isolated parietal lobe disease, however, aphasia is never found, but two distinct types of alexia without aphasia occur. Lesions in the area of the angular gyrus produce *alexia with agraphia.* Such patients are truly illiterate, perhaps retaining only recognition of isolated letters or numbers; such patients usually experience great difficulty in writing or reading even when the words are spelled aloud or written on the palms of their hands. Surprisingly, affected patients have little insight into their disability and claim their reading glasses are at fault. Thus, symbolic defects may represent focal neurologic symptoms and not just the effects of advancing age.

Alexia with agraphia may occur with or without a field defect. When accompanied by right-left confusion and contralateral finger agnosia (e.g., patient can't tell when fingers are being passively moved up or down) it is termed a *Gerstman syndrome.* This should be checked for in severely dyslexic children, as its existence implies a poor prognosis for reading.

The second more common form of acquired pure alexia is *alexia without agraphia,* usually caused by dominant-sided posterior cerebral artery occlusion. This lesion involves destruction of the splenum of the corpus callosum near the parietal-occipital juncture. This produces an occipital lobe hemianopia on one side combined with an interruption of the crossing visual output to the angular gyrus from the intact occipital lobe. In a right-handed person then, such an infarct would involve the left, literate, hemisphere to produce a right-field defect. While the left, illiterate field sees, it cannot transmit its information across to the left angular gyrus, and symbolic decoding of visual material cannot occur. Thus, these patients are visually alexic, but can produce written speech and are not truly illiterate since they recognize words spelled aloud or written on their skin. Color-naming errors are also common in this syndrome.

Patients with devastating nondominant or bilateral parietal lobe lesions are often visually incapacitated despite reten-

tion of good visual acuity, and even an intact hemifield or more (see Figure 32.19). Such patients are visually inattentive, may not look at someone entering the room, and may seem blind. This false impression is reenforced by spatial agnosia that may be profound, such as repeatedly getting into another patient's bed in the nursing home or misreaching for objects on the food tray. Patients with this Balint's syndrome may show extremely inaccurate and ill-sustained EOMs or pointing move-

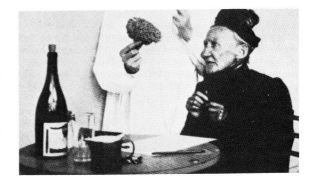

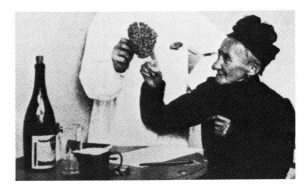

**FIGURE 32.19.**
Inability to recognize common objects despite good acuity in a case of visual agnosia (*above*). Note the change of expression in the elderly woman when she recognizes the sponge by touch (*below*).
Reprinted by permission of the publisher, from von Stauffenberg W: Arb hirnanat Inst Zurich 8, 1914.

ments to visually presented objects. Occasionally, they may demonstrate a complete visual agnosia. Since a brain tumor can produce what seems to be a dementia in such patients, it is again important to recognize such a presentation as a focal neurologic syndrome.

# EXAMINATION

The examination of the patient with potential parietal lobe disease has two related goals. The first is to recognize when a plotted defect might reflect parietal lobe disease by awareness of key symptoms and tests discussed in the preceding section. The second is simply to recognize subtle hemispheric symptomatology suggesting the need for a field exam in the first place. In practice, the two aspects are often interrelated.

Lesions in the parietal lobe are more common causes of field defects than tract or temporal lobe lesions, but less common than occipital lobe lesions. The major defect is complete homonymous hemianopia, which is said often to split rather than to spare the macula, but this cannot be relied upon. Large test objects, such as an index card, should be used to test for some residual sight in the upper quadrants as this favors a parietal lobe origin. When parietal lobe disease is suspected, the field must always be checked for extinction using simultaneous presentation of the target in both hemifields. Patients showing even full fields on a standard tangent screen exam may be totally unaware of one of the examiner's hands in the "inattentive" field, thus strongly suggesting a parietal lobe lesion.

Patients with parietal lobe disease may show cogwheel pursuits toward the side of the lesion. If not, pursuit pathology should still be tested for using the OKN tape, as lack of crisp nystagmus only when the tape is passed toward the suspect hemisphere represents *asymmetrical optokinetic nystagmus*, a cardinal ocular sign of parietal lobe disease. This response is unrelated to the hemianopia as it occurs when the stimulus is moved toward the intact field and may exist even in the absence of a field defect.

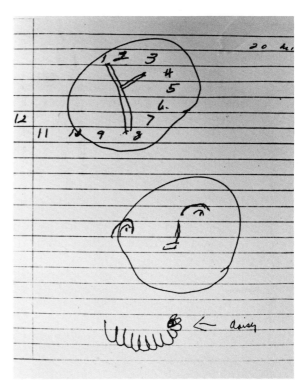

**FIGURE 32.20.**
**Constructional apraxia and inattention to the left visual field in a 66-year-old man who suddenly lost his way while driving on familiar roads. Patient suffered a nondominant perietal lobe infarction on the right side.**
Reprinted by permission of the publisher, from Cogan D. Neurology of the visual system. Springfield, Ill.: Charles C Thomas, 1966.

In patients volunteering minimal symptoms with field defects, it is important to probe for lateralized signs of parietal lobe disease. The skin of face and hands can be easily tested for extinction or finger agnosia. Dysgraphesthesia is tested for on each side by having the patient close his eyes and attempt to identify numbers traced on the palms held up so as to face the eyes. Astereoagnosia is easily tested for by having the patient attempt to recognize common objects placed in each hand with the eyes closed (safety pin, rubber bands, coin, etc.). Obviously, a diagnosis of such cortical defects presumes the patient has normal sensation.

Dominant parietal lesions affecting reading obviously should be manifest in the routine exam and need not be discussed except to point out that they have been overlooked or misinterpreted by "eyeball" oriented practitioners. Nondominant function should also be tested for. While spatial agnosia may be painfully obvious, it occasionally will be manifest only in having the patient draw objects such as a clock dial (constructional apraxia as in Figure 32.20). A convenient office test for spatial agnosia is available for patients complaining of insecurity in space. In this case, loss of global stereopsis may be readily manifest by total lack of appreciation of Random Dot Stereogram despite near perfect performance on the Wirt Circles test. Such a finding strongly suggests a nondominant hemispheric lesion.

Ideomotor apraxia can be tested by asking the patient if he has had difficulty with common tasks such as getting dressed or by asking him to follow directions: "take this cup and fill it at the sink and bring it back here." Obviously some of these tasks will be more difficult to interpret if the patient is also aphasic.

# CLINICAL SIGNIFICANCE

The significance of a field defect or other symptomatology suggesting parietal lobe dysfunction depends on its mode of onset. The patient who becomes aware of a field defect because of a realization of close calls on the left side while driving may be suffering from any number of lesions, often vascular, at any site from the rear of the chiasm to the tip of the occipital lobes. On the other hand, such a field defect, with an onset and progression not ascertained, has a more restricted interpretation when, for example, a right-handed patient has recently begun to find himself lost while in the car and for the last several days has been inattentive to one side and arrives at the office with only the right side of the face properly shaved. Here the origin is right parietal lobe; the history suggests steady progression, and a tumor is expected.

While field defects from parietal lesions are less common than occipital-vascular insults of the elderly, they are much more likely to represent a mass lesion.

# The Occipital Lobes

*The final segment of the optic radiations passes through the occipital lobes to synapse on primary visual cortical cells, which lie in a small wedge of (striate) cortex just above and below calcarine fissure.*

## BACKGROUND

The occipital radiations and visual cortices are supplied by the two posterior cerebral arteries, which represent end arteries of the vertebrobasilar system. Because of its watershed location, and possibly also because of its high metabolic rate, the occipital cortex is commonly affected by vascular insults, usually thromboembolic disease, but occasionally AV malformation or irreversible ischemia from hypotensive crises such as shock or cardiac arrest. The cortical macula representation is at the occipital poles, with more peripheral visual fields being represented deeper, the superior field below the fissure (lingual gyrus), the inferior fields above (cuneate gyrus).

Depending on the individual, there may be a dual arterial supply of the macula's representation via middle cerebral artery anastomosis. Occipital lobe stroke often shows retention of 5° or more of central vision in the blind hemifield. Such macula sparing may reflect this dual supply and is quite suggestive of occipital lobe disease, but far from definitive. Occipital field defects are always rigorously congruous.

When a thrombus forms at the origin of both posterior cerebral arteries, complete cortical blindness may result. If some central vision remains, its extent often tends to improve over several weeks to months. The sensitivity of occipital cortex function to anoxia/ischemia is suggested in common experience by the circular collapse of the visual fields that often attends syncope. Interestingly, the toxic mercury variety of tunnel vision, such as that from eating industrially contaminated fish, also represents focal occipital lobe damage.

## EXAMINATION

The occipital lobes are the most frequent site responsible for homonymous hemianopia. Except for variable macula sparing, which may also occur with lesions elsewhere in the radiations, there are no specific aspects of a field defect usually present that strongly suggest an occipital focus (Figures 32.21 and 32.22). Rather, it is the absence of the neurologic company typical of tract, temporal lobe, and parietal lobe disease that tends to incriminate the occipital lobes. When these associated defects are looked for and specifically ruled out, the onset of a hemianopia in elderly patients generally reflects occipital lobe infarct. In cases of

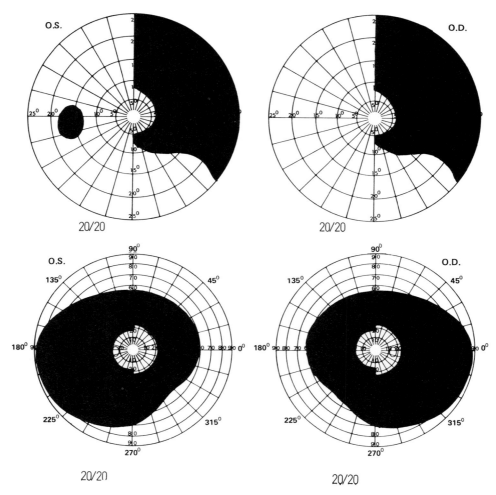

**FIGURE 32.21.**
Occipital lobe field plots. *Above.* Macula sparing greater than 5 degrees suggests occipital lobe disease, especially with an upper quadratic defect, as temporal lobe field cuts generally extend to fixation. *Below.* Bilateral homonymous defects are almost pathognomonic of basilar artery insufficiency. Such constricted fields with vertical stepping are never psychogenic.

bilaterally severely restricted fields of occipital origin, there often is some vertical stepping to indicate that the defect actually reflects bilateral homonymous hemianopia with macular sparing, and, of course, pupillary reactions will be brisk. Such patients may read 20/20 but have difficulty recognizing family members by sight (prosopagnosia) and often will do poorly on office color plates.

Although occipital masses are uncommon relative to stroke, it must be appreciated that they may remain clinically occult for long periods. Because of this neurologic silence, occipital masses have an unfortunate tendency to present finally

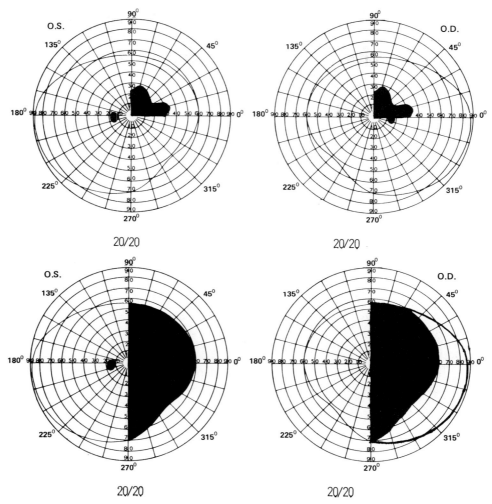

**FIGURE 32.22.**
Occipital lobe field plots. *Above.* Perfectly congruous homonymous
hemicentral scotomas are characteristic of trauma to the occiput.
*Below.* Sparing of the temporal crescent in OD is always occipital in
origin, with or without macula sparing.

with signs of parietal lobe extension or even increased intracranial pressure. Youth, progression, headache, early involvement of the central isopters, or photopic seizures tend to suggest a mass. Such photopic episodes may mimic migraine, especially when caused by AV malformation (see Chapter 9).

In the elderly, vertebrobasilar TIAs often are accompanied by headache, and these patients often may claim that the transient loss of a hemifield was a loss of vision in the right or left eye, incorrectly suggesting carotid artery disease. Often such patients have had other spells that indicate the vertebrobasilar origin of the symptoms (i.e., blackouts, vertigo, diplopia, loss of equilibrium, memory disturbances, bilateral motor or sensory symptoms, etc.) Such spells generally last only a minute or two. A recent history of such spells in a patient with hemianopia strongly suggests posterior cerebral artery infarct.

Patients with occipital lobe field loss sometimes give evidence of seeing by looking toward moving targets even when they are unable to verbalize seeing the target and give absolutely no evidence of seeing a stationary one: the *Riddoch phenomenon*. Even in cases of demonstrable total cortical blindness, the patient may claim to be able to see, called *Anton's phenomenon*.

Although denial is common to the early stages of all severe visual disability, there is some evidence that these patients may retain some "subcortical" sight. In forced choice experiments, some patients with no other evidence of vision point to flashed targets quite accurately, can even distinguish shapes and colors, and walk more hesitantly in the dark.

The key point in accepting occipital lobe disease is the ruling out of alternate sites for the hemianopia. The distinguishing features of disease at each level are highlighted in Table 32.1.

# CLINICAL SIGNIFICANCE

The significance of an occipital field defect is its cause. If sudden in onset without any company in the elderly, a vascular origin is probable; it is almost certain if alexia without agraphia coexists. Here the focus is on preventing further morbidity by study of the heart and great vessels for sources of embolization, treating hypertension, hyperlipidemias, and often antiplatelet therapy.

The most common mass in this region is the glioma, which tends to remain silent until significant size is attained. Meningiomas are the second most common tumor and may be suggested by insidious onset and slow progression of a defect with sloping edges, especially in middle-aged women. Meningiomas of the falx separating the two hemispheres may present early with homonymous hemicentral scotomas or quadrantanopias in one or even both hemifields. In such cases, the headaches may be referred to the periorbital area. The usual cause of paracentral homonymous field defects is trauma to the occipital poles, however.

Other lesions are much less common, but AV malformation should be suspected when a field defect is found in the area of an atypical migraine photopsia. A bruit may be auscultated over the occiput or retromastoid space in some of these cases, and is a significant indicator of this important diagnosis prior to subarachnoid hemorrhage. Trauma to the occiput is also not rare, and cortical blindness has also followed aggressive manipulation of the cervical spine in cases where bony abnormalities surrounding the vertebral arteries or atheromatous plaques have preexisted.

Finally, cortical blindness is occasionally congenital and is suggested by parental history, lack of optically elicited eye movements, but retention of good pupillary responses. In these patients the VER usually is extinguished, despite a normal ERG. If it is not, consider congenital oculomotor apraxia (Chapter 19); however, at least one case is on record with true cortical blindness from destruction of areas 18 and 19, but with preserved area 17 and intact VER.

# References

Cogan, DG. Neurology of the visual system. Springfield, Ill.: Charles C Thomas, 1966.

Denny-Brown, D. Handbook of neurological testing and case recording. Cambridge, Mass.: Harvard University Press, 1974.

Glaser, JS. Neuro-ophthalmology. Hagerstown, Md.: Harper & Row, 1978.

Harrington, DO. The visual fields: a textbook and atlas of clinical perimetry. St. Louis: C.V. Mosby, 1981; 5th ed.

Huber, A. Eye signs and symptoms in brain tumors. St. Louis: C.V. Mosby, 1976; 3rd ed.

Matthews, WB. Practical neurology. Oxford: Blackwell Scientific, 1975; 3rd ed.

Raeder AL, Harper DG. Confrontation visual field testing. JAMA 1976;263:250. (Letter)

Tate GW, Lynn JR. The principles of quantitative perimetry: testing and interpreting the visual field. New York: Grune & Stratton, 1977.

Thompson, HS. Topics in neuro-ophthalmology. Baltimore: Williams & Wilkins, 1979.

Volpe BT, Soave R. Formed visual hallucinations as digitalis toxicity. Ann Intern Med 1979;91:865–866.

Walsh TJ. Neuro-ophthalmology: clinical signs and symptoms. Philadelphia: Lea & Febiger, 1978.

## Chiasm

Burde RM, Karp JS. Clinical neuro-ophthalmology: the afferent visual system. Int Ophthalmol Clin 1977;17(1):1–173.

Cooper TD, Jun CL. Diencephalic syndrome of emaciation in infancy and childhood. In: Smith JL, ed. Neuro-ophthalmology update. New York: Masson, 1977;253–260.

Glaser, JS. Topical diagnosis: the optic chiasm. In: Glaser JS, ed. Neuro-ophthalmology. Hagerstown, Md.: Harper & Row, 1978;133–153.

Graham MG, Wakefield GT. Bitemporal visual field defects associated with anomalies of the optic discs. Br J Ophthalmol 1973;57:307–314.

Hoff J, Patterson R. Craniopharyngiomas in children and adults. J Neurosurg 1972;36:299–302.

Kohler PO, Ross GT. Diagnosis and treatment of pituitary tumors. Proceedings New York: Elsevier, 1973.

Lindenberg R, Walsh FB, Sachs JG. Neuropathology of vision: an atlas. Philadelphia: Lea & Febiger, 1973;230–235.

Post KD, Jackson IMD, Reichlin S, eds. The pituitary adenoma. New York: Plenum, 1980.

Reichlin S. Diagnosis and treatment of the prolactinoma problem. N Engl J Med 1979;300:313–315.

## Tracts

Bell R. Relative afferent pupillary defects in optic tract hemianopias. Am J Ophthalmol 1978;85:538–540.

Paul TO, Hoyt WF. Fundoscopic appearance of pappilledema with optic tract atrophy. Arch Ophthalmol 1976;94:467–468.

Savino PJ, et al. Optic tract syndrome. Arch Ophthalmol 1978;96:656–663.

Vedel-Jennsen N. Optic tract neuritis in multiple sclerosis. Acta Ophthalmol 1959;37:537–545.

## Parietal Lobe

Bender MB. Phenomenon of visual extinction in homonymous fields and psychological principles involved. Arch Neurol & Psychiatry 1945;53:29–33.

Benson DF, Geschwind N. The alexias. In: Vinken PJ, Bruyn GW, eds. Handbook of clinical neurology. New York: Elsevier, 1969;4:112–140.

Cogan DG. Visuospatial dysagnosia. Am J Ophthalmol 1979;88:361–368.

Hamsher K deS. Stereopsis and unilateral brain disease. Invest Ophthalmol Vis Sci 1978;17:336–343.

Katzman S. Clinical approach to dementia. In: Smith JL, ed. Neuro-ophthalmology, focus 1980. New York: Masson, 1979;341–346.

Lessel S. Disorders of higher visual function. In: Glaser JS, Smith JL, eds. Neuro-ophthalmology: symposium of the University of Miami and the Balscom Palmer Eye Institute. St. Louis: C.V. Mosby, 1975;8.

Smith JL, Cogan DG. Optokinetic nystagmus: a test for parietal lobe lesions. Am J Ophthalmol 1959;48:187–193.

Tyler HR. Abnormalities of perception with defective eye movements (Balint's syndrome). Cortex 1968;4:154.

## Temporal Lobe

Glaser JS. Topical diagnosis: retrochiasmal visual pathways. In: Glaser JS, ed. Neuro-ophthalmology. Hagerstown, Md.: Harper & Row, 1978;154–167.

Jensen I, Seedorff HH. Temporal lobe epilepsy and neuro-ophthalmology; ophthalmological findings in 74 temporal lobe resected patients. Acta Ophthalmol 1976;54:827–841.

Kay ME, Levin HS. Prosopagnosia. Am J Ophthalmol 1982;94:75–80.

Trobe JD, Lorber ML, Schlezinger NS. Isolated homonymous hemianopia: a review of 104 cases. Ophthalmology (Rochester) 1973;89:381–399.

## Occipital Lobe

Bodis-Wollner I, et al. Vision association cortex and vision in man: pattern evoked occipital potentials in a blind boy. Science 1977;198:629–631.

Cogan DG. Visual hallucinations as release phenomena. Albrecht von Graefes Arch Klin Exp Ophthalmol 1973;188:139–150.

Hoyt W, Walsh F. Cortical blindness with partial recovery following acute cerebral anoxia from cardiac arrest. Arch Ophthalmol 1958;60:1061–1069.

Riddoch G. Dissociation of visual perception due to occipital injuries with especial reference to appreciation of movement. Brain 1917;40:15.

Weiskrantz L, et al. Visual capacity in the hemianopic field following a restricted occipital ablation. Brain 1974;97:709–728.

# INDEX